Everyone's Guide to
CANCER THERAPY

*W*hat must I do to be saved?

ACTS 16, 30

*I*t is knowledge that ultimately gives salvation.

MOHANDAS GANDHI

CANCER THERAPY

MALIN DOLLINGER MD
ERNEST H. ROSENBAUM MD
AND GREG CABLE

A Somerville House Book
◆
Andrews and McMeel
A Universal Press Syndicate Company
Kansas City

For information, please write to: Andrews and McMeel, a Universal Press
Syndicate Company, 4900 Main Street, Kansas City, Missouri 64112.

Produced by Somerville House Books Limited.
3080 Yonge Street, Suite 5000
Toronto, Ontario
Canada
M4N 3N1

Interior design of book: Falcom Design and Communications Inc.
Medical illustrations: Kam Yu

Library of Congress Cataloging-in-Publication Data

Dollinger, Malin.
    Everyone's guide to cancer therapy : how cancer is diagnosed, treated, and man-
aged day to day / by Malin Dollinger, Ernest H. Rosenbaum, and Greg Cable : pref-
ace by Samuel Broder. — Rev. 2nd ed.
p   cm
"A Somerville House book."
Includes bibliographic references and index.
ISBN 0-8362-2428-0 (hd) : 29.95. — ISBN 0-8362-2427-2 :19.95
1. Cancer—Popular works. I. Rosenbaum, Ernest H. II. Cable, Greg, 1946-   . III.
Title
[DNLM: 1. Neoplasms—therapy—popular works. QZ 201 D666e 1994]
RC263.D59 1994 616.99'406—dc20
DNLM/DLC for Library of Congress 94-268

CIP

To our wives, Lenore and Isadora

and

*To Vincent DeVita, Jr., MD, Susan Molloy Hubbard, RN,
and Richard A. Bloch for their vision, ingenuity and dedication
in creating PDQ – The Physicians Data Query.*
MD and EHR

*To Diana Darroch, a kind-hearted, loving, compassionate nurse who
knows the challenge and the victory.*
GC

To Agnes Thomson (Tommie) Somerville.
JS

CONTENTS

$\diamond$

PART I: DIAGNOSIS AND TREATMENT

ACKNOWLEDGMENTS

The successful completion of such a complex and comprehensive book depends upon the support, assistance and help of a great number of people.

A very special word of gratitude goes first and foremost to our editor and co-writer Greg Cable. We wish to acknowledge the hard work, dedication and enormous effort he put into making highly complex medical information comprehensible to the general public. His contribution was essential in the successful completion of this book.

We are especially indebted to Jane Somerville, whose creative instincts and dedication to addressing an important need in our society have been singularly important in the creation of *Everyone's Guide to Cancer Therapy*. Her able and effective co-workers, including Patrick Crean, Keith Dundas, Kathy Legris, Dawn Arnold, Vivien Clark and Elizabeth Sherman have been of invaluable assistance. Thanks are warmly extended as well to Shaun Oakey for his skillful copy-editing, Fortunato Aglialoro for designing this book, and Voirrey Broe for her editorial comments. We are also grateful for the skill and artistic talent of medical illustrator Kam Yu. We are grateful to Ruth Chernia, who carried out the important task of coordinating the production of the second edition, to Michelle Bennett at Somerville House, to Heather Ebbs for creating a new index, and to Peter Scaggs for managing the production.

We extend warm thanks to our American publisher Tom Thornton of Andrews and McMeel, and his Editorial Director Donna Martin and Promotion Director Kathy Hilliard for their tremendous support and enthusiasm.

Our contributing authors generously gave to the project the extremely important gifts of their time and energies, sharing with us their expertise in their particular fields. Their contributions were critical to ensuring that the information presented here would be as complete, comprehensive and up-to-date as possible. We hereby acknowledge and express our gratitude to them all for their excellent work, especially Carlos A. Pellegrini, MD (Surgical Oncology), T. Stanley Meyler, MD, and Lawrence Margolis, MD (Radiation Oncology), for their comprehensive review of chapters dealing with specific tumors. John Hayward, MD, reviewed the entire book and offered invaluable advice and criticism.

In medicine, as in any scientific endeavor, peer review of published material is not only valuable but essential. Many people expert in the treatment of cancer and the care of cancer patients reviewed the manuscript and gave us the benefit of their knowledge and insights. We would like to express our thanks to:

Arthur Ablin, MD, Frederick Aronson, MD, Orlo Clark, MD, Lloyd Damon, MD, Jerry Finklestein, MD , Bruce Friedman, MD, Gary Friedman, MD, Anthony Giorgio, MD, Francine Holberg, MD, Robert Ignoffo, MD, Phil Kivitz, MD, Benjamin Landau, MD, Kenneth McCormick, MD, Eugene Morita, MD, Joyce O'Shaugnessy, MD, Jacob Rajfer, MD, Arthur Rosenbaum, MD, J.C. Rosenberg, MD, PhD, Gene Sherman, MD, Thomas Simko, MD, James Tamkin, MD, Frank Valone, MD, Kenneth A. Woeber, MD.

We owe our special thanks for valuable assistance to:

Mary Arnold, Tina Anderson, Bernadette Bell, Jeanine Bernet, Denise

Boland, Barry Bowman, Sharon Buckeridge, David Chan, MD, Paula Chung, Carmel Finigan, Lowell Greenberg, MD, Chester Gottlieb, MD, Sue Harmon, Jean Jenkins, Melinda Johnson, Liz Jorgensen, Anita Klecker, Diane McElhiney, Dottie Miller, Patty Mullins, Carol Richardson, Brett Ringler, Elaine Ryan, Beth Silverstein, Carolyn Small, Gail Sorrough, Teresa Squires, Jill Sternthal, William Sundbeck, Kathleen M. Thompson, Celeste Torrens, Ted Wilden, Arthur Wisot, MD, Gloria Won and Stuart Wong, MD.

A very special acknowledgment is due the National Cancer Institute Information Center for providing the Physician Data Query (PDQ) database and literature updates. This book is a knowledge link to PDQ, since much of the information in it is taken from PDQ sources. We want to express our appreciation and thanks to the National Cancer Institute for the concept of carrying the message of modern comprehensive cancer care to the practicing physician and the public, and to the staff of the Institute's PDQ Section for their cooperation in making the database available and for the time and attention they devoted to our needs. In so many ways they facilitated our use and understanding of the PDQ material, which was of great help in preparing the manuscript in a format suitable and useful to the general reader.

We thank David Bull, publisher of Bull Publishing Co., for drug and nutritional data. We would also like to express our appreciation to the University of California, San Francisco/Mt. Zion Medical Center, specifically Louis Giancola, Director, Martin Diamond, the Arseny Olga Koushar Memorial Foundation and the Ernest H. Rosenbaum Research Fund for support of this endeavor. We are equally indebted to American Medical International, Inc., South Bay Hospital, Redondo Beach, California, and its CEO, Dennis Bruns, for major support and assistance, and the Better Health Foundation.

We would like to express our gratitude for inspiration and guidance early in our careers to Arthur C. Giese, PhD, Laurance V. Foye, Jr., MD, Arthur Furst, PhD, Norman J. Sweet, MD, and Thomas Chiffelle, MD.

We owe a tremendous personal debt to our teachers, David Karnofsky, MD, Joseph Burchenal, MD, Irwin Krakoff, MD, William Dameshek, MD, Harris Fishbon, MD, John J. Sampson, MD, Sidney Levin, MD, and Russell Tat, MD, who cared about the advance of knowledge, about their patients and about us.

We also now understand why authors thank their spouses. Their acceptance and tolerance of the many hours, days, weeks and months of time devoted to "The Book" is an all-important ingredient in any manuscript's completion.

In our case, there is an even more important contribution. Our professional lives have been devoted to the care of seriously ill patients who often seemed like "family" too. Our wives, Lenore Dollinger and Isadora Rosenbaum, have understood and accepted the many demands created by our professional relationships, and they have freely given us the support, the time and the inspiration to continue.

Finally, we are grateful to our patients who have shared with us some of the most important and difficult struggles of their lives. They have allowed us to play a part in their struggle and in many cases to feel like one of the family. We have learned much from them over the years, not only about cancer and its treatment but about hope, courage and the indomitable human spirit.

In a larger sense, we want to express our appreciation to all cancer patients. Most of the current research on cancer treatment has been obtained through the clinical trial programs where promising new treatments can be compared with either a standard treatment or another promising treatment. Virtually all advances in cancer therapy have emerged from these extremely important clinical investigations and literally thousands of patients have consented to participate in them. We, and society, owe them a great debt and thanks.

Malin Dollinger, MD
Ernest H. Rosenbaum, MD
California, 1994

PREFACE TO THE FIRST EDITION

by Samuel Broder, MD, Director, National Cancer Institute, Bethesda, Maryland

—————◇—————

If people with cancer are to become full partners with their doctors and health care teams in their recovery from the disease, then it is critical that they have an understanding of the illness and of the kinds of treatments that might be recommended.

Everyone's Guide to Cancer Therapy offers an excellent step-by-step approach to this process. It explains what is currently known about the early detection of cancer, how a malignancy develops, how and why the correct stage of the cancer is determined and how each tumor is best treated. The book explains the basis for the many tests all cancer patients must undergo. It explains clearly and simply what to expect from the various forms of therapy and outlines the many ways individuals can cope and contribute to their own well-being during the period of recovery.

I would like to highlight one critical aspect of this book that I especially applaud—the central role that clinical trials play in cancer care. The National Cancer Institute (NCI) in the United States sponsors clinical trials all over the country aimed at improving the best currently available therapy for each type of cancer.

This clinical research process is vital. It is the mechanism by which advances are made in the treatment of cancer. All NCI-sponsored clinical trials undergo vigorous scientific and ethical review so that all participants can be assured that the therapy they receive in a clinical trial is at least as good as—and perhaps better than—standard treatment. They are fully informed of all their options and are kept abreast of any developments in the treatment of their disease.

It is important for those with cancer and their families to understand that for a tumor for which no highly effective therapy exists, investigational therapy within the context of an NCI-sponsored clinical trial represents the very best therapy available. Clinical cancer research is first and foremost treatment. It is state-of-the-art therapy that defines and builds upon the standard of care.

PREFACE TO THE SECOND EDITION

The wide public acceptance of *Everyone's Guide to Cancer Therapy* over the past few years has been very gratifying. Medical and other health care professionals, as well as cancer patients and their families, have welcomed the book as a valuable resource in the fight against cancer. We are very pleased to have been awarded an Honorable Mention from the American Medical Writers Association in the Trade Category of the 1992 Medical Book Awards Competition.

It has also been extremely gratifying that this acceptance has spread beyond the United States. Separate editions have been published in Canada (1992) and Greece (1993), and new editions are planned for Poland, France and Italy, and in Serbo-Croatian.

We hope this revised edition finds similar favor around the world.

Cancer therapy is a dynamic, ever-changing field. In the years since the first edition was published, there have been many impressive advances in cancer diagnosis and treatment. There have been important discoveries in biological therapy, as well as in the choice, rationale and timing of new chemotherapy programs. Novel and aggressive techniques in surgery and radiotherapy have been developed. New diagnostic studies have emerged. The use of bone marrow and stem cell protection is a rapidly evolving discipline that allows trials of very high dosage chemotherapy programs to attempt to cure otherwise incurable forms of cancer. Not least, we are making our first advances in the use of gene therapy to treat cancer.

All these discoveries have been incorporated into this revised text. And we have added seven new chapters that focus on areas worthy of more detailed discussion than was possible in the first edition.

♦ A day rarely goes by without significant articles appearing in the popular press about some aspect of cancer diagnosis and treatment. The importance of cancer research and care has assumed great attention around the world. In Chapter 34, Vincent DeVita Jr., MD, provides an overview of the worldwide effort to control the disease.

♦ New anticancer drugs have been tested and introduced in the past few years. In Chapter 36, Franco Muggia, MD, describes those that are most likely to prove useful.

♦ Chapter 27 is an excellent discussion about palliative care. Written by Margaret Fitch, RN, PhD, and Leslee J. Thompson, RN, MScN, it first appeared in the Canadian edition of *Everyone's Guide*.

♦ Whether or not they are cured, cancer patients experience unique anxieties. In Chapter 29, Malin Dollinger, MD, and Bernard Dubrow, MS, furnish a new way of thinking about "Living with Mortality: Life Goes On."

♦ The emotional needs of cancer patients are always of critical importance. Ernest Rosenbaum, MD, offers new insights into these needs in Chapter 28, "The Decision to Live."

♦ Cancer patients often encounter significant problems with employment, discrimination and social acceptance, and Susan Nessim and Diane Shader Smith provide insights into this vital area in Chapter 31.

♦ Payment for cancer care is an area of great concern. Joseph Bailes, MD, Barbara Quinn and Malin Dollinger, MD, discuss these issues in Chapter 32.

Our contributing authors, each an authority in his or her field, continue to provide diligent overviews of their areas of expertise. We are pleased that a number of new contributors have joined us for this edition. Our contributors now number 76, compared with 42 for the first edition. We welcome them all.

We are indebted to Andrew Kneier, PhD, Mary Pat Dorr, June Peters, MS, Marcee Vincent, Ellen Tronolone, Helen Hardy and Bernadette Bell, RD, for their valued assistance.

We are grateful to Ruth Chernia, who carried out the important task of managing editor; to Michelle Bennett at Somerville House; Heather Ebbs, who created the index; and to Peter Scaggs, who managed production.

We are grateful to our publishers, Somerville House, Toronto, and Andrews and McMeel, Kansas City, for their enthusiasm, their support and their continued devotion to producing this book as a vital aid in the battle against cancer.

FOREWORD

⬦

In 1978, I was diagnosed with terminal lung cancer. I was given three months to live and told there were no treatments that could help me. The following week, I went to a major cancer center in another state where the doctor told me I could be cured.

Over the next three years, I learned a great deal about cancer. It is an extremely complex disease. There are hundreds of types and stages, with numerous treatment methods available. Progress in finding more effective treatments is being made at a staggering rate, and I soon came to realize there is no conceivable way any single human being could know the latest and most appropriate treatment for every kind of cancer. It is difficult to keep up with every current treatment for even one kind of cancer. Yet if cancer is to be beaten, it must be treated promptly, properly and thoroughly. There is often no second chance.

I also came to realize that if a doctor is unaware of the latest and best treatment for an individual patient, all the research—all the work done and all the money spent—is wasted as far as that patient is concerned. Many lives can be lost not because treatments to cure or control a cancer haven't been discovered, but because the physician may be unaware of them.

In 1981, I was Chairman of the Board of H & R Block, Inc., my family's income tax firm. We had acquired a computer service company in Columbus, Ohio, named CompuServe. One of its services was a network whereby anyone with a computer could call a local telephone number, be connected with the huge mainframes in Columbus and get all kinds of information instantly. One kind of information service offered was news.

When a newspaper is set today, it is done on a computer and CompuServe had arrangements with eleven major newspapers in the United States to have their articles fed into the company's mainframes as they were set. At night, I could contact CompuServe with my home computer and read the next morning's New York Times, Los Angeles Times, Washington Post or Chicago Tribune. I could read the front page, the editorial page, the sports, financial columns or whatever I selected. And I could read it before the people in those cities could get their paper locally.

It seemed obvious that, in the same way, a continually updated computer database of the latest cancer treatments could instantly deliver state-of-the-art information to any practicing physician in his or her own office.

The National Cancer Institute (NCI) had been working along similar lines. The Institute had the task of developing effective methods to prevent, diagnose and treat cancer, and was given additional resources by Congress to develop a program to disseminate cancer information.

First, an International Research Data Bank had been established, and in 1974 NCI began developing specialized systems to aid in collecting information to be made available to the scientific community. Mary Lasker, a member of the National Cancer Advisory Board at that time, requested that the NCI publish a book of treatment protocols to help practicing physicians find out about promising investigational therapies. She also asked that the book be updated every six months, but it wasn't feasible to prepare the equivalent of a textbook on clinical cancer research and change it semi-annually.

In response, Dr. Vincent T. DeVita, Jr., then the Director of NCI's Division of Cancer Treatment, decided to develop a computerized database called CLINPROT (Clinical Protocols) containing information on protocols supported by the Institute. By 1980, Dr. DeVita, now director of the NCI, had established a working group to expand the database with state-of-the-art treatment information and make it available to the growing number of physicians with personal computers.

In 1981, I communicated to Dr. DeVita my idea of having an easily accessible database of cancer therapies. He heartily agreed about how important it was to communicate fresh information directly to physicians and explained that NCI was developing such a database in two stages. The first stage involved adding a geographic matrix to CLINPROT, allowing physicians to identify investigational studies by area and other factors. This new file would be called PDQ1. The second stage involved adding state-of-the-art treatment information to PDQ1 and developing a comprehensive directory of physicians and treatment facilities that could be contacted for cancer care. This expanded database was named the Physician Data Query system, but came to be known simply as PDQ.

I was so enthusiastic about this project that I assembled a group of donors to purchase a building just off the NIH campus to house these activities. And in 1982 I became a member of the National Cancer Advisory Board. Throughout my six-year term on the Board, I continued to support the development and refinement of the system.

PDQ is now available instantly to physicians in the United States as well as in many other parts of the world through their personal computers, their hospital computers or the facilities of any medical library. And it is available absolutely free to any individual by calling 1-800-4-CANCER.

Everyone's Guide to Cancer Therapy continues this important work in making the most up-to-date cancer information as widely available as possible. In its tumor treatment sections, it expands on the PDQ database and translates the information into clear, easily understood terms. It is hoped that the *Guide* will serve as a critical resource for cancer patients, their families and anyone else whose life has been or might be affected by this disease. It is also hoped that it will serve health professionals who want additional information about cancer and supportive care techniques for themselves and for their patients.

The NCI has stated that if physicians used the latest recommended therapy, cancer mortality would be reduced 10 percent, saving some 40,000 lives annually.

Considering that the proper information can now be had so rapidly and easily, can there be any excuse to lose lives by failing to get it for every patient?

Richard Bloch
Kansas City, 1991

TO THE READER

When your life has been touched or, rather, grabbed by cancer, many things change. Whether it has happened to you, a member of your family, or a friend, the impact of a cancer diagnosis is always the same. It's like being hit by a truck.

New emotions suddenly crop up, the greatest being the cold fear of a new and unknown disease. New questions arise. What can be done to cure me? What medical and psychological help is available? Will I suffer? Will there be pain? How can I live with this disease? Do I have to die?

Your life and the lives of those around you are affected in many significant ways. You have likely had no preparation for these sudden, drastic changes.

It is our wish and purpose to give you as thorough, as careful and as complete an understanding as possible of what you are facing and what you can expect. Our aim is to describe in easily understood language the details and consequences of the particular cancer you or someone close to you may be confronting. We'll explain what treatments are available, what they involve and what you should do to get the best treatment in the shortest time with the least worry, discomfort and uncertainty.

Cancer comes with its own vast vocabulary, most of it probably unfamiliar to you. Many new words and complicated descriptions will become part of your everyday thinking. The extensive glossary of medical terms will help you keep your bearings as you travel through this strange new world.

Important questions will arise. How should you choose a cancer physician or an appropriate hospital? What tests will be done and what is their significance? What treatment options are available?

What are their risks and side effects? Who is involved in the treatment plan? How can open and clear communication be maintained? We have included a general guide to the cancer treatment system that will help you find answers to these questions.

Cancer can also be an emotionally devastating issue, not only to you as a sufferer but to your family and friends. So we have included a section on living with cancer and how you can work to improve your physical and mental well-being.

Cancer treatments are continually changing, and this book is a guide to diagnosis and treatment, not a collection of definitive medical opinions suitable for everyone. Each person with cancer is a unique individual in a unique situation.

Your physician has the role and responsibility of making diagnostic and treatment decisions, discussing them with you, giving you the benefit of his or her medical opinion and devising together with you the treatment plan most appropriate to your situation.

We have attempted to present the most current and accurate information about cancer, but it is not possible to convey all possible approaches to diagnosis and therapy. Although we have tried to reflect the treatment guidelines listed by the information services of the National Cancer Institute, there may in some cases be alternative approaches or even newer methods of diagnosis and treatment that your physician may discuss with you.

This book is to help you get more out of these discussions by helping you understand the complex problems of cancer treatment, ask the right questions and search for and obtain the best medical care.

CONTRIBUTORS

Malin R. Dollinger, MD
Clinical Professor of Medicine, University of Southern California, Los Angeles, CA

Vice President of Medical Affairs, John Wayne Cancer Institute, affiliated with Saint John's Hospital, Santa Monica, CA

Malin Roy Dollinger's lifelong dedication to the field of oncology and patient education has included a patient care and research position at the Memorial Sloan Kettering Cancer Center for Cancer Research in New York and a post as Director of Medical Oncology at Harbor General Hospital/ UCLA Medical Center in Los Angeles. He has written over 60 articles and contributed to a number of books about cancer and is a member of the editorial advisory board of *The Medical Letter* (New York), *Annals of Internal Medicine* and *The New England Journal of Medicine.*

In addition to his extensive patient care activities, he teaches at the University of Southern California School of Medicine, has lectured extensively to medical professionals and the public and has helped to educate the public about cancer in radio and TV appearances. He is especially interested in improving communication with cancer patients and their families and in the emotional issues associated with the disease.

Ernest H. Rosenbaum, MD
Clinical Professor of Medicine, University of California, San Francisco, CA

Associate Chief of Medicine, University of California, San Francisco/Mt. Zion Medical Center

Founder of the Medical Oncology Service, University of California, San Francisco/Mt. Zion Medical Center

Associate, Cancer Research Institute, University of California, San Francisco, CA

Medical Director, Better Health Foundation, San Francisco, CA

Ernest H. Rosenbaum's career has included a fellowship at the Blood Research Laboratory of Tufts University School of Medicine (New England Center Hospital) and MIT. He teaches at the University of California, San Francisco/Mt. Zion Medical Center, and was the co-founder of the Northern California Academy of Clinical Oncology.

His passionate interest in clinical research and good communication with patients and colleagues resulted in over 50 articles on cancer and hematology in various medical journal. He has participated in many national radio and television programs and frequently lectures to medical and public groups.

He has co-authored *Nutrition for the Cancer Patient* and has written numerous books, including *Living With Cancer, A Home Care Training Program for Cancer Patients, Decisions for Life, You Can Live 10 Years Longer With Better Health*, and *A Comprehensive Guide for the Cancer Patients and their Families*. For the latter work, he received Honorable Mention from the American Medical Writers Association for Excellence in Medical Publications.

Greg Cable, BA
A writer since 1970, Greg Cable has worked in publishing, television, film and education. He has co-authored several books, including *Catch: A Major League Life, Player Productions* and *Everyone's Guide to Outpatient Surgery*. He lives in Kitchener, Ontario.

Arthur Ablin, MD
Professor of Clinical Pediatrics, Emeritus, University of California School of Medicine, San Francisco, CA

David Alberts, MD
Professor of Medicine and Pharmacology;

Director, Cancer Prevention and Control Programs and Clinical Pharmacology Programs, Arizona Cancer Center, University of Arizona College of Medicine, Tucson, AZ

Robert Allen, MD
Professor of Clinical Surgery, University of California, San Francisco/Mt. Zion Medical Center

James Armitage, MD
Professor of Medicine, University of Nebraska School of Medicine; Director, Bone Marrow Transplantation Center, University of Nebraska, Omaha, NE

Kenneth A. Arndt, MD
Professor of Dermatology, Harvard Medical School, Boston, MA; Chief of Dermatology, Beth Israel Hospital, Boston, MA

Josefa Azcueta, RN, OCN
Director, Oncology Nursing, Cancer Care Associates, Torrance, Redondo Beach, San Pedro, and Gardena, CA

Joseph Bailes, MD
Clinical Assistant Professor of Medicine, University of Texas Health Science Center, San Antonio, TX; Member, Board of Directors, and Chairman, Clinical Practice Committee, American Society of Clinical Oncology

Harold Benjamin, PhD
Founder and Executive Director, Wellness Community, Santa Monica, CA; Author of *From Victim to Victor*

Christopher Benz, MD
Associate Professor of Medicine, Cancer Research Institute and Division of Hematology-Oncology, University of California School of Medicine, San Francisco, CA

Richard Bloch
Founder, H & R Block, Kansas City, MO

Mary Buller, MA
Research Specialist, University of Arizona Cancer Center, Tucson, AZ

David G. Bullard, PhD
Associate Clinical Professor of Medicine and Medical Psychology (Psychiatry), University of California, San Francisco, CA

David Byrd, MD
Assistant Professor and Acting Chief, Surgical Oncology, University of Washington School of Medicine, Seattle, WA

Barrie R. Cassileth, PhD
Adjunct Professor of Medicine, University of North Carolina at Chapel Hill; Consulting Professor, Community and Family Medicine, Duke University Medical Center, Durham, NC

Raphael Catane, MD
Professor and Head, Division of Oncology, Shaare Zedek Medical Center, Jerusalem, Israel. Formerly Director, Clinical Cancer Research, Bristol-Myers Squibb Co., Pharmaceutical Research Institute, Wallingford, CT

Orlo H. Clark, MD
Professor and Vice-chair of Surgery, University of California School of Medicine, San Francisco, CA; President, International Association of Endocrine Surgeons; Chief of Surgery, University of California, San Francisco/Mt. Zion Medical Center

Patricia Cornett, MD
Assistant Clinical Professor of Medicine, University of California School of Medicine; Chief of Hematology/Oncology, Veterans Administration Medical Center, San Francisco, CA

Vincent T. DeVita, Jr., MD
Director, Yale Cancer Center; Professor of Medicine, Yale University School of Medicine, New Haven, CT; Formerly

Physician-in-Chief, Memorial Sloan-Kettering Cancer Center, New York, NY; Director, National Cancer Institute, Bethesda, MD

Lenore Dollinger, PhD, RN
Certified Health Consultant, Palos Verdes Estates, CA

W. Lawrence Drew, MD, PhD
Associate Clinical Professor of Laboratory Medicine and Medicine, University of California School of Medicine, San Francisco, CA; Director of Microbiology and Infectious Disease, University of California, San Francisco/Mt. Zion Medical Center

Bernard Dubrow, MS
Retired Scientist and Technical Manager, Redondo Beach, CA

Frederick Eilber, MD
Professor of Surgery, University of California, Los Angeles, CA; Associate, Jonsson Comprehensive Cancer Center, Los Angeles, CA

James Fick, MD
Brain Tumor Research Center, Department of Neurological Surgery, University of California Medical Center, San Francisco, CA

Jerry Z. Finklestein, MD, CM
Adjunct Professor of Pediatrics, University of California, Los Angeles, CA; Medical Director, Jonathan Jaques Children's Cancer Center, Miller Children's Hospital, Long Beach, CA

Margaret I. Fitch, RN, PhD
Oncology Nurse Researcher, Comprehensive Cancer Program, Toronto-Bayview Regional Cancer Centre, Sunnybrook Health Science Centre; Assistant Professor, University of Toronto, Toronto, Ontario, Canada

Gary D. Friedman, MD
Clinical Instructor of Plastic Surgery, St. Francis Hospital, San Francisco, CA

Michael A. Friedman, MD
Associate Director, Cancer Therapy Evaluation Program, Division of Cancer Treatment, National Cancer Institute, Bethesda, MD

Timothy S. Gee, MD
Associate Professor of Clinical Medicine, Cornell University Medical College, New York, NY; Attending Physician and Acting Chief, Leukemia Service, Memorial Hospital for Cancer and Allied Diseases, New York, NY; Clinical Member, Sloan-Kettering Institute for Cancer Research, New York, NY

Alan B. Glassberg, MD
Clinical Professor of Medicine, University of California School of Medicine; Chief, General Oncology, University of California, San Francisco/Mt. Zion Medical Center; Associate, Cancer Research Institute, University of California, San Francisco, CA

William H. Goodson, III, MD
Professor of Surgery, University of California Medical Center, San Francisco, CA

Mark Greenberg, MB, ChB
Head, Division of Oncology, The Hospital for Sick Children; Professor of Paediatrics and Surgery, University of Toronto, Toronto, Ontario, Canada

John D. Hainsworth, MD
Associate Medical Director, Sarah Cannon (Minnie Pearl) Cancer Center; Professor of Medicine, Division of Oncology, Vanderbilt University Medical Center, Nashville, TN

Deborah Hamolsky, RN, MS, OCN
Case Manager, Home Care, University of California, San Francisco/Mt. Zion Medical Center, San Francisco, CA

Russell Hardy, MD
Hematology/Oncology Group, Santa Rosa, CA

James Helsper, MD
Associate Clinical Professor of Surgery, University of Southern California School of Medicine, Los Angeles, CA; President, Society of Head and Neck Surgeons

I. Craig Henderson, MD
Professor of Medicine, University of California School of Medicine, San Francisco, CA; Chief, Clinical Oncology Programs, University of California, San Francisco Clinical Cancer Center, San Francisco, CA

Sandra Horning, MD
Associate Professor of Medicine, Stanford University School of Medicine, Palo Alto, CA

Susan Molloy Hubbard, RN, BS
Co-creator of PDQ; Director, International Cancer Information Center; Associate Director, National Cancer Institute, Bethesda, MD

Eliot S. Krames, MD
Medical Director, San Francisco Center for Comprehensive Pain Management, University of California, San Francisco/Mt. Zion Medical Center

Larry K. Kvols, MD
Director of Clinical Research, Mallinckrodt Medical, Inc., St. Louis, MO; Formerly Professor of Medicine, Mayo Medical School

Robert Kyle, MD
Professor of Medicine and Laboratory Medicine, Mayo Medical School; Chairman, Division of Hematology, Mayo Clinic, Rochester, MN

Pamela Lemkin, RN, BSN, OCN
President, Board of Directors; Administrator of Doctor's Home Technologies for Torrance Memorial Medical Center, Torrance, CA

Stephen Lemkin, MD
Medical Director, Doctor's Home Technologies for Torrance Memorial Medical Center, Torrance, CA; Clinical Assistant Professor of Medicine, UCLA School of Medicine; Member, Cancer Care Associates, Torrance, Redondo Beach, San Pedro, and Gardena, CA

Alexandra Levine, MD
Professor of Medicine; Chief, Department of Hematology, USC School of Medicine, Los Angeles, CA

Michael W. McDermott, MD
Assistant Clinical Professor, Department of Neurological Surgery, University of California School of Medicine, San Francisco, CA

Kerry Anne McGinn, RN, BSN, MA
Coordinator, Breast Health Resource Center; University of California, San Francisco/Mt. Zion Medical Center

Francine Manuel, RPT
Physical Therapist, Manuel, Richardson & Hauser, San Francisco, CA

Lawrence W. Margolis, MD
Clinical Professor and Vice Chairman, Department of Radiation Oncology, University of California Medical Center, San Francisco, CA; Chief of Radiation Therapy, Zellerbach Saroni Tumor Institute, University of California, San Francisco/Mt. Zion Medical Center

Stanley Meyler, MD
Clinical Professor of Radiation Oncology, University of California, San Francisco; Associate Chief of Radiation Therapy, Zellerbach Saroni Tumor Institute, University of California, San Francisco/Mt. Zion Medical Center

Lawrence Mintz, MD
Clinical Professor of Medicine, University of California School of Medicine, San Francisco, CA; Co-Director of Infectious Disease; Epidemiologist, University of California, San Francisco/Mt. Zion Medical Center

Malcolm S. Mitchell, MD
Professor of Medicine; Director, Center for Melanoma Research and Biological Therapy and Director of Melanoma Treatment and Biological Therapy, Scripps Clinic and Research Foundation, La Jolla, CA/University of California, San Diego and the UCSD Cancer Center. Formerly, Professor of Medicine and Microbiology, University of Southern California, Los Angeles, CA

Franco Muggia, MD
Director, Division of Medical Oncology and Clinical Investigations, Kenneth Norris Jr.–USC Comprehensive Cancer Center, Los Angeles, CA; Professor of Medicine, University of Southern California; Formerly Director for Cancer Therapy Evaluation, Division of Cancer Treatment, National Cancer Institute

Sean J. Mulvihill, MD
Associate Professor of Surgery; Chief, Division of General Surgery, University of California School of Medicine, San Francisco, CA

Susan Nessim
Founder, Cancervive, Los Angeles, CA; Co-author of *Cancervive*

Guy Newell, MD
Mesa Petroleum Co. Professor of Cancer Prevention, University of Texas, Houston, TX; Chairman, Department of Cancer Prevention and Control, M.D. Anderson Cancer Center, Houston, TX; Formerly Interim Director, National Cancer Institute

Carlos Pellegrini, MD
Professor and Chairman, Department of Surgery, University of Washington School of Medicine, Seattle, WA

Herbert Perkins, MD
Clinical Professor of Medicine, University of California School of Medicine, San Francisco, CA; Senior Medical Scientist, Formerly Director, Irwin Memorial Blood Centers, San Francisco, CA

Barbara F. Piper, RN, OCN, DNSc
Oncology Nurse Specialist, University of California, San Francisco/Mt. Zion Medical Center

Margaret Poscher, MD
Assistant Clinical Professor of Medicine, University of California, San Francisco; Attending Physician, Dept. of Infectious Disease; Director, Clinical HIV Services, University of California, San Francisco/Mt. Zion Medical Center

Barbara Quinn
Manager, Insurance Department, Cancer Care Associates, Torrance, Redondo Beach, San Pedro, and Gardena, CA

Isadora R. Rosenbaum, MA
Medical Assistant, San Francisco Hematology Oncology Medical Group, San Francisco, CA

Diane Shader Smith
Director of Communications, Cancervive; Free-lance Multimedia Writer and Author

Edward Sickles, MD
Professor of Radiology and Chief, Breast Imaging Section, University of California School of Medicine, San Francisco, CA

Ivan Silverberg, MD
Associate Professor of Medicine and Radiation Therapy, University of California School of Medicine, San Francisco, CA

Jill Slater-Freedberg, MD
Chief of Dermatology, Boston Veterans
Administration Medical Center; Instructor
in Dermatology, Boston University School
of Medicine

Penny Sneed, MD
Assistant Professor, Radiation Oncology,
Department of Radiation Oncology,
University of California School of
Medicine, San Francisco, CA

Jeffrey Stern, MD
Associate Clinical Professor, Obstetrics
and Gynecology, and Reproductive
Services; Director, Division of Gynecologic
Oncology, Department of Obstetrics and
Gynecology and Reproductive Services,
University of California School of
Medicine, San Francisco, CA

Jean M. Stoklosa, RN, MS
Formerly Clinical Specialist, Veterans
Administration Hospital, San Francisco,
CA; Lecturer, Department of Nursing, San
Francisco State University, CA

Leslee J. Thompson, RN, MScN
Director of Nursing, Comprehensive
Cancer Program, Toronto Bayview
Regional Cancer Centre, Sunnybrook
Health Science Centre; Assistant
Professor, University of Toronto, Toronto,
Ontario, Canada

Alan Venook, MD
Associate Professor of Medicine, and Chief
of Gastrointestinal Oncology, University of
California School of Medicine, San
Francisco, CA

Charles B. Wilson, MD
Chairman, Department of Neurosurgery;
Professor of Surgery, University of
California School of Medicine, San
Francisco, CA

Alan Yagoda, MD
Professor of Clinical Medicine, Division of
Medical Oncology; Associate Director for
Clinical Research, Columbia University
Cancer Center, New York, NY

Norman Zinner, MD
Adjunct Associate Professor of
Surgery/Urology, University of California,
Los Angeles, CA; Private practice, Doctor's
Urology Group, Torrance, CA; Formerly
Professor and Chairman, Department of
Urology, Charles R. Drew Postgraduate
Medical School, Los Angeles, CA;
Formerly, Boorhaare Professor, University
of Leiden, The Netherlands

PART I:
DIAGNOSIS AND TREATMENT

1
UNDERSTANDING CANCER

Malin Dollinger, MD, and Ernest H. Rosenbaum, MD

———————◇———————

Cancer is a general term for the abnormal growth of cells.

Our bodies are vast collections of cells, and every one of them contains 23 pairs of chromosomes. Winding through each pair is the double spiral of the DNA molecule, the genetic blueprint for life. DNA is the controller and transmitter of the genetic characteristics in the chromosomes we inherit from our parents and pass on to our children.

Our chromosomes contain millions of different messages that tell the body how it should grow, function and behave. One gene tells our stomachs how to make gastric juice; another tells the glands to secrete this juice when food lands in the stomach. Other genes determine the color of our eyes, tell injured tissues how to repair themselves and direct the female breasts to make milk after a baby is born. Most of the time these genes function properly and send the right messages. We remain in good health, with everything working as it should.

But there are an incredible number of genes and an unimaginable number of messages. And since the chromosomes reproduce themselves every time a cell divides, there are lots of opportunities for something to go wrong. Sometimes something does go wrong in the process of cell division—a mutation that alters one or more of the genes.

A cancer cell has an abnormal chromosome from genetic change or damage. The altered gene starts sending the wrong message or at least a message different from the one it should give. A cell begins to grow rapidly. It multiplies again and again until it forms a lump that's called a malignant tumor. Or cancer.

Uncontrolled Growth Rapid cell growth is not the same as malignancy. We all experience two normal situations in which our body tissues grow much more rapidly than they usually do. We grow from a single cell to a perfectly formed human being in nine months. Then we grow into a normal-sized adult human being over the next 16 years or so. As well, when we are injured and need rapid repair, restoration and replacement of damaged tissues, our bodies can produce many new cells in a very short time.

When either of these processes—growth or healing—is completed, a set of genes tells the body that it is time to "switch off." We don't continue growing throughout our lives, and the scar we have after a cut has healed remains just that—a scar. Those are the rules.

But a cancer cell doesn't obey the rules. The change in its genetic code makes it "forget" to stop growing. Once growth is turned on, cancer cells continue to divide in an uncontrolled way. It's as though you set the thermostat in your house for a certain temperature, but no matter how hot your house gets the furnace keeps running. No matter what you do to turn it off, it produces heat as if it had a mind of its own.

Doubling Times Cancer starts with one abnormal cell. That cell becomes two

———
3
———

abnormal cells that become four abnormal cells and so on. Cells divide at various rates, called doubling times. Fast-growing cancers may double over one to four weeks; slow-growing cancers may double over two to six months. It may take up to five years for the duplication process to happen 20 times. By then the tumor may contain a million cells yet still be only the size of a pinhead.

So there is a "silent" period after the cancer has started to grow. There is no lump or mass. It's too small to be detected by any means now known. What is not commonly appreciated is that the silent period is considerably longer than the period when we do know a tumor is present.

After many months, usually years, the doubling process has occurred 30 times or so. By then the lump may have reached a size that can be felt, seen on an x-ray or cause pressure symptoms such as pain or bleeding. To be able to see a tumor on an x-ray, it usually has to be about half an inch (1 cm) in diameter. At that stage, it will contain about 1 billion cells. When it is smaller, x-ray imaging techniques are not usually sensitive enough to detect it, although some newer imaging methods— especially computerized tomography (CT) and Magnetic Resonance Imaging (MRI)— may sometimes detect such small tumors.

Benign and Malignant Tumors Tumors are not always malignant. Benign tumors can appear in any part of the body. Many of us have them—freckles, moles, fatty lumps in the skin—but they don't cause any problems except (sometimes) cosmetic ones. They can be removed or left alone. However they are treated, they stay in one

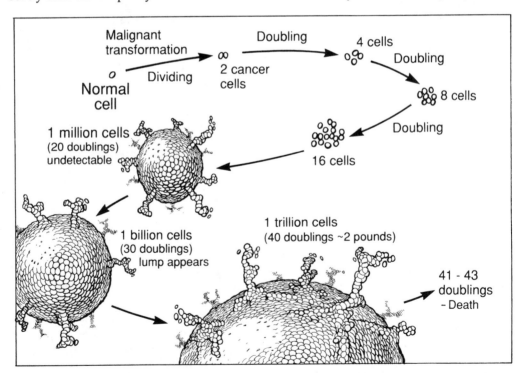

The malignant transformation of a normal cell and subsequent doublings. After 20 doublings (one million cancer cells) the cancer is still too small to detect.

place. They do not invade or destroy surrounding tissues.

Malignant tumors, on the other hand, have two significant characteristics:

♦ They have no "wall" or clear-cut border. They put down roots and directly invade surrounding tissues.

♦ They have the ability to spread to other parts of the body. Bits of malignant cells fall off the tumor, then travel like seeds to other tissues where they land and start similar growths. Fortunately, not all the many thousands of cancer cells that break off a tumor find a place to take root. Most die like seeds that go unplanted.

This spreading of cancer is called metastasis. And doctors are always concerned about whether the cancer has metastasized during the silent period. If it has, then the migrating cancer cells have begun to go through their own silent period. They too are too small to detect for many months or years.

Almost all cancers share these two properties, although cancers arising in various organs tend to behave differently. They spread to different parts of the body. They grow in very specific ways that are characteristic of that cancer. The consequence is that there is a specific method of diagnosis, staging and treatment for each kind of cancer. One set of principles governs diagnosis and treatment of breast cancer, for example, while the rules for lung or colon cancers are just as complex but somewhat different.

WHAT CAUSES CANCER

Although cancer is usually thought of as one disease, it is in fact more than 200 different diseases. For many of these cancers, no definite cause is known. There is no one single cause. In fact, cancer remains something of a mystery. But new clues and solid research are greatly increasing our understanding.

The Role of Oncogenes One of the most

exciting and important developments has been the recent discovery that some normal genes may be transformed into genes that promote the growth of cancer. These have been called oncogenes, the prefix onco meaning tumor. This discovery has led to much research, better understanding of how cancer develops and insights into methods of prevention, detection and treatment.

What usually stops the normal genes from being transformed are other genes called suppressor genes. If they don't do their job properly or are missing altogether, the cancer-producing action of the oncogene may not be suppressed (*see* Chapter 37).

The Implications for Screening All this new information raises the possibility that we may soon be able to test individuals, for example with a blood test, to discover whether a specific oncogene is present and if the suppressor gene is defective or absent. The presence of certain oncogenes may even give us information about how likely it is that a cancer will spread. We soon may be able to identify people with a higher risk for cancer and possibly carry out other intensive detection and screening methods. Techniques for testing for oncogenes have been developed recently and are beginning to be available for general use. This new knowledge is already used in the study of familial (inherited) polyps of the colon. (See Chapter 35 for additional screening information.)

How the Process Works There are anywhere from 50,000 to 100,000 genes within a human cell. But research suggests that not more than a hundred regulate cell growth or division. It is now also thought that we all carry normal cells that contain oncogenes in the chromosomes but that these oncogenes are never activated. They simply lie dormant throughout our lives.

In other cases, a mutation may occur because of some assault on the cell struc-

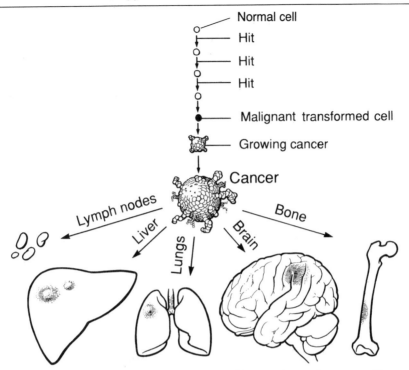

Normal cell

Hit

Hit

Hit

Malignant transformed cell

Growing cancer

Cancer

Lymph nodes

Liver

Lungs

Brain

Bone

After two or more "hits" a transformed malignant cell grows into a lump we call cancer. Cells may eventually break off and spread (metastasize) via lymph vessels or blood vessels.

ture. Some stimulus or chemical agent turns on a "switch," several oncogenes are activated, and they set to work together to transform a normal cell into a cancer cell. This is thought to be at least a two-step process. First, the DNA must go through an initial change that makes the cell receptive. Then a subsequent change or set of changes in the DNA transforms the receptive cell into a tumor cell.

The big question is, what causes these changes in cellular DNA in the first place? There are several theories. One focuses on viruses, which can insert their own DNA into a cell's DNA and make the cell produce more virus-containing cells. Viruses may insert a viral oncogene or they might simply act as a random mutating agent.

There is also some evidence that an assault by a "single carcinogenic bullet" hitting the cell at just the right spot can

make a cell become cancerous. But the theory that has gained a lot of support focuses on multiple "hits."

The Multiple Hit Theory According to this theory, all cancers arise from at least two changes or "hits" to the genes in the cell. These hits build up and interact over time. Eventually, a breaking point is reached and cancerous growth is switched on.

The hits may come from chemical or foreign substances that cause cancer, called carcinogens. These initiate the cancer process. Or the hits may be promoters that accelerate the growth of abnormal cells. What is critical is the number and types of hits, their frequency and their intensity.

Initiators include:
♦ Tobacco and tobacco smoke carcinogens. Lung cancer was a rare disease before cigarette smoking became widespread.

◆ X-rays. It is well known that there is an increased incidence of leukemia among atomic bomb survivors. This same increase has been noted in radiologists, the doctors who specialize in the use of x-rays. It should be pointed out that the average diagnostic use of x-rays does not increase the chance of getting cancer enough to rule out their use as a valuable health care tool. The risk of not having an x-ray may far outweigh the risk of cancer being caused by the use of x-rays for diagnosis. Used properly, x-rays are of great benefit in finding cancer at an early, curable stage.

◆ Certain hormones and drugs, such as DES, some estrogens (female hormones) and some immunosuppressive drugs.

◆ Excessive exposure to sunlight.

◆ Industrial agents or toxic substances in the environment, such as asbestos, coal tar products, benzene, cadmium, uranium and nickel.

◆ Excesses or deficiencies in diet, particularly high-fat and low-fiber diets.

◆ Obesity.

◆ Sexual practices, including the age of a woman when she first had intercourse and first becomes pregnant. Certain sexually transmitted viruses can cause cancers, and the risk of catching one of these viruses increases with unprotected sexual contact and with the number of sexual partners. This is particularly true for AIDS-related cancers such as Kaposi's sarcoma.

Promoters include:

◆ Alcohol, which is a factor in 4 percent of cancers, mainly in cancers of the head and neck and the liver.

◆ Stress, which may weaken the immune system. Stress is also relieved all too often with cigarettes, alcohol, rich food and drugs.

Miscellaneous Factors include:

◆ Heredity.

◆ Weaknesses of the immune system. When two or more hits are combined—

tobacco smoke and asbestos exposure, or cigarette smoking and alcohol, for example—the chance of getting cancer is not the sum of the individual risks. Rather, the chances are multiplied. Cancer is an additive process with many different hits occurring and interacting over many, many years.

What it comes down to is that the risk of developing cancer depends on:

◆ who you are (genetic makeup);

◆ where you live (environmental and occupational exposures to carcinogens); and

◆ how you live (personal lifestyle).

Now that so many factors in our daily lives that affect the risk of getting cancer can be identified, cancer risk assessment has become increasingly vital to our continued good health. Risk assessment screening of apparently healthy people is now used in many cancer centers (*see* Chapter 35).

HOW CANCER SPREADS

Although tumors can start to grow in several places simultaneously, that is unusual. They usually grow at a single site. So if cancer spreads, it is usually because small bits of cancer cells are cast off the original, or primary, tumor and travel to other parts of the body. There are three ways for the cancer to spread.

Direct Extension As the tumor mass grows, it invades the organs and tissues immediately next to it. It tends to form roots, growing into the layers of surrounding tissue like carrots growing into the earth.

Through the Blood (Hematogenous Spread) Tumors have a blood supply. Arteries pump blood into the malignant cells and veins take it away. Pieces of the tumor can grow through the walls of these blood vessels, enter the bloodstream and circulate around the body until they land in various organs. Fortunately, very few

CANCER RISK FACTORS, WITH PERCENTAGES

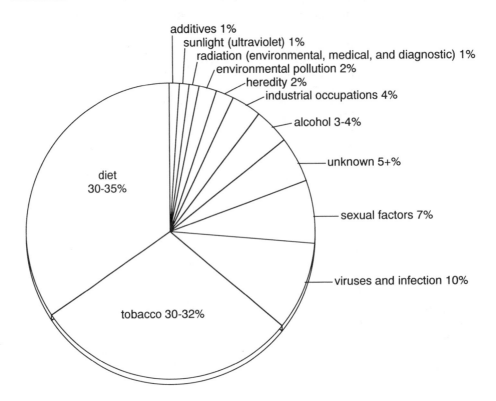

additives 1%
sunlight (ultraviolet) 1%
radiation (environmental, medical, and diagnostic) 1%
environmental pollution 2%
heredity 2%
industrial occupations 4%

alcohol 3-4%

unknown 5+%

diet
30-35%

sexual factors 7%

viruses and infection 10%

tobacco 30-32%

of these circulating cells actually find a place to grow.

Through the Lymphatic System There are two blood vessel systems in the body. One consists of arteries that move blood to all parts of the body, veins that return the blood to the heart, and small capillaries around the organs and tissues that allow oxygen to be transferred.

The second is the lymphatic system. This is a separate system of tiny blood vessels—called lymphatics—under the skin and throughout the body. These vessels carry a liquid called lymph. The purpose of lymph is to drain waste products such as infectious, foreign or otherwise toxic materials.

Lymph Nodes Stations along these vessels, called lymph nodes, trap these materials. Tonsils, for example, are lymph nodes. When you have tonsillitis you have a high temperature, you have trouble swallowing and you generally feel awful. But you feel that way because the tonsils are doing their job by trapping bacteria and preventing them from getting into your body. If they weren't doing their job, you might develop a bloodstream infection—"blood poisoning."

The lymph system begins with very small tubes that drain into lymph nodes at different levels of the body. Eventually the system feeds into the thoracic duct in the left side of the neck. That duct drains into the venous system, which returns the lymph fluid to the heart. From there it is pumped through the body.

Tumor cells can easily spread into the lymphatic system. Breast cancer, for example, often spreads initially via lymphatic vessels to the lymph nodes in the armpit (axillary nodes). If not stopped there, the cancer cells continue traveling in the lymphatics to other locations in the body. In this situation, a doctor can sometimes feel the axillary nodes during a physical examination. But just to be sure, the nodes have to be examined under a microscope after they are surgically removed.

When breast cancer spreads to the lymph glands under the armpit, we hope the glands did their job and prevented the cells from spreading any farther. You might visualize these lymph glands as train stations and the lymph blood vessels as tracks. We hope the cells behave like a local train, stopping at the next lymph node station, and don't behave like an express, scooting past several nodes and getting directly into the body.

THE DIFFERENT KINDS OF TUMORS

Treating cancer properly depends on defining each and every tumor very precisely. All kinds of characteristics are taken into account when coming up with this definition, but all these characteristics essentially fit into three broad categories. The three key questions that have to be answered are: where is the tumor growing, how fast is it growing, and how big has it already grown?

The first of these questions is critical because, again, cancers that develop in different tissues tend to behave differently. There are generally three types of malignant tumors, which develop in the three kinds of tissues.

Carcinomas These develop in the tissues that cover the surface or line internal organs and passageways (epithelium). Most epithelial cancers—carcinomas—develop in an organ that secretes something. For example, lung tissue secretes mucus, breast tissue secretes milk, and the pancreas secretes digestive juices.

Sarcomas These are soft tissue or bone tumors. They develop in any supporting or connective tissues—muscles, bones, nerves, tendons or blood vessels. Since supporting or connective tissue is found throughout the body, sarcomas can be found anywhere.

The same organ that develops a carcinoma can also develop a sarcoma, since the organ also has connective tissue in it. There are blood vessels in the pancreas, for example, and if a cell in the wall of the blood vessel develops a tumor, the tumor is a sarcoma even though it's in the pancreas.

Lymphomas and Leukemias These tumors develop in the lymph glands or arise from the blood-forming cells in the bone marrow.

Lymphomas (lymphosarcomas) are the tumors that develop in the lymph glands, the small, round or bean-shaped structures found throughout the body. These tumors are almost always malignant. One specific kind of tumor in this broad class is called Hodgkin's disease, and all the other ones have come to be referred to as non-Hodgkin's lymphomas. To make things more complicated, there are many sub-varieties of both Hodgkin's disease and non-Hodgkin's lymphomas.

The leukemias are cancers of the white blood cells and are named after the type of white blood cell affected. Plasma cell myeloma (multiple myeloma) is a cancer of the plasma cells in the bone marrow.

Understanding Tumor Names There are many different names for the various cancers and it's easy to get confused. There are tumors in each of the three tumor categories that are named after the doctors who discovered them—Hodgkin's disease, Ewing's sarcoma of the bone, Kaposi's sarcoma or Wilms' tumor of the kidney. Tumors may also be named after the tissue of origin, such as a schwannoma, which is a tumor that develops in the Schwann cells surrounding nerves.

For the most part, there is a method to this confusing terminology. Every tissue or body part has a specific name. We all know these names in English. Bone is bone and fat is fat. But scientific medicine usually uses the Greek or Latin name for a body part and then adds a helpful tag onto the end of it. The rule for naming sarcomas, for example, is that if the tumor is benign, *oma* is usually added to the Greek or Latin name. If the tumor is malignant, *sarcoma* is added.

The term for bone, for example, is *osteo*, so a benign tumor in the bone is an osteoma and a malignant tumor is an osteosarcoma. The term for fat is *lipo*, so there are lipomas and liposarcomas.

There are also different names for some organs, so a carcinoma of the stomach may be called a gastric carcinoma and a carcinoma of the kidney may be referred to as renal carcinoma. There are also alternative designations. For example, since the glands in the lung usually line the air passage (bronchus), carcinomas of the lung are sometimes called bronchogenic carcinoma (*genic* being the Latin way of saying "formed from").

MEASURING THE RATE OF GROWTH

The second way to classify tumors is according to how fast they are growing. It would be nice if there were a simple way of doing this, like pointing a radar gun at the tumor and getting a read-out of the speed. But what usually has to happen is that a piece of the tumor is surgically removed and examined under a microscope, a process known as a biopsy. Its appearance and behavior can reveal a lot of information.

Well-Differentiated Tumors Under the microscope, some tumor cells look very much like the normal tissue they came from. If they do, they are called well-differentiated. A normal pancreas has a characteristic look, for example. A pathologist can look at a slide of tissue and see that it's a pancreas even if it is cancerous. Similarly, a follicular carcinoma of the thyroid resembles normal thyroid tissue rather well, so it is not difficult for a pathologist to know where that tumor comes from.

Undifferentiated Tumors Other tumors don't particularly look like the normal tissues they come from. They resemble the tissue of origin only slightly or not at all. They look more primitive or immature. Sometimes they don't really look like any specific tissue. These are called undifferentiated or poorly differentiated.

Looking at a piece of undifferentiated tissue under the microscope, a pathologist will probably not be able to tell where the tissue was taken from. An undifferentiated tumor of the pancreas may look the same as an undifferentiated tumor of the lung, so the pathologist has to rely on the surgeon to say what area the tissue is from.

Undifferentiated or poorly differentiated tumors tend to be more aggressive in their behavior. They grow faster, spread earlier and have a worse prognosis than well-differentiated tumors. But there are exceptions for both types of tumors. Some poorly differentiated tumors grow no faster than well-differentiated ones.

High-Grade and Low-Grade Tumors There is another classification system that sometimes overlaps with the system based on differentiation. This system refers to tumors as "high-grade" or "low-grade." A high-grade tumor is immature, poorly differentiated, fast growing and aggressive. A low-grade tumor is usually mature, well-differentiated, slow growing and less aggressive. The grading of tumors is used to help determine cancer prognosis.

DEFINING THE STAGE OF CANCER

The third classification used in cancer treatment is called the staging system. Staging has a number of purposes.

♦ It is a useful way of identifying the "extent" of the tumor—its size, the degree of growth and spread. Obviously, if a tumor is found in only one place it is in an early stage. If it has spread to some distant part of the body or is found in several places, it is in an advanced stage.

♦ It provides an estimate of the prognosis since the chance of cure decreases as you move across the categories into more advanced or extensive stages.

♦ It provides a common and uniformly agreed upon set of criteria against which doctors around the world can compare treatments for a specific stage of tumor. They can then know that if one treatment has better results than another, the difference is really due to the treatment and not to differences between patients or the stages of the disease.

♦ It is generally the most important factor in deciding on the appropriate treatment.

The TNM System All kinds of staging systems have been developed for different kinds of cancer. But in the past few years a lot of thought and effort has been going on around the world to develop a relatively uniform classification system.

This system is known as TNM. T stands for the size of the tumor, N for the degree of spread to lymph nodes, and M for the presence of metastasis. A number is added to each of these letters to indicate degrees of size and spread.

Greatly simplified:

♦ T0 means the tumor was completely removed by the biopsy used to establish the diagnosis. T1 indicates the smallest tumor. T2, T3 and T4 indicate larger tumors that may have grown into surrounding tissues.

♦ N0 means that the nearby lymph nodes are free of tumor. N1, N2 and N3 signify increasing degrees of involvement of these regional nodes. An N2 tumor is more serious than an N1 tumor.

♦ M0 means that no distant metastases (cancer cells) have been found. If there are metastases, the classification is M1.

This seems simple enough. But the system is actually quite complex. The classifications are defined differently for each kind of cancer and each stage can include variations to the basic TNM classification. Here are the staging categories and stage grouping for breast carcinoma, for example (*see* page 12).

A breast cancer might be classified as a T2 N1 M0 lesion. This could represent a tumor 1 inch (2.5 cm) in diameter removed from the breast with some involvement of lymph nodes in the armpit but with no evidence of metastasis.

The TNM system has two overlapping classifications, the second having to do with the stage of cancer that represents a composite of the TNM classification. You will see in the tumor section that each tumor is grouped usually in one of four stages. Since there are many possible further TNM subdivisions, these are lumped together. You have to refer to the specific table for each cancer to be sure of the specific stage. For example, the T2 N1 M0 breast cancer described above is a Stage IIB cancer. A T3 N2 M0 cancer is Stage IIIA.

Staging and Treatment The significance of this classification is that treatment depends on the stage of the disease as defined by the TNM system. Your doctor has to know the stage to decide on appropriate therapy and to interpret the always evolving guidelines for treatment produced by major cancer centers and research groups.

This system has to be understood precisely so that very critical decisions can be made. Some stages of cancer are best treated surgically, others with radiotherapy, still others with chemotherapy. It is also becoming more and more common to use two of these treatment methods together and sometimes all three. Occasionally, they are given in sequence.

All these decisions are closely correlated with the stage of the tumor. In treating colon cancer, for example, chemotherapy with the drugs 5-fluorouracil and lev-

amisole may be given for Stage III cancer, but not for Stages IA or IIB. Similarly, Stage I prostate cancer may be treated surgically. But surgery is not usually an option by Stage III, when the tumor has extended beyond the prostate.

Although the TNM system is not applicable to all cancers—it is not used with lymphomas, for example—it has now replaced earlier classification systems for tumors in the colon and rectum and is used to stage many other kinds of cancer. As of 1994, it is the recommended staging system for most cancers.

AMERICAN JOINT COMMITTEE ON CANCER

Staging for Breast Carcinoma

T = Primary Tumor   **N** = Regional Tumor   **M** = Distant Metastasis

PRIMARY TUMOR (T)

TX	Primary tumor cannot be assessed
T0	No evidence of primary tumor
Tis*	Carcinoma in situ: Intraductal carcinoma, lobular carcinoma in situ, or Paget's disease of the nipple with no tumor
T1	Tumor 2 cm or less in greatest dimension
T2	Tumor more than 2 cm but not more than 5 cm in greatest dimension
T3	Tumor more than 5 cm in greatest dimension
T4†	Tumor of any size with direct extension to chest wall or skin

*NOTE: Paget's disease associated with a tumor is classified according to the size of the tumor.

†NOTE: Chest wall includes ribs, intercostal muscles, and serratus anterior muscle but not pectoral muscle.

REGIONAL LYMPH NODES (N) (CLINICAL)

NX	Regional lymph nodes cannot be assessed (e.g., previously removed)
N0	No regional lymph node metastasis
N1	Metastasis to movable ipsilateral axillary lymph node(s)
N2	Metastasis to ipsilateral axillary lymph node(s) fixed to one another or to other structures
N3	Metastasis to ipsilateral internal mammary lymph node(s)

DISTANT METASTASIS (M)

MX	Presence of distant metastasis cannot be assessed
M0	No distant metastasis
M1	Distant metastasis (includes metastasis to ipsilateral supraclavicular lymph node[s])

© 1989, American Cancer Society, Inc.

STAGE GROUPING

Stage 0	Tis	N0	M0
Stage I	T1	N0	M0
Stage IIA	T0	N1	M0
	T1	N1*	M0
	T2	N0	M0
Stage IIB	T2	N1	M0
	T3	N0	M0
Stage IIIA	T0	N2	M0
	T1	N2	M0
	T2	N2	M0
	T3	N1, N2	M0
Stage IIIB	T4	Any N	M0
	Any T	N3	M0
Stage IV	Any T	Any N	M1

*NOTE: The prognosis of patients with pN1a is similar to that of patients with pN0.

2

HOW CANCER IS DIAGNOSED

Malin Dollinger, MD, and Ernest H. Rosenbaum, MD

———————◇———————

Cancer can be treated. But if it is going to be treated with any degree of success, it has to be detected in its early stages and a diagnosis quickly made. This isn't always easy because of the silent period of tumor growth—the months or years when the malignant cells are quietly doubling again and again. There may be absolutely no indication that this process is going on.

So how do we discover that the tumor is there? Your own complaint may be the tip-off. Or your doctor might pick up on some clue that appears during a physical. Whatever sets off the search for cancer, the investigative process that leads to a definitive diagnosis follows a standard pattern. Suspicions are aroused. Questions are asked. Doctors try to find answers through examinations, tests, images of body organs and analysis of tissues under a microscope.

SYMPTOMS

When a lump has grown to a certain size, its presence is signaled in a number of ways.

♦ It presses on nearby tissue, which sometimes produces pain.

♦ It grows into nearby blood vessels, which may produce bleeding.

♦ It gets so large that it can be seen or felt.

♦ It causes a change in the way some organ works. Trouble swallowing (dysphagia), for example, might be the sign of a tumor involving the esophagus, the passage between the throat and stomach. Hoarseness or change of voice might indicate a tumor in the larynx, or voice box.

These symptoms—pressure, bleeding, a mass or interference with function—are reflected in the American Cancer Society's list of *Seven Early Warning Signals*:

1. **C**hange in bowel or bladder habits.
2. **A** sore that does not heal.
3. **U**nusual bleeding or discharge.
4. **T**hickening or lump in breast or elsewhere.
5. **I**ndigestion or difficulty in swallowing.
6. **O**bvious change in wart or mole.
7. **N**agging cough or hoarseness.

Recognizing a symptom is the first critical step in the search for cancer. Unfortunately, many people don't pay any attention to these warning signals. They wait and wait, sometimes for months, before getting the medical attention that could save their lives.

The best chance of diagnosing cancer early depends on someone's thoughtful and perceptive awareness that something new has happened to his or her body—especially the appearance of one of these symptoms.

THE PHYSICAL EXAMINATION

The suspicion that a cancer is growing is often aroused during a routine physical examination, the major part of what should be a yearly checkup of your general health. The physical examination is a thorough, systematic and progressive search throughout your body for signs of disease or abnormal function. To make sure that no significant area is missed, each physician generally develops his or her own standard pattern or sequence. Some start with the head and work down the body, others examine each organ system as a unit.

Whatever the pattern, a good physical examination with a view to detecting cancer involves a search of the entire body with a special emphasis on the parts that are most prone to malignancy.

♦ The nose and throat are examined. There is a quick and painless mirror examination of the larynx.

♦ The lymph node–bearing areas—such as the neck above the collarbone, under the arms and in the groin—are checked.

♦ Specific attention is paid to the breasts in women and the prostate gland in men.

♦ The abdomen is carefully pushed and probed to detect enlargement of any of the abdominal organs, especially the liver and spleen.

♦ Examination of the pelvic area in women, including a Pap smear, is essential to detect cancers of the cervix, uterus and ovaries.

♦ A probing of the rectum with a gloved finger is an essential part of the physical for both men and women.

During the examination, your doctor will ask you a lot of questions about various body functions. There will be specific questions about hoarseness, signs of gastrointestinal bleeding, constipation, swallowing problems, coughing up blood and so on. A "yes" answer to any of these questions leads to more detailed questions, more specific physical examinations and possibly to blood tests, x-rays or other studies.

You might also be asked questions about any family history of cancer, particularly among close relatives—parents, grandparents, aunts, uncles, brothers and sisters. Detailed answers to these questions will help in the search for any cancers with a genetic basis, such as some breast and colon cancers.

Suspicious findings in any part of the physical examination will lead to further tests. An enlarged lymph node in the neck, for example, might indicate a cancer that has spread from somewhere else. This will set off a vigorous search for the primary site. Persistent coughing, especially with blood, might lead the doctor to look directly inside your lungs with a special instrument (a bronchoscope) to detect tumors (see page 20).

BLOOD TESTS

The next level of the diagnostic process involves a laboratory analysis of blood samples. Two categories of blood tests are used to help in the diagnosis of cancer.

Non-Specific Tests Most blood tests are non-specific. This means they can reveal an abnormality in the blood that indicates some illness, but not which one.

A blood count, for example, may show anemia. Why would you be anemic? Lots of reasons, including cancer. But the anemia may not be related to a tumor unless you have a history of bleeding in the bowel and x-rays show a cancer of the colon. Similarly, there are tests for liver function that indicate abnormalities in that organ. But the problem might be caused by gallstones, hepatitis, tumors or drug toxicity. Certain patterns in the test results will suggest tumors or some other cause of bile obstruction. Other patterns suggest hepatitis. But essentially these patterns are only important clues. They are not solutions to diagnostic questions.

There are so many tests used to detect abnormalities in different organ systems that physicians usually obtain a whole panel of them—blood counts, tests of metabolism (including levels of minerals such as calcium) and tests for the liver, kidneys or thyroid. The test results may suggest certain types of tumors, but no

Table 1: Blood Tests Useful in Cancer Diagnosis

Non-Specific Tests

Alkaline phosphatase	elevated in bone and liver disease
SGOT and SGPT	elevated if there is liver damage
Bilirubin	elevated in liver disease, especially with bile obstruction
LDH	elevated in many diseases, including cancer
Uric acid	elevated in gout, cancers of the blood and lymph nodes, and after cancer treatment
Creatinine and BUN	elevated in kidney disease
Calcium	elevated in cancer that has spread to the bone, with tumors that produce parathyroid hormone-like protein and in multiple myeloma, as well as in some non-malignant diseases
Electrolytes (sodium, potassium, carbon dioxide, chloride)	these levels are useful in metabolic and endocrine disease, and for monitoring both nutritional status and the effects of treatment
Amylase	used to assess pancreatic disease

Specific Tests and Markers

Not all cancers produce these markers

CEA (carcinoembryonic antigen)	elevated in cancers of the colon, rectum, lung, breast and pancreas
CA-125	elevated in cancers of the ovary and uterus
CA 19-9	elevated in cancers of the colon, pancreas, stomach and liver
CA 15-3	elevated in breast cancer
Alpha-fetoprotein (AFP)	elevated in primary liver cancer and some cancers of the testis
HCG (human chorionic gonadotropin)	elevated in some cancers of the testis and ovary and some lung cancers; also elevated in pregnancy
Prostatic acid phosphatase (PAP)	markedly elevated in some cases of prostate cancer
Prostate specific antigen (PSA)	helpful in diagnosing prostate cancer, in detecting recurrent disease and in guiding treatment
Serum protein electrophoresis	abnormal gamma globulin (monoclonal "spike") is found in multiple myeloma
Serum protein immunoelectrophoresis (IgG, IgA, IgM)	similar to above, but can classify the type of abnormal gamma globulin present

specific diagnosis can be made on the basis of these tests alone.

Specific Tests Other blood tests are fairly specific for particular kinds of cancer, often several kinds. These tests will be ordered if your doctor strongly suspects one of these cancers.

Tumor Markers The most important are tests for chemicals called tumor markers. These are produced by various types of tumors. Breast, lung and bowel tumors, for example, produce a protein called the carcinoembryonic antigen (CEA). Some inflammatory diseases may produce low levels of this chemical, but some tumors in these areas produce very high levels. If a very high CEA level is found, then a tumor is assumed to be present until proved otherwise. Similarly, prostate cancers and many cancers of the testicles and ovaries produce known chemicals.

Some very exciting research is now being done to find more and more accurate markers for different types of cancer. We can now envision the day in the not-too-distant future when specific blood tests will identify most human cancers. But at the moment, the few tests we do have are invaluable. They not only help make the diagnosis but are especially useful for keeping track of the cancer after treatment. If the marker is elevated at the time of diagnosis, then successful treatment should result in the level falling or disappearing altogether. The reappearance of the marker often signals a relapse. If that happens, even if no other sign or symptom appears, there would be a search for a new tumor and consideration would be given to retreatment.

Other Blood Tests When a cancer is in the blood cells themselves, tests of the blood and the blood-forming organs may be all that's needed to make the diagnosis. Cancer of the white blood cells—

leukemia—can often be diagnosed by looking at a sample of blood taken from the finger or arm. The diagnosis can be confirmed by examining cells from the bone marrow, where these cells are made. Bone marrow analysis will also diagnose multiple myeloma, which is basically a malignancy of plasma cells in the marrow.

TESTS OF FLUIDS AND STOOLS

Our bodies produce wastes—urine and stools—that can reveal clues about disease. But there are also other fluids that can be analyzed to detect cancer cells.

♦ The most familiar test of body fluids is the urinalysis that is part of a regular checkup. Analyzing the urine's composition can reveal all kinds of abnormalities. The presence of protein might indicate kidney disease. The level of sugar might indicate diabetes. Too many white blood cells can indicate an infection. Too many red blood cells could indicate bleeding, maybe because of a tumor, maybe from some other cause. If tumor cells are found, other tests will be done.

♦ A physical or x-ray examination may reveal the presence of fluid in the chest cavity, abdomen or joints. A needle can be inserted into these areas and the fluid drawn out for examination.

♦ A lumbar puncture, also known as a spinal tap, is a special procedure to remove fluid from the spinal canal. It involves the insertion of a needle between the vertebrae, after you've been given a local anesthetic. Tests can identify any infection, inflammation or cancer.

The Hidden Blood Stool Test Blood in the stools is always a sign of something going wrong in the digestive tract. Sometimes this blood can be easily seen in a bowel movement; most of the time it's all but invisible. One simple procedure to find out whether there is blood in the stools is called the occult (hidden) blood test. A small amount of stool is smeared on specially treated paper, then chemicals that will reveal blood are added. If blood is found, the upper and/or lower bowel will be examined with scopes or barium x-rays.

Blood in the stools is often caused by hemorrhoids, but a benign or premalignant tumor (a polyp) or a hidden cancer is always a possibility.

IMAGING TECHNIQUES

Any suspicious findings in the physical exam or the lab test results will make your doctor want to find out what is going on inside your body. He or she could just look inside directly, either with special instruments or by opening up some area. But the first step usually involves the use of one or more devices that produce images of suspicious areas.

These "imaging studies" may show a tumor in a specific organ and the image will help your doctor assess its size and whether it has involved surrounding tissues.

If you complain of indigestion, for example, your doctor may suspect stomach cancer. This would lead to an x-ray or endoscopy of the upper gastrointestinal tract. Lower digestive tract complaints such as constipation or bleeding might lead to an x-ray or endoscopy to diagnose a possible carcinoma of the colon. Blood in the urine may lead to an x-ray of the kidneys to confirm a suspected tumor in the kidneys or bladder. And complaints of severe headaches, together with other symptoms of increased pressure in the head, may result in a CT scan of the head in search of a brain tumor.

Until fairly recently, radiography (x-ray) was the only imaging technique available. If x-rays couldn't answer critical questions in the diagnostic investigation, then a surgeon would have to open up the body to take a direct look. But new techniques have revolutionized the art and science of diagnosis. Some of the new techniques involve the use of x-rays, others do not.

X-rays This familiar imaging technique involves passing a small dose of electromagnetic radiation through a specific area of the body and onto a film. This produces a two-dimensional picture of the structures inside.

Bones and some other dense substances absorb more x-rays than other tissues, so they show up on the film as shadows that your doctor can interpret. But soft tissues can't be seen very well on x-rays. It is impossible to see the inside of a stomach, for example, without adding a substance that will prevent the x-rays from penetrating.

If your stomach is going to be x-rayed, you will have to swallow a barium "meal." The barium will improve the contrast and so produce a better picture. If your bowel is going to be seen, you will be given a barium enema. If your kidneys are going to be examined, another type of "contrast agent" may be injected into a vein to fill the kidneys, which will allow them to be seen.

A fluoroscope might also be used. This lets the doctor see a continuous, moving image. In this procedure, the x-ray beam strikes a small fluorescent screen and the image is amplified through a video system.

Nuclear Scans Radioactive isotopes that emit gamma rays can produce an image on photographic film or on a scintillation detector. Some of these isotopes, generally given by injection, are organ-specific, which means that they concentrate in that part of the body suspected of harboring cancer.

Different organs react to the isotopes in different ways. The isotopes used for liver scanning concentrate in normal tissues but are not taken up by cancer cells. So the image shows "cold spots" that may be cancerous areas. The isotopes used for bone scans, however, work in the opposite way. Cancer cells make the bone react to the isotope to a greater degree than normal bone, so "hot spots" light up the image of the skeleton. Hot spots can be produced by diseases other than cancer, however, such as bone injury or arthritis.

Angiography This is a very useful way to study the blood vessels in a specific area of the body. Angiography is sometimes used to diagnose and precisely locate tumors in the pancreas, liver and brain, especially when surgery is being considered.

Angiography is also used in some chemotherapy treatments, when a plastic tube (catheter) is placed in an artery to deliver anticancer drugs to the tumor. It is especially important in those cases to know the exact size of the tumor to make sure all of it is treated. It makes no sense to insert the catheters and then miss a portion of the tumor not supplied by the blood vessel being used. Angiograms safeguard against this problem by defining the blood vessels within the tumor, which have a different quality and appearance than the arteries next to the tumor.

CT Scans For the past several years, computerized tomography (CT) scans have made it possible to see parts of the body that are difficult or impossible to view any other way. The images produced are far superior to those obtained by traditional

x-rays. And the images are even clearer if you drink a contrast agent or get an injection before the scan is done.

The CT machine scans the area being investigated—chest, brain, abdomen or any other part of the body—by taking x-rays of one thin layer of tissue after another. A computer puts the images together to create a cross-section of the area. Total-body scans are also done.

Although there is higher x-ray exposure with CT scans than with conventional x-rays, *not* undergoing the procedure is much riskier if cancer is strongly suspected. The information from the scan is not only useful for diagnosis but is very helpful in planning treatment.

Magnetic Resonance Imaging (MRI) The MRI scan can complement or even supplant the CT scan in some cases. The images look similar to CT scan images, but there are no x-rays involved. The MRI scanner uses a powerful magnetic field to make certain particles in the body vibrate. Extremely sophisticated computer equipment measures the reaction and produces the images.

MRI has a few important advantages apart from no risk of x-ray exposure. Cross-sections can be obtained not only across the body, as in CT scanning, but also from front to back and from left to right. This lets your doctor see your body

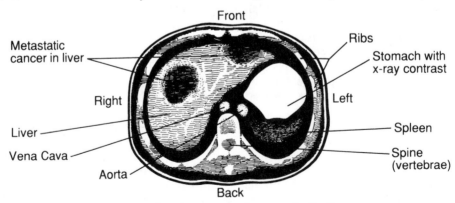

CT image of the upper abdomen, showing metastatic cancer in the liver.

from all three directions. In some cases, the images provide more information and are superior to those obtained by CT scans. This is especially true for images of the central nervous system and the spine. In some other cases, CT scanning is more useful than MRI scanning.

MRI is not suitable under certain conditions. Implanted devices such as a pacemaker, clip or pump can be affected by the strong magnetic field.

Ultrasound This is a harmless and painless imaging technique. It is "non-invasive," meaning that nothing enters your body except sound waves.

The technique involves spreading a thin coating of jelly over a particular area of the skin, then bouncing high-frequency sound waves through the skin onto internal organs. It works basically on the same principle as the sonar used by the navy to detect submarines, where sound waves are sent through the water and the "ping" of the sound bouncing back is analyzed. In a similar way, the complex ultrasound scanning apparatus draws a picture of whatever organ the sound waves are bouncing off. This picture can reveal a lot of information.

Many people are aware of ultrasound as a safe way to examine a fetus to search for abnormalities. But it is also useful for detecting possibly malignant masses or lumps without the need for x-rays.

Ultrasound is used to examine the neck for tumors of the thyroid gland or of the parathyroids. It is the standard method to diagnose gallstones, since the sound waves bounce quite nicely off the stones. And it is often used in the pelvis to study possible enlargement of the prostate or an ovary. Benign ovarian cysts are common, and other ways of examining this part of the body are not very precise. It has also recently been adapted to help stage rectal and esophageal cancers.

ENDOSCOPY

Sometimes images are not enough. The use of direct visualization has become more and more important in recent years, not only for diagnosing malignancies but in some cases as an aid in treatment (*see* Chapter 9).

Rigid, thin telescopes have been used for years to look inside body cavities with natural openings. A bronchoscope inserted into the mouth or nose and through the windpipe (trachea) can be used to look inside the lungs. A cystoscope inserted into the urethra can be used to examine the bladder. Sometimes mirrors are used with these rigid scopes to examine, for example, the nasal passage and the back of the mouth (nasopharyngoscope) and the larynx (laryngoscope).

Flexible Scopes Lately, flexible fiber-optic "telescopes" have come into widespread use. These scopes use bundles of glass fibers that can bend around corners and form perfect pictures of the tissues at their far ends. Doctors looking through one end of the scope can look into many areas of the body safely, often with a minimum of sedation or local anesthetic. Not only can your doctor see exactly what's going on in these areas but he or she can also take photographs or remove cell samples.

The inside of the lung passages can be examined easily and quickly with the fiber-optic bronchoscope. A diagnosis of lung cancer can often be made by this method alone, without resorting to the surgical procedures that used to be necessary.

Similar instruments have revolutionized the diagnosis of tumors in the stomach and bowel. With a flexible gastroscope or colonoscope, the entire stomach or colon can be clearly seen and pieces of tissue can be collected. Similar specialized instruments for other body cavities have made diagnostic procedures much safer. And the procedures can be repeated after treatment to see how effective the treatment has been.

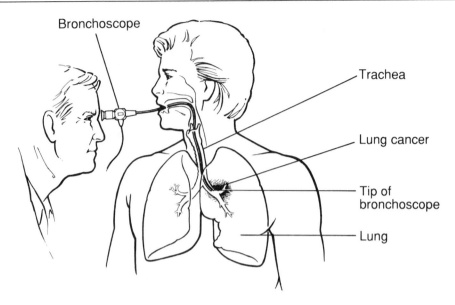

Bronchoscope

Trachea

Lung cancer

Tip of bronchoscope

Lung

Lung cancer can often be diagnosed and biopsied through a bronchoscope.

ERCP Clever adaptations of these endoscopic methods and tools are sometimes used for specialized diagnosis and therapy. In a procedure called endoscopic retrograde cholangiopancreatography (ERCP), for example, a doctor can pass a flexible fiber-optic telescope into your stomach, visualize the opening of the ducts releasing bile from the liver, insert a tube (stent) into these ducts from inside the stomach either to provide drainage or to take pictures showing the exact location of tumors in the bile ducts and exactly how involved the ducts are.

A new technique is used when lung cancers partially or completely block air passages or when a tumor blocks the esophagus or colon. A beam of laser light can be passed through a flexible scope to create or enlarge an opening in the center of the tumor (*see* Chapter 9).

CYTOLOGICAL STUDIES

Cytology is simply the study of cells. In cancer diagnosis, the term cytological studies means the examination of cellular material removed from the body. The cells might be removed by natural means, such as coughing up sputum (phlegm). They might also be removed by washing a body cavity with a salt solution—the inside of the abdomen after abdominal surgery, for example—or by scraping the surface of an organ or a suspected cancer.

The best-known cytological test is the one developed by George Papanicolaou—the Pap smear. The cervix is scraped and brushed to remove for analysis cells that could be abnormal or cancerous. In the same way, the tongue, esophagus, stomach or the lung's air passages can be easily scraped using a small brush through a scope.

The removed cells are put on slides, stained with dyes and examined under a microscope. The cytologist will look for the characteristic appearance of malignant or premalignant cells. A pathologist will also examine the slides and either diagnose cancer or report a strong suspicion of cancer. In many cases, a conventional surgical biopsy will usually be done to confirm the diagnosis.

Tumor Tests Several new techniques for cell analysis have been developed recently. These techniques improve doctors' ability to diagnose cancer, help determine the likely clinical course and help guide the choice of treatment options.

♦ Special stains. There are now a large number of special ways to stain cancer tissue in the laboratory. These stains are often of great help in determining the type of cancer when there is some uncertainty. They also provide helpful information about prognosis and treatment.

♦ Flow cytometry. This technique analyzes a tumor's DNA content to find out whether the cancer cells contain the normal number of chromosomes (diploid) or an abnormal amount (aneuploid). Aneuploid tumors tend to be poorly differentiated and aggressive.

♦ S-phase testing. This technique measures how fast a tumor is growing. In the S-phase of a cell's growth cycle, new DNA is synthesized to prepare for the division of one cell into two. A tumor that is growing slowly may have less than 7 percent of cells in the S-phase. A rapidly growing tumor has 8 percent or more. Tumors with higher rates of growth have a poorer prognosis and may need more aggressive treatment.

BONE MARROW ANALYSIS

Bone marrow is analyzed to diagnose blood or bone marrow cancers and to find out if a malignancy from somewhere else has spread to the bone marrow.

The procedure is simple and brief. It can be done in a doctor's office using a local anesthetic similar to the one used by your dentist. In much the same way as blood is taken from your arm, a needle is inserted into either the breast bone or the pelvic bone, both of which are just under the skin and are easily entered. A small amount of liquid bone marrow is drawn into a syringe, placed on slides and examined under a microscope for evidence of leukemia, lymphoma or any other cancer cells.

Sometimes a bone marrow biopsy may be done. A special cutting needle can be put into an anesthetized area of the pelvic bone and tiny bone chips can be removed. This procedure may be necessary for several reasons—to diagnose certain types of blood and bone marrow malignancies, to see if other cancers involve the marrow or as part of the staging process.

Bone marrow examinations are also sometimes done to check for infections, follow up the effectiveness of treatment or discover how well the bone marrow could produce blood cells if really aggressive chemotherapy were to be given.

BIOPSIES

Ultimately the diagnosis of cancer depends on examining a small bit of tissue to see if it has the characteristic patterns and cell types defined as cancer. The definitive way to diagnose a suspicious area is to perform a biopsy. Sometimes this is done even before doing other tests.

This microscopic examination is carried out by a pathologist who is expert in the very exact criteria that separate malignant cells from normal or benign ones. It is essential to obtain a specimen of tissue to do this examination. The biopsy is the procedure for obtaining the tissue (*see* figure on next page).

There are two types:

♦ an incisional biopsy involves cutting into a portion of the tumor, then stitching the area closed;

♦ an excisional biopsy involves removing the entire tumor.

The excisional biopsy is often done with tumors that are easily accessible, such as those involving the skin, the mouth or nasal cavity, lymph nodes or a woman's reproductive system.

Biopsies are often done during the surgery that may be needed to expose the tumor. In such cases, it's customary to take tissue samples not only from the apparent site of the tumor but also from the lymph nodes or other tissues in the neighborhood. This will help measure the tumor's potential or actual spread. This defines the stage of the cancer, so the staging process may be carried out at the same time as the diagnostic process. Of course, the surgeon may also try to carry out the most appropriate therapy at the same time by removing all the visible tumor.

Needle Biopsies For easily accessible tumors and also for some tumors inside the body—in the kidney or pancreas, for example—needle biopsies have become quite common. In this procedure, an anesthetic is placed both in the skin and in the soft tissues under the skin. A very thin needle is then directed into the tumor, and a small bit of tissue is withdrawn for examination. This is called fine needle aspiration (FNA).

It's very important to be sure the needle is actually in the tumor, so needle biopsies of internal areas are often done in the x-ray department, where an x-ray machine or CT scanner can show the needle's position accurately.

Tumors in the lung and the liver can be diagnosed by a needle biopsy. Even a tumor involving a deep organ like the pancreas can be diagnosed in this way about 80 percent of the time. But the amount of tissue obtained through a needle is not usually enough to diagnose cancers of the lymph glands accurately.

A needle biopsy is not always advisable. When there are vital structures in the area—over the collarbone, for example—there is a risk of complications such as bleeding or nerve damage.

The Next Step Once the biopsy is performed and the diagnosis confirmed, the medical evaluation should be rapidly completed. At this point, treatment planning can begin.

Types of biopsy for cancer diagnosis

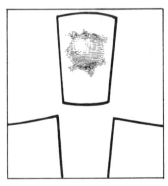

Excisional biopsy
Complete removal of tumor

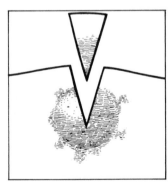

Incisional biopsy
Remove part of tumor

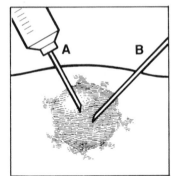

A
Fine needle
aspiration

B
Cutting needle
(core) biopsy

3
WORKING WITH
THE HEALTH CARE TEAM

*Ernest H. Rosenbaum, MD, Malin Dollinger, MD, Lenore Dollinger, RN, PhD,
and Isadora Rosenbaum, MA*

◇

After you've been diagnosed with cancer, you enter a world that is probably unfamiliar to you. The cancer treatment system is large and complex. Many different kinds of health care facilities and institutions are involved, and the system is populated by a bewildering array of professionals.

You may feel like you are being processed, sent from one place to another for tests or other procedures for reasons you don't quite understand. And at every turn, you meet new people who seem to speak a different language. It's easy to feel lost and disoriented in such a large system.

But it doesn't have to be that way. You simply have to remember that *you* are the one fighting for your life. And all the people and facilities are there to help you in your battle. Fighting cancer is fighting a war, and the more highly trained forces you can gather to attack the invader the more successful you are likely to be.

WHO DOES WHAT IN THE CANCER TREATMENT SYSTEM

Cancer treatment today is very much a team effort that emphasizes total care. A wide range of medical specialists, therapists, technicians, counselors, social workers and others become involved in your treatment and your rehabilitation.

Diagnosis If you have been diagnosed as having cancer, you have already come in contact with several members of the health care team, even if you haven't met them all personally.

♦ Your cancer symptom may have been detected by your internist or primary physician—whoever it is you call when you have a fever, a pain you think should be looked at or when you're just feeling generally sick. If you are a woman, the primary physician may have been a gynecologist. If your child has the cancer, the primary physician may have been a pediatrician. Or it may have been a specialist in family practice, still fondly remembered by some as a GP, or general practitioner.

♦ A laboratory technician may have drawn your blood for tests.

♦ The tissue for a biopsy may have been taken by your primary physician, by a general surgeon or possibly by a radiologist or medical oncologist doing a fine needle aspiration.

♦ Your tissue sample was then examined under the microscope by a pathologist, an expert in the analysis of tissue to identify disease.

Treatment Planning Once the diagnosis is made, the treatment team is assembled. Depending on the most appropriate kind of treatment for your particular tumor, you may deal with internists, surgeons or medical or radiation oncologists.

♦ Internists are specialists in many fields

of internal medicine. They may specialize, for example, in the blood (hematologists), cancer (oncologists), the endocrine system (endocrinologists), the gastrointestinal or GI tract (gastroenterologists), kidneys (nephrologists) or the brain and nervous system (neurologists).

♦ Medical oncologists—internists with additional training in the treatment of cancer—prescribe chemotherapy drugs as well as hormones and other biological agents.

♦ Surgeons—who cut out as much cancerous tissue as possible, ideally before it has a chance to spread—also often specialize, operating only on specific areas of the body. But you should be aware that medical practices aren't always the same in all communities. Most general surgeons, for example, will operate on organs in the abdomen. Most will operate on the colon and rectum, although in larger cities there are usually surgeons who specialize in this area of the body (proctologists). Some general surgeons do chest surgery, others don't. Some back operations will be done by neurosurgeons in some communities but by bone and joint (orthopedic) surgeons in others.

♦ Radiation oncologists are specialists in the use of high-energy x-rays to cause tumors to shrink. Within the radiation department, the radiation oncologist is supported by diagnostic radiologists, who interpret x-ray studies, and radiotherapy technologists and radiation physicists, who check the radiation dosage to make it as safe as possible.

Support Many other health care professionals work as a united team to help you through your cancer treatment and recovery.

♦ Oncology nurses play an essential role on the health care team. They have specialized knowledge and skill in giving chemotherapy and in meeting the special needs of cancer patients. They may specialize even further, as radiation oncology nurses, for example (*see* Chapter 15).

♦ Nutritionists evaluate any deficiencies in your diet and prepare individualized plans that take your condition into account and make sure you get enough nutrients.

♦ Physical therapists can make sure you maintain proper muscle tone and adapt to any changes to your body that result from treatment.

♦ Occupational therapists help teach activities of daily living—how to eat, swallow and use your body efficiently.

♦ Enterostomal therapists specialize in the care of ostomies.

♦ Respiratory therapists help you keep your lungs and breathing passages clear.

♦ Speech therapists work with people who have lost their voice box (larynx) and have to learn to speak in a new way.

♦ Psychologists, psychotherapists and other emotional counselors such as clergy and social workers help you through depression, fear or other emotional problems you may have because of your cancer or its treatment.

♦ Dentists evaluate the state of your mouth before treatment and help you deal with treatment side effects such as mouth sores.

♦ Cosmeticians ensure proper skin care during treatment and help you cope with physical changes.

♦ Laboratory technologists perform specialized blood tests.

♦ Pharmacists prepare complicated medications and ensure correct dosages.

♦ Technologists make sure that breathing machines, chemotherapy pumps, home oxygen equipment and other mechanical devices work properly at all times.

Direction As with any effective team, one person usually takes charge of the overall direction of the team's efforts. He or she is essentially the commander of the forces brought to bear on your cancer. He or she decides what "intelligence" information is needed, delegates specific tasks to the people best able to perform them, analyzes all the options and makes the key decisions.

Most important, he or she is the one who reports to you on your situation. How do things look? What can be done? What are the risks? What are the odds? What are the alternatives?

In some cases, the overall direction will be the responsibility of your primary physician. But since cancer treatment is so complex and so many specialists may be called in at various times, direction is now more often in the hands of an oncologist. And because medical oncologists are also specialists in internal medicine, they often assume overall responsibility.

There are many advantages to this chain of command. Medical oncologists see many cancer patients and are knowledgeable about the effects and likely results of the most up-to-date treatments. Oncologists also tend to do a lot of talking with you because cancer is serious business. Drugs are serious, radiation and surgery are serious, side effects are serious and so is the prognosis. Nothing is trivial.

CHOOSING AN ONCOLOGIST

There are several straightforward ways that an oncologist can become involved in your care. The most common is through a referral from your primary physician, who may recommend a specialist he or she has worked with before, has confidence in and is an expert in the specific kind of cancer care you need. Sometimes you may know a specialist yourself, either because of your own experience or the experience of a family member or friend.

It is unusual these days that you have to choose a specialist without any help from family, friends or general physicians. But if you do have to start from scratch, the American Cancer Society or other medical societies in your area can supply you with names of several qualified physicians.

When you are choosing an oncologist, you can look into his or her credentials in a number of ways, the easiest being to check the *American Medical Directory* or the *Directory of American Specialists* at your local library. The latter lists doctors who have had special training and have demonstrated their competence to a recognized medical certification board (such as the American Board of Surgery or the American Board of Internal Medicine). You can also call PDQ (Physicians Data Query) or, from within the U.S., 1-800-4-CANCER, a National Cancer Institute resource, for a list of specialists. There are excellent oncology specialists who have had full training and are competent and up to date yet are not board-certified. But if you are starting from scratch, the board certification may give you a little extra reassurance that you are in good hands.

UNDERSTANDING WHAT YOUR DOCTOR IS SAYING

Right from the time you hear the cancer diagnosis, the medical team has to get a lot of new information across to you and your family. This isn't always an easy process, either for you or for your doctor. Each stage of cancer care involves a tremendous amount of information that is generally unknown to the lay public. And all too often doctors use technical terms that any non-medical person has trouble understanding. Yet open and clear communication has become an essential part of a good medical relationship.

Cancer is a family affair. One member gets the disease, but the whole family goes through the experience. So it is very important that both you and your family know and understand all aspects of your disease. You should know how it is treated, what side effects there might be and how you best can cope. Trying to learn how to deal with your new life situation may improve how you cope with your treatment program.

The Initial Visit Exactly where and how you find out about the diagnosis isn't always up to you. Yet this first confrontation with the fact that you have cancer can affect your relationship with the disease, your doctor and the medical system.

Most doctors realize that difficult problems come up when someone is told he or she has cancer right in the recovery room after biopsy surgery. No one can fully appreciate what's going on in those circumstances. Most doctors also dislike telling someone he or she has cancer over the phone. It's very traumatic and it doesn't help the relationship. So doctors often try to make sure you are in a proper emotional state and have time to ask questions and discuss various aspects of treatment.

The proper emotional state is hard to achieve, though. Your initial visit to an oncologist's office can be a very trying experience. Fear and anxiety about cancer, no matter how controllable or curable it might be, often limit the effectiveness of the visit. And the diagnosis, once made, often makes you unable to concentrate on the information being given. Faced with a serious, life-threatening illness, it is often difficult to express feelings, ask questions or assimilate all the new information.

When you are under such emotional stress you often cannot think clearly. In our experience, one woman—a medical social worker—walked out of the office and her sister asked, "What did the doctor say?" She said, "I forgot." She hadn't even made it to the reception area.

Sharing the Information For this reason, many doctors encourage family members or close friends to come to the consultation. For this reason too, some doctors record the initial consultation and dictate the letter to the referring physician in front of the patient during the office visit. A separate tape to "translate" the technical letter and to explain the disease, treatment and side effects, along with pertinent questions and answers,

can also be very helpful. In a study at Minnesota's renowned Mayo Clinic, it was found that patients had to listen to a taped explanation at least three times before understanding the whole message.

If your doctor tapes your initial consultation, you will find it very beneficial to take the tape home, listen to it as often as you need to, review it with your family and friends in a calm, relaxed atmosphere or even send copies to family members in other cities who wish to be informed.

Ignorance, confusion and unspoken fears can isolate people from one another. In a situation filled with anxiety, the isolation can be especially severe and painful. When family and friends share information about treatment plans, medications and side effects, cancer becomes more understandable and bearable for everyone concerned.

Besides reducing misunderstandings and improving communication, the use of audiotapes has the advantage of making the doctor's explanations more organized and concise. For the doctor, it will also mean fewer unanswered questions and fewer calls from family members trying to find out what's going on.

Getting More Information Besides the discussion and the audiotapes, your doctor may provide you with information in the form of handouts, pamphlets or recommended reading. These are available free from the National Cancer Institute, the American Cancer Society and many support organizations.

Pamphlets and books have their place in giving you both general and detailed information about your cancer and its treatment, but videotapes can accelerate the learning process. Videotapes may be especially important in the period just after your diagnosis because the emotional adjustment you have to make to having cancer can interfere with the concentration necessary for reading. A decrease in attention span and comprehension—a kind of emotional or mental paralysis, really—is not unusual. So videotapes to explain CT scans, radiation therapy, good nutrition, exercise or any other aspects of cancer and cancer therapy can be very helpful.

Videotapes also bring the family together to watch and learn and talk about the procedures shown. Videotapes can present helpful ideas on how to cope and how to solve simple problems such as how to set up a bedroom or tackle more serious problems. This can become a "quickie course" for family members to learn their role in supportive and home care.

The Doctor's Responsibility Doctors are well aware of the problems you and your family go through when you get the diagnosis of cancer. And your doctor does have a responsibility to reduce fears and confusion and to make it as easy as possible for you to understand what he or she is saying.

But not all doctors have learned to communicate effectively. If your doctor doesn't use techniques such as audio- and videotapes, ask about them. With your doctor's permission, perhaps you could take your own tape recorder into your consultations. Experience has shown that this technique promotes active discussion and doesn't intimidate physicians, patients or families.

COMMUNICATING WITH YOUR DOCTOR

When you have cancer, the worry, fears and concerns never stop, even after treatment. If your cancer is cured or permanently controlled, you always have that nagging fear that it might come back with a vengeance sometime in the years ahead. If it is not completely controlled, you worry that the treatment won't work, that you'll be a burden to your family or friends or that you'll suffer pain and disability. No matter how hard you try to put these fears to rest, they reawaken and rise

back up with each visit to the doctor.

You don't know whether you should be reassured by having extra tests or reassured by not having extra tests. You are always waiting for clear, definite answers to all the questions bombarding your brain. Am I really in remission? Is the cancer really gone? Will the pain go away? Can I go back to work? Will I ever feel safe? How long will I live?

While you are trying to understand everything your doctor is telling you, you may feel at a loss about how to get your concerns across. After all, you've had no training in how to deal effectively with specialists or even deal with that nagging voice in your head that keeps whispering all the questions and fears.

What Helps and What Blocks Communication Two main factors affect the way you communicate with your doctor. Both can either help the process along or block effective communication.
♦ Your attitudes and feelings about yourself and about your illness.
♦ Your need to be realistic, to understand your expectations and to express your needs clearly.

The attitudes and feelings that help communication are easy to list—openness, honesty, respect, clarity, responsibility, accountability and a willingness to listen and to learn.

What blocks effective communication are anger, resentment, dishonesty, intimidation and holding back information. And unless you do something to remove these blocks, you won't be receiving the best care your doctor can offer you.

Anger It isn't the anger you might feel about having cancer or anger over a test result that can hinder communication. It is a generalized anger that some people feel toward doctors, an anger that says "they earn too much, they never listen, they're insensitive, they don't really care, they think they're God."

You may have good reason to feel angry. Your doctor may keep you waiting for an hour and then spend only five minutes with you. It may take forever for your calls to be returned. Whether your anger is justified or not, communicate how you feel. If you don't say it openly, the anger will be communicated anyway and will always be a barrier to openness and honesty.

You can express your anger and still be respectful. Write down how you feel clearly and concisely. If you write it down it will be easier to speak without resentment. Then respect your doctor's time. Let the appointment desk know you want extra time during the next visit to talk about things that are bothering you and interfering with your ability to have a good working relationship.

When you tell your doctor how you feel, give him or her reasonable suggestions for resolving the problems, such as getting the first appointment of the day so you won't have to wait. Ask him or her what time calls are usually returned and say that you will call only at those times unless there's an emergency. Then stick to it.

Doctors know that anger is a secondary feeling, rising up in response to fear, anxiety or frustration. But doctors are also human and under a lot of pressure. So it might be difficult for your doctor to respond to you in a supportive way if you confront him or her only with anger. Ask yourself what lies beneath the anger—fear? rejection? disappointment?—and express those feelings. If it's emotional support you want and your doctor doesn't seem to have the time or compassion to meet your needs, ask if there is someone else who can. You have to be willing to accept your doctor's limitations but be unwilling to accept less than *you* need.

Intimidation This is a two-way street. Many patients feel intimidated by their doctors. Patients can be afraid that doctors will think they're stupid if they ask too many questions or not like them for taking up so much time. This is fear, pure

and simple. Make it work for you. Simply say, "I'm afraid to take up your time but I'm more afraid for myself." You'll be amazed how that kind of honesty can work for you.

The other side to intimidation is when the patient intimidates the doctor. If you think to yourself—or say right out (in a joking way, of course)—"I know as much as you do, so don't try to talk down to me," again recognize the fear at the source of this need to intimidate. Express this fear openly and honestly. If you really think your doctor is doing less than he or she should, talk about it and listen to how the doctor responds. Only then can you make a rational decision about what action you should take.

Withholding Information Holding back or not being completely honest and clear about how you feel not only blocks good communication, it puts your doctor at a terrible disadvantage and doesn't serve your best interests at all.

If you have a lot of new symptoms, you may be afraid of sounding like a hypochondriac or appearing to be too emotional. So when the doctor asks you how you are, you reply, "Just fine." When you say that, you lose a golden opportunity to communicate your needs. These new symptoms may be causing you all kinds of worry and distress, but by your two little words you've made sure that your doctor will not be able to put your mind at ease. You can only hope your doctor doesn't believe you.

And when your doctor explains a procedure, treatment or test result and asks if you understand, don't just automatically say, "Sure. Got it." If you don't really understand, say so. All pretending can do is add to your confusion and increase your anxiety.

Dealing with Fear It should be clear by now that the feeling of fear can block communication. If fear stops you from asking perfectly reasonable questions or accepting needed treatment or if it comes out as anger, it can badly damage your relationship with someone who is doing his or her best to make you well again.

But fear can also work for you in communicating with your doctor. Fear can make you stop and think for yourself. It can make you think seriously about all the alternatives before you and ask for explanations and support. Only then can you realistically evaluate the risks you have to take.

Talking About "What If. . .?" There is one subject that many cancer patients don't want to talk about. Sometimes this is called the "what if. . .?" scenario. What if the treatment doesn't help? What if everything that might help has already been done? What if the only goal now is to try to stay comfortable, physically and mentally?

It is hard to talk about all the aggressive treatments that might be used, the side effects and your critical need to always have hope, and at the same time discuss "what if?" You may not want to talk about it at all. You don't always need to. And your doctor will respect your wishes. But if you do want to discuss it, let your doctor know.

There is one aspect of "what if . . .?" that really should be discussed. If your situation does become grave, your doctor will need some guidance on how you want things handled. How heroic do you want your doctor to be, especially if the end seems near? If the situation does reach that stage, you may not be in any condition to discuss the question rationally. Your doctor may be able to talk it over with your family, but it is *your* wishes that are most important (*see* Chapter 31).

HOW YOU CAN HELP YOURSELF GET AN EFFECTIVE REVIEW

Fifteen minutes may not seem like a lot of time to cover critical information that may be important to your very survival. But a lot can happen during a fifteen-minute office visit. Unfortunately, a lot of time can also be used up by relatively trivial matters.

From the doctor's point of view, it sometimes may take about three minutes to cover the strictly medical procedures. A schedule for a chemotherapy program, the dosage and the side effects can be covered quickly. But a doctor has to deal with what happened last week, how you felt about things, what your hopes and fears are—all the secret things going on beneath the surface that might be important. So the other 12 minutes are often given to psychological evaluation and counseling, rather than purely technical matters.

All questions and problems are in some way important, but some are more important than others. And if you want to help yourself get the best chance of an effective review, there are certain rules or guidelines you should be aware of.

♦ *Focus on the matter at hand* Doctors try to take care of the most pertinent issues first. The doctor's most important questions will be about what's happening with you right now. Do you have a sore mouth? Are you losing weight? Do you have any major complaints? Do you have diarrhea? What's new since your last visit? The doctor then has to try to analyze and make sense of what's changing. Doctors are always trying to anticipate changes so they don't have to play "catch-up." Until you have a problem, your doctor can't solve it. So give the clearest, most detailed answers you can without holding anything back. It might help if you keep notes of significant symptoms or events that you noticed between visits.

♦ *Be cooperative* Every doctor has seen patients who, because of anxieties—the fear of illness or death—simply aren't cooperative. They object to having extra blood tests or doing things that are sometimes necessary but that they simply don't want to do. When they come into the office, they should undress for an examination, yet some say, "I don't want to get undressed today." That's not the best way to get help. You have to follow certain patterns and be cooperative if you expect results.

♦ *Avoid raising irrelevant problems* Your doctor is always ready to deal with important problems like weight loss or nausea or a swollen arm or leg. When all that has to be covered during the office visit, it's hard to deal with a stubbed toe or whether the pimple on your backside has to be removed. Talking about a half-dozen minor problems can use up half the appointment. Of course, the doctor realizes that what you are really saying is, "I'm scared. I'm frightened for my life." But still, discussing extraneous problems is not the most effective use of office time.

♦ *Ask the pertinent questions* Unless you try to limit your questions to the most essential problems, you lose both focus and the chance for better explanations. All questions are relevant, but if you take a long list of questions you're going to defeat yourself before you begin. As a patient, you have an obligation to be practical and to do your best to work with your physician rather than frustrate each other.

4
DECIDING ON THE APPROPRIATE TREATMENT

Malin Dollinger, MD, and Ernest H. Rosenbaum, MD

"Cancer is one of the most curable chronic diseases in this country today."
—*Vincent T. DeVita, Jr, MD*

◇

Medicine has now reached the stage where almost half of all diagnosed cancers are cured. Of course, this statistic is an average. The cure rate for some cancers is much higher than for others. And some cancers can come back even after the "five years cancer-free" that is used to define "cure."

But even with cancers still considered incurable, proper therapy often yields tremendous benefits. Treatment can add months or years to a reasonably normal life. It can also greatly improve the quality of your life by relieving pain or ensuring the relatively normal functioning of your body processes. Many people live a normal life span with chronic cancer before succumbing to some other disease.

Unfortunately, far too many people still think a cancer diagnosis is a death sentence. Far too many take the attitude that if it can't be cured there's no point in undergoing treatment. What is even more unfortunate is that this attitude is found not only among people with cancer and the lay public but within the medical community.

In many cases, cancer truly is an incurable disease. But it's not the only one. Diabetes and heart disease can't be cured, but they can be treated on an ongoing basis. They're treated all the time. Few people take the "why bother?" attitude with either of them. Why? Because they know both can be managed day by day and that people with either disease can

lead long, active and productive lives. The same can be true for cancer patients.

The key to getting the chance for cure or successful management is getting the best treatment as soon as possible after your diagnosis. What that treatment is, you will have to help decide. Yes, you should rely on experts with training and experience in fighting cancer. But it's your life on the line, and ultimately, the decisions must be yours. And you will have to base those decisions on a detailed analysis of your disease and the recommendations of your primary physician or cancer specialist.

WHAT ARE THE OPTIONS? A TREATMENT OVERVIEW

The three mainstays of cancer therapy over the years have been surgery, radiation and chemotherapy. These have now been joined by biological therapy, which uses the body's immune system to combat growing cancer cells. The goals, procedures, risks and side effects of each of these four kinds of therapy (sometimes referred to as modalities) are detailed in the next four chapters. Here, the treatment options are briefly reviewed.

 Surgery This is the oldest and most successful approach to cancer treatment. If it is possible to "cut it out" safely and there is no residual disease, you may be cured. Two key questions have to be answered when deciding if surgery is the right thing to do.

♦ Is the tumor just in one place (localized)? Once the cancer has spread, surgery may or may not be appropriate.

♦ Can the tumor be removed without damaging vital organs or causing major functional problems? A cancerous lung or a kidney can be removed because everyone has a spare. But a surgeon can't cut out the whole liver or vital parts of the brain.

There are two surgical approaches. In the one-stage approach, the diagnostic biopsy might be followed immediately by the removal of the tumor while you are still under anesthesia. After the operation, you can discuss whether you need additional therapy and what the most effective method or sequence would be, particularly if several therapies might be realistic alternatives.

In the two-stage approach, only the biopsy is done. You then discuss the results with your doctor. If the biopsy shows cancer, you and your doctor plan the definitive cancer treatment. If surgery is an option, the operation to remove the tumor will then be carried out.

 Radiation Therapy The purpose of radiation is to make tumors shrink or disappear. Radiation does this by damaging the genetic structure (DNA) of the tumor cells so they can't grow or divide. The damage is done by a beam of x-rays, gamma rays or electrons aimed directly at the tumor from a high-energy x-ray machine set up at a specific distance from your body or by radioactive materials placed inside or close to the tumor.

There is no pain or discomfort during radiation therapy. Undergoing treatment is much the same as having a chest x-ray, except the machine is left on for several minutes instead of a second or two. Radiation may be the only treatment needed for some localized cancers, or it might

be used along with other kinds of therapy.

 Chemotherapy This term is often misunderstood. What it means is treating some medical condition with chemicals (drugs). Treating cancer with 5-fluorouracil is chemotherapy. So is treating an infection with penicillin or a headache with two aspirins.

Yet when chemotherapy is mentioned in connection with cancer, the term generates a lot of fear. Almost everyone has heard horror stories about serious side effects. These side effects can be unpleasant, but they are in general greatly exaggerated. It's true that a few people cannot tolerate chemical therapy at all. But most can tolerate it reasonably well. Others have moderate to significant reactions. When approaching the subject, also keep in mind that many drugs are used in chemotherapy and not all of them have serious side effects. The side effects themselves can often be reduced or controlled by antinausea drugs or other medications.

While surgery and radiation treat cancers that are growing in one particular place, chemotherapy is generally used for cancers that have traveled through the blood and lymph systems to many parts of the body. In the past, chemotherapy was used only when surgery and radiation were no longer effective. But now it is the treatment of choice for some kinds of cancer and is often used in combination with surgery and radiation, especially for localized cancers.

 Biological Therapy This is a relatively new way to treat cancer. It takes advantage of recent research that shows that the immune system may play a key role in protecting the body against cancer. The immune system might even play a part in combating cancer that has already developed.

The immune system consists of white

blood cells called lymphocytes that act as a defense system against foreign organisms such as bacteria and viruses. One type of lymphocyte—the T cell—is formed in the thymus gland and is a natural killer of foreign cells, including cancer cells. Another lymphocyte—the B cell—is produced in the bone marrow and lymph nodes and makes antibodies in response to stimulation by a foreign protein. B lymphocytes can also kill cancer cells. Another white cell—the monocyte—interacts with T and B cells.

Biological therapy consists mainly of using highly purified proteins—interferon and interleukin-2 are the best known—to activate the immune system. In many different ways, they boost the lymphocytes' cancer-killing properties.

COMBINATION AND ADJUVANT THERAPIES

Five or 10 years ago it was common to think about treating cancer only by surgery *or* radiation *or* chemotherapy, depending on the stage of the disease. Two or all three therapies might be used, but usually only one at a time and in the sequence mentioned—surgery if the tumor was localized, then radiation if there was an actual or potential recurrence, then chemotherapy if the cancer involved vital organs or had spread so far that surgery or radiation had to be ruled out.

Recently there has been great interest in using what is called combination or multimodality treatment. Many aggressive forms of cancer therapy incorporate two or three of the standard treatment methods. There is no universal agreement yet on what the best combination or best sequence is for most malignancies. But broad principles have emerged.

♦ When tumors are large, locally aggressive and touch adjacent structures, radiation or chemotherapy might be given before surgery. This will shrink the tumor and make the surgical procedure much

simpler. This is called neo-adjuvant therapy. In hospitals with special radiotherapy equipment, radiation will sometimes be given during surgery to kill invisible or microscopic tumor cells that might cause the cancer to come back in the future.
♦ Both radiation and chemotherapy may be given after surgery. Radiation will usually be used if the surgeon finds during the operation that the tumor is invading nearby tissues that couldn't be removed.
♦ Radiation and chemotherapy have also been combined in an attempt to produce a more powerful antitumor effect than either treatment can produce alone. Radiation, for example, has a more powerful killing action against smaller tumors, so chemotherapy is sometimes used to shrink the tumors before radiotherapy.

A number of procedures (clinical protocols) use both methods—together or in sequence—to take advantage of the increased sensitivity a tumor may have when both treatments are used. The combined therapy does not usually produce more toxic effects, side effects or complications than each treatment produces on its own. But the dosages of both may sometimes have to be reduced to prevent really major side effects.
♦ The new biological therapies—interferon alpha, beta and gamma, interleukin and other investigational programs—are being blended with standard radiotherapy and chemotherapy. But research on these combinations is still in a fairly early stage. We are still in the process of testing this form of therapy to discover what sequence, dosage or combination is the most helpful or even whether adding biological therapies to the others is more effective than today's standard treatments.

Adjuvant Chemotherapy The purpose of giving chemotherapy after surgery—called adjuvant therapy—is to wipe out tumor cells that may be invisible to the surgeon's eye but that might cause a recurrence later on. There has been a great deal of interest in using chemotherapy after surgery because studies of experimental tumors in animals have shown that chemotherapy can cure very small tumors. In fact, chemotherapy is most effective when tumors are so small that they are invisible. Adjuvant radiation therapy is also given after surgery to kill remaining cancer cells.

The interest in adjuvant therapy has been especially high in the treatment of breast cancer. Women whose breast cancer has spread to the lymph glands under the armpit (axilla) have a high probability of cancer showing up in other parts of the body within 10 years after surgery. Studies have now shown that almost half the premenopausal women who otherwise would have a recurrence can be cured by adjuvant therapy.

HOW YOUR PHYSICIAN DECIDES ON THE BEST TREATMENT

Making the decision on which treatment to use is a stepwise process. It really begins with the suspicion of cancer aroused by signs or symptoms, then proceeds through the diagnostic process outlined in Chapter 2. Once the diagnosis is confirmed by a positive biopsy, several factors have to be considered.

The Stage How far along the tumor is in its development is the most critical factor. Sometimes the stage isn't known until a surgeon actually has a look at the tumor. But there are other ways to find out what stage the malignancy has reached.

During the staging process many parts of the body will be searched for evidence of cancer. Tests will discover the extent of the spread and the involvement with other tissues at the primary site. This will involve blood tests to see how organs such as the kidneys and liver are functioning. Imaging techniques such as chest x-rays and CT scans will be used to see if there is any involvement of the lungs either directly or by spread.

Other specialized tests will be ordered according to the primary site and the type of tumor being investigated. Each type of cancer has a typical pattern of spread, so different specific areas of the body will be investigated in each case.

Prostate cancer, for example, usually spreads to bone, so bone scans, bone x-rays and blood tests will be quite important. Lung cancers can spread to the center of the chest (mediastinum), an area that can be mapped with a CT scan and looked at directly through a scope (mediastinoscopy). Cancers of the stomach and bowel commonly spread to the liver, so liver scans and blood tests will be needed to be sure about those areas.

It is important to understand that *when a cancer spreads, it remains the same cancer.* A breast cancer that spreads to the bone does not become bone cancer. If it spreads to the lung, it does not become lung cancer. Wherever it lands, it grows as breast cancer. It's like blowing the seeds off a dandelion—whether the seed lands in a field, a forest or a crack in a sidewalk, what grows is still a dandelion.

This is important because cancer treatment depends mainly on where the tumor starts, *not* where it lands.

The Biology of the Disease An analysis of the disease—its cell type, biology and expected behavior—is an important factor to consider. The tumor's biology strongly affects the likelihood of a particular therapy slowing down or stopping the disease process.

State-of-the-Art Alternatives Once the staging process is completed, your doctor has to consider all the treatments that might be appropriate considering the type of tumor, the site of origin and the stage of spread. In some cases, only one specific therapy may be generally accepted as appropriate. But in many cases, a variety of approaches might be used.

Cancer treatment is always evolving. Every year new discoveries are made and old methods are modified or discarded. It's hard even for specialists to keep up with all the developments in the field. But there are several ways your primary physician can find out about the most current treatment methods that are considered state-of-the-art.

♦ Tumor specialists (medical oncologists) are often consulted at this stage. So are surgeons or specialists in radiotherapy.

♦ The most recent medical literature can be reviewed, perhaps along with a computer search of your disease via a database like PDQ (*see* Chapter 38).

♦ Physicians and specialists attend many of the hundreds of cancer meetings that take place every year where important research findings and other cancer information are presented.

Tumor Boards Another way for your doctor to review your case, get information and discuss the best treatment, especially with unusual types of cancers, is to attend a meeting called a Tumor Board. These boards are held frequently in all hospitals where cancer treatment is offered. They allow a group of doctors specializing in cancer to meet, discuss particular cases and give their opinions about the advantages and disadvantages of treatment alternatives. It is very common at this meeting for biopsy results to be presented and explained by the pathologist and for the radiologist and nuclear medical specialists to present all the x-rays and scans.

Your primary physician or oncologist will present your case (anonymously) so that each physician there has the same information your doctor has in making his or her decision.

In many larger hospitals there are specialty Tumor Boards that review cases in one particular field—breast cancer, urologic cancer, gynecologic cancers or head and neck cancers, for example.

When it comes to recommending treatment then, your doctor has had the benefit of input and ideas from a wide range of professionals.

Personal Factors: Benefits and Risks Which treatment is finally recomended will also depend on such personal factors as your age, other medical problems (which might make surgery risky) and especially the possibility of significant side effects with one or another treatment.

Age comes into the decision because the patient who is forty years old may be able to tolerate the aggressive chemotherapy drugs that bring about a substantial rate of remission. The same drugs given to an eighty-year-old could be risky. At that age the kidneys don't function as well as they do earlier in life and the risk of therapy could outweigh the potential benefit. But each case has to be decided on its own merits.

Both you and your doctor have to consider the relative advantages and disadvantages of each therapy. You have to weigh the chances of achieving remission or cure with the risks and side effects of treatment. You and your family are partners with your physician in this decision-making process.

Your Decision In making the final decision on treatment, nothing replaces a good discussion between you and your doctor. He or she should be able to explain to you the staging process, the tests that were done, their results and all the available methods of treatment.

He or she may present the information from any Tumor Board that was held. Or he or she can sometimes pass on the consensus of the informal consultations with other doctors that often take place in medical groups having several physicians involved in the cancer field. Your doctor should also have alternative forms of therapy in mind and should outline what could be done if your tumor doesn't respond to treatment or if some other problem comes up.

Informed Consent There may be legal principles regarding "informed disclosure" that come into play during these discussions. In the State of California, for example, patients with breast cancer must be given a pamphlet published by the State describing the various methods of primary treatment and the advantages and disadvantages of each. Although this document appears to be comprehensive, its coverage of many important areas is incomplete and outdated.

A brochure certainly cannot replace the important and key discussion between physician, patient and family. Nothing can. This initial comprehensive discussion about deciding on therapy is *the most important single meeting* that you have with your physician. It forms the basis for all of the decision-making that follows.

WHEN AND HOW TO ASK FOR A SECOND OPINION

As noted, by the time your doctor explains the recommended treatment to you, he or she has probably already reviewed the literature, consulted other doctors, met with pathologists and radiologists, drawn on his or her own experience and perhaps met with a Tumor Board.

Nevertheless, you may still feel insecure about the treatment options you've been given. You might want to discuss them with another physician. This is a perfectly acceptable, rational and appropriate thing to do.

There should be no hesitation on your part in asking your doctor if he or she would have another specialist review all the material relating to your case. Second opinions are not unusual. They are actually required by some insurance companies.

In view of your need for a continuing relationship with your primary physician or specialist, it would be helpful to express your satisfaction with his or her

decision and care. You can simply say that you wish to have someone else review the case to assure yourself that your decision to accept treatment will be made on the most thoroughly informed basis possible.

Who to Consult You may have a certain consultant in mind or you might ask your doctor to select a senior specialist in your city or at a major medical center, depending on your diagnosis. Many times your oncologist may recommend a second opinion and refer you to a local specialist or a specific cancer center where researchers with a special interest in your disease are working. Your doctor should have no hesitation in making your case material, including slides and x-rays, available to the second opinion consultant. This consultation is generally done fairly quickly so it does not delay treatment.

It is not a good idea to get a second opinion "in secret." Ultimately, it is not in your best interest. Second opinion consultations are done by physicians for physicians. They are done to review and help improve your medical care. Consultants cannot really evaluate your case properly unless they have at least the same information your primary doctor has, including the slides, x-rays and results of laboratory tests and other procedures.

Don't think your doctor will take offense or feel hurt. Your doctor should welcome the opportunity to satisfy your need for a second opinion.

CONSIDERING A CLINICAL TRIAL

Depending on the type and stage of your cancer, your doctor might recommend a new kind of treatment. The word investigational might come up. Or experimental might be the term used. If the standard treatment options available to you aren't likely to be effective, your doctor might simply suggest that you take part in a "clinical trial."

All these terms might make you feel

more than a little anxious. They shouldn't. Investigational treatments that are being given a clinical trial are used only under very stringent conditions. They wouldn't be used at all if there wasn't some hope they would be more effective than other treatments.

What a Clinical Trial Is Advances in cancer treatment are rarely made by one scientist or physician working with a single or even a few patients. Advances usually come about because of some clever idea or concept for a new therapy proposed by a cancer research physician. This idea is eventually tested in a large number of patients to find out two things: Is it effective? And is it as good as or better than conventional treatments?

It takes several hundred and sometimes several thousand patients to prove quickly and reliably whether a new treatment will work and is worthwhile. It is almost impossible to conduct a trial in any single hospital or cancer center. The concept of cooperative clinical trials was developed for just this reason. The rules and procedures for clinical trials are standardized and quite specific.

The Clinical Protocol A clinical trial consists of an exact written description of a treatment program that is called the clinical protocol. This is formulated and written with great care. Not only do the researchers need to be sure that the trial will answer the two main questions about effectiveness, but the rights of the patients being treated have to be safeguarded too. The risks involved have to be minimized and disclosed.

The clinical protocol outlines the criteria for patients who might participate in the trial. It also describes what tests will be done and how the researchers will determine if a tumor is responding. Systems for monitoring the patient and checking for any adverse effects will be detailed. And there will be provisions for "informed consent."

Who Approves the Trial The entire project has to be approved by a Human Use Committee made up of physicians and non-physicians who have no relationship with the study. The members of this committee certify that the patient's rights are protected, that the trial is reasonable and logical and that the study will answer the question it is supposed to answer. These same committees review the studies again during and after completion of the trial as originally proposed. The Cancer Therapy Branch of the National Cancer Institute also keeps watch on these investigational studies.

The Importance of Clinical Trials Almost every advance in cancer treatment over the past 20 years has come about because of clinical trials. In fact, just about every chemotherapy drug and radiation treatment now considered standard therapy was first given in a clinical Phase I trial. These treatments were given to patients who were willing to be in the forefront of advances in medical knowledge.

The willingness of thousands of women to participate in clinical trials by the National Surgical Adjuvant Breast Project (NSABP), for example, has resulted in answers being given to extremely important treatment questions. These trials have formed the basis for adjuvant chemotherapy in breast cancer patients with a high risk for recurrence even though no apparent tumor is left after surgery. This has saved many lives. All because of the usefulness of these clinical trials.

The Three Phases of Clinical Trials Whether for surgery, chemotherapy, radiotherapy or biological therapy, clinical trials are always conducted in three phases.

A chemotherapy clinical trial, for example, proceeds this way:
♦ *Preliminary* After a new anticancer drug has been found to be effective against one or more experimental tumor systems in the lab, it is tested in rats or other small animals to find out which dosage might

be both effective and reasonably safe.

♦ *Phase I* About 20 human patients are treated with the same drug. There is no assurance or certainty that a significant tumor response will occur, although, again, every single anticancer drug now useful in therapy was initially a Phase I agent.

Patients selected for these trials are almost always in cancer research centers and have already received all known effective anticancer therapy. After the proposed treatment is explained to them, they may volunteer to receive the new treatment. There is, therefore, no moral objection to giving this new treatment. Since there is "nothing to lose," it is hoped that a specific new agent may in fact prove effective.

This phase is completed when no unusual problems or toxic effects have been found and the dose necessary to produce a biologic effect has been determined. The study can then move to the next phase.

♦ *Phase II* Ten to 20 patients are treated, each with various types of tumors known to be responsive to chemotherapy. These might include lymphomas, breast cancer or colon cancer. Since these tumor types are known to be responsive, the patients will be those who have already received all standard forms of therapy that seem reasonable. The use of a Phase II trial does not deprive anyone of any therapy known to be effective. If a significant number of patients with each type of tumor respond to the therapy, the trial moves to the next level.

♦ *Phase III* In this phase the new therapy is compared with standard treatment to see if there is an improvement in the response or if the same response rate is achieved but with less-toxic side effects.

A therapy tested in a clinical trial does not necessarily involve a drug not already in clinical use. A new treatment often consists of standard drugs used in a new combination or a new sequence, in new dosages or even simply given in a new

way. But if a new drug is involved and the Phase III trial is successful, the National Cancer Institute will approve the drug for general use. Eventually, the new therapy might become the standard therapy.

Clinical Trials and the "Approved" Uses of Drugs When using anticancer chemicals, it is important for both you and your doctor to be aware of how the pharmaceutical industry works. Once drug companies have fulfilled the lengthy and complex testing—and the drawn-out legal procedures—required to market a new drug, they tend *not* to devote a lot of effort to discovering new uses for that drug. They more or less delegate this responsibility to the cancer physicians conducting clinical trials.

But every drug comes with an official "package insert" detailing what dose to use for what illness. This information is also listed in the *Physician's Desk Reference*. These summaries usually contain only the information "passed" by the government's approval agencies. Why this is important is that many drug programs in standard use are not listed as "approved." They are used because experience with patients has shown they are effective. About *half* of all the current uses of anticancer drugs in the United States and Canada are for indications and schedules *not* given in the official inserts.

Since the inserts do not necessarily reflect the most up-to-date cancer research, the current standard use of these drugs, nor even their optimum use, your doctor should not be restricted to printed drug-listing materials. In fact, appropriate use of anticancer drugs may be for indications *not* listed in such official sources.

This is another reason why an oncologist can be a useful member of your health care team. Cancer physicians are up to date on the most recent research findings and important advances in treatment even though that information may not appear in the drug-related literature.

5

WHAT HAPPENS IN SURGERY

Carlos A. Pellegrini, MD, and David Byrd, MD

◇

If you have cancer, there is a very good chance that you will see a surgeon during the course of your treatment. Surgery plays a crucial role in treating the disease. It is the oldest form of treatment and also the most effective. More cures are achieved by surgery than by any other form of therapy.

Surgery's role in cancer treatment has expanded considerably over the past few years. Better understanding of the natural history of many tumors, safer anesthetic techniques and improved pre-operative and post-operative care have led to better immediate and long-term survival rates. Surgeons can now also plan operations more effectively because a tumor's size and location can be determined more precisely with modern imaging techniques.

Surgery can support other treatment methods too. For example, the development of pumps and similar devices that allow precise, continuous and comfortable delivery of drugs has added a new dimension to cancer treatment. So has the implanting of radioactive seeds to deliver measured doses of radiation to internal tumors. Surgery is critical to the effective use of these techniques.

WHY SURGERY MIGHT BE RECOMMENDED

Since surgery is used in the diagnostic, treatment and post-treatment phases of cancer management, your primary physician or oncologist might suggest surgery in a variety of circumstances. The many different types of surgery each have their own goals. In general, there are eight reasons why surgery might be recommended.

♦ *To prevent or lower the risk of developing cancer* Some benign diseases associated with a high risk of developing cancer are commonly referred to as pre-cancerous conditions. To avoid the risk of cancer, therefore, it may be beneficial to remove an organ affected by one of these diseases.

Ulcerative colitis, for example, is a benign inflammatory condition of the large bowel. Colon cancer develops in about 40 percent of people whose large bowel has been affected by the disease for over 20 years. If a younger person has ulcerative colitis affecting the entire colon, then it *may* be appropriate to remove the colon before cancer appears.

Any operation performed to prevent cancer—commonly called prophylactic surgery—must be discussed in detail by both you and your doctor. The risks of developing cancer have to be weighed carefully against the risk of surgery itself and the permanent changes that surgery will cause. The situation may not always be clear and options may be possible. In such cases, you, the surgeon and your oncologist have to study all the facts and decide on a course of action that takes your preferences into account.

As an example, consider that several risk factors significantly increase the chance that some women will develop breast cancer. A prophylactic mastectomy would prevent the breast cancer but would also result in the loss of the breast.

Whether to perform the surgery is up to the woman. Some women may feel more comfortable avoiding surgery at an early stage and living with the risk. Others may feel otherwise.

♦ *To diagnose or stage the disease* Although many non-surgical techniques can diagnose cancer accurately, in most cases it is still necessary for an oncologist planning therapy to have a sample of tissue to analyze. A surgeon can remove a small amount of tissue by inserting a very fine needle into the area of the tumor and drawing out a few cells to be examined under a microscope. This needle aspiration—or aspiration cytology—is the easiest and most comfortable technique used to obtain sample cells, but the very small amount of tissue involved may not be enough for an accurate diagnosis.

When more tissue is needed, a larger needle can obtain a "core" of tissue for microscopic examination. If that sample is still not enough, a small operation—an incisional biopsy—may be performed to remove a portion of the tumor. When the tumor is small, the surgeon might do an excisional biopsy, meaning that the entire lesion is removed rather than just a sample of it. This is very common with skin lesions, where the doctor has to know whether the lesion is a benign condition, malignant melanoma or some other skin cancer.

To stage the disease properly a more formal operation may be needed to obtain tissue from several areas of the body. This is common with lymphomas, where a staging laparotomy—opening and examining the abdomen—may be required to remove sample tissues from the liver and lymph nodes and to remove the spleen.

It is important to remember that diagnostic surgery is just that—an operation designed merely to obtain tissue to confirm a diagnosis or to help plan adequate treatment. The goal is not to cure the cancer.

There has been a recent explosion in the development of minimally invasive surgery in both the diagnosis and treatment of solid malignancies. Videoendoscopic surgery is now frequently used to stage cancers in the abdomen (laparoscopy) and the chest cavity (thoracoscopy), and often eliminates the need for a major exploration of the abdomen or chest when unsuspected disease is found by these techniques. These procedures are most commonly performed under general anesthesia, and involve small incisions, which allow rapid recovery and return to normal activity. This technology is rapidly evolving and is under evaluation for the resection of some solid tumors.

♦ *To remove the primary tumor* For many cancer patients, removal of the tumor may be the best form of treatment. In some cases, surgery might lead to a cure. This form of surgery is referred to as surgery for the primary lesion. For this to be possible, the tumor has to be localized in an organ or area of the body that can be safely removed.

This type of surgery generally involves a major operation requiring admission to the hospital, general anesthesia and several days for recovery. The surgeon will try to remove the affected organ or area along with an adjacent area—called the margin—of normal-looking tissue. This is done because cells and small parts of the tumor may extend beyond what the surgeon can see as obvious cancer.

The lymph glands connected to the organ with the tumor might also be removed, since most tumors spread to lymphatic glands quite early. Removing the nodes along with the tumor improves the chance of removing all the cancer and, therefore, the chance of cure.

After the operation, the surgeon passes the entire specimen—the "gross" (visible) cancer, the margin and the lymphatic glands—to a pathologist for examination under a microscope. The pathologist will be able to find out the exact kind of tumor involved and how far it extends into normal tissues and glands. As always, the extent of the tumor determines the prognosis and the need for additional forms of therapy. It usually takes two or three days for a specimen to be processed and examined, so the surgeon will not usually be able to discuss the final diagnosis or prognosis with you or your family for a few days after surgery.

♦ *To remove other tumors* Besides removing the primary tumor, surgery may also be performed for residual, metastatic or recurrent lesions. Surgery for "residual" tumors means that the operation has been preceded by radiation therapy or chemotherapy. The idea is that certain tumors shrink or even disappear with radiation or chemotherapy and that the surgeon can then remove the rest of the affected organ.

In other cases, after the original tumor is removed the surgeon may remove the metastases, those small cancer cells that have broken off the tumor and spread to other organs. Patients with colon cancer, for example, who develop a single metastasis to the liver and in whom there is no other evidence of disease can benefit from the removal of the metastatic tumor.

Finally, if the tumor has returned at the original site—"recurrent" disease—the surgeon may attempt a second removal of the tumor. This operation may be performed with some melanomas or breast cancer, for example.

♦ *To relieve symptoms* Some tumors produce mechanical problems in the body. If the tumor becomes large enough to block some part of the gastrointestinal tract, food cannot move properly through the system. A large tumor could also block the biliary tract so that bile could not get into the intestine. Or a tumor could press on a nerve and cause pain. When the tumor cannot be removed safely, surgery can still be useful to bypass an obstruction or relieve the compression on a nerve. This kind of surgery is referred to as palliative.

Other symptoms caused by tumors can also be palliated. A cancer of the stomach may bleed a lot, for example. If the tumor is extensive and the presence of metastases makes surgery for cure impossible, the tumor may still be removed solely to stop the bleeding. In that case the operation would be considered a palliative one.

♦ *To reconstruct or rehabilitate* Removing an organ or tumor can sometimes produce some deformity or functional problem. When that happens, surgery can

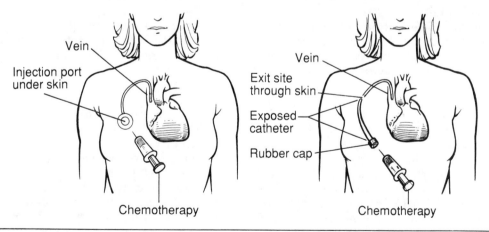

Implanted port for intravenous infusion.   *Implanted external catheter for intravenous infusion.*

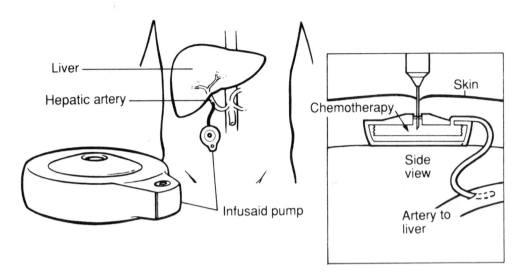

Infusaid pump for prolonged internal infusion.

often improve appearance, function and the quality of life. Excellent techniques provide reconstruction for women who have had a radical mastectomy. There are also ways to restore appearance and function after head and neck surgery.

It is not unusual for both doctor and patient to focus so sharply on treatment that they simply accept some of the crippling results of major surgery and overlook alternatives that can improve the quality of life. So be aware of this form of surgery and discuss the alternatives for reconstruction with your oncologist, surgeon or other doctor involved in your treatment.

♦ *To support chemotherapy and radiation therapy* Surgery is often used to support other forms of cancer therapy. If you need to have drugs administered intravenously, for example, you may have a port, catheter or pump surgically implanted. Ports and catheters are implanted under local anesthetic in an operating room, although general anesthetic can be given to people who prefer less discomfort.

A port is essentially a small chamber placed under the skin, usually near the shoulder. The chamber connects to a small tube inserted in a vein and threaded through it into larger veins. Access to the port is easy for the person injecting the drug and avoids the pain and discomfort often associated with intravenous injections.

Catheters may sometimes need to be placed into large veins through the skin. The catheter differs from the port in that its end is left outside the skin; the tube enters the body through a small puncture. Catheters usually have up to three inner lines so that different solutions—medication or nourishment, for example—can be given.

Pumps are more sophisticated devices. They have a large chamber that is filled with a drug, usually 1 to 1 1/2 ounces (30 to 50 mL). The pump has a mechanism, driven by the body's heat, that allows the drug to be delivered constantly through a small catheter inserted into a vein or artery without the need for a stay in the hospital. It is sometimes possible to target a specific organ such as the liver and deliver large amounts of chemotherapy drugs directly to it through an artery.

To support radiation therapy, an operation can be performed to implant catheters that are subsequently loaded with a radioemitter. Surgery is also used to expose a tumor so that a large dose of radiation can be given directly to the tumor or the tumor bed (*see* "Intraoperative Radiation" in Chapter 6).

♦ *To treat complications* Tumors or their treatments often suppress the immune system. This can lead to infections, bowel perforations or obstructions that may require surgical treatment.

PREPARING FOR SURGERY

Before you have surgery, your doctors will study the kind and extent of the tumor involved, then discuss what kind of surgery you need. The intensity of preparation for the surgery will depend on the kind of operation planned. If the surgery is for diagnosis and will involve a needle biopsy, there may only be a need to make sure your blood will clot so that bleeding from the needle puncture will stop quickly.

Preparation is much more elaborate for a major operation. Assuming that the tumor has already been studied thoroughly, two areas will be given special attention—the identification of any abnormalities or associated diseases and their correction before the operation. Patients are examined less or more comprehensively depending on the type of operation planned and their age. As people get older they tend to develop diseases of the heart, lungs and other organs that can jeopardize their recovery from an operation.

Diagnosis of Associated Diseases It is important for a surgeon to know if you have diabetes, if you are being treated for some other disease, what medications you are taking, how many white and red blood cells are in circulation, how well your blood clots and so on. Much of this information can be obtained through blood tests. Blood-clotting abnormalities can be

discovered with tests, but the best indicator of an increased risk of bleeding during surgery is a history of bleeding problems.

Similarly, a chest x-ray will give the surgeon an idea of the state of your lungs and an electrocardiogram (ECG) will help evaluate the state of your heart. Tests of lung (pulmonary) and heart function may also be performed. These will not only help evaluate the overall risk of surgery but also help determine the kind of anesthetic and other drugs you may need.

Correction of Associated Diseases Once problems have been identified, as many abnormalities as possible should be corrected. High blood pressure (hypertension), for example, should be treated before the operation. Infections can be treated with antibiotics, blood can be replenished if the blood counts are not high enough, and there may be ways of improving pulmonary function.

One of the most common problems people with cancer have is malnutrition. It is very important to correct this before the operation, since good nutrition gives your body the strength to get through the trauma of the operation and to heal properly. If necessary, additional feedings through a small tube in the stomach or an intravenous line can provide your body with an extra 2,500 to 3,000 calories a day.

WHAT YOU CAN DO TO PREPARE

While your doctor will look after most of the abnormalities noted above, there is a lot you as a patient can do to improve the outcome of the operation.

First, if you smoke, stop. Whether or not you intend to stop forever (which is always beneficial), you should stop as soon as the decision to operate is made. Lung and breathing problems are the most common type of complication after surgery and they can be minimized if the pulmonary system is working well. Clearing the lungs for as many days as possible before surgery will significantly improve your chances of not developing these problems.

Second, become as physically fit as possible. This will make both the operation and your recovery a lot easier. Eating appropriately and losing weight if you are overweight will also help. And any form of exercise, including walking, will be beneficial because it improves both circulation and pulmonary function.

Third, make sure to discuss with the surgeon the details of the operation and what you can expect afterward. Knowledge of the hospital, the intensive care unit, the staff and the procedures to be followed will help you prepare for the operation emotionally.

Fourth, discuss the use of blood. Most major surgery requires administering blood and there is some risk involved, albeit a small one. That risk can be completely abolished if you use your own blood. If your blood count is high enough and the state of your tumor permits, it may be appropriate to store your own blood two weeks before surgery so it can be returned to you if needed (*see* Chapter 14).

ANESTHETICS

Modern anesthetic techniques have greatly increased the safety of major cancer surgery and the ability of surgeons to combat cancer. Anesthesia is safe and comfortable. Each form of surgery requires a different form of anesthetic, the major kinds being local, regional and general.

♦ *Local anesthesia* is used for procedures that are short and superficial, in other words, near the skin. A biopsy or catheter placement, for example, can be performed under local anesthetic. The surgeon injects a drug such as lidocaine that numbs the site. You will remain awake and will usually feel some pressure as well as minor pulling of tissues in the area. If you do feel any pain, tell the surgeon so you can get additional anesthetic.

♦ *Regional anesthesia* involves giving the anesthetic agent near the spinal cord. The drug may be given by a single injection (called an epidural) or continuously through a small catheter tube placed directly into or near the spinal canal (peridural).

This form of anesthesia is excellent for operations in the lower part of the body, especially the lower extremities and the pelvis. The main advantage of regional anesthesia is that it gives you complete pain relief for many hours and that it wears off slowly, allowing you to take other forms of pain relief as needed after the operation. Another advantage, especially if you have lung problems, is that you stay awake throughout the operation, eliminating the interference with breathing that takes place with general anesthetic. Remaining awake, however, may be considered a disadvantage by some people.

♦ *General anesthesia* is normal in most major operations for cancer. Anesthetic agents are given by intravenous injection, through a breathing mask or both. They act directly on the brain to produce a temporary loss of consciousness. In most cases, the anesthesiologist will also use muscle relaxants to produce a profound relaxation of the body. This will make the surgery easier to perform and will mean less pain afterward. Because your muscles will not be functioning, you won't be able to breathe spontaneously. But a tube will be placed in your windpipe (trachea) and connected to a machine (ventilator) that will deliver air to your lungs every few seconds.

The anesthesiologist monitors breathing by periodically checking the concentration of oxygen in the blood. The anesthesiologist is also in charge of administering fluids intravenously, including blood when needed. The amount and the quality of the fluids are regulated carefully to maintain adequate blood pressure, an adequate amount of circulating blood and adequate blood flow to the body's organs.

AFTER THE OPERATION

Contrary to popular belief, waking up from general anesthesia is not always unpleasant. In fact, it is not too different from waking up from any deep sleep. You will usually wake up in a recovery room, although you may not remember the experience.

Depending on the operation, you may find upon awakening that one or more intravenous lines are running into your body. You may also find drains in some body cavities. You may feel some discomfort and not be able to eat for a few days. The surgeon will have covered all these points with you before the operation.

Pain Control Most patients worry about pain after the operation, but there are several relatively easy ways to control it. If low-level pain relievers (analgesics) like aspirin and codeine won't do the job, pain can be controlled by the injection of stronger analgesics, the most potent being narcotics like morphine. These drugs provide relief from pain for three to four hours and should be readministered by the clock or as soon as the pain reappears.

Traditionally, patients have had to call a nurse each time they felt the need for an injection, but patients themselves can now activate devices that deliver the analgesic. The "patient controlled analgesia" (PCA) device has a compartment for the morphine, a trigger button to press and a small computer that delivers a fixed dose of the drug. There is also a lock-out period set by the doctor and nurse—usually at 20 minutes—to make sure the drug isn't administered too often. The main advantage of this form of pain control is that the pain can be relieved as soon as it felt, which usually means that smaller amounts of medication are needed.

Another way to control pain is with morphine or a local anesthetic administered into the spinal canal, just like the epidural given during the operation. This will control the pain completely, but usually causes bladder malfunction. A catheter, therefore, will be needed to drain the bladder of urine.

These options should be discussed and a basic plan devised before the operation. The main point to remember is that pain can be controlled and that there is no need to suffer. It's also useful to note that taking liberal doses of morphine or other analgesics in the post-operative period *does not* lead to drug addiction.

WHAT ARE THE RISKS?

It is important for you to discuss with the surgeon before the operation the risk of anesthesia, the risk of the surgical procedure itself and any potential complications. You should also discuss the operative mortality—usually defined as a death that occurs within 30 days of an operation—that can result either from the underlying disease or from complications that develop during the operation.

♦ *The risk of anesthesia* is related to your age, the magnitude of the operation and the presence of associated diseases. The American Society of Anesthesiology has devised a formula to classify the status of patients, divided into five classes. As the age or the associated diseases increase, the number of the class increases to indicate a greater risk. Class 1, for example, is a middle-aged patient with no significant associated disease who has a localized process requiring a limited operation. Class 3 patients have severe systemic disturbance from other diseases, such as low pulmonary function, vascular complications or heart disease. The overall risk of anesthesia, however, is very small.

♦ *The operative risks* vary greatly with the kind of operation performed. They are usually divided into immediate risks (occurring within a few days or weeks of surgery) and late risks (occurring months or years after the operation). Just as in the case of anesthesia, the immediate risks are increased by the presence of other diseases.

Bleeding is usually quoted as a common risk of surgery, but very few patients suffer much from it. The most common immediate complications are pulmonary and usually result from earlier lung disease, a history of smoking or the fact that postoperative pain and being in bed prevent the lungs from expanding. These complications can be prevented or minimized by vigorous coughing, as a nurse may request, and by getting up and walking around as soon as possible.

Another complication that may occur after a prolonged period in bed is the development of a clot in the legs brought on by poor circulation. The major risk is that part of the clot might break loose and lodge in the lungs. This is called a pulmonary embolism and is a potentially serious complication that can be prevented by walking or by moving your legs, particularly the calf muscles, while in bed.

Other common complications in the postoperative period have to do with the operative wound. Infection can set in around the incision, but infections can be easily treated and shouldn't cause you much physical or emotional discomfort.

Late complications of surgery have to do with the scarring that is an inevitable part of the healing process. Scarring in the abdomen can occasionally lead to a bowel obstruction or some other form of mechanical blockage.

CHOOSING A SURGEON AND A MEDICAL FACILITY

This is not usually an overwhelming problem. In most cases, your oncologist or the general physician who diagnosed your cancer will recommend someone whom he or she knows and has worked with before. In other cases, you may know of a surgeon personally or by reputation and can either use him or her directly as the surgeon or as a source of information.

If you want to make the choice yourself, it is a good idea to get information from the local medical society about doctors who are Board-certified in surgery. While certification by the American Board of Surgery does not necessarily mean outstanding performance, it does have implications about a surgeon's level of knowledge and adherence to certain standards.

Most reputable surgeons are also Fellows of the American College of Surgeons, which can also help you with names of surgeons practicing in your community. Write to American College of Surgeons, 55 E. Erie Street, Chicago, IL 60611 or telephone (312) 644-4050.

When the procedure you are facing is minor or has to do with one of the more common forms of cancer, chances are that the operation can be performed successfully by most surgeons. But if your oncologist says your disease is out of the ordinary or if the operation you need is a major or complex one, it is usually best to seek out the services of an experienced surgeon working in a sizable hospital or other medical institution. His or her experience is an important asset, but more important is that the specialists, sophisticated equipment and advanced techniques that may be needed to react to problems during and after an operation are available only at large medical centers.

Once you have made a preliminary decision about a surgeon, it is a good idea to arrange a meeting. Decide for yourself whether he or she is the kind of person you want to entrust your life to. If you feel positive about it, follow through. If not, it is easy enough to find another surgeon who can perform the operation just as well.

At this point you might also want to get a second opinion. Another opinion can be very useful, especially with a case that is difficult, complex or uncommon. You will be able to compare the two approaches to the disease, and that may give you more confidence as you face your operation.

When all this has been done, you are ready for surgery.

6
WHAT HAPPENS IN RADIATION THERAPY

Lawrence W. Margolis, MD, and T. Stanley Meyler, MD

About half of all people with cancer need radiation therapy as part of their overall treatment plan at some point in their illness. It is often recommended as the primary treatment, but can also be used along with chemotherapy or surgery. When used with surgery, it might be given before, during or after the operation. When used with chemotherapy, it may be given before or after the program begins or at the same time as chemotherapy.

There are two main goals in radiation therapy:
♦ Cure the cancer. This usually requires a long and complex course of treatment.
♦ Relieve symptoms (palliation). Treatment to achieve this goal is usually less complex and takes less time.

HOW IT WORKS

Radiation therapy—which is also called radiotherapy—uses high-energy x-rays, electron beams or radioactive isotopes to kill cancer cells without exceeding safe doses to normal tissue.

Radiation accomplishes its purpose by killing cancer cells through a process called ionization. Some cells die immediately after radiation because of the direct effect, though most die because the radiation damages the chromosomes and DNA so much that they can no longer divide.

The key to successful treatment is getting the appropriate amount of radiation to the tumor in the most effective way. There are several technical ways of doing this. The most common way is by external

radiation in which a radiation beam is directed at the tumor from a machine. Internal or systemic radiotherapy delivers radiation by giving a radioactive source intravenously or by injection—intravenous radioactive iodine or radioactive gold into the abdominal cavity, for example. With intracavity radiotherapy, an applicator containing radiation seeds is placed into an organ such as the uterus. In interstitial radiotherapy, the sources are placed directly into the tumor. These methods are usually used in combination with external radiation.

PLANNING THE THERAPY

All radiation treatment is supervised by physicians who are generally Board-certified specialists trained to evaluate and treat cancer patients using radiation. Your specialist may be called a radiation oncologist, radiotherapist, radiation therapist or therapeutic radiologist.

Whatever the term used in your particular hospital, this specialist is an important member of your cancer team. He or she may be consulted at any time during your treatment, from immediately after the diagnosis to well along in your therapy. At whatever stage the radiation oncologist joins your team, the treatment planning process follows several standard steps.

The Goal The first thing the radiation oncologist has to do is thoroughly evaluate your case. He or she will give you a physical examination, review all scans, diagnostic x-rays, pathology slides and operative reports, then will discuss your case with your primary physician, medical oncologist or possibly a surgeon. After the evaluation has been completed, a decision will be made on what role radiation therapy will play—will the goal of treatment be curative or palliative? At this point, the radiation oncologist will also decide on the method of radiation to be used—external, the various internal methods or a combination. Then the detailed planning starts.

The Simulation If external radiation is going to be used, the first step in the detailed planning stage is called a simulation, performed on a special x-ray machine built to resemble the machine that ultimately will be used. Certain "contrast agents" or probes may be used to aid in the simulation. The point of the exercise is to make all the necessary measurements to fix the precise location of the tumor. Marks will be made on your skin with a colored ink to outline the target the radiation oncologist will be aiming for—the "radiation port"—which has to be the same every day.

While the simulation is being done, the radiation oncologist may use the services of a clinical physicist and dosimetrist. The physicist is specially trained in the clinical application of radiation therapy and will give advice on technical matters that the radiation oncologist will incorporate into the plan. A dosimetrist is a person who, with the use of computers, helps design the specialized treatment plan developed for each individual.

Following the simulation, you will be ready to start treatment either that day or possibly several days later if your case is complex. The reason for the delay is that all the data from the simulation will be fed into a computer. The treatment team will need time to study the various plans and tailor-make any shielding or blocking devices that may be needed to keep radiation away from your healthy tissues.

The Dosage The amount of radiation you receive is measured in units that used to be called rads. The term used now is centigray (cGy), but since one gray equals 100 rads the two terms are interchangeable.

Deciding what dosage of radiation to give is a critical part of the treatment plan. Careful planning allows the radiation oncologist to deliver the maximum effective dose to the visible tumor and any invisible tumor cells that might be nearby while protecting the surrounding normal tissues as much as possible.

Calculating a dosage figure that balances these two goals can be complex, since the size and stage of the tumor have to be taken into account and since different tissues tolerate different levels of radiation. The liver, for example, will tolerate 3,000 cGy, the lungs 2,000 and the kidneys 1,800. Higher doses can be delivered to small parts of one of these organs, but if the entire organ is given higher doses than these, normal tissues will be harmed.

The radiation oncologist prescribes the total dose necessary to destroy the tumor, then calculates the daily dose over a specific period. This is called the fractionation schedule. Throughout, the radiation oncologist works with a figure called the therapeutic ratio, defined as a comparison of the damage to the tumor cells compared with normal cells. The therapeutic ratio can be enhanced in a number of ways—by using altered time fractionation schedules, careful treatment planning, selection of the optimum radiation energy for the specific problem and by the use of experimental techniques such as high LET radiation or chemical modifiers that either make the tumor cells more sensitive to radiation or better protect normal tissues.

The Number of Treatments Radiation is usually given daily five days a week. That schedule can continue for two to eight weeks depending on the tumor, the kind of treatment being used and the dosage required. The point of using multiple treatments instead of a single treatment is to give normal cells a chance to recover and repair themselves.

TYPES OF EXTERNAL RADIATION

Radiation oncologists now have a variety of ways to deliver the most effective amount of radiation to specific tumor cells. Which method to use is based on many factors, including the biology of the tumor involved, the possibility of side effects or complications, the physical characteristics of the various sources of radiation and how these different sources affect the body's many different cells, tissues and organ systems. The methods can be broadly divided into external and internal radiation, with several options available within each category.

External radiation—the delivery of the dosage from a source outside the body—can vary according to the photon energy of the machines involved, the type of beams produced (electrons, x-rays, gamma rays), when the treatment is given and the number of beams involved in the treatment procedure.

High and Low Energy Radiation External beam treatment uses special equipment that uses either low energy (orthovoltage machines) or high energy (megavoltage machines). All the machines used today are quite precise about where they deliver the radiation dose.

Orthovoltage Equipment Orthovoltage x-rays are produced in a tube in which a filament is heated to a high temperature. Electrons are emitted and strike a tungsten target, producing x-rays with energies up to 300 kilovolts. This type of machine delivers its maximum dose on the surface of the skin and has a very lim-

ited range of penetration. These days, orthovoltage machines are used only for surface tumors such as skin cancers.

Megavoltage Equipment These are high energy machines with energies greater than 1,000 kilovolts. Megavoltage machines let the radiation oncologist treat internal tumors without giving an excessive dosage to the skin. Commonly used megavoltage machines include Cobalt 60 and Linear Accelerators that produce the maximum dose at an internal depth determined by the energy of the machine. A 25-megavolt Betatron, for example, delivers its maximum dose almost 2 in. (4.5 cm) beneath the skin.

♦ Cobalt 60 became available in the 1950s and is still used. This machine contains a radioactive source housed in a specially designed lead container. As the cobalt isotope decays over time, it produces a beam in the megavoltage range.

♦ The Linear Accelerator, one of the most popular machines now being used, is available in energies ranging from 4 to 35 megavolts. Many of these machines can treat patients with x-rays or electrons or a combination of both. The combination is called a mixed beam and allows the radiation oncologist to tailor the treatment to a specific tumor and reduce the dose to surrounding tissues.

The machine works by producing electrons that are accelerated along a wave guide to a high velocity. These electrons can be directly used for treatment in the electron mode or they can be directed at a target within the machine to produce the x-rays that are then used for treatment. The high energy electrons used in the electron mode have a specific range of penetration into tissue, determined by the energy of the beam selected. The higher the megavoltage, the greater the penetration. Because an electron therapy beam produces a high skin dose, the whole course of treatment will seldom be given with only the electron beam unless you are being treated for cancer near or involving the skin.

Intra-Operative Radiation Therapy (IORT) People with localized tumors that can't be completely removed or have a high risk for a local recurrence—carcinoma of the pancreas, for example—may be candidates for IORT, a treatment carried out during surgery. The surgeon localizes the organ containing your tumor and removes as much of the tumor as possible. He or she then moves the normal tissue out of the path of the radiation beam. Radiation equipment may then be brought into the operating room or you may be wheeled to a radiation department. A treatment cone connected to a Linear Accelerator is placed directly over the tumor, which is then treated with a single high dose. Normal tissues are spared since they are outside of the beam.

Stereotactic (Stereotaxic) Radiosurgery
This was introduced in the 1950s by Dr. Lars Leksell of Sweden who found that he could treat deep-seated blood vessel malformations within the brain by using a number of cobalt sources. This is sometimes called a gamma knife.

If you are receiving this treatment, your head will be placed in a special frame that helps to maintain alignment and localize the treatment volume. With the frame in place, you will have a CT or MRI scan or an angiogram study. Technical information from the scan is then fed into a treatment-planning computer and a dose distribution is calculated for the Linear Accelerator. You will then be transported to the Linear Accelerator, which will direct high doses of radiation from specific angles outside your head so that they converge on the target area. Surrounding tissues are for the most part spared.

The computer revolution and the availability of Linear Accelerators has made this form of treatment especially useful for vascular malformations, meningiomas, acoustic neuromas and some malignant brain tumors.

TYPES OF INTERNAL RADIATION

Modern radiation treatment makes extensive use of methods that deliver radiation to cancer cells not from a distance but by being inserted directly into or around the tumor. Radioactive sources can be injected, housed in special applicators or implanted in the form of needles or seeds.

Internal (Systemic) Radiation Therapy
With this type of treatment, radioactive isotopes are given intravenously or placed in an organ such as the bladder or abdomen.

♦ One of the most common forms of systemic treatment involves the use of radioactive iodine (I-131), which is sometimes used for carcinoma of the thyroid. Its use in thyroid cancer is limited because many thyroid cancers fail to take up iodine. But if a thyroid cancer does show iodine uptake in preliminary tests, then by giving I-131 the isotope will be concentrated in the gland, thereby administering a high dosage of radiation to the organ while sparing other tissues.

♦ At one time, radioactive phosphorus isotopes were placed within an abdominal cavity to treat malignant fluid (ascites) or to prevent reaccumulation of that fluid. But its use today is quite limited.

♦ An agent called strontium 89 (Metastron) is currently used for treatment of bone metastases from prostate and breast cancer. Given intravenously, this isotope shows promising preliminary results.

Interstitial Radiation Therapy This method, also called brachytherapy, places the sources of radiation directly into the tumor and surrounding structures. It's most commonly used in tumors of the head and neck, the prostate and the breast. It is also usually used in combination with external radiation.

There are two types of implants:
♦ A permanent implant involves small

radioactive seeds such as gold or iodine placed directly into the affected organ. I-125 seeds, for example, are used for prostate cancer. Over several weeks or months, the seeds slowly deliver a specific dose of radiation to the tumor.

♦ A removable implant is the most common method of interstitial radiation therapy. The operation, usually carried out under general anesthesia, involves placing narrow, hollow stainless steel needles through the tumor. Once the placement seems satisfactory, Teflon tubes are inserted through the needles and the needles are then removed, leaving the tubes in place. The operation is then terminated and you return to your room, where a small ribbon of radioactive seeds will be inserted into the tubes in a procedure called afterloading.

With computerized treatment planning, the specific strength of each seed can be selected, thereby providing the desired dose to the tumor volume over a specific period. Once the dose is reached, the tubes and the seeds are removed. This type of implant is commonly used for tumors of the head and neck or as a boost after external beam radiation of breast cancer after a lumpectomy.

Intracavitary Radiation The most common use of this method is in gynecologic tumors, such as carcinoma of the uterus. Specially designed hollow applicators are placed into the uterus under general or spinal anesthesia. X-rays are taken in the operating room to determine correct positioning, and once the placement is satisfactory the operation is ended. After you return to your room, a small plastic tube containing the required number of sources of radioactive isotope of a specific strength are inserted into the hollow applicators. The sources and applicators are left in place for 48 to 72 hours, during which time you have to stay in bed. The seeds deliver the dose over the specified time, and once the dose is reached, the applicator and the sources are removed.

The advantage of this method is that a very high dose of radiation can be delivered to the tumor while the rapid fall-off in the dose gives maximum protection to the surrounding structures.

Intraluminal Radiation Therapy This method has limited use with some tumors in hollow organs like the esophagus and biliary tract. In esophageal carcinoma, for example, a specially designed tube is placed into the opening (lumen) of the esophagus. Then under x-ray visualization—fluoroscopy—several small radioactive sources are placed into the tube opposite the tumor. The tumor receives a high dose of radiation while the dose to the surrounding structures is minimized. Intraluminal therapy is often used in combination with external radiation.

NEW TECHNIQUES TO IMPROVE RADIOTHERAPY

Today's researchers are exploring several ways to make radiation therapy more effective, building on important advances in biology, physics and engineering. Some have already produced significant results.

Hyperthermia The effect of heat on some types of cancer has been observed for more than 100 years. In 1893, W. B. Cooley reported that high temperatures had an effect on 38 patients, 12 of whom had a complete regression of their cancers. Many malignant cells show a therapeutic response to high temperatures. And even moderate hyperthermia (108°F/42°C) can cause destruction of malignant cells.

Compared to radiotherapy alone, the combination of heat plus radiation has increased the response rate of certain tumors such as melanoma, and there are also promising preliminary results from treating brain tumors using interstitial implants plus heat.

Researchers are now studying the use of a new "multimodality" treatment—the

combination of radiation therapy, chemotherapy and heat—which may increase
the response rate for some tumors (*see*
Chapter 11).

Clinical Modifiers Research continues in
the hope of finding chemical compounds
that will modify radiation effects. Since
radiation is more effective in cells with a
good oxygen supply, one of the first
approaches to modifying radiation sensitivity was through the use of hyperbaric
oxygen chambers. Patients were placed in
a closed chamber so they could breathe air
with a higher than normal concentration
of oxygen.

More recently, radiation sensitizing
agents that have an effect similar to oxygen have been developed. Other compounds now being investigated are
"radioprotectors" that may decrease damage to normal tissues.

**High Linear Energy Transfer (LET)
Radiation** Radiation with accelerators that
use heavy particles or subatomic particles
rather than electrons, x-rays or gamma
rays is now being studied in many centers.
Several types of heavy particles are under
investigation, including protons, helium
ions and neutrons. Two features seem to
make this type of radiation—called High
Linear Energy Transfer (LET) heavy particle radiation—more effective. First, it can
kill poorly oxygenated cells better than
standard radiation can. Second, tumor
cells are less able to repair sublethal damage from high LET radiation.

Several tumors have been identified
that may benefit from high LET particle
radiation—including sarcomas of bone
and soft tissue, salivary gland tumors,
some head and neck tumors and
melanomas of the eye—and the search is
on to find others. In the past few years,
high LET radiation has been used with
patients with advanced malignant disease.
But it is still an investigational treatment
and is available only in a few facilities in
the United States.

Hyperfractionation In recent years there
has been considerable interest in hyper-
fraction, in which patients are given radiation treatment twice daily rather than the
conventional once daily. By using multiple smaller doses of radiation, a higher
overall dose can be delivered. The treatments are usually given at least 6 hours
apart to allow for tissue repair.
Preliminary data suggests an improvement in the control of head and neck
tumors without significant difference in
acute toxicity. These altered fractionation
schemes are being extensively studied in
head and neck, brain and lung tumors.

DEALING WITH SIDE EFFECTS
The common side effects of radiation therapy can be divided into generalized (systemic) and localized effects. What the
effects are and how severe they become
generally depend on the area treated, the
size of the radiation port, the daily dose
rate and the total dosage delivered.

Not everyone who has radiation therapy suffers side effects. Many people go
through treatment experiencing only minimal effects or none at all. But for some
people, the side effects can be significant
and uncomfortable.

Systemic Effects One of the most common systemic side effects is fatigue or
malaise. This is especially common among
patients receiving treatments to large
areas, such as the whole abdomen or total
lymph node radiation.

A lot of people associate nausea and
vomiting with x-ray treatments, but both
these symptoms are unusual in radiotherapy patients. Again, it depends on the
area being treated. Nausea and vomiting
may occur in patients receiving radiation
to the upper abdomen, but it is rare in
patients getting radiation to the head and
neck, chest or pelvis. Even when you are
receiving treatment to the abdomen, nau-

sea and vomiting can usually be controlled by adjusting the dosage, changing the diet or using antinausea medications.

Localized Side Effects As certain parts of your body are treated, you may experience several common localized side effects. Your radiation oncologist will go over these with you before treatment and will give them individualized attention if they occur.

♦ *Skin* All radiation has to pass through the skin, but with today's high energy machines and daily treatment techniques using multiple ports, the side effects on the skin are seldom a problem unless the treated area actually involves the skin.

Most skin reactions appear as a redness called erythema. This is similar to sunburn and goes through the same stages—redness, gradual tanning, then peeling. Once the condition is treated, the reaction will usually go away within a week or 10 days. If the dose has been high, late skin changes may appear in the form of increased pigmentation, which may be more noticeable in people of dark complexion.

If you develop any of these symptoms, it is important not to put any creams or lotions on your skin without your radiation oncologist's approval.

♦ *Head and neck* One of the most significant side effects is irritation of the membranes lining the body cavities, such as the lining—or mucosa—of the mouth. If you are being treated for a cancer of the head and neck, the mucosa surrounding the tumor may become red. And as treatment progresses, quite a few small superficial ulcers may develop. This can cause a lot of discomfort and will probably interfere with swallowing and nutrition. Fortunately, the effect is temporary and will disappear as soon as the treatment is finished.

Radiation to the head and neck may also interfere with taste if your tongue is in the primary radiation beam. And the amount of saliva produced can be significantly reduced if the salivary glands happen to be in the treatment beam (*see* "Special Problems of Radiation Patients" in Chapter 17).

♦ *Chest* Most patients receiving chest radiation will not have any local symptoms. But the esophagus, which carries food from the mouth to the stomach, passes through the chest and may develop a mucosal reaction similar to that described for the mouth. If this happens, you may develop heartburn-type symptoms, which can be relieved by taking liquid antacids such as Amphogel, Gelusil, Maalox, Mylanta or Riopan.

♦ *Abdomen* The most significant side effects of radiation are associated with treatment to the abdomen. The larger the radiation port and the higher the dosage, the more likely you are to experience these effects.

Radiation to the upper abdomen can cause nausea and vomiting, usually during the first few days of treatment. As the treatment progresses the symptoms often diminish.

Treatment to the pelvis can be associated with cramps, perhaps followed by diarrhea during the second and third weeks of treatment. A low residue diet or antidiarrhea medications such as Lomotil, Imodium or Kaopectate will usually control the problem.

Most patients getting radiation treatment to the pelvis do not develop any significant bladder problems. But it is not unusual to have to urinate often, to feel an urgency to urinate or to feel some pain when urinating. Fortunately, these symptoms are usually temporary and will go away soon after the treatment course is completed. In the meantime, medications such as Pyridium or Urispas will usually ease the problem.

♦ *Hair loss* Only hair within the radiation port will be affected by treatment. So you will lose scalp hair only if you are receiving radiation to your head, usually for tumors involving the brain. If the entire brain needs to be treated, the radiation can affect the entire scalp. But only a part of the scalp might be affected if a smaller portion of the brain is radiated.

Whether the hair loss is temporary or permanent depends on the dosage (*see* "Hair Loss" in Chapter 17).

7
WHAT HAPPENS IN CHEMOTHERAPY

Malin Dollinger, MD, and Ernest H. Rosenbaum, MD

———————◇———————

The idea of treating cancer with chemical agents or medications has been around since the days of the ancient Greeks. Yet the practice of cancer chemotherapy as it's known today really only began in the 1940s. Near the end of that decade, nitrogen mustard became the first drug approved to fight tumor cells. Over the next 20 years, chemotherapy was essentially an investigational treatment.

But in the last 30 years, more effective antitumor drugs have been developed, and other new drugs and supportive techniques have come along to reduce the side effects of the cancer-killing agents. Now, with greater understanding of the nature of cancer and of how chemicals interact, chemotherapy has become a standard therapy. Either alone or in combination with other treatments, chemotherapy can now cure some common forms of cancer—testis cancer, leukemia, choriocarcinoma, many cases of Hodgkin's disease and non-Hodgkin's lymphomas and some cases of ovarian cancer.

The Range of Drugs For many years, researchers looked hard for one single drug—a "magic bullet"—that would cure cancer. This has yet to be found, if it exists at all. Today, about 50 anticancer drugs are available on the market. About a dozen others have not yet been approved for general distribution but have proved to be useful in some forms of cancer. These experimental or investigational drugs are supplied to clinical trial investigators under a special government license. To make drugs available earlier for

therapy, some drugs with an established role in treatment are also made available to practicing oncologists, even though they are not yet on the retail market. In 1989, for example, a year before it was released to the general market, the National Cancer Institute made the drug levamisole available to be used in combination with 5-fluorouracil for treatment of Dukes' Stage C carcinoma of the colon. This new policy may mean earlier release of new drugs in the future.

THE GOALS AND POSSIBLE RESULTS OF THERAPY

Your doctor might recommend chemotherapy for several reasons. The goal might be:
♦ to cure a specific cancer;
♦ to control tumor growth when a cure isn't possible;
♦ to relieve symptoms such as pain;
♦ to shrink tumors before surgery or radiation therapy; or
♦ to destroy microscopic metastases after tumors are removed surgically.

While surgery and radiation therapy are used to treat localized tumors, chemotherapy treats the whole body. It destroys malignancies of the blood, bone marrow and the lymphatic system (leukemias and lymphomas). It destroys cancer cells that have broken off from solid tumors and spread through the blood or lymph systems to various parts of the body.

Adjuvant Therapy When chemotherapy is

used to eliminate small invisible metastases after surgery or radiation therapy, it is known as adjuvant therapy. This is given when there is a high risk of a cancer recurring because small cells that couldn't be detected during surgery or any other way may remain and later grow back.

Adjuvant chemotherapy usually involves combinations of drugs known to be effective against particular tumors. They are given in the highest dosages the patient can tolerate. And they will usually be given as soon as possible after surgery or radiotherapy since the longer the delay, the less chance of cure. In some cases, chemotherapy is given *before* surgery or radiation therapy, and is then called neoadjuvant therapy.

What Chemotherapy Can Achieve There are four possible results of chemotherapy given for visible or known areas of cancer.
♦ *Complete remission* The tumor may seem to disappear completely, meaning that there is a complete response to the drugs. This clearly indicates the treatment is working, though it has to continue for a while so any "hidden" cancer cells will be destroyed. Current detection methods can miss an internal tumor smaller than half an inch (about 1 cm) and if treatment is stopped too soon there is a high chance for a relapse.

Some remissions, especially for very responsive tumors, may be permanent. Others are temporary, lasting for months or even years. But then the tumor reappears or begins to grow again. Complete remission, therefore, is not necessarily the same as a cure. "Cure" usually means the lack of any sign of cancer for at least five years, but how it's defined really depends on the kind of cancer being treated and on the individual patient.
♦ *Partial remission* The tumor may shrink by more than half its size but not disappear. This is obviously a good result, but therapy has to be continued until the tumor either completely disappears or

stops shrinking. If it simply stops shrinking, the drug program may be changed or surgery or radiotherapy may be used to try to wipe out the remaining tumor cells.
♦ *Stabilization* The tumor may neither shrink nor grow. This can be looked on as a favorable result of therapy, but doctors tend to be nervous when this happens. They basically worry that the effect may be brief and the tumor will start growing again. The period of stabilization can sometimes last months or years.
♦ *Progression* The tumor may keep growing despite therapy. The doctor's task is to discover this as soon as possible after the therapy has had a fair trial. Then a different treatment program can be worked out.

HOW ANTICANCER DRUGS WORK

Like normal, healthy cells, cancer cells go through a continuous process of change. Each cell divides into two daughter cells. These cells grow, rest and then divide again. The drugs used in chemotherapy are powerful chemicals designed to interrupt this cycle and stop the cells from growing.

Several different types of drugs are used in chemotherapy. Each type kills cells at a different stage of the cell's life cycle. Each does its job in a different way.

Antimetabolites attack the cells during the process of division, when they are more easily killed. The antimetabolites imitate normal cell nutrients. The "antivitamin" methotrexate, for example, resembles the normal B vitamin, folic acid. The cancer cell consumes the drug— "thinking" it's getting a good meal—and starves to death.

Alkylating agents attack all the cells in a tumor whether they are resting or dividing. These drugs bind with the cells' DNA in various ways to prevent reproduction.

Antitumor antibiotics insert themselves into strands of DNA. They either break up the chromosomes or inhibit the DNA-directed synthesis of RNA that the cell needs to grow.

Alkaloids prevent the formation of chromosome spindles necessary for cell duplication.

Hormones such as estrogen and progesterone inhibit the growth of some cancers, although how they do it is not clearly understood.

Drug Combinations It used to be that anticancer drugs were given one at a time. But now combinations of drugs are usually given, all according to a plan designed to inhibit or kill as many cancer cells as possible.

Drugs that attack tumor cells at every stage of their life cycle—called non-cell-cycle-specific drugs—may be given first to reduce the size of the tumor. This may activate the remaining cells to divide. When they do, cell-cycle-specific drugs that attack dividing cells will be given. Other sequences of other drugs can also be devised to maximize the therapeutic effect.

This is much like fighting a war, making sure you use all your forces on several fronts with repeated attacks. Your chances of winning the battle are greatly improved.

Drug Resistance There's another good reason for giving drug combinations: it reduces the chance that you'll develop a resistance to any one drug.

Resistance is one very common reason why these agents fail to do what they're supposed to. A course of chemotherapy is often quite successful at first. The cancer responds, leading to a remission. But then, even though the drugs are still being given, there is a relapse and the cancer starts to grow again. A resistance to therapy has developed just like the resistance to penicillin or other antibiotics that can develop when treating an infection.

When this happens, the drugs in the treatment program have to be changed.

Unfortunately, if you develop resistance to one drug or group of drugs there may be less chance that your body will respond to another drug program.

Why Resistance Develops One of the mysteries of cancer therapy is why some people respond really well to a treatment while others have problems. About 10 years ago, research on drug resistance led to speculation that multiple resistance developed during therapy and that this was responsible for progressive and uncontrollable metastatic disease.

More recent research has begun to explain how cancer cells become resistant to drugs. There is a protein called P-glycoprotein on the surface of a cancer cell. This protein acts like a pump, regulating the passage of drugs into and out of the cancer cell. Tumor cells with larger amounts of P-glycoprotein may not allow any drugs to enter. This, of course, makes chemotherapy ineffective.

There are now ways to measure the amount of this protein, so it can often be predicted whether a cancer will be resistant to chemotherapy. P-glycoprotein genes have also been discovered, which may explain why some cells in a tumor are resistant to drugs while others are not. This in turn may explain why some drugs are not effective when administered even when a drug sensitivity test indicates that the tumor *should* be sensitive to a certain drug. Researchers are now trying to overcome drug resistance related to P-glycoprotein.

HOW THE DRUGS ARE GIVEN

The drugs used in chemotherapy are very powerful. The line between a therapeutic and a toxic dose is so fine and the consequences of the wrong dose so severe that general physicians without special training don't prescribe them. So chemotherapeutic agents are usually given only by oncologists, usually medical or pediatric oncologists (specialists in the medical treatment of cancer) and hematologists (specialists in diseases of the blood), although some surgical and gynecological oncologists also give chemotherapy.

Delivery Routes and Methods The drugs can be delivered to your circulatory system by many different routes. They can be taken orally in capsule, pill or liquid form. They can be injected through a syringe into a vein, artery or muscle. Or they can be given intravenously through an IV drip device.

Single or multiple drugs can be injected directly into organs such as the liver, using a small pump to ensure a constant flow. An external pump might be used, although internal pumps can now be surgically implanted and remain in the body for several weeks or months or permanently (*see* Chapter 5 for illustrations of catheters, ports and pumps).

Each delivery route has its advantages and disadvantages.

♦ *Intravenous* For intravenous delivery, you have to have a vein that can be entered easily and without causing a lot of discomfort. This isn't always easy. Some people naturally have small veins. Sometimes the veins get "used up" after several chemotherapy sessions.

If a vein isn't easily accessible, a temporary plastic tube can be implanted under the skin in the chest or in an arm or leg. These catheters, or central lines, as they are called, extend into larger veins. They provide an access point either for injections or for the slow drip (continuous infusions) of therapy over hours or even days. All kinds of fluids can enter the vein through the catheter—chemotherapy drugs, nutritional formulas, antibiotics, blood or platelet transfusions, antinausea drugs or morphine or other pain-killing narcotics.

The catheters avoid any discomfort from vein "sticking" and also any worry about having shots of irritating drugs that might leak out into the tissues. They can't be pulled out with an average pull or jerk, so they are quite safe. And they are simple to care for. They just need occasional cleaning and changing of the injection cap and periodic injections of heparin, a drug that prevents blood clotting in the catheter.

♦ *Implanted infusion ports* Another type of catheter is completely under the skin. It is called a port, and it's filled by placing a special needle through the skin into the chamber. The chamber contains a rubber or Silastic cover that can be punctured thousands of times with a special needle to deliver therapy, antibiotics or nutrients directly into a large vein.

The advantage of the implanted system is that since it is completely under the skin, no dressings or cleaning are needed and care is much simpler. Heparin injections won't be needed so often either. The disadvantage is that there is a slight risk of the drug leaking out. Also, a port can occasionally get out of position and become more difficult to enter.

♦ *Ambulatory pumps* Small portable pumps that deliver chemotherapy while you go about your normal activities are called ambulatory pumps. ("Ambulatory" just means you can walk around.)

These devices are often about the size of a deck of cards. They hold the drug supply, a mechanism for injecting it slowly and smoothly into an attached catheter, a battery to power the mechanism and controls for regulating the rate of drug delivery. Many of the pumps have become very sophisticated. Some have alarms to alert you to problems. One of the newer systems can deliver four separate drugs in a preset time sequence.

Several types are available. The balloon pump (Travenol infuser) is the cheapest and simplest, consisting basically of a large plastic reservoir. The pump is filled, then attached to a port or catheter. The pump empties automatically when it's connected.

◆ *Central nervous system delivery* Some patients, such as those with acute leukemia, need chemotherapy drugs injected into the spinal fluid. This can be done by repeated lumbar punctures (spinal taps), but the preferred method is to use an Ommaya reservoir. This is a rubber bulb usually placed under the scalp. A tiny tube connects the reservoir to the spinal fluid compartment. This requires a minor operation for placement of the reservoir and tube. Drugs are injected through the skin into the reservoir. Infection in the reservoir area is a possibility, so patients are usually monitored for side effects such as tenderness, inflammation, fever, stiff neck and headaches.

◆ *Intraperitoneal* This technique which involves delivering drugs directly into the abdominal cavity is sometimes used for ovarian or abdominal metastatic cancer. A catheter is connected to a chamber, usually on the chest or abdominal wall. The drugs are injected into the chamber, which releases them into the abdominal cavity. This eliminates the need to put a new tube into the abdomen every time drugs have to be given. High dosages can be given this way, higher than would be possible with any other method of delivery.

◆ *Intra-arterial* Drugs are often given to specific areas such as the liver, head and neck, or pelvis through the artery supplying that area. This is usually done in the hospital, where the delivery system can continuously infuse chemotherapy over a specific time. The drugs are given through a pump that can overcome arterial pressure.

◆ *Infusaid pumps* This special pump was developed to be surgically implanted within the abdomen. The pump is shaped like a hockey puck and has two chambers—one for the drug, the other for a fluid that forces the drug into the catheter. It also has a side port for chemotherapy injections. The pump can deliver a drug for as long as two weeks, then the chemotherapy solution can be replaced with salt water to give your system a rest.

Which Route to Use This decision depends on several factors, mainly the type of tumor and the drug being used. There are many questions to answer. Can the drug be absorbed in the stomach? How big a dose is required? What are the side effects? Are they tolerable?

Ultimately, the decision will be made on the basis of what is the most effective way to get the highest dosage of the right drug to the right place. Whichever route is chosen, your doctor will give you and your family or friends complete information on the usual effects of the drug, its side effects, any safety precautions to take and what reactions to report.

Where the Drugs Are Given Intravenous administration of some drugs requires a stay in the hospital for a few days. Injections are usually given in a hospital or in the doctor's office, although oncology nurses can give the drugs as part of a home care service.

If pills, liquids or capsules have been prescribed, you can take them at home or at work. Even if you are taking the chemotherapy orally, however, you will still have to visit your doctor's office every so often so the tumor's response can be monitored and your blood counts analyzed. Some drug programs require more frequent office visits because the schedule can be fairly complex.

HOW LONG TREATMENT LASTS

Cancer therapy is a fast-changing field with new treatment schedules always being tested in clinical trials. Although new chemotherapeutic drugs are being developed, it is often the same standard drugs in new combinations or given on different schedules that make the difference between success and failure in destroying cancer cells.

So there are few hard and fast rules on how often drugs are given or how long treatment lasts. Apart from the ever-changing recommended treatments, every person is different, every tumor is different, and every chemotherapy program is tailored to fit the situation.

Just as an example, a cycle of therapy may consist of one drug being given every day for two weeks with other drugs being given on particular days in the two-week period. After a rest period to allow normal tissues to recover, the entire cycle might be repeated every few weeks for six months or longer.

The length of treatment varies with different treatment programs.

♦ For programs that may be able to cure certain forms of cancer, even if widespread, the therapy is typically given for no more than about six months or up to a year in a few cases. This is true of Hodgkin's disease, some lymphomas, cancer of the testis and adjuvant therapy for breast and colon cancer.

♦ Where a remission has been achieved in various forms of metastatic cancer, treatment will be given until the maximum effect has been observed and then for a little while longer in an attempt to destroy hidden tumor cells. If therapy is stopped—unmaintained remission—it may be a long time before the tumor begins to grow again and more therapy is needed. But sometimes chemotherapy is continued indefinitely—maintained remission—until a relapse occurs, at which time the drug program will be changed.

♦ For programs in which chemotherapy is combined with radiotherapy, specific rules and formulas apply to each treatment protocol—prescribed doses, schedules and drug combinations—which are generally followed exactly.

♦ There are similar standards for adjuvant chemotherapy programs for patients who have a high risk for recurrence. The therapy to wipe out small nests of cancer cells that cannot be detected is generally given for six months to one year.

SELECTING THE RIGHT DRUGS

Which drugs to use, alone or in combination, is decided on the basis of many factors, including the extensive guidelines for treatment in the cancer literature. Yet each treatment program is, in a sense, an experiment, since the results in a particular patient cannot be predicted. There are no guarantees. It is not possible to state ahead of time whether a certain drug or combination of drugs will stop or slow down tumor growth in a certain individual.

Doctors are able to estimate, for example, that perhaps 30 or 55 or 73 percent of patients can be expected to respond to a particular drug program for a particular tumor. But they cannot know until they conduct the treatment trial whether any one individual will respond with the hoped-for tumor shrinkage.

What "Response Rate" Means A misconception often arises when a doctor says that a drug has, say, a 60 percent response rate. Patients sometimes think this means that the drug will be at least partly effective against tumors in all treated patients. But to say a drug has that response rate is like saying that a diaphragm or condom is a 95 percent effective way of preventing conception. That figure doesn't mean that all women will become 5 percent pregnant. It means that those contraceptives work 100 percent of the time in 95 percent of the people who use them and don't work at all for the other 5 percent.

Similarly, a drug with an average response rate of 60 percent means that 60 percent of the patients receiving it will respond. But 40 percent will not, although tumor growth might be delayed in some of them.

Devising the Plan As with any plan for cancer treatment, the chemotherapy program your doctor recommends will be tailored to the precise stage of your particular kind of tumor, your age, physical condition and any other medical problems. He or she will be generally guided by some specific information.

♦ *What's worked in the past* Oncologists rely primarily on experience from clinical trials involving many patients with similar tumors. They will usually consult reports in medical journals and the research findings presented at cancer meetings. Since more and more literature on drug treatment is being produced every month, the updated cancer information provided by the Physician Data Query (PDQ) system of the National Cancer Institute should also be consulted. Such computer databases are now essential for physicians who want to keep track of the rapid changes in the field.

Many state-of-the-art treatments are part of clinical trial protocols available at major cancer centers as well as some community hospitals.

♦ *Drug sensitivity* A lot of research over the past 15 years has been devoted to finding ways of predicting which drugs would kill which tumor cells most successfully. This research has involved growing an individual patient's cancer cells in the laboratory and testing a whole battery of anticancer agents on them.

This drug sensitivity test program— called a clonigenic assay—may give a doctor some guidance on which drugs to use. But it's especially useful for indicating which drugs *not* to use. If a drug doesn't kill single cancer cells in the lab, then it probably won't be effective in the body. So any drugs that are inactive in a laboratory test of a patient's tumor cells would not usually be used with that patient.

These tests may be useful in selected patients, but are not yet the final solution to the problem of drug selection. Their usefulness is limited by a number of factors:

♦ The tumor may not grow in the laboratory, or only certain drug-sensitive cells may grow.

♦ There may be differences between the way the drug works in the body and the way it works in a test tube. In the body, the drug can be bound and inactivated, eliminated by the kidneys or not be allowed to get through the P-glycoprotein "gate" on the cell surface.

♦ These test procedures apply only to one or, at most, two drugs tested one at a time. But chemotherapy cures are generally produced only by combinations of many drugs.

♦ *The possibility of using other therapies* There is no one absolutely right choice in cancer therapy, and the treatments recommended can change over the course of the illness. One reasonable choice at a particular time may not be appropriate at a later time.

A woman whose breast cancer recurs in a non-vital place, for example, may have several options. Her doctor may recommend: surgery, radiation treatment to the region to possibly control the cancer for years, hormone treatments, simple chemotherapy, complex chemotherapy or even doing nothing until the cancer grows and starts to bother her in six months' or a year's time.

Each treatment option has advantages and disadvantages, and there may be more than one option that is sensible.

SELECTING THE RIGHT DOSAGE

Larger doses of chemotherapy drugs do result in more cancer cells being killed. But a balance has to be struck between improved therapeutic effects and unacceptable toxic effects.

It may *not* be a kind act for your doctor to limit the dosage to avoid toxic effects. For those tumors that can potentially be cured with chemotherapy or have a good chance of going into remission, reducing the dosage to minimize toxicity will also reduce the possibility of cure or remission. The kindest act is to provide the maximum safe dose for cure, even at the cost of some toxicity. When the risks are weighed against the benefits, it doesn't make sense to take all the risks yet fail to get the benefits because the dosage was too low.

When Therapy May Be Stopped Because of Side Effects There is no reason to stop therapy when the drugs produce few problems and the control of the tumor is very satisfactory or even barely satisfactory. But major or objectionable side effects or complications can only be justified by a very significant and pronounced antitumor response.

The decision to stop therapy really depends on how you and your doctor define "objectionable" and what you are willing to put up with. Most men with metastatic testis cancer, for example, can be cured with less than six months of chemotherapy. Naturally, both doctors and patients are usually willing to put up with more discomforting side effects in that case because of the improved chance of cure. The alternative would be fatal.

What is important is for the doctor to give an adequate dosage of drugs—one that would be expected to produce results if that particular tumor in that particular patient happens to be sensitive. Then, after waiting an appropriate time—often about two or three months—tests will show if the tumor is shrinking.

High-Dosage Chemotherapy Several new and exciting programs for high-dosage chemotherapy are now being tested in major cancer centers. The hope is that greatly increased dosages may cure some malignancies that may not be curable with standard dosages. Various supportive measures may be used with these programs to decrease the toxic effects of the higher dosages, although in some cases, it is known that increased dosages may be given without the need for additional measures.

A very aggressive supportive measure is removing early blood-forming cells—called stem cells—from the body before very high dosage chemotherapy is given. These stem cells are preserved, then reinjected to re-establish normal blood production and blood counts. This procedure used to be called bone marrow transplantation. A more appropriate term is bone marrow protection.

In cases of heart, liver or lung transplants or in the case of bone marrow transplanted to patients with acute leukemia, the transplanted tissue takes over and replaces the diseased tissue or cancer-affected normal organ. In the case of high-dosage chemotherapy, the early blood-forming cells do not replace any diseased tissue. The anticancer treatment is the chemotherapy, not the removal and reinjection of early blood cells.

With special equipment, stem cells can now be removed from veins. Although bone marrow may also be collected as a backup, many high-dosage chemotherapy programs depend primarily on stem cell protection. Research is determining the role of high-dosage chemotherapy with stem cell protection in treating several potentially curable malignancies. (*See also* Chapter 12.)

MEASURING THE RESPONSE

There are several ways to tell if a tumor is responding to treatment. They are pretty much the same methods used to diagnose the tumor in the first place—physical examination, x-rays, blood tests and scans. These same tests will have been done before treatment to establish a baseline for future comparisons.

♦ A lump or a tumor involving lymph nodes can be felt and measured directly. The size of the liver, spleen and other organs can also often be determined by physical examination. Your doctor will record these direct measurements in your chart and compare them from time to time to see if the size of the tumor is decreasing.

♦ Some tumors, such as those involving the lungs, show up on x-rays. If new x-rays are taken at one-, two- or three-month intervals, the size of the tumors on the x-ray film can be measured directly with a ruler.

♦ Internal tumors, such as those involving the liver or other organs, are more difficult to measure. So special techniques have to be used—scanning using radioactive tracer isotopes, CT or MRI. Again, the size of the tumor as shown on the image can be measured directly at various intervals.

♦ Sometimes blood tests provide a clue to tumor response. Both non-specific tests, such as liver function tests, and tests for specific tumor markers may be used.

MONITORING BLOOD COUNTS

The drugs used in chemotherapy are growth inhibitors. They are especially good at turning off cells that are growing very quickly. Unfortunately, the drugs are not selective in their action. They turn off every fast-growing cell. There's no way the drug can tell an abnormal cell from a normal one.

The most important rapidly growing normal cells affected by the drugs are the blood cells. The red cells that carry oxygen are not usually affected very much. But the levels of the white cells that fight infection and the platelets that stop bleeding usually fall during chemotherapy.

There are no signs or symptoms of a minor decrease in blood counts. A slight decrease isn't harmful anyway. In fact, blood counts are expected to fall. This ensures that the drugs are being given in the maximum possible safe dosage. The lowered counts also show your doctor that the drugs are doing what they are supposed to do—stop fast-growing tissues from growing. If there is enough drug in your system to stop white blood cells, then there is enough to have a poten-tial effect on other rapidly growing cells, namely the cancer cells.

Still, it is very important that your doctor keep a close watch on the blood cells. The blood counts have to be measured regularly, usually before each chemotherapy treatment. If the counts are normal, it may be safe to give the standard dose or even increase the drug dosage. If one of the counts is too low, a drug dose can be modified or even put off for a while. When a therapy session is skipped because of low counts, this does not mean that the cancer cells will get out of control. The rest period is a normal part of the therapy, done for safety reasons.

The Danger of Infection A very low white blood cell count could lead to serious infections, and a very low platelet count could lead to bleeding. If the white blood count or platelet count falls lower than is safe, a rest period will allow the blood counts to recover. If you have fever, chills or any other sign of infection, like a cough or sore throat, during chemotherapy, call your doctor so therapy can be stopped until the infection has been treated effectively. Chemotherapy may suppress your immune system, making it harder for you to fight off infections. Any infection might spread and could become serious.

Minimizing Infection To lessen the chance of a serious infection developing, it is sometimes useful to administer colony-stimulating factors (CSFs) such as G-CSF (Neupogen) or GM-CSF (Leukine). This practice minimizes the time when the white blood cell count is low. These agents are also used to improve a low white blood cell count after an infection has already developed.

New aggressive chemotherapy programs may incorporate CSFs into the treatment plan. This may allow for the safer use of higher dosages of chemotherapy. It may also increase what is called dose intensity. This means that the chemotherapy schedule can be completed without any delays caused by low white blood cell counts. Improved dose intensity has improved the remission rate in a number of responsive cancers. (*See also* Chapter 8.)

DEALING WITH SIDE EFFECTS

The prospect of chemotherapy can be frightening. This is not surprising, seeing as how the side effects have been portrayed so horrifically in the popular press. Word of mouth hasn't helped either. Everyone seems to know an uncle of a friend of someone at work who had just a terrible time. But the side effects are usually not nearly as bad or troublesome as your friends may have told you or as you may have read about or seen on TV.

Many people tolerate chemotherapy very well and have few negative reactions. The person who visits the doctor's office, gets a shot for colon or breast cancer, then goes home or back to work and functions fairly well rarely appears on television or gets written up in the papers (*see* Chapter 17).

Taking the Right Approach You should bear in mind that more than 50 drugs are used in cancer chemotherapy. Some produce very few side effects and are easy to take. Others have major problems that have to be combated with appropriate medications. It is also important to remember that some of the most active drugs against cancer are also the ones that provoke the most side effects.

You should try hard to put any fears behind you. Fear of treatment and fear of side effects is a major problem, for anxiety can make the reaction worse. Supportive care, counseling and anti-anxiety drugs may became vital to making sure therapy continues. A more relaxed attitude toward chemotherapy may well lead to fewer bad experiences.

You should approach chemotherapy with the knowledge that it is impossible to attack cancer cells with drugs without also affecting normal tissues. As mentioned earlier, the drugs are most effective against rapidly growing cells. Tumor cells grow rapidly. So do hair follicles, the bone marrow and the cells in the lining of the gastrointestinal tract— mouth, stomach and bowels.

There are basically two kinds of side effects of chemotherapy, immediate and chronic.

Immediate Side Effects These are mainly nausea and vomiting. Both can occur soon after treatment, but both usually go away fairly quickly. Fortunately, a number of very effective antinausea medications have been developed over the past few years. They are often given two, three or four at a time, sometimes intravenously, and can usually prevent major problems with both nausea and vomiting. Very often your doctor will have to try different combinations of antinausea medications if the first combination isn't working as well as you both would like.

Sometimes these nausea medications produce their own side effects, mainly sleepiness or general fatigue. But these minor effects are well worth the trade-off if you can avoid feeling sick. Treatment schedules can also be arranged so that the medication does not disrupt your life too severely. Chemotherapy may be given on a Friday, for example, so that any tiredness will wear off enough by the following Monday that you can return to work.

Chronic Side Effects Since fast-growing cells are affected most, there may be some hair loss, sore mouth, nausea and diarrhea or depressed blood counts.

Hair Loss This problem occurs with some chemotherapeutic drugs, but not all. The amount of hair loss can vary from a slight thinning to baldness. The loss may be gradual or sudden. Sometimes all body hair—head, eyebrows, legs, armpits and pubic areas—may be lost. Depending on the drug used (and on the individual), hair loss on the head can be reduced by using a tourniquet or an ice cap. These narrow the blood vessels in the scalp so that less drug reaches the hair follicles.

The hair loss will be less upsetting if you plan ahead. Before treatment, get a short haircut so the loss won't be so noticeable. Get fitted for a scarf, turban or wig. And keep in mind that hair loss is always temporary. Many people find that their hair starts growing back while they are still getting chemotherapy.

Sore Mouth Sores in your mouth or a sore mouth are side effects of some drugs, but last only a few days. Your doctor can prescribe medication to relieve any pain. Choosing soft, bland foods, rinsing frequently with mild mouthwashes and using a soft toothbrush will help.

Low Blood Counts Depressed blood counts can have several effects, depending on which blood component is low.

♦ Low red cell counts may lead to a general feeling of weakness. You can offset this effect by making sure you get enough rest and not overtaxing yourself in your daily activities.

♦ Low white cell counts leave you vulnerable to infection, so it will be important to avoid people with colds or the flu and to take other preventive measures (*see* Chapter 20).

♦ Low platelet counts may lead to easy bruising and bleeding, so you'll have to take care to avoid cuts, burns or injuries and to avoid aspirin and alcohol. If the platelet count is very low, you can get a transfusion. The bone marrow will usually return to normal in two or three weeks.

Some drugs have very specific side effects. Your doctor can spell these out for you, indicate your chance of having them and outline special measures you can take to minimize or prevent them (*see* Chapter 17). For information on the latest drugs being used in clinical trials, *see* Chapter 36.

If you need additional information, several excellent books can be consulted, including *Coping with Chemotherapy*, by Nancy Bruning, *Nutrition for the Cancer Patient*, by Janet Ramstack and Ernest H. Rosenbaum, and *A Comprehensive Guide for Cancer Patients and Their Families*, by Ernest H. Rosenbaum and Isadora Rosenbaum.

8
WHAT HAPPENS IN BIOLOGICAL THERAPY

Raphael Catane, MD, and Malcolm S. Mitchell, MD

Biological therapy is a relatively new way to treat cancer. It is based on the idea that the human immune system, which is designed to eliminate and destroy any foreign substance found inside the body, can play a role in destroying cancer cells.

There are several problems with this approach. One of the biggest is that the immune system doesn't always treat cancer cells as "foreign." It is easy for the system to recognize bacteria or viruses, since they are completely different from normal human cells. But the difference between a tumor cell and a normal cell is small.

Great strides have been made, however, and biological therapy is now an accepted treatment for some cancers. The therapy consists mainly of treating the immune system with highly purified proteins that help activate the system or help it do its job more effectively. Interferon and interleukin-2 are the best known of these proteins. Many others are being evaluated.

HOW YOUR IMMUNE SYSTEM WORKS

To understand the role biological agents play in cancer treatment, you have to know how the normal immune system works.

When something foreign, such as a bacteria, virus or tumor cell, gets into your body, several kinds of cells go into action in what is called the immune response.

♦ *Macrophages* These are the body's front line of defense. They are the first cells to recognize and engulf foreign substances (antigens). They break down these foreign substances, then present the resulting smaller proteins to the T lymphocytes (which results in the production of antibodies and T cell-mediated immune responses).

Macrophages produce substances called cytokines that regulate the activity of lymphocytes. They can also act as nonspecific "soldiers" under the direction of the T lymphocytes, attacking tumor cells when attracted by substances called lymphokines made by specific antitumor T cells.

♦ *Lymphocytes* These small round cells are the most important immune cells. They are divided mainly into B and T cells.

B lymphocytes produce antibodies—proteins (gamma globulins) that recognize foreign substances and attach themselves to them.

T lymphocytes are the cells programmed to recognize, respond to and remember antigens. When stimulated by the antigenic materials presented by macrophages, the T cells make lymphokines that signal other cells. The T cells are also able to destroy cancer cells on direct contact.

Subsets of T cells—called helper or suppressor T cells, depending on their function—are involved in stimulation or inhibition of antibody production in collaboration with B lymphocytes.

♦ *Polymorphonuclear leukocytes (PMNs)* This is a general name for a group of white blood cells consisting of neutrophils, basophils and eosinophils.

Neutrophils are the most common immune cells in the body. If you have an infection, their number increases rapidly. They are the major constituents of pus and are found around most common inflammations. Their job is to "eat" (ingest) and destroy foreign material.

Basophils and eosinophils are PMNs that contain large granules—storage sacs—inside the cell. They interact with certain foreign materials. Their increased activity may lead to an allergic reaction.

How the Cells Interact The immune response is a coordinated effort. All these immune cells have to work together, so they have to communicate with each other. They do this by secreting a large number of special protein molecules called cytokines that act on other cells.

There are many different cytokines—interleukins 1 through 12, interferons alpha, beta and gamma, tumor necrosis factors alpha and beta, prostaglandins and colony-stimulating factors, for example. Some immunotherapy strategies involve giving large doses of these proteins, either alone or in combination. This is done in the hope of stimulating the cells of the immune system to act more effectively or of making the tumor cells more recognizable to the immune system.

TYPES OF IMMUNOTHERAPY

There are really five ways to improve the workings of an immune system. They are analogous to ways you could make an army more effective if it was fighting a battle in the field. You could increase the number of your troops, both foot soldiers and more specialized units. You could help the troops focus their efforts more

effectively by helping them communicate with each other. You could quickly replace any troops already lost in the fight. You could give them more precise weapons. Or you could make sure their efforts aren't wasted in a scattershot way by clearly identifying or highlighting the targets they're shooting at.

In a similar way, cancer immunotherapy can be conveniently characterized by five broad strategies.

♦ *Active stimulation* This is based on the idea that everyone has some intrinsic anti-tumor immunity and that if the defensive cells can just be aroused in some way they may have an effect against cancer cells. There are both non-specific and specific strategies involved.

The non-specific strategy uses bacterial or chemical booster substances (adjuvants) to "turn on" a whole range of immune cells—macrophages, natural killer cells and other non-specific killer cells. One effect of stimulating macrophages is that T cells are activated too.

The specific strategy uses the tumor cells themselves or tumor-associated antigens to trigger specific "effector" cells such as killer T cells. These are often called tumor vaccines.

♦ *Adoptive* This strategy involves transferring immunological cells or molecules that carry information (especially lymphokines, the cytokines secreted by lymphocytes) that will help the immune system do its work in a more coordinated way.

♦ *Restorative* Cancer itself and treatments like radiation and chemotherapy can decrease the number of immunological cells available to take part in the immune response. The restorative strategy involves replacing these cells or accomplishing the same goal indirectly by inhibiting the action of suppressive influences on the immune system, such as suppressor T cells.

♦ *Passive* This strategy involves giving the immune system specific "weapons" such as antibodies or short-lived antitumor "factors," that can attack specific cells. Special kinds of antibodies can also be programmed to deliver killer molecules such as radioactive isotopes or toxins to tumor cells.

♦ *Tumor cell modulation* This category isn't formally recognized yet, but "tumor cell-modulating immunotherapy" is really the most appropriate term when talking about biological agents such as the interferons. All types of immunotherapy depend on the immune cells recognizing the tumor cells. The only way they can do this is by spotting certain antigens on the surface of these cells, which is not always an easy thing to do. "Cell modulation" means that the tumor-associated antigens are highlighted, giving the immune cells a cleaner target to aim for.

BIOLOGICAL AGENTS

Over the past few years, many biological agents and many approaches to biological therapy have been investigated. Most clinical trials originally concentrated on one or another of the strategies outlined above, trying to understand and exploit individual approaches to improving the immune response of cancer patients.

With the data from these trials in hand, it is now becoming possible to design useful combinations of strategies and agents. At the moment, a range of biological agents is being researched. These include biological response modifiers that have no direct antitumor effect but are able to trigger or stimulate the immune system and so indirectly affect tumors.

The Interferons (IFN) There are several interferons. One of them—interferon-alpha—was the first of the cytokines shown to have an antitumor effect, both a direct effect and indirect effects through a more active immune system.

So far, studies have shown that interferon-alpha causes tumors to shrink 15 to 20 percent of the time in patients with kidney cancer (renal cell carcinoma) and melanoma. Other studies have shown it to have a major effect in 90 percent of patients with the rare hairy cell leukemia and with the more common chronic myelocytic (myelogenous) leukemia. Interferon-alpha is also occasionally effective in people with indolent non-Hodgkin's lymphoma and in some people with AIDS who develop Kaposi's sarcoma.

Researchers are now investigating interferon-beta and interferon-gamma, both of which have some similar antitumor effects. And all the interferons are being evaluated in combination with other cytokines or in combination with chemotherapy. What isn't understood very well yet is the exact mechanism that makes the interferons effective. They may make the tumor cells seem more foreign (increase the antigenicity), which makes them more vulnerable to attack by antibodies or by the various immune cells.

Interleukins There are many interleukins (IL-1 through IL-12). The one most intensively investigated by the National Institutes of Health and many universities is interleukin-2, which increases the activity of lymphocytes. The lymphocytes that have been non-specifically activated by IL-2 are called LAK cells (lymphokine-activated killer cells), and these do a much better job of identifying and destroying tumor cells than ordinary lymphocytes. All the other interleukins are still in an early investigational stage, but several will soon be studied in cancer patients.

Some researchers have tried to make IL-2 treatment more effective by collecting lymphocytes from a patient's blood with a special machine, activating them with IL-2 in the laboratory, then returning them to the patient as LAK cells along with more IL-2. An alternative is to activate lymphocytes from a patient's tumor, producing what are called tumor infiltrating lymphocytes (TIL cells).

Studies of treatment with IL-2 show a

response rate of 20 to 25 percent in patients with kidney cancer. IL-2—with or without the addition of LAK or TIL cells— also produces a response rate of about 20 to 25 percent in cases of advanced malignant melanoma. These responses are usually partial; complete responses are rare.

Colony-Stimulating Factors (CSFs) The CSFs are not directly effective against tumors, but they do play a major role in increasing the number and the activity of neutrophils and/or macrophages.

What makes research with CSFs particularly exciting is that high-dose chemotherapy dramatically reduces the number of white blood cells (including neutrophils) that fight infection, making chemotherapy patients vulnerable to various infectious diseases. It is for this reason that the dosage of chemotherapy often has to be kept low, thwarting any attempts to give higher and potentially more effective doses. Today the number of neutrophils can be increased by using colony-stimulating factors (such as G-CSF and GM-CSF), so both the severity and the duration of low white blood counts can be reduced. Infections are therefore less common and less severe. The CSFs allow greater doses of chemotherapy to be given, which in turn may lead to more complete remissions.

T Cells Some investigators are studying the use of T cells rather than less specific cells in the fight against cancer. The T lymphocyte is a very important component of the immune response. It recognizes tumor cells and either makes helper factors that stimulate the rest of the immune system or makes killer factors that destroy tumor cells.

Tumor vaccines depend on stimulating T cells in the body. But another approach is to take T cells *out* of a patient's body— either from the bloodstream or from within the tumor itself—make more of them and at the same time stimulate them with

IL-2, then return them in greater numbers than the patient could generate by himself or herself.

Although this approach is in its early stages, there have been some promising results in animals and in early studies with humans. Once again, melanoma and kidney cancer seem to be the most readily affected. As additional T cell growth factors are produced by genetic engineering, it should be possible to do a better job of growing T cells outside the body and causing them to be more highly activated than is now possible with IL-2 alone.

Tumor Vaccines One type of immunotherapy that has been studied for years and is only now coming of age is "active specific immunotherapy," more commonly known as the use of tumor vaccines. These would in theory work the same way as vaccines for measles, smallpox or other diseases.

The major difference in cancer treatment is that vaccines are used *after* someone has cancer. The vaccines are given to prevent recurrences or to get the body to reject tumor lumps, both of which are more difficult than preventing a viral infection. Nevertheless, encouraging results have been obtained in melanoma, colon, ovarian, breast and kidney cancers and in lymphomas.

In melanoma, when there is some degree of clinical response, survival has increased even in patients with widespread disease. Improved survival, even with persistent cancer, may be the most important effect of biological treatment. This is in contrast with chemotherapy, where survival is usually unaffected except by complete remissions.

Although vaccines alone have not been effective in more than 20 percent of patients with melanoma or kidney cancer, higher response rates have been suggested when vaccines are used in combination with other agents such as interferons and interleukins.

The National Cancer Institute has made tumor vaccines a priority area of research, so this type of immunotherapy will receive a great deal of attention over the next decade, specifically with altered tumor cells and purified tumor antigens.

Tumor Necrosis Factors (TNFs) Tumor necrosis factors alpha and beta (also called lymphotoxin) are cytokines produced by both macrophages and lymphocytes. TNFs can stimulate immune cells, damage tumor cells directly, influence the blood vessels around tumors and make tumors more recognizable to the immune system.

Unfortunately, high doses of TNFs are very toxic and have not been useful against tumors. Smaller doses or doses administered at the tumor site may prove to be beneficial in combination with other treatments.

Gene Therapy The technique of inserting genes into tumor cells or into the cells of the immune system has made headlines in the past few years. The promise of this approach is that tumor vaccines can be made more potent by attracting more T cells and macrophages to the site of injection and by stimulating them more strongly when they arrive.

T cells, which have a long lifespan in the body, can also carry genes around the body for a long time. If the genes make the T cells better able to recognize tumor antigens or to multiply more rapidly, the immune response can be augmented for a long period.

In colon cancer—and probably in other cancers—an abnormal (transformed or mutated) gene or the absence (deletion) of a gene cause the cancer to develop. Replacing defective or absent genes with properly working ones in susceptible people could prevent the disease from occurring.

Gene therapy is in its infancy. As it matures, it will influence not only immunotherapy and cancer prevention but a host of other disorders caused by abnormal genes.

ANTIBODY THERAPY

Antibodies are proteins (gamma globulins) that are produced by B lymphocytes. Every B lymphocyte produces one kind of antibody that recognizes the foreign structure, or antigen. If the antibody can make contact with the antigen, it will become attached to it. This is important because a tumor cell surrounded by antibodies is more vulnerable to destruction by some cells of the immune system.

The antibodies have two parts—a variable part and a constant part.

♦ The variable part recognizes the antigen, or the specific structure of the "foreign" invader.

♦ The constant part, or the "tail," is recognized by the effector cells of the immune system such as monocytes, macrophages, neutrophils and LAK cells. So this constant part attracts the working immune cells, which then attack and destroy the structure to which the whole antibody is attached.

Monoclonal Antibodies A very modern and sophisticated way to use antibodies is to produce them in the laboratory as monoclonal antibodies (MAbs).

What makes MAbs different is that the antibodies produced naturally in the body by the many different B lymphocytes are always a mixture of different antibodies. But antibodies produced in a lab by a colony of B lymphocytes are all derived from the same parent cell (from the same "clone"). These antibodies won't be a mixture, but a pure accumulation of the specific antibody of the parent cell. The goal of this procedure is to produce a large culture of antibody-producing cells and then to select from the culture only the clones of those cells that make the specific antibodies against the antigens found on the surface of the cancer cell being treated.

How the Clones Are Made Live human cancer cells carry the antigens that are going to be the targets for the antibodies. So the cancer cells (or their tumor-specific antigens alone) are injected into mice. The immune systems of the mice are activated, and the mice produce lymphocyte colonies in their spleens. Each of these lymphocytes has reacted to an antigen from the cancer cell. These activated B lymphocytes are then removed from the spleens and "immortalized" by fusion with a special B cell. This produces a "hybridoma"—basically, a factory that can indefinitely manufacture antibodies against a specific antigen of the original cancer cell.

The Effect on Normal Cells One problem with monoclonal antibodies is that while many MAbs can be produced to recognize tumor-associated antigens, most tumor antigens are not specific for the tumors. This means that these antigens may also be found on some normal cells. This could create problems, but many antigens are found in large quantities on tumor cells and only in very limited amounts on normal cells. So an antibody designed to react against such an antigen will be able to destroy quite a few tumor cells without causing too much harm to normal cells.

Programming MAbs MAbs can be programmed to serve purposes other than reacting against specific cancer cells.

♦ MAbs can be programmed to be specific against cell growth factors, for example. This will interfere with the growth of cancer cells, which are frequently dependent on such factors.

♦ MAbs can be very helpful in some cases of bone marrow transplantation. Often, a cancer patient will donate his or her own marrow before heavy radiotherapy or chemotherapy, with the idea that it will be returned after treatment. But one problem with this kind of procedure (called an autologous transplant) is that cancer cells might be in the bone marrow. If the marrow is removed, stored and reintroduced, the cancer cells would be put right back and the cancer would recur. MAbs can be effective in purging the bone marrow cells of any cancer cells if the marrow is treated while it is outside the body.

♦ MAbs against a specific cancer cell can also be programmed to carry a radioisotope source to the tumor. This "radioactive-labeled" antibody will find the cancer cell and attach to it; the radioactive particles then destroy the tumor cells.

One problem is that the therapy requires an isotope strong enough to kill cells in the area of the target cancer cell. With radioactive iodine (I-131)-labeled antibodies, this treatment has been used successfully in cases of lymphomas, which are very radiosensitive tumors. But it is hard to deliver enough radiation to kill cells when treating many other kinds of tumors. Cancers of the colon, pancreas, stomach and esophagus, for example, are not very sensitive to radiation. With more research it is hoped that this technique may soon have better success.

♦ In the same way, MAbs that are specific against a certain cancer can be programmed to deliver other anticancer agents such as chemotherapy drugs or cell toxins like ricin to the tumor. As with the radioactive-labeled therapy, this is really antibody-guided treatment. The monoclonal antibody homes in on the cancer cell, latches on to it and lets the payload of drugs or toxins do their work.

Problems and Promise Antibodies—plain or bound to radioactive materials or other toxic substances—are being evaluated as therapy for cancer in clinical trials. The verdict on their usefulness isn't in yet, though theoretically they have a potential for specifically targeting and destroying many tumor cells.

What is clear so far is that the success of antibody therapy depends on how specific the monoclonal antibody is against the target antigen on the surface of the tumor cell, on the blood supply to the cancer and on how any one person's system handles the antibody. Unfortunately, there are still many problems to be overcome.

The major ones are damage to normal cells and the failure of MAbs to reach the tumor in sufficient amounts to destroy it. Repeated courses of MAbs can also cause allergic reactions, with symptoms including fever, chills, itching, skin rashes, nausea, vomiting and flushing. A severe form of hypersensitivity known as serum sickness has also been reported.

SIDE EFFECTS

All cytokines are proteins, which means they can be destroyed by stomach enzymes. So they cannot be taken orally. They have to be given by injections into a vein, into a muscle or under the skin. Antitumor antibodies—polyclonal or monoclonal—are also given by injection.

There can be side effects at the site of the injection such as redness or swelling. But since biological agents are getting into your system, the side effects can also be generalized, or systemic.

♦ Tumor vaccines have few or no side effects except muscle aches or, on occasion, low-grade fever.

♦ Most of the cytokines cause fever, fatigue and occasionally chills and a skin rash. They may cause changes in blood pressure, usually decreasing it.

♦ Interferons and TNFs cause general malaise, sometimes called flu-like syndrome.

♦ IL-2 can give rise to extremely severe and life-threatening side effects. IL-2 causes the peculiar capillary leak syndrome. If this develops, you may rapidly gain weight, experience a drop in your blood pressure and find it difficult to breathe. Tissues become swollen as fluid accumulates and there are sometimes toxic effects on the heart. Unless treatment is discontinued at this stage, IL-2 may cause kidney shutdown or respiratory arrest and death.

For these reasons, high-dosage IL-2 is usually given in an intensive care unit, where blood pressure, urine output and breathing can be closely monitored and side effects treated promptly to avoid failure of a vital organ. However, it is possible to achieve responses with low dosages of IL-2. Patients receiving such low dosages do not require hospital admission, and can sometimes continue working part time.

♦ Antitumor antibodies—polyclonal or monoclonal—can cause an allergic reaction varying from a mild skin rash, coughing and wheezing to an acute and severe reaction called anaphylaxis. With a full-blown anaphylactic reaction, blood pressure drops, various parts of the body swell, a severe skin rash breaks out and breathing can become difficult. This reaction can be fatal unless it is treated promptly with epinephrine and corticosteroids.

The possibility of allergic reactions to antibodies (or to any foreign substance) increases markedly with every additional injection, because eventually you become immunized against the foreign molecules. Your immune system will rapidly destroy these molecules, with the allergic reaction being a sign of your immune cells' increased activity.

♦ The side effects of antibodies vary with their target. An antibody aimed at a colon antigen may cause diarrhea. One directed against white blood cells will cause low white blood cell counts.

WHEN BIOLOGICAL THERAPY IS APPROPRIATE

A role for biological therapy has been established for melanoma, kidney cancer and some cancers of the blood such as chronic myelogenous leukemia and hairy cell leukemia. There is also some evidence of its effectiveness in treating breast, ovarian and colon cancer, as well as Kaposi's sarcoma.

The FDA has officially approved giving interferon-alpha for hairy cell leukemia, giving IL-2 for kidney cancer and Kaposi's sarcoma and giving the colony-stimulating factors for minimizing the period of low white blood cell counts caused by chemotherapy. In practice, physicians use these approved agents for other conditions as well.

Yet biological therapy is still in the early phases of development. These therapies should be used when there is no effective standard treatment, generally in clinical trials performed at qualified cancer centers, or when known treatments have failed to work or have stopped working. In diseases for which no useful chemotherapy programs exist, such as melanoma and kidney cancer, biological therapy is often given as a first-line treatment.

Caution and Hope Many promoters of unproven and useless anticancer treatments claim that their product or therapy improves the immune system and so will probably cure cancer. As an educated consumer of health care services, you should beware of any such false claims about new agents that augment the immune system. Except for some rare tumors such as Kaposi's sarcoma and some lymphomas that often result from immune suppression, there is as yet no definite proof that cancer is caused by failure of the immune system.

This does not mean, however, that stimulating the immune system will not treat cancers effectively. The limited success of single agents such as interferon, IL-2 and vaccines suggests that immunological therapies will be useful for many cancers, particularly when given in combination with one another and with chemotherapy. Physicians are still learning how to use individual substances and combinations most effectively.

Precisely how the body rejects cancer is still not understood, and many substances, such as interferon, have a variety of actions in the body. Perhaps because of these factors, many agents with a proved capability of stimulating the immune system have failed to produce a long-lasting antitumor effect. Nevertheless, while avoiding unrestrained optimism and blind trust in the "miracle breakthroughs" that seem to occur every week, you should be aware that biological therapy is a new approach to controlling tumor growth that holds considerable promise.

9
LASER THERAPY

Carlos Pellegrini, MD, Ernest H. Rosenbaum, MD, and Malin Dollinger, MD

---◇---

Laser therapy involves the use of high-intensity light to destroy tumor cells. Lasers are fairly new weapons in the anti-cancer arsenal, and their role is still limited. In a few select cases laser therapy can cure a cancer. But the technique is now used mainly to relieve serious symptoms such as bleeding or obstruction, especially when the cancer can't be cured by surgery, radiation or chemotherapy or when standard treatment can't be used because of advanced age, malnutrition or heart or pulmonary disease.

The verdict isn't in yet on whether laser treatment can truly be a curative procedure or if it is useful only for palliation. The final answer will have to await results from more studies.

HOW LASERS WORK

The word *laser* is an acronym for "light amplification by stimulated emission of radiation." The light is produced by devices that can "excite" substances such as carbon dioxide, argon and neodymium:yttrium-aluminum-garnet (Nd:YAG) to a higher energy state. As these substances return to their "resting" state, they release their extra energy in the form of a powerful light with a special "energy" that is capable of vaporizing human tissue, including tumor cells.

What makes this type of energy so useful in cancer treatment is that it can be aimed so precisely. Lasers focus on very small areas with extreme accuracy.

Endoscopic Laser Therapy Laser therapy is usually given by activating the special light beam through a flexible tube called an endoscope, the same instrument used to diagnose many cancers. The scope can be passed through any opening in the body—the mouth, nose, anus or vagina.

A laser operator looking through the scope can see the tumor directly and aim the light beam precisely into the target tissue. The operator then activates the device and the energy is produced. On contact with the tissue, the laser beam produces an intense heat. At 60°C (140°F), this heat can coagulate protein. At 100°C (212°F), it can vaporize tissue. The tissue usually burns for just a few seconds, giving off a bit of smoke and leaving a hole or ulcer.

Removing a tumor with a laser beam is not as effective as removing it with conventional surgery. A surgeon removes all the visible tumor, the tumor below the surface of the organ and a wide margin of tissue on each side. The laser operator removes only the visible tumor on the organ's surface. But tumors are like icebergs. What is visible is simply the tip of a much greater mass below the surface. After laser treatment, the bulk of the tumor is still in place.

Photodynamic Laser Therapy In some cases, laser therapy can be made more effective by the use of photodynamic therapy. This involves injecting a chemical before the laser treatment that can make tissue more sensitive to light. Malignant tissues have a special affinity for light with a specific wavelength. After a tumor is sensitized by hematoporphyrin, for example, the laser is more selective in its cell-destroying action.

WHEN LASER THERAPY MIGHT BE RECOMMENDED

Laser therapy is used primarily to treat cancers of the skin, trachea, lungs, esophagus, stomach, colon, rectum and anus. It can't replace surgery, radiation or chemotherapy as a definitive cancer treatment, but it can complement these therapies in a variety of ways.

Direct laser therapy to the skin or cervix can be very successful. But the usual objective of laser therapy is to help relieve an acute obstruction. This might be done so that surgery, radiotherapy or chemotherapy can be used effectively. Or it may be done to keep some vital body tube open—the esophagus for swallowing, the trachea for breathing or the colon, rectum and anus for eliminating stool.

The benefits are usually short-term, however, and there are technical limitations. The best results are usually obtained in centers where the procedure is performed frequently by highly experienced endoscopists.

Planning the Treatment Before laser therapy is even attempted on the trachea, bronchi or gastrointestinal tract, the first thing to decide is whether an endoscopic biopsy needs to be done to verify the diagnosis.

The next step is a thorough clinical assessment. This may involve specific kinds of x-rays (such as a barium swallow or barium enema), CT or MRI scans and ultrasound. These imaging studies are needed to estimate the risk of bleeding and to map the exact shape and size of the tumor and any sharp angles (as in the colon or esophagus) that will have to be dealt with.

Endoscopic ultrasonography may help, since it allows the tissue beneath the surface to be assessed. It is very important to know how much of the tumor is within the opening, or lumen, of the body tube and how much of it has extended through the wall of the lumen into surrounding tissues. The status of the lymph nodes is important too, and this staging can be done quickly if an emergency arises.

Treating an Obstruction in the Trachea Tumors in the windpipe (trachea) can't be treated very successfully with standard treatments. Less than 30 percent of patients are candidates for surgical removal of the tumor, and radiotherapy has few long-term survivors. Yet if the goal of treatment is palliation, laser therapy is a reasonable alternative.

Tracheal and endobronchial cancers can be directly seen through an endoscope and can be treated with a YAG laser, with or without the light-sensitizing hematoporphyrins. The tumor usually grows back and another treatment will be needed in four, eight or twelve weeks. With intrabronchial lesions, this interval can be stretched out by "afterloading" iridium-192. This involves placing empty catheters next to the tumor through an endoscope, then inserting the radioactive materials into the catheters to deliver a specific dose of radiation.

TREATING COLORECTAL AND ANAL CANCER

Laser treatment might cure a few cases of colorectal and anal cancer, though surgery along with radiation therapy is considered the primary treatment, with chemotherapy for certain stages. So the goal of laser therapy once again is usually palliation.

Colorectal Cancer If the purpose of laser treatment is to reduce or stop bleeding or to reduce the bulk of a tumor, one or two treatments will usually be enough.

When the obstruction is large, it may be hard to get the endoscope into the tumor.

It may be necessary to pass a guidewire through the tumor mass and use a smaller scope. An alternative is to use a guidewire to insert a balloon to dilate the constricted area, which will also allow a small scope to be passed to accomplish laser treatment.

♦ The most successful treatments occur when the tumor is growing inward, extending into the bowel lumen rather than outward toward the layer of the colon or rectum beneath the inner surface (submucosa).

♦ Short or smaller tumors and straight rather than curved or angulated areas of the colon are more successfully treated.

♦ The treatment is not curative and will require follow-up treatment to keep the lumen open every four, eight or twelve weeks, depending on how fast the tumor is growing.

♦ In rare instances, an obstruction of the bowel from colorectal or anal cancer may be decompressed by endoscopic laser therapy. This may allow surgery or other therapies to be planned on an elective rather than an emergency basis.

Anal Cancer What is often treated is a growing adenoma or an obstructing cancer when surgery, radiotherapy and chemotherapy are not appropriate treatments. Again, the best results from laser treatment are when the tumor is within the lumen rather than extending through the wall to adjacent tissues. A well-differentiated cancer that is small (less than 1 in./2.5-3 cm), non-ulcerating and growing into the lumen may have the best results.

The procedure is the same as for colon cancer and can be repeated after about 48 hours if you are in the hospital or about a week later if you are being treated as an outpatient. Several treatments might be needed to completely remove the obstruction.

♦ Fluid might accumulate in the tissues, which may temporarily intensify the obstruction or require pain-relieving medications.

♦ Retreatment is usually necessary four, six or twelve weeks after the obstruction is first removed.

♦ Many studies have shown that the obstructed lumen can be kept open in approximately 90 percent of cases. Bleeding can be controlled in over 85 percent of cases.

LASER THERAPY AND ESOPHAGEAL CANCER

Theoretically, laser therapy might be the only form of treatment needed for a very small tumor in the esophagus that could be completely vaporized.

Still, if the tumor can be cured with surgery, laser therapy isn't recommended for esophageal cancer. For one thing, tumors that small are very, very rare. For another, your doctor could never be sure the tumor hadn't invaded the wall of the esophagus beyond the laser's reach.

But if the cancer can't be cured by surgery (and esophageal cancer can seldom be cured), lasers can still help relieve the symptoms. When the tumor becomes so large that the opening of the esophagus—the lumen—gets blocked, you can't swallow food or even saliva. About 50 percent of patients can maintain their ability to swallow throughout their illness when a laser restores the lumen by vaporizing the tissue blocking it.

Laser vs Prosthetic Placement There are alternatives to laser therapy to treat swallowing problems. A tube, or prosthesis, placed in the esophagus can achieve an esophageal opening for swallowing in 95 percent of patients. But the procedure has a 13 percent complication rate and a 4.3 percent mortality.

Prostheses have a number of problems. They tend to get out of position and may block the esophagus on their own. They also don't propel food down to the stomach, so you may be limited to fluids or semi-solids. In general, they are not good for palliation of swallowing problems.

Laser therapy, on the other hand, offers 100 percent chance for success, with a 3.6 percent complication rate and approximately 1 percent mortality when performed by experienced practitioners. Laser is also considered better for high esophageal obstruction, where plastic prostheses such as Celestin's tubes cannot be fitted.

Endoscopic Laser Treatment Pretreatment evaluation will again involve mapping the exact geometry of the tumor and staging the disease. The size, depth of penetration of tumor invasion and lymph node status will determine whether the tumor is operable.

In the procedure itself (YAG laser with or without hematoporphyrin), the endoscope will be passed through your mouth and down the esophagus to the tumor site. Only the top layers of the treated area will be affected and only small pieces of tissue will evaporate. Three or more sessions might be needed to achieve an opening. These sessions are often spaced at 48-hour intervals to allow tissue breakdown to be more complete and to give the patient a rest. The technique varies and is decided upon by the operator. He or she will usually treat the lowest part of the tumor first, then come higher with each treatment session.

◆ Lasers are most useful in the middle and lower esophagus, which is straight, and least valuable for tumors outside the esophageal wall.

◆ It is difficult to know how deep to go into the submucosa since there are no good landmarks.

◆ There may be very narrow spaces (strictures) involved, which makes laser treatment more difficult. Dilating the esophagus first may help.

◆ There is acute angulation—a corner—at the junction of the esophagus with the stomach that makes laser therapy in this area very difficult.

◆ Since only the tumor within the lumen is removed, tumors usually come back quickly. The therapy will have to be repeated every two to eight weeks to keep the passage open.

◆ Laser therapy can help control bleeding as well as open a passageway to allow foods to be swallowed.

Combining Lasers and Other Treatments Different degrees of swallowing difficulty merit different approaches. Dilation of the esophagus before using chemotherapy or radiotherapy to help shrink the tumor may be the best way to get a functional esophageal opening that will improve the quality of life.

◆ Obstruction may occur with squamous cell esophageal cancer or with an adenocarcinoma of the stomach that grows upward to obstruct the esophagus. Lasers might be used in combination with standard treatments for these cancers.

◆ There may be a longer survival for squamous cell carcinoma with laser and radiation therapy. Squamous and adenocarcinoma have the same results for laser treatment, with tumors on the surface (Stage I) being easier to treat than tumors under the surface (Stage II).

◆ Results are better if the lesions are less than 2 in. (5 cm) in diameter. In one study, lasers gave almost all the patients (97 percent) an open passageway, but only 70 percent could eat satisfactorily.

◆ After the obstruction is removed, radiotherapy with afterloaded iridium-192 seeds can help prolong the swallowing interval.

10
HYPERTHERMIA

Penny K. Sneed, MD

———◇———

The idea of using heat to help destroy tumors has been around for a long time. In the early 1800s, there were medical reports that some people with cancer showed signs of tumor shrinkage after they developed high fevers. By the end of the last century, there were reports of some complete remissions because of high body temperatures.

But hyperthermia—the word means elevated temperature and refers to the use of heat in the treatment of cancer—has only recently been added to the arsenal of anticancer weapons. It is a specialized weapon, since hyperthermia techniques are still not applicable to all types of tumors. But in certain cases, when heat is applied for about an hour once or twice a week in conjunction with radiotherapy or sometimes chemotherapy, the results have been very promising.

HOW IT WORKS

When temperatures rise above 106°F (41°C), the heat starts to damage cells. How much damage is done depends on the temperature and how long the exposure lasts. The temperatures now used range from about 106 to 113°F (41 to 45°C).

Combining Hyperthermia with Other Therapies Heat is particularly effective when combined with radiation, for heat is especially destructive to two types of cells that tend to be resistant to radiation:
♦ cells making DNA in preparation for division; and

♦ cells that are acidic and starved for oxygen (poorly oxygenated). Unlike normal tissue, many tumors are likely to have poorly oxygenated cells that are particularly susceptible to hyperthermia, and tumors can often be heated to higher temperatures than surrounding normal tissues.

Heat also makes cells more sensitive to radiation by preventing them from repairing radiation damage. Heat and radiation work best together when the two treatments are given simultaneously or within perhaps an hour of each other. Hyperthermia treatments are usually given only once or twice weekly, because after cells are exposed to heat, they become somewhat resistant to subsequent exposures for about three days.

Heat also seems to improve the effect of some of the drugs used in chemotherapy, such as bleomycin, cisplatin, cyclophosphamide, melphalan, mitomycin-C and the nitrosoureas.

Heating Techniques During the past 15 years devices have become available to heat tumors directly and safely.

Hyperthermia treatment techniques can be divided into three broad categories—localized, regional, and whole body heating.
♦ Localized heating of tumors in or near the skin is often performed using an external applicator. This square or round box is placed on the outside of the body over the tumor. The applicator is connected to equipment that supplies different types of energy—microwave, radiofrequency or ultrasound—that will heat the tumor cells.

Localized heating can also be accomplished internally in a process called interstitial (inside the tumor) hyperthermia. Under anesthesia, needles or plastic tubes are placed into the tumor. Heat sources are then inserted directly into the plastic tubes or radiofrequency current is passed through the needles. Interstitial techniques often raise the tumor temperatures much higher than could be done with external techniques and without doing much damage to surrounding normal tissues.

♦ Regional hyperthermia involves using microwave or radiofrequency applicators to heat large volumes of tissue deep inside the body.

♦ Whole body heating can be accomplished by using hot water blankets, specialized oven-like devices or other methods. This procedure is safe, using temperatures up to about 107°F (41.8°C). This temperature may not be high enough to be effective in combination with radiation therapy alone, but may become useful with chemotherapy. Whole body and/or regional hyperthermia can also be combined with localized hyperthermia to improve results.

Although the hyperthermia treatment may be given externally, the temperatures inside the tumor usually have to be carefully monitored to control the treatment properly. This often means that tiny thermometers have to be placed into the tumor region, usually inside one or more small needles or tubes that are gently inserted through the skin under a local anesthetic.

Side Effects Hyperthermia does not cause any marked increase in radiation side effects or complications. Superficial hyperthermia by itself, however, can cause discomfort or even significant local pain in about half the patients treated. It can also cause blisters, which generally heal rapidly. Less commonly, it can cause burns, which tend to heal very slowly and occasionally need surgical repair.

How often blisters and burns occur depends on whether the tumor involves the skin and on the degree of skin cooling used during the treatment. In one study, heat blisters occurred in 10 percent of the superficial areas treated, but normal tissue ulceration occurred in less than 1 percent of cases. This indicates that burns can normally be avoided with careful monitoring and control of surface temperatures.

WHEN HYPERTHERMIA IS APPROPRIATE

As a form of treatment, hyperthermia has had very limited success when used by itself. In one study, only 13 percent of superficial tumors treated with hyperthermia alone had a "complete response"—in other words, disappeared completely. But many studies in patients with superficial malignancies have shown benefits when hyperthermia is added to radiation therapy.

A review of 15 studies revealed a complete response rate of 37 percent for tumors treated with radiation alone, and 63 percent for tumors treated with radiation and hyperthermia. The tumor response was often evaluated by comparing the results with different tumors in the same patients. In these same-patient comparisons, the complete response rate was 31 percent for tumors treated with radiation alone versus 71 percent for tumors treated with radiation and hyperthermia.

Superficial hyperthermia has been used successfully in combination with radiation therapy to treat:

♦ chest wall recurrences of breast cancer after a mastectomy and/or radiation therapy

♦ advanced primary breast cancer

♦ advanced or recurrent tumors involving lymph nodes containing metastatic cancer

♦ recurrent primary or metastatic melanoma in the skin or in tissues just under the skin

- primary cervix cancer
- melanomas in the eye
- soft tissue sarcomas

Interstitial hyperthermia—applying heat with probes inserted into the tumor—has been used for some tumors in the head and neck, breast, pelvis (such as cervix and prostate cancer) and skin or soft tissues. There is also now a lot of interest in using interstitial hyperthermia and radiation for brain tumors.

New Directions Many exciting areas of investigation could make clinical hyperthermia much more useful in the near future. Studies are in progress to find out just how much hyperthermia is needed to improve the results of radiation treatment. Several methods may soon be available to help predict a tumor's response to hyperthermia based on small samples of the cancerous cells.

It may also soon be possible to improve results by manipulating the flow of blood to the tumor or by manipulating its sensitivity to heat. Computer-based treatment planning, incorporating knowledge of blood flow in tumors and normal tissue, could be used for more effective hyperthermia treatment planning.

Some investigators have reported exciting preliminary results using continuous heating over many hours simultaneous with interstitial hyperthermia. This long-duration hyperthermia may be much more effective than standard one-hour hyperthermia sessions by continually sensitizing tumor cells to the radiation and by allowing accumulation of a greater "heat dose" over time.

Although many tumors are unfortunately still difficult to heat with available devices, great improvements are being made in technology and treatment techniques that will allow hyperthermia to be applied to many more tumors.

11
HYPERTHERMIC PERFUSION THERAPY

Robert E. Allen, Jr, MD

Regional perfusion is a way to deliver chemotherapy drugs to tumors in parts of the body that can be isolated from the circulatory system. The arms and legs are most frequently isolated. Techniques of isolation of the liver and lung recently have been developed.

The first reported use of this technique was in 1950, when nitrogen mustard was infused into the arteries supplying blood to tumors while the veins returning the blood were blocked. This maximized the exposure of the tumor to the chemotherapy drug.

The technique was refined in 1957 by using a tourniquet to isolate an extremity and adding a heart-lung machine to the process. The machine supplied oxygen and circulated the mixture of blood, drug and mineral solution (the perfusate) throughout the isolated limb. This method allowed an increase of 6 to 10 times the normal dosage of drug that could have been given locally to the cancer. The drug's toxic effects to the entire body were reduced and the rate of response was increased. The first report of a large number of patients treated with isolated limb perfusion at normal body temperature showed they had a survival rate 20 to 25 percent better than those treated in the conventional way.

A later development added heat to the perfusion system. Heat will kill tumor cells more often than normal ones at certain critical temperatures. The tumor-killing effect depends on the amount of heat used and the length of time it is applied. Using a heated perfusate improved the response rate in a 1967

study and heat has played a role in the procedure ever since.

What makes isolated limb perfusion particularly effective is that it delivers high-dose chemotherapy not only to the tumor but to the entire limb below the tourniquet, including potential sites of metastases. All that limits the dosage of the chemotherapy drug to be given is local tissue toxicity.

WHEN THE PROCEDURE IS APPROPRIATE

Perfusion can be used to treat a variety of cancers in the arms and legs. Melanomas, sarcomas and some localized cutaneous lymphomas have been treated with this method, but it has been most widely and effectively used to treat cutaneous malignant melanoma. (*See* "Melanoma".)

This cancer can be cured surgically if the tumor is discovered at an early stage, but isolated heated limb perfusion is suggested for people with extensive local tumors. And perfusing may be the treatment of choice for those who have melanomas involving the palms of the hands, the soles of the feet and the fingernails and toenails (subungual areas). Melanomas in these locations tend to have a poor prognosis.

People who have locally recurrent melanomas or spreading melanomas that are traveling away from the primary site toward nearby lymph nodes—the prognosis is very grave in both situations—are best treated by perfusion.

Results of Treatment Whether the treatment leads to a beneficial outcome depends on the stage of the cancer. There is some controversy about whether people with high-risk Stage I melanoma should have prophylactic perfusion or just surgery alone. One report has shown increased disease-free survival for Stage I patients treated with perfusion.

The five-year cure rate for acrolentiginous melanomas treated with perfusion ranges from 70 to 78 percent; the cure rate for the same lesions treated without perfusion ranges from 38 to 50 percent. On the average, perfusion offers people with Stage II or III melanomas a 20 to 25 percent increased survival over other treatment methods.

The following survival rates have been reported for the various stages as defined by the staging system developed at the M. D. Anderson Tumor Institute, the system most often used to stage melanomas of the extremities.

STAGE	FIVE-YEAR SURVIVAL AFTER PERFUSION
♦ **Stage I**	
Localized primary melanoma	89-94 percent
♦ **Stage II**	
Local recurrence within or adjacent to the scar	74-77 percent
♦ **Stage III**	
Regional metastases	
IIIA In-transit metastases	70-81 percent
IIIB Positive regional lymph nodes	48-54 percent
IIIAB In-transit metastases with regional nodes	30-45 percent
♦ **Stage IV**	
Systemic metastases, positive iliac lymph nodes	20-25 percent

WHICH DRUGS ARE USED

Alkylating agents are the most effective drugs to be perfused. They react with DNA, altering the nucleic acid and eventually killing the cell.

Melphalan (L-phenylalanine mustard) has been the drug most extensively used, either alone or in combination. Other drugs—cisplatin, thiotepa, dactinomycin and dacarbazine—are also used, but melphalan has many of the qualities of the ideal agent for isolated limb perfusion. It is the least toxic single drug, with low toxicity to soft tissues and blood vessel linings. It has a short half life (meaning that it disappears quickly) and its action isn't limited to specific phases of the cancer cell's life cycle.

A new agent, tumor necrosis factor (TNF), injures the small blood vessels supplying the cancer. It has produced over 90 percent complete tumor responses against melanoma and some sarcomas when used in the isolated perfusion circuit. TNF is very toxic, and leakage into the general circulation can cause toxic shock syndrome and death. Constant monitoring for leakage with radioisotopes is required.

Whatever anticancer drug is used, its effectiveness is enhanced by two aspects of the perfusion procedure. The use of high oxygen concentrations magnifies the effects of the drugs by sensitizing tumor cells and has a tumor-killing effect of its own. Heat opens the blood vessels so that there is a more even and thorough perfusion.

HOW IT WORKS

There are several steps in the regional hyperthermic perfusion procedure.

Isolating the Limb The technique begins with the process called cannulating, which means that small tubes are inserted into the arteries carrying blood to the limb and the veins carrying blood out. This means placing tubes into the axillary artery and vein when treating an arm and into the external iliac artery and vein when treating a leg. The blood vessels in the thigh (femoral) and behind the knee (popliteal) have also been used when treating a leg.

To make the isolation complete, a rubber tourniquet is placed at the top of the arm or leg and held in place with a mechanical device. The blood vessel tubing is then connected to a heart-lung machine.

Preparing the Circuit The complete perfu-

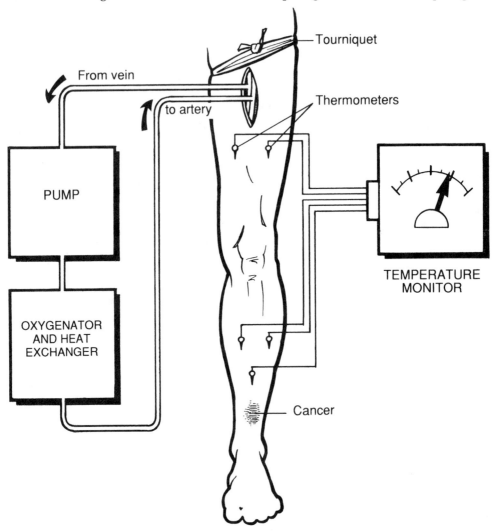

System used for hyperthermic perfusion therapy.

sion circuit consists of a low flow modular pump, arterial and venous tubing, an oxy-generator with an arterial line filter, a heating and cooling unit and an arterial blood temperature probe.

The circuit is primed with a mixture of your own blood and an electrolyte (mineral) solution, which circulates through the isolated limb with very high concentrations of oxygen. Heparin, a substance that prevents blood from clotting, is added. Leakage of the perfusate into the general circulation is checked by injecting fluorescein dye into the mixture, and any leakage is monitored and corrected during the operation.

Special thermometers (needle thermistors) are placed in the soft tissues at strategic locations to record the temperature of the limb during the procedure.

Giving the Drug The perfusate temperature is raised to 107.6°F (42°C). The temperature of the extremity is raised to 104°F (40°C) and is not allowed to rise beyond that.

When the average temperature near the tumor is 102.2°F (39°C), the chemotherapy drug is added to the solution and the perfusion continues for one hour (tourniquet time is limited to a maximum of two hours). Flow rates are in the range of 400 to 600 cc/min. for a leg and 250 to 350 cc/min. for an arm, with perfusion pressures never allowed to exceed the average blood pressure in the body.

When the procedure is complete, the drug is drained from the arm or leg and the limb is washed out with a mixture of dextran-40 and a balanced salt solution.

After the Procedure You will have to stay in bed with the extremity elevated for three days after the procedure, during which time you will be given low doses of heparin, the anticoagulating agent.

The oxygen saturation of the perfused limb has to be continuously monitored for four days after the operation. A fall in the saturation usually signals the start of what is called the compartment syndrome, meaning that the limb swells so severely that it may interfere with circulation.

Complications About 30 percent of people who have perfusion will experience complications, but most of them are minor and pass quickly.

♦ Severe bone marrow toxicity occurs in about 5 percent of patients, but this is usually temporary.

♦ The compartment syndrome occurs in 3 to 4 percent of patients. This is an emergency situation and if proper treatment is not given promptly, the limb may have to be amputated.

♦ There is always a buildup of fluid in the tissues (edema), but this does not last long if it is properly treated.

♦ Since anticoagulation is used, there is an increased risk of postoperative bleeding.

♦ Inflamed veins and blood clots in the legs (thrombophlebitis) occur in 10 to 15 percent of patients, but the clots rarely travel to the lungs (pulmonary embolism).

♦ Mortality from the procedure is variously reported from 1 in 2,000 (0.05 percent) to 3 in 200 (1.5 percent).

12
BONE MARROW TRANSPLANTATION

James O. Armitage, MD

———◇———

Bone marrow contains immature (or stem) cells that are capable of continuously producing new cells. This is what helps make bone marrow the "factory" for normal blood cells—the red cells that carry oxygen, the white cells that fight infections and the platelets that help blood clotting.

Bone marrow can sometimes be defective—for example, not producing enough normal blood cells. Red cells, white cells and platelets are necessary for life, so this is obviously a serious situation. Doctors long ago realized that if defective bone marrow could be replaced with normal marrow from another individual, a potentially critical situation like that could be resolved. But only in the past 20 years has medical knowledge advanced to the point where effective bone marrow transplantation techniques could be developed.

These techniques involve the intravenous administration of immature blood cells capable of reproducing themselves and repopulating an empty or defective bone marrow.

WHY A TRANSPLANT MIGHT BE RECOMMENDED

Replacing the defective bone marrow of an otherwise healthy person is one use of transplantation techniques. But at least 90 percent of all bone marrow transplants are performed to treat cancer.

Direct Benefit Transplanted bone marrow can have a direct effect against a cancer like leukemia. The transplanted marrow—which represents the immune system of another person—can recognize cancer cells as abnormal and destroy them. Unfortunately, this same phenomenon is thought to be related to an unwanted side effect known as graft-versus-host disease. Ideally, it would be possible to have only the effect against the cancer and avoid damage to normal tissue.

To Support Other Therapies A number of cancers are very sensitive to chemotherapy and radiation, but they cannot quite be cured with conventional doses. Unfortunately, the high drug or radiation doses that might cure the cancers can irreversibly damage other tissues.

Bone marrow is the organ generally most sensitive to the toxic action of chemotherapy and radiation. There is a wide difference between the intensity of therapy that leads to lethal toxicity in bone marrow and the higher intensity that leads to lethal toxicity in other organs. So, if the bone marrow could in a sense be written off and replaced after therapy, higher doses of chemotherapy and radiation could be administered without irreversibly damaging other major organs. Assuming the cancer cells are sensitive to treatment, the increased intensity of therapy should lead to higher cure rates.

When a Transplant Is Appropriate Bone marrow transplantation is not a procedure that can be recommended lightly. It is a dangerous treatment and is not appropriate in every case. If a patient can be cured with therapy that does not require bone marrow transplantation, that is obviously the easiest approach. If a patient can be cured only with therapy so intense that other organs as well as the bone marrow are lethally damaged, there is no advantage to having a bone marrow transplant, for survival is unlikely anyway because of the organ damage.

But bone marrow transplantation can be uniquely curative for a patient whose cancer could be cured with high-dose therapy that irreversibly damages bone marrow but does not fatally damage any other organ. Some patients who can almost but not quite be cured with standard therapies could cross the "cure threshold" with increased amounts of therapy. With certain malignancies sensitive to chemotherapy and radiation, it is clear that this "window of opportunity" does exist.

TYPES OF TRANSPLANTS

Transplanting any organ—a heart, a kidney, a lung or bone marrow—from one person to another is a complicated procedure. The immune system is designed to destroy foreign tissues, and "graft rejection" is always a possibility. The risk of rejection can be reduced by matching as much as possible the tissues of the donor and the tissues of the person receiving the transplant.

Depending on the availability of appropriate donors, there are three types of bone marrow transplantation that can be attempted.

Allogeneic This type involves the transfer of marrow from one individual to a completely different individual. The marrow donor is selected through a process known as HLA typing.

Matched vs Unmatched Each individual has genes on one chromosome that code for proteins that appear on cell surfaces and are involved in cell self-recognition. These bits of information, or antigens, can be identified in the laboratory. It is also becoming possible to directly compare the genes themselves. This makes it possible to tell whether bone marrow from two individuals would be "matched" or "unmatched."

Usually allogeneic transplants are between brothers and sisters. This can be done when all the known antigens are matched or if there is a mismatch at only one site. The treatment will be equally successful in either case. But, in general, the better the match, the better the outcome.

Related vs Unrelated Allogeneic transplantation between unrelated people can be done. But given the extraordinary complexity and diversity of HLA antigens—there are more than a billion possible combinations—finding matched but unrelated individuals is very difficult.

The National Marrow Donor Bank now operates in the United States to try to find unrelated donors. This registry has made it possible to identify donors for most patients with common HLA antigens. Yet it is still hard to find donors for patients with uncommon antigens. Adding to the problem is the uneven distribution of HLA antigens among people with different genetic backgrounds. Because most of the volunteer donors so far are of European ancestry, it is especially hard to find donors for patients with African, Asian or other ancestry. (If you are interested in participating in the National Bone Marrow Donor Program, contact your local Red Cross Blood Center for information about how to volunteer.)

Syngeneic The best donor for any bone marrow transplant is an identical twin. Since identical twins share all the same genes they have exactly the same HLA antigens, so there is no risk of rejection. This is called a syngeneic transplant and, of course, is uncommon.

Autologous A somewhat similar situation arises if someone receives his or her own bone marrow after high-dose chemotherapy and/or radiotherapy. This can be done by removing marrow before therapy and keeping it in cold storage (cryopreserving) until treatment is complete. This procedure—called an autotransplant or autologous bone marrow transplantation—should avoid the problems associated with introducing cells with different HLA types. There should be no risk of rejection. But it adds the risk of possibly reinfusing cancer cells that were inadvertently stored along with the marrow.

There are small numbers of cells circulating in the blood that are capable of replenishing the bone marrow just like cells from the bone marrow itself. A transplant using these cells is often called an autologous peripheral stem cell transplant.

HOW BONE MARROW IS OBTAINED

In newborn children, essentially all bones have active marrow. In adults, active marrow is found mainly in the center of the pelvic bones, ribs, spine and collarbones. When an appropriate donor is identified, active marrow usually is removed from these bones with needles and a syringe. In some circumstances, it is possible to remove stem cells from blood.

Needle Aspiration Most bone marrow transplants involve extracting bone marrow from the bones of the pelvis by repeated needle punctures. The donor is usually under anesthetic during this process, which is a good thing, for it takes 150 or 200 needle punctures to remove enough marrow for a transplant—about 500 to 1,000 cc (one or two pints).

How the bone marrow is handled after it is removed depends upon the type of transplant to be done.
♦ If the transplant is allogeneic and the

donor and the recipient have the same ABO red blood cell type, the marrow is immediately given intravenously.
♦ If the red blood cells of the donor and recipient are incompatible, the red cells can be separated and discarded.
♦ If an autotransplant is planned, the cells have to be stored. This requires mixing them with a substance to prevent ice from forming and then freezing the cells in liquid nitrogen. The cells are sometimes also treated with chemicals or antibodies—in a process called marrow purging—to try to remove potentially contaminating cancer cells. It is not yet known how effective this is.

Getting Cells from the Blood If you are going to have an autologous transplant, immature blood cells can be obtained from your blood by repeated separating (apheresis) procedures. This involves drawing blood into an apparatus that works like a cream separator. The same type of cells obtained by needle aspiration are collected and the remainder returned to you. The procedure has to be repeated several times to get enough cells for transplantation. Each procedure usually lasts two to four hours. The number of immature cells in the blood might also be increased by the administration of various chemicals, allowing more rapid collection.

COMPLICATIONS AND RISKS

The transplant procedure is fraught with risk. Anyone undertaking this risky venture usually does so because the alternatives are so much worse. In general, anyone who undergoes a bone marrow transplantation is someone who will certainly die soon without one.

The specific risks are related to the phase of the procedure and can be divided into effects that are delayed or immediate.

Delayed Effects Long-term toxic effects of high-dose therapy can include cataracts in people receiving total body radiotherapy. Exposure to irradiation also increases the chance of developing other cancers. Delayed effects can also include sterility, although people who've been extensively treated for their cancer before a transplant are often already sterile. But there have been cases where women who have had a bone marrow transplant have conceived and borne healthy children.

Immediate Risks Much more threatening are the risks during and soon after the transplant procedure. The high-dose therapy itself, the damage to the immune system and the reaction of the immune system to the transplanted marrow can all cause dangerous complications.

♦ *Toxic reactions from drugs and irradiation* High-dose therapy occasionally has an acute toxic effect on the heart that can be lethal, although this is quite rare.

♦ *Infections* After the transplant, there will be a period of two to six weeks during which the new bone marrow cannot manufacture red cells, white cells or platelets. Though it is fairly easy to transfuse red cells and platelets, it is nearly impossible to transfuse white cells. Going without them for any time is dangerous because the risk of infection is high when blood counts are very low. So anyone getting a transplant will usually be given liberal amounts of antibiotics. Sometimes these are given before any signs of infection appear and are usually not discontinued until the blood counts have returned to a more normal level. They are always given at the first sign of a fever. Most of the time infections can be controlled until normal white cells return. But certain infections—such as fungal infections—can still prove fatal.

It is now possible to reduce the period of low white blood cell counts by using agents called hematopoietic growth factors (such as G-CSF or GM-CSF). These normally occurring products can be isolated and administered in doses that accelerate the return of white blood cells after a transplant. These agents shorten the period of hospitalization and reduce the cost of the procedure.

♦ *Bleeding* Platelets can usually be transfused easily, but for a few patients it is difficult to transfuse enough of them. For these patients, serious bleeding is a possibility.

♦ *Graft rejection* This is a major risk, particularly for people having an allogeneic bone marrow transplantation for aplastic anemia. The risk seems greater for those who have unrelated or less well matched allogeneic transplants. What usually happens is that the marrow function starts to come back, but then it disappears. This is a serious complication, but it can sometimes be overcome by a second transplant.

♦ *Pneumonia* The lung seems to be the organ most sensitive to the adverse effects of transplantation. It has been suggested that the lung is to bone marrow transplantation what the quarterback's knee is to the football game. A lot can go wrong. The lung can be injured because of infection, because of the toxic effect of high-dose chemotherapy and radiation or because of some unknown cause.

When severe pneumonia develops after a bone marrow transplant, death often—but not always—results. The most common pneumonia in these cases is caused by cytomegalovirus, a particularly severe pneumonia that can develop several months after the transplant. If it does develop, it is often in association with another serious complication, graft-versus-host disease.

♦ *Graft-versus-host disease* After an allogeneic bone marrow transplant, the immunologically active cells in the new marrow can recognize the "host" organism—the patient receiving the transplant—as foreign and go on the attack. The most commonly damaged organs are the skin, liver and intestines.

Medicines can be given after the transplant to reduce the possibility of graft-versus-host disease. The marrow can also be treated outside the body to remove the cells that cause graft-versus-host disease (T cell depletion). If the condition nevertheless develops, it can occur soon after the return of white cells (acute graft-versus-host disease) or much later (chronic graft-versus-host disease).

The two types are similar in some ways, though each has distinctive features. The acute form often doesn't last long but can be quite severe. If it is severe, the prognosis for survival is very poor. Chronic graft-versus-host disease almost always requires therapy, and most patients recover. One positive note is that when patients develop chronic graft-versus-host disease after an allogeneic transplant for leukemia, they are less likely to have recurrent leukemia.

CHOOSING A TRANSPLANT CENTER

If you are told that you might be referred for a bone marrow transplant, it is usually at a time when things aren't going too well. If there were a simpler way to cure your cancer, there would certainly be no call for bone marrow transplantation.

Having the procedure will sometimes involve traveling a considerable distance to a marrow transplant center. Which center to choose is often a difficult decision, with such factors as convenience, the center's experience with the disease and insurance issues all affecting the decision.

♦ *Experience* When facing a treatment as dangerous as bone marrow transplantation, most people want to be sure they are treated at a highly experienced center so the risk can be minimized. With certain cancers, it might be appropriate to choose a transplant center that has a special interest and extensive experience with your particular type of tumor.

You and your doctor may want to consult the American Society of Clinical Oncology and the American Society of Hematology, which have made joint recommendations for the *minimal* criteria for a center to perform the procedure.

♦ *Costs* Bone marrow transplantation is expensive and, in the United States, all transplant centers, before they will allow admission, will want some guarantee that the cost of the treatment will be reimbursed. Most health insurance companies in the United States now reimburse the cost for transplantation for leukemia and lymphoma, but how willing they are to reimburse for other diseases varies widely. It's unfortunate, but some patients will be denied this treatment because their insurance company will refuse to pay for it.

Securing a Bed If you are referred to a particular transplant center, you will usually have to go to the facility for a "transplant interview." The center has to decide whether you are a good candidate for the treatment. You have to decide whether you feel comfortable undergoing treatment at that center.

Once this decision has been jointly made, there will be other decisions such as whether more "traditional" therapy might be done to improve the chance for success. An allogeneic donor may have to be found or stem cells will have to be taken and stored for an autotransplant. Then it will be necessary to secure a bed in the transplant unit. Keep in mind that some centers have long waiting lists. Once a bed has been secured, you enter the hospital and begin therapy.

A SUMMARY OF THE STEPS TO A SUCCESSFUL TRANSPLANT

For a successful bone marrow transplant to be performed, your medical team will have to complete a number of steps in sequence. Each step involves critical decisions and potential risks.

1. Determine that the cancer is sensitive to high-dose therapy and cannot be cured with simpler treatment.
For both doctor and patient this is the

hardest part of the procedure. The candidate for a transplant has to have a disease serious enough that a treatment as risky as bone marrow transplantation is a reasonable option.

What makes the decision particularly difficult is that transplants are much more useful when patients are referred for treatment early in the course of their disease. Then they are more likely to be healthy. There is less cancer and it hasn't become highly resistant to therapy after repeated treatments. But transplant-related deaths are least acceptable in these early stages. The easiest course would be to refer a patient for transplantation when he or she is almost dead from cancer and all other therapies have failed. Unfortunately, at that point we know bone marrow transplantation is not likely to be beneficial.

The best approach, then, is to identify those who might benefit from the procedure and refer them for the treatment as soon as it seems clear that they cannot be cured with a simpler therapy.

2. Identify a source of marrow stem cells.
Once the decision to have a transplant is made, the possibility of your being able to use your own marrow cells or blood stem cells has to be evaluated. If your bone marrow is extensively involved by tumor, an allogeneic or syngeneic transplant or peripheral stem cell transplant will be the only choices. A bone marrow donor will have to be found—an HLA-matched brother or sister or a partially matched relative for an allogeneic transplant, a matched but unrelated donor for an allogeneic transplant or an identical twin for a syngeneic transplant—or it must be confirmed that there are no tumor cells circulating in your blood.

Allogeneic transplantation is more effective in younger people. The incidence of graft-versus-host disease rises rapidly in those over 30, occurring most often in people older than 40 to 55.

3. Administer high-dose chemotherapy—with or without radiotherapy—to kill the cancer and, in an allogeneic transplant, destroy your own immune system.
The purpose of the high-dose therapy is to destroy the cancer, suppress the immune system if necessary and empty the marrow to provide space for the new bone marrow cells to grow. If an allogeneic transplant is being performed, your own immune system must be destroyed. If it isn't, your immune cells will reject the donor's bone marrow cells and leave you without a functioning bone marrow.

4. Infuse the marrow stem cells intravenously.
In a typical bone marrow transplant unit, the day on which the marrow is given is referred to as Day 0. The other days you spend in the hospital are numbered as either a plus or minus, counting from the day the marrow is infused.

5. Manage the complications until the marrow produces enough normal blood cells and, in an allogeneic transplant, until graft-versus-host disease is controlled.
While the high-dose therapy is often uncomfortable, the period after the marrow infusion is the most dangerous. This is when the bone marrow cells begin to proliferate, ideally to the point where the marrow will produce enough red cells, white cells and platelets. This is when you run the risk of infections and bleeding problems. Most patients who don't survive long after a bone marrow transplant die from infections or the effects of graft-versus-host disease after the new marrow starts to grow.

Until you recover adequate white blood cell and platelet counts, you will be kept under close medical observation, usually in a special hospital room. After the marrow starts to grow, you will stay under close medical supervision until it is clear that the new marrow is functioning properly, that there has been no serious graft-versus-host disease and that your cancer has been controlled.

EFFECTIVENESS WITH DIFFERENT CANCERS

The table below summarizes the results of allogeneic and autologous bone marrow transplantation as a treatment for a variety of cancers. These results are only summaries and certainly vary with specific clinical situations.

It is also important to recognize that bone marrow transplantation as a treatment for cancer is a fast-changing field. New high-dose therapies or improved transplant techniques might change the results with a particular disease in a very short time.

Leukemias The first common cancer to be treated with bone marrow transplantation was acute leukemia. Even patients with "end stage leukemia" could sometimes be cured when they had allogeneic bone marrow transplantation, although there were better results when it was used early in the treatment of the disease.

Acute Leukemia The results for allogeneic transplantation in acute leukemia seem to depend very much on age. Patients who have a transplant as part of their initial therapy have a cure rate of more than 50 percent if they're under 20. But as age increases, the cure rate decreases. Results in patients over 40 are much poorer, although successful transplants can still be performed. But the fact that regular-dose chemotherapy also has better results in younger patients—and can sometimes cure them—makes the use of marrow transplantation in the initial control of the disease (first remission) very controversial.

In patients who are initially treated with other therapies for acute leukemia and then relapse, bone marrow transplantation is usually the treatment with the best chance for cure. Though the cure rate is less than 50 percent, it has become the generally accepted form of therapy.

The transplantation can be either allogeneic or autologous in acute leukemia. But if autologous transplantation is the choice, there has to be a source of uncontaminated bone marrow cells for reinfusion after high-dose therapy. This is usually accomplished by trying to eliminate—purging—contaminating leukemia cells from bone marrow collected during a period of remission.

CURE RATES WITH BONE MARROW TRANSPLANTATION

Type	Late in the Disease	Early in the Disease
Leukemias ◆Acute Lymphoblastic and Acute Myeloblastic	10 percent	50 percent
◆Chronic Granulocytic	10 percent	50 percent
Lymphomas ◆Hodgkin's Disease	10 percent	40–60 percent
◆Large Cell Non-Hodgkin's	10 percent	30–60 percent
◆Low-Grade Lymphoma	uncertain	uncertain
Neuroblastoma	less than 10 percent	30 percent
Breast Cancer	occasional prolonged remissions	studies too early to determine cure rate

Chronic Leukemias Bone marrow transplantation has only recently been used in cases of chronic granulocytic leukemia, a disease that occurs in young adults and is always fatal with standard therapy. During the late 1970s and 1980s, quite a few patients with this cancer underwent allogeneic bone marrow transplantation and a promising number of them were cured. Allogeneic transplantation has now become the treatment of choice for patients of an appropriate age with chronic granulocytic leukemia and who have an HLA-matched brother or sister. Cure rates of over 50 percent have been reported.

Non-Hodgkin's Lymphomas and Hodgkin's Disease Lymphomas are among the tumors most responsive to chemotherapy and radiation. Hodgkin's disease was the first commonly occurring solid tumor shown to be curable with combination chemotherapy, and all types of lymphomas can be cured with radiation when they haven't spread. So it is not surprising that these tumors are among those most likely to respond to very high-dose therapy accompanied by a bone marrow transplant.

Aggressive Non-Hodgkin's Lymphomas
These can be cured between one-third and one-half of the time with primary therapy. But if there is a relapse after initial therapy, bone marrow transplantation can cure a significant percentage of patients.
♦ It apparently can cure about a third of patients who are treated early after relapse when their disease is still sensitive to chemotherapy at lower doses (they have at least a partial response to chemotherapy at lower doses but cannot be cured by it).
♦ It can cure 10 to 15 percent of patients who have relapsed after primary chemotherapy but whose tumors are no longer sensitive to lower-dose chemotherapy or whose tumors have never responded to chemotherapy.

There is now considerable enthusiasm for testing the use of bone marrow transplantation even earlier in the course of aggressive lymphomas, perhaps incorporating it into the initial therapy for patients who aren't likely to be cured with standard treatments. As we become better at identifying patients with a poor outlook with primary therapy, this might become an important use of bone marrow transplantation.

Low-grade Non-Hodgkin's Lymphomas
These malignancies are rarely cured with standard therapies, although they are associated with a long average survival. But an average survival of even 10 years is not good enough for people who are 30 or 40 years old at the time of diagnosis. For this reason, several centers have recently begun to treat low-grade lymphoma patients with high-dose therapy and bone marrow transplantation early in the course of their disease. The results so far show that these patients tolerate the transplant process well and a large proportion of them stay in remission for extended periods. It is still too early to know if this treatment can actually cure the disease.

Hodgkin's Disease Patients with this cancer do so well with standard treatment approaches that physicians in the past have been reluctant to refer them for transplantation early enough in their disease for a transplant to be beneficial. But patients who relapse after high-quality combination chemotherapy have a poor outlook with more standard therapy. And when these patients are referred for high-dose therapy and bone marrow transplantation soon after their relapse, 50 percent or more seem to be long-term, disease-free survivors—in other words, probably cured. The cure rate is much less (10 to 20 percent) when they have the transplant after failing many chemotherapy regimens.

Other Blood Cancers A number of other hematologic malignancies have occasionally been treated with bone marrow transplantation, and some patients with hairy cell leukemia and chronic lymphocytic leukemia have been cured.

More recently, bone marrow transplantation has been used to treat patients with multiple myeloma. Although many patients with this disease are past the age at which bone marrow transplantation is usually attempted, there are still many who might benefit from the treatment. The results aren't conclusive, but it appears that both allogeneic and autologous bone marrow transplantation can bring about complete remissions in some multiple myeloma patients.

Solid Tumors in Adults Bone marrow transplantation has been used in a wide variety of so-called solid tumors—carcinomas and sarcomas—in adults. It can cure some men with advanced testicular cancer, for example, a predictable result given the extraordinary responsiveness of testicular cancer to chemotherapy. A small number of patients with soft tissue sarcomas have also had long remissions after high-dose therapy and a bone marrow transplant.

Unfortunately, many common solid tumors such as lung cancers and gastrointestinal cancers aren't sensitive enough to high-dose chemotherapy and radiation to make the bone marrow procedure beneficial.

One of the most common carcinomas in the United States—breast cancer—*is* reasonably sensitive to chemotherapy and radiotherapy. Recent clinical trials with high-dose therapy and autologous bone marrow transplantation suggest that increased doses of drugs active against breast cancer can dramatically increase the response rate. Some women have had complete remissions and some of these remissions have lasted several years. It will be a while before long-term results on large numbers of patients are available. Yet investigators are encouraged that bone marrow transplantation might be able to cure some breast cancer patients who have a poor prognosis with standard therapy.

Solid Tumors in Children Most pediatric solid tumors are sensitive to chemotherapy and can sometimes be cured by chemotherapy without bone marrow transplantation. But, as might be expected, high-dose therapy and autologous or allogeneic transplantation can cure some children who can't be cured with standard therapy.

Neuroblastoma is the pediatric cancer in which the procedure has been most carefully studied. It appears that some children can have long-lasting remissions—in other words, can probably be cured—with high-dose therapy and bone marrow transplantation. But, as with many other diseases, the optimal timing and treatment procedures haven't been identified yet.

Another common group of solid tumors in children—brain tumors—are also undergoing clinical trials with bone marrow transplantation. How useful the technique is in these cases will have to await further studies.

THE FUTURE OF TRANSPLANTATION

Bone marrow transplantation is a rapidly evolving field that is likely to become more important in cancer treatment. The advances over the past 20 years have been remarkable.

The first attempt at allogeneic bone marrow transplantation was reported in the 1930s. It didn't work because the scientific advances that led to HLA typing had not yet been made. Autologous bone marrow transplantation was first tested in the 1950s. Once again, the attempt failed, this time because the techniques for cryopreservation of bone marrow cells had not been perfected.

The development of HLA typing in the 1960s made allogeneic transplantation a reasonable possibility, and the first successful transplants were performed at the end of that decade. Through the 1970s, allogeneic bone marrow transplantation gradually became an accepted form of therapy. The successful cryopreservation of bone marrow cells was perfected in the late 1970s, making autologous bone marrow transplantation a widely available therapy in the 1980s.

Now the future for the use of bone marrow transplantation in cancer treatment is optimistic. It is likely to be used for some time to treat leukemia and lymphoma. It also appears that more patients with carcinomas or sarcomas—solid tumors—will be identified who can benefit from, and possibly be cured by, the procedure. The increased use of hematopoietic growth factors to accelerate marrow regrowth after transplantation will likely make the technique safer and more widely available.

Also very exciting is that the ability to use peripheral blood stem cells has increased the number of patients who might benefit from autologous transplants, while the National Marrow Donor Program for identifying unrelated donors has greatly increased the number of patients who might benefit from allogeneic transplants.

13
QUESTIONABLE AND UNPROVEN CANCER THERAPIES

Barrie R. Cassileth, PhD

◇

Surgery, radiation therapy and chemotherapy have been "accepted" cancer treatments for a long time. They are accepted because they were developed after years of study with animals and then humans. The studies were based on logical, scientific principles, and the treatments were then shown to be effective against the growth of tumors in thousands of people.

These conventional cancer treatments are responsible for dramatic improvements in survival over the past few decades. Where few people used to survive for long after a cancer diagnosis, about half of all diagnosed patients are now cured.

Every few years or so, the media present a startling report on some new way to treat cancer. The treatment is typically described as resulting in "miraculous cures" or as being able to prolong lives in some extraordinary fashion. The exact formula or chemical content is usually unknown or is kept secret by the practitioner promoting this new method. Knowledge of the treatment often spreads only by word of mouth or by being publicized in certain types of popular magazines and tabloid papers.

These "cures" are not reported in the scientific literature, however, nor are they backed by the extensive data and research information that accompany reports of new medical tests and therapies. There are two reasons why reports on these cures never show up in scientific journals:

♦ The most common reason is that the practitioners promoting the unorthodox method did not actually study it and so never prepared any report to send to scientific publications. Typically, these practitioners say they are too busy treating patients to spend time on evaluation or research, even though it is only through rigorous evaluation and research that the worth of a treatment can be known.

♦ The other reason is that a report may have been sent to a journal's editorial board, but that its publication in a medical journal was considered not warranted because the quality of its data was so poor or because it lacked accurate information.

Most unproven methods have never been studied at all. The only "proof" their developers usually offer is the display of people who—the practitioners say—have been cured by their therapy. The "beneficiaries" of the miracle treatment may be displayed live during some publicity event. Or they may testify to the worth of the treatment in writing, often in a brochure. Of course, it is not possible to know from these kinds of displays whether people were cured by the unproven method, whether they received conventional treatment before or at the same time as receiving the unproven treatment or if they were, in fact, ever diagnosed as having cancer at all.

Stories told by or about a patient are called anecdotal reports, and they can sound very impressive and persuasive. Even assuming they are true, however, no faith can be placed in anecdotal reports about one or even a few patients. Careful study of many clinically similar patients is required before a legitimate conclusion can be drawn about any new therapy.

The Appeal of New Methods To people with cancer and their families, unproven treatments can look very appealing, especially when no conventional treatment is left to be tried. They may be drawn to some unorthodox remedy even if there is no solid evidence that a product or procedure is beneficial. Patients and families may be ready to try anything, feeling that they have nothing to lose.

But there *is* something to lose. The financial losses can be considerable for anyone who pursues a useless treatment, usually at an expensive private clinic. For those who are terminally ill and beyond the help of conventional treatment, false hope can also rob them of the good use of what time they have left. When patients can still benefit from conventional treatment and there is a possibility of a long remission or even cure, what can be lost is a life.

It is understandable that you or your family may be attracted to some unproven therapy. The best physical and financial protection, however, is to become an educated health care consumer. Develop a basic understanding of medical procedures and services, including unproven methods.

THE ROOTS OF UNPROVEN METHODS

Unproven remedies for cancer and other serious illnesses have been with us for centuries. They have taken many forms, including:
♦ liquefied grasses to drink
♦ small wooden objects with magical properties to hold in the hand
♦ pastes to rub on the skin
♦ radio waves and magnetic forces to direct at various parts of the body
♦ potions made from many different natural and unnatural items to take

And many others. None has survived very long. These remedies usually enjoyed a brief popularity, then faded from view. But they were soon replaced by some other questionable cure. Understanding the roots and sources for these questionable remedies will help you understand the role questionable remedies play today.

Parallel Medicine in the Nineteenth Century Unproven cancer treatments have typically mimicked or paralleled developments in scientific medicine. The promotion of unproven methods in the nineteenth century arose in response to the development of modern clinical methods and the emphasis on local pathology. In the early 1800s, medical efforts began to be devoted to finding and treating a specific source or cause of illness. At the same time, advocates of questionable remedies began working to make "every man his own doctor" and to develop a "holistic" self-care alternative to a medical system oriented toward disease.
♦ In the early 1880s, the hot/cold theory of diseases—Thomsonianism—gained a wide following. This theory promoted hot baths and emetics (to induce vomiting) while opposing "mineral" drugs and the "tyranny of doctors."
♦ Around 1850, homeopathy became popular. This was based on its Law of Similia, which stated that disease results from suppressed itch ("psora"). Over 3,000 drugs, each a highly distilled organic or inorganic substance, were used for cures.
♦ Naturopathy, a belief system that gained popularity about 1890, was another alternative. In opposition to scientific medicine, it held that disease results not from external bacteria but from violation of the "natural laws" of living. Its cures involved diets, massages and irrigation of the colon.

Twentieth Century Alternatives After these approaches were tried and failed to demonstrate any benefit, there was a shift in the early 1900s to quasi-medicines in pill or liquid form. All kinds of these nostrums appeared, including Radol and Chamlee's Cancer-Specific Purifies-the-Blood Cure.

During the 1920s, in the exciting early days of the electronic age of radio, telephone and other miracles produced by energy, "energy" cancer cures appeared. "Cosmic energy treatment" and "light therapy" became the rage.

Koch's glyoxilide (distilled water) cure of the 1940s was followed in the 1950s by the Hoxsey Treatment in pill and extract form. Injectable krebiozen—which turned out to be essentially mineral oil—was popular in the 1960s and was followed in the 1970s by Laetrile, a substance prepared from apricot pits and often referred to as vitamin B_{17} even though it is not a vitamin. Like all the others, Laetrile was shown upon investigation to have no effect against cancer.

The long history of unproven methods and the fact that few survived for more than a few months or years indicate their lack of usefulness. Still, there is a natural human tendency to respond to claims for new cures, especially cures promoted as more effective or less difficult than existing scientific treatments. This is a major reason that unproven therapies persist.

Today, the concerns of the medical counterculture mirror the nineteenth-century perspective. Just as the "natural" whole-body treatments arose then in response to modern clinical methods, so the currently popular unproven methods stem partly from a reaction to today's technologic, heroic medicine. The very specialization and sophistication that offer clinically optimal care also create dissatisfaction and unease among some patients. Many people are uncomfortable seeing a series of specialists rather than being cared for by a single physician. Many find the marvels of current diagnostic and treatment equipment too technical, cold and mechanical.

It is not surprising that contemporary unproven treatments represent a throwback to nineteenth-century beliefs in disease as a systemic, total-body phenomenon, in demystification and simplification of illness, in self-care and in "natural" cures. Now, as 150 years ago, the medical counterculture is firmly rooted in a political anti-authority context. Now, as then, ambivalence or hostility toward the medical profession is clearly evident.

The cycle of popular unproven approaches has gone full-circle—from the natural, holistic alternatives of the 1800s, through the quasi-medicines of the early and mid-twentieth century, back to the natural, holistic, dietary regimens of today.

TODAY'S POPULAR ALTERNATIVES

The questionable cancer remedies now getting the most attention range from those that are based on misinterpretations of scientific data to those that are downright fraudulent. All are good examples of why cancer patients and their families must become *educated* health care consumers. The principles or concepts on which unproven methods are based must be reviewed critically so that their logic and accuracy can be evaluated.

Adjunctive Therapies Promoted as Cures

The standard treatments—surgery, chemotherapy, radiation therapy and biological therapy—are all designed to remove or kill tumor cells. But cancer specialists and other doctors may also recommend other types of treatment that are not designed to kill tumor cells. Instead, these treatments aim to bring about some overall improvement in general health and well-being. They are often called complementary or adjunctive treatments because they are used along with the standard therapies.

Nutritional therapy, relaxation therapy, a focus on emotional well-being, the provision of effective support systems, yoga and so on all fit into this category. When used in conjunction with standard therapies, these are legitimate therapeutic approaches. They are helpful in recovery or rehabilitation.

But sometimes these adjunctive or complementary therapies are advertised as having the power to cure cancer on their own. Nutritional programs are promoted as dietary "cures." Relaxation therapy or imagery are promoted as essential to developing the right attitude that will make cancer go away.

Many people are drawn to these "cures" because they are claimed to be free of the sometimes unpleasant side effects of conventional treatments. But this is a very destructive and unfortunate misuse of otherwise helpful activities. When cancer patients look on these complementary therapies as cures, they may decide—or even be encouraged—to stop their conventional treatments. Some may assume that they no longer have to see their oncologist or receive chemotherapy. If that happens, they may lose their chance for remission or cure.

Immune-Enhancing Therapies After a long period of intense and well-publicized scientific study of the immune system, a number of unorthodox practitioners developed therapies aimed at improving cancer patients' immune systems. Several unorthodox approaches work toward this goal. One aims to stimulate immune function through injected vaccines. Another aims to enhance the immune system through mental imagery and attitude.

These therapies sound legitimate because they address an issue—the immune system—that is a subject of legitimate scientific investigation. Because the terminology sounds scientific and the rationale appears to be a great deal more accurate than it really is, it is important to understand some background information before evaluating these therapies.

There is some scientific experimental evidence showing that the immune system plays a role in the body's defenses against cancer. There is very little evidence indicating that the system is helpful against metastatic disease once cancer has developed. But there is no scientific proof that mental imagery or adopting a new emotional attitude influences the immune system in a way that affects the growth of tumors.

Many immune-stimulating agents have been studied in clinical trials. These include the tuberculosis vaccine, BCG, as well as a variety of chemicals that have been shown to stimulate immunity in animals. One immune stimulant—Levamisole—was approved by the National Cancer Institute in late 1989 for use in combination with standard chemotherapy for one stage of colon cancer because this combination produced better results than chemotherapy alone. BCG has also been approved for the treatment of early bladder cancer. Yet very few immune-enhancing substances are known to improve disease in humans. Ongoing studies with other cancers have not yet shown much benefit from immune-enhancing techniques.

Metabolic Treatments These are offered by many practitioners and clinics in the United States and in Tijuana, Mexico. Metabolic procedures vary according to the practitioner, but they generally include:

♦ "detoxification," typically through cleansing of the colon
♦ special diets
♦ vitamins
♦ minerals
♦ enzymes

Metabolic treatments sound appealing. They emphasize "natural" therapy with treatment directed at "cellular detoxification and restoration." But these treatments are neither natural nor safe. Many people have been harmed by them. Like most unproven treatments, metabolic therapy is based on an invented principle: that toxins and waste materials in the body interfere with metabolism and healing. Cancer and other chronic illnesses are seen as the result of degeneration of the liver and pancreas or of the degeneration of the immune and "oxygenation" systems.

The educated consumer will know that there is no such thing as an oxygenation system. Nor is there any such thing as cellular detoxification and restoration.

Special Diets The "miracle diet" that cures cancer is a staple of the tabloid press. You can read about these diets at the checkout counter of any supermarket, but not in many other places.

Such diets are a good example of the faulty logic that often accompanies a misunderstanding of scientific information. People read or hear that low-fat diets may help prevent some cancers. Eating a low-fat, high-fiber diet, for example, can lower the risk of developing some kinds of cancer. But some people then make an illogical leap from prevention to cure and assume that these same dietary measures can cure a cancer once it has started to grow.

Following a special diet or eating certain foods will not make cancer go away. Yet many dietary "cures" are promoted in North America today and they are often accepted at face value. Little attention is paid to how they may rob the body of necessary nutrients or that they may be based on false, illogical concepts. The popular macrobiotic diet, for example, is based on a fanciful and completely faulty concept of how the human body works.

The special diets are usually "practitioner-specific." This means that each promoter offers a different approach to cancer therapy through a different type of diet. Oriental herbal remedies recently joined various diets as popular cancer treatments or cures.

None is known to be helpful. Many result in nutritional deficiencies, a situation cancer patients should avoid at all costs. Moderation is still the best approach to diet for all medical problems. Taking excessive amounts of vitamins, minerals or "health food" substitutes may do more harm than good.

The Newest Fads Consistent with the shifts and trends that characterize unconventional cancer medicine, several products and approaches recently have attained special prominence. Among the most popular are two very different methods: efforts to harness mind-body power, and the use of shark cartilage as a cancer cure.

Advocates of the first method claim that happiness, positive attitudes, a strong will, meditation, mental imagery and other psychological or mental efforts can cause cancer to regress or disappear. These claims are groundless. Emotions do not influence cancer outcome (nor is there any evidence that they play a role in the development of cancer in the first place). Attitude, meditation and so on can enhance quality of life—an important goal in itself—but they do not cure cancer.

The shark cartilage cancer cure fad stems from a recent book with an untrue title, *Sharks Don't Get Cancer*. Powdered cartilage is sold in health food stores, thus avoiding the clinical proof of effectiveness and safety that proper research provides, and to get around the FDA review necessary before a product or treatment can be approved for use as medicine. There is no acceptable evidence to show that shark cartilage works.

HOW TO TELL WHEN A THERAPY IS QUESTIONABLE

To make educated decisions about a treatment, it is necessary to go beyond testimonials and promises. You have to understand what the unproven method is all about, the concepts on which it is based and what its track record is.

A legitimate treatment method meets the following standards. A dubious or questionable treatment does not meet any of them.

♦ The method was studied scientifically and shown to be more effective than no treatment at all.

♦ The benefits of the method clearly exceed any harm it might do.

♦ Studies of the method have been properly conducted. That is, an appropriate research design has been used, the studies have been subject to review by others knowledgeable in the field and a human studies committee has given the study its approval.

If you have any doubt about a therapy, examine it critically against these three standards. Check the brochure or any other available literature to see if the method was studied and found to be better than nothing. The brochure will certainly note the "benefits" of the method, but you will have to look for or ask about any problems.

The third point is the easiest to determine. Legitimate treatment methods are *always* evaluated with the participation of other scientists. They are *always* reviewed and approved by a human subjects committee in an established, reputable medical institution.

"Secret" cures or treatments that are said to work only in the hands of one practitioner are questionable by definition. New scientific therapies are always made available through meetings, talks and publications to the entire community of scientists and researchers. The worth of the treatment can be confirmed only when the results of research can be reproduced by others.

An in-depth, critical evaluation of an unproven program can tell you whether the "cured patients" offered as proof of its worth actually had a diagnosis of cancer confirmed by a tissue biopsy. It can tell you whether the "cured patients"

received conventional treatment along with the questionable therapy, even if all credit is given to the unproven method. It will indicate what the problems and toxicities associated with the unproven treatment might be.

Your oncologist can help supply this information and should be your major source for information and assistance. He or she best understands your illness and knows which treatments are useful for you. You can also contact your local offices of the American Cancer Society or the American Medical Association.

Other sources of information include:

National Council Against Health Fraud
PO Box 1276
Loma Linda, CA 92354

Consumer Reports Health Letter
PO Box 52145
Boulder, CO 80321-2148

In 1991, the Office of Alternative Medicine was established by the United States Congress. Part of the National Institutes of Health, the major goal of this new office is to evaluate the merits of complementary techniques and promising alternatives in effecting cure or alleviating the symptoms of illnesses, including cancer. A range of alternatives, including homeopathy, meditation and other mind-body techniques, and acupuncture, will be evaluated. Regardless of their outcome, such investigations will provide extremely important information.

That eventual information, your physician's advice and the resources noted above will help you and your family become educated health care consumers able to consider helpful adjunctive or complementary therapies and avoid treatments that have no benefit. You will certainly save financially. You will spare yourself much anguish. You may gain yourselves precious moments together. And, if there is still a chance for remission or cure, you may also prevent a tragedy of the highest order.

14
BLOOD TRANSFUSIONS AND CANCER TREATMENT

Herbert A. Perkins, MD

◇

Blood is a complex living tissue. It is made up of three kinds of cells that are manufactured in the blood cell "factory"—the marrow cavity of our bones. All these cells are suspended in a liquid called plasma, and each cell plays a critical role in keeping us alive.

♦ Red blood cells carry oxygen to our tissues.

♦ White blood cells—leukocytes—help us fight off infections.

♦ Platelets are necessary to form the blood clots that stop bleeding.

Blood transfusions play a crucial role in cancer treatment. The disease can reduce the marrow's ability to produce blood cells, sometimes so severely that the cells have to be replaced by transfusion. Some forms of cancer—leukemia and multiple myeloma—grow in the marrow cavity, leaving no space for the development of normal blood cells. These normal cells will then have to be provided by transfusion.

But most of the people with cancer who need blood transfusions need them because of the aggressive approaches used to treat the disease. If blood transfusions weren't available, most of the remarkably effective cancer treatments available today could never have been introduced—the chemotherapy used to kill cancer cells, for example, which may also kill developing blood cells in the marrow. Many cancers can also be cured or at least helped by surgery and that surgery may result in loss of blood by hemorrhage to the point where it has to be replaced. No other form of medical treatment can make such a difference between life and death as blood transfusions can.

WEIGHING THE RISKS

In the vast majority of instances, blood transfusions are very safe, and the benefit far outweighs the risks. However, as with other forms of treatment, transfusions can bring about complications. Most of these are not serious and are easily controlled. Rarely, however, serious and potentially fatal complications may occur.

Infection Unless you donate blood to yourself, there is always a very slight risk that you could be infected by some organism.

AIDS The risk foremost in everyone's mind lately is the possibility of being infected with the HIV virus that can lead to Acquired Immune Deficiency Syndrome (AIDS). But the risk of getting AIDS from a transfusion is now so low—one in 225,000, and possibly lower—that it should have almost no effect on the decision to have a transfusion that is medically indicated.

Hepatitis The number-one infectious risk associated with transfusion is, and always has been, the serious infection of the liver called hepatitis. The risk has been markedly reduced in the past 15 years, decreasing from one in ten in the 1970s to one in 6,000 in 1993.

Other Infections Blood banks test for syphilis and HTLV I and II (HTLV I is a virus that may occasionally cause leukemia). Other infections are rarely transmitted.

Reactions to Differences in Donor Blood
Unless you are transfused with your own blood or have an identical twin who donated blood for you to use, the blood you receive will contain many things that are foreign to you. This is true even when the blood is correctly cross-matched.

The donor's blood—the red and white blood cells, platelets and even plasma proteins—will all have antigens (proteins) your body will have never come in contact with before. What usually happens when you are exposed to foreign antigens is that your immune system reacts. After all, the system is designed to recognize and try to destroy anything foreign that gets into our bodies, especially invading germs such as bacteria or viruses. Fortunately, the immune system rarely recognizes most of the differences between a donor's blood and your own.

Differences in Red Blood Cells These are the most critical. While there are more than 400 recognized differences, only three are of practical importance. These have to do with certain antigens, namely the A, B and D antigens that determine your ABO and Rh blood types.

Antibodies are part of the immune response to foreign antigens. If you have type B blood, you have anti-A antibodies, so if you are transfused with Type A red cells, those cells will be destroyed. Not only will the transfusion not accomplish its purpose but you may experience chills, fever, aches and pains and in rare cases shock, bleeding, even death. Blood banks and hospital transfusion services do repeated tests and checks to be sure patients don't receive blood with the wrong ABO type.

Red blood cells are also either Rh positive or Rh negative, depending whether you have one of the Rh antigens called D.

The D antigen is easily recognized as foreign by an Rh-negative patient whose system then makes an antibody against it.

Blood banks always test red blood cells from donors and transfusion patients to see if they contain A, B and D. They also test the serum (a form of plasma) to see if it contains antibodies to these antigens. The hospital transfusion service also checks the serum of each patient who will be transfused to see if it contains antibodies to other red cell antigens. If it does, the blood bank must provide donor blood lacking these antigens. As a final check, the transfusion service does a cross-match, a test to see if the serum of the patient recognizes anything in the donor blood cells as foreign.

Differences in White Blood Cells The white cells have an entirely different set of foreign antigens than the red cells do. The most important are called HLA antigens. These are the same antigens that a laboratory looks for when tissue typing to select an organ donor for a transplant.

Antibodies to white blood cells develop fairly easily through transfusion or pregnancy. They rarely cause serious harm, but they do explain the chills and fevers experienced by about 3 percent of patients receiving transfusions. If you have such reactions to an uncomfortable degree, your doctor can prevent or minimize them in future transfusions by ordering red blood cells from which most of the white cells have been removed (leukocyte-poor red blood cells) or by transfusing blood through a filter that removes white cells.

Differences in Platelets Donor platelets have the same HLA antigens as the white blood cells, plus they have antigens unique to platelets. If you have to have repeated platelet transfusions, your immune system may form antibodies that will attack and destroy the donor platelets, making the platelet transfusions useless. These antibodies can also cause chills and fever when they react with donor platelets.

Differences in the Plasma Reactions to donor plasma in the form of hives happen in up to 5 percent of patients. Hives can sometimes be severe to the point of generalized swelling and, in rare cases, the reaction can result in a life-threatening obstruction to breathing. Allergic reactions to plasma can usually be simply treated or prevented with antihistamines. And if you do have a severe reaction, future transfusions can be given without causing a reaction by washing the blood cells with salt solution to remove the plasma.

WHAT GETS TRANS-FUSED AND WHEN

When someone donates blood, about a pint of blood is usually drawn into a plastic bag. The bag contains a solution that keeps the blood from clotting and helps preserve the red cells. Each bag, with its attached tubing and the needle that goes into the donor's arm, comes as a sterile unit in a sealed pouch and is used only once.

The blood is stored in a refrigerator under carefully controlled conditions until it's used. If it isn't used within five or six weeks, the blood has to be discarded because changes in the red blood cells during storage make it less effective and possibly dangerous, although in special circumstances, red blood cells can be frozen and stored for years. What part of this stored blood is transfused depends on your condition and your needs.

Whole Blood This is used only when a patient is hemorrhaging large amounts of blood in a short time. Almost always, the blood bank separates each unit of blood into red cells, platelets and plasma.

Red Cells Because of your cancer or your treatment, you may become anemic to the point where breathing becomes difficult,

your heart pounds or you become very weak. If that happens, red blood cells will be transfused. If your marrow is not doing its job, it may be necessary to transfuse red blood cells every three to four weeks. Red blood cells will also be transfused when there is a lot of bleeding, as there may be during surgery.

Platelets When your marrow can't produce enough platelets on its own, a platelet transfusion might be necessary to prevent bleeding. Moderate drops in the platelet count do not need treatment. But very low counts—less than 10,000 or 20,000 without bleeding, a little higher with—will require platelet transfusions, often every two to three days.

At least 70 percent of patients who get repeated platelet transfusions will make antibodies to foreign platelet antigens, making the transfusions less and less effective. Blood banks can solve this problem by providing platelets that have the correct HLA type and by doing many cross-matches with donor platelets.

The Apheresis Technique Modern cancer treatment has led to such a voracious need for platelets that the need cannot be met just by making a platelet component from each whole blood donation. So blood banks have turned to a procedure known as apheresis. In this process, a donor's blood is taken from a vein, passed through an apheresis (or separating) device and returned to the donor through another vein. The device skims off and saves the blood platelets while the red blood cells and plasma are returned. When patients no longer respond to the platelets of random donors, family members are often asked to donate platelets by apheresis, since they are much more likely than a random donor to have the same platelet antigens as the patient.

Plasma The plasma component of whole

blood is used in a variety of ways.

♦ It may be immediately frozen (fresh frozen plasma) and then used to transfuse missing plasma proteins into patients with unusual deficiencies of clotting factors.

♦ It can be processed into cryoprecipitate, a special product used to treat hemophilia.

♦ It can be made into albumin to treat shock, gamma globulin to prevent hepatitis, and clotting factors.

DONATING BLOOD TO YOURSELF

Since any blood bank component can transmit infections or cause reactions, the safest blood donor is yourself. Getting your own blood is called an autologous transfusion. It is not always possible for people with cancer to donate blood, since it is certainly not appropriate if you are likely to have cancer cells in your blood. But it is worth asking your surgeon whether any of the following approaches are possible or advisable.

Pre-Deposit Donation Many cancer patients can provide their own blood before surgery if time permits and a few basic conditions are met. In this "pre-deposit autologous donation," your blood is taken exactly as it is from a standard blood donor. The usual age limits for donors don't apply, but you can't be too anemic or have certain types of serious heart disease. It is usually possible to collect two, three or four units of blood in the five-to-six-week period that blood can be stored. Since you will be giving blood much more often than is permitted for the usual blood donor, your doctor will usually prescribe iron so that red cell production is not slowed down by iron deficiency.

Hemodilution This is another approach to autologous transfusion. Instead of blood being gradually donated before the operation, several pints are taken in the operating room just as surgery is about to begin. A saline (salt) solution is transfused at the same time so that your total blood volume doesn't change. Your blood is then transfused during the surgical procedure or after the operation as the salt solution escapes from your circulation.

Cell Salvage This approach is possible when fairly large amounts of blood escape into a body cavity during surgery. The blood can be removed, washed with a saline solution, and later returned to you. Cell salvage may not be possible, however, if there is a risk that cancer cells will be returned to your system.

BLOOD FROM OTHER DONORS

If you can't donate blood for your own use, you will have to rely on blood supplied by volunteer blood banks or on blood donated from a relative or friend.

Directed or Designated Donations Directed donors may be selected by a patient or a patient's family in the belief that their blood will be safer than that from the usual blood bank volunteer. Usually, this belief is not correct. Although positive tests for AIDS are rare among both directed and routine donors, directed donations have a *higher* frequency of positive hepatitis tests. In some areas, directed donors also have a higher frequency of positive AIDS tests.

Why Directed Donors Are Riskier There are logical reasons why directed donors are less safe on the average.

♦ People asked to donate for a relative or friend may, because of embarrassment or for reasons they wish to keep confidential, not want to confess that they are ineligible.

♦ Directed donors are usually first-time donors, while more than two-thirds of routine donors have given in the past, most on many occasions. With each donation there was a chance that the medical history or laboratory tests would uncover some reason for ineligibility or that an investigation of an infection in a transfused patient would identify the donor as a possible source.

Despite the arguments against the use of directed donors, most patients and families are convinced that *their* relatives and friends are safer than routine donors. For the peace of mind of the patients and families, most blood banks accept requests for directed donations. In some states they are required by law to do so.

Community Blood Bank Donors These donors are volunteers who have no reason to donate their blood other than the pleasure it gives them to help their fellow humans.

Each blood donor (and this applies to directed donors as well) must read an information sheet that details reasons why a person should *not* donate blood. If the donor concludes that he or she is eligible, a medical history is then obtained using a series of very detailed questions, a number of which are specific about sexual practices.

The donor is also given the opportunity to indicate confidentially that the blood he or she donates should not be transfused. This procedure takes care of situations in which the donor knows he or she is not eligible but does not wish this to become apparent to relatives, friends or co-workers. Finally, the blood donated is tested for

a whole series of infectious agents—AIDS, hepatitis B, hepatitis C, HTLV and syphilis, as well as CMV in special circumstances. The result is the safest blood supply by far that this country has ever known.

The Need for More Donors Eighty-five to 90 percent of transfusions use blood from volunteer donors in the community. The rest are autologous or directed. If blood isn't available when a patient needs it, that patient could die. Yet serious blood shortages, which require rationing of the available supply, are frequent in many communities.

There are many reasons for the shortage of blood donors. Most people who do not give blood fail to do so because they just ignore the need or assume someone else will do it. A quarter of the population has the completely mistaken notion that it is dangerous to donate blood, that one might become infected with AIDS. And a very large number of people are not eligible to be blood donors anymore, based on the strict criteria used and tests performed.

People with cancer cannot donate blood for others. Yet cancer patients should have an unusual awareness of the need for an adequate blood supply. Carry the message to your relatives and friends to become regular blood donors. Then, if you need a transfusion in an emergency, the blood will be there waiting for you.

15
THE ONCOLOGY NURSE

Josefa Azcueta, RN, OCN, and Deborah Hamolsky, RN, MS, OCN

Margaret was a 42-year-old mother of two. She discovered a lump in her breast a few months after she had learned Breast Self-Examination techniques from Nancy, a nurse at the local Breast Examination Training (BET) center. After mammography and fine needle aspiration of the lump, she saw her doctor, who confirmed the diagnosis of cancer. After a Tumor Board presentation, her oncologist reviewed and explained all the options to Margaret and her husband. The decision was made to go ahead with surgery, chemotherapy and radiation.

After her mastectomy, Margaret met nurses like Maria who changed her dressings, gave her medications and sat on the bed and held her hand when she cried in the middle of the night.

After Margaret was discharged, Louise and Joe came to her home for follow-up visits. And when chemotherapy was started in the oncologist's office, nurses like Judy, Irene and Nancy taught her about the effects of different chemotherapy drugs. They gave her both the chemotherapy injections and emotional support.

After four months of chemotherapy, Margaret started on radiation. Mary helped explain the treatments to her, drew blood for tests and was always ready with a much-needed hug.

Then, to help them both cope with cancer, Margaret and her husband attended weekly cancer support group meetings, led by Kate, at the local hospital. There they could share their feelings and fears with others who really knew what they were going through.

This story is just one illustration of how many different oncology nurses touch the lives of so many people with cancer.

From before the diagnosis, through the course of treatment and beyond to supportive care, you will continually meet these specially trained nurses. They will share their knowledge and expertise with you. They will help you with their support and understanding when you need it most.

PROFESSIONAL TRAINING

Many nursing studies have shown that people with cancer want and expect many things from nurses. Competency is the most important expectation. People care that the nurse can start the IV and give chemotherapy, change a dressing, insert a catheter and know how to respond to an emergency.

When you are getting treatment for your cancer, you obviously want to know without any doubt that you are in the hands of someone who is an expert, aware of the most up-to-date treatment methods.

Professional Organization In the United States, the national organization of oncology nurses is the Oncology Nursing Society (ONS). Founded in 1975, it is now a large national organization with many local chapters. ONS is dedicated to professional development, promotion of excellence in clinical practice, research, education and political influence. Many oncology nurses belong to local chapters and attend yearly meetings where they learn about medical or other advances that can improve the care they give you and your family. There is also an organization of cancer nurses who specialize in the care and treatment of children, the Association of Pediatric Oncology Nurses (APON).

Specialized Education Oncology nurses have special training in the care of cancer patients within the hospital, the doctor's office, at home or in special facilities such as radiation therapy units. Oncology nurses build on their basic medical knowledge with additional training in:

♦ Giving chemotherapy and managing side effects such as nausea, vomiting and hair loss.
♦ Controlling cancer pain.
♦ Managing cancer emergencies.
♦ Providing emotional support to patients and their loved ones.
♦ Postoperative care.
♦ Care and teaching of long-term intravenous (IV) devices such as Hickman catheters, Groshong catheters and ports.
♦ Participation in clinical research teams or independent nursing research.
♦ Managing new technology and treatments—such as bone marrow transplants or biological therapies—as they evolve.

Nurses can also develop their knowledge in several subspecialties such as radiation oncology, surgical oncology, medical oncology, palliative (comfort) care, cancer prevention and early detection, in-patient nursing, hospice, home care, patient education, research, and ambulatory and office nursing. Some nurses, particularly in large regional cancer centers, may develop an even more specific area of interest such as breast cancer, immunotherapy or pain control.

Radiation Therapy As one example of further education, nurses who specialize in radiation oncology work primarily in radiation therapy departments, either in hospitals or with independent practices. Their specialized knowledge of radiation treatment for cancer includes

♦ how the machines work
♦ what can be expected from the treatment planning, treatment and follow-up care, which treatment courses are expected to cause side effects
♦ managing side effects—fatigue, skin changes, diarrhea, sore mouth—when they do occur
♦ radiation safety
♦ emotional support and education
♦ nutrition.

The nurses work in collaboration with radiation oncologists, radiation physicists, radiology technicians, social workers and dietitians to carry out the treatment plan prescribed by the radiation oncologist for each individual patient.

If you need a radiation implant, you would be hospitalized, usually in an oncology unit, for as long as the implant is in place. But other types of radiation can be given on either an in-patient or outpatient basis. In either case, oncology nurses can help you and your family with information and coping strategies during the course of your treatment.

HOW NURSES WORK WITH YOUR DOCTOR

Treating cancer is very much a team effort these days. And, working closely with other members of the team, oncology nurses are becoming more and more closely involved with the care of people with cancer.

Although your primary physician or oncologist is responsible for the diagnosis and planning of effective treatment, there is now more of a professional collaboration between oncology physicians and nurses than there used to be. The oncology nurse will make decisions about your care within her or his scope of practice. The physician encourages and values the nurses' recommendations and contributions.

♦ In the hospital, it is the nurses who will be with you 24 hours a day, seven days a week. So your doctor will often ask the nursing team for updates on your condition. Nurses may make "walking rounds" with the doctor to find out how you are doing and to make plans for the upcoming day. It is the oncology nurse at the hospital who monitors your vital signs, assesses lab work and physical findings, evaluates your needs and calls the physician when necessary.

♦ On an out-patient basis or in the office, the nurse will work with you at a more independent level. Your doctor still maps out the treatment plan, but the oncology nurse is an invaluable colleague in carrying it out. Nurses may help the doctor plan and decide the most effective way to deliver chemotherapy drugs. And the nurse's opinion will be especially valuable in, for example, choosing the antinausea medications most likely to be effective for your particular chemotherapy treatment.

♦ Nurses and doctors will usually hold patient care conferences to discuss your treatment. Nurses can often point out subtle changes in your condition that your doctors might not be aware of, some of which could possibly change the treatment plan.

♦ In the research field, oncology nurses may work independently or collaborate with physicians, but most of the time, physician and nurse work very closely together. The nurse is a member of the research team that conducts clinical trials of new therapies, collecting data and assessing responses and side effects. When the data are all collected and the analysis done, the nurse's name appears on the published work alongside the physician's.

♦ Because you usually spend many more hours with a nurse than you do with your doctor, a special relationship often develops. Sometimes you can become so overwhelmed with new terms and complex treatment schedules that the nurse may take extra time to explain the information your doctor gives you. Often the nurse will follow up the next day in the hospital or by telephone to make sure you understand and feel comfortable about your treatment.

Your care and treatment is truly a team effort by your oncologist and the oncology nurse. And it is you who benefits most from this collaboration.

NURSING IN THE HOSPITAL, CLINIC AND OFFICE

While there are many nursing roles in the office, hospital, home and hospice, the majority of cancer nurses work in hospitals. Most cancer centers and many community hospitals have wards devoted to cancer treatment—oncology units—staffed by oncology nurses.

Hospital staff nurses provide direct care to patients over eight-, ten- or twelve-hour shifts. During your hospital stay you will probably come in contact with a great variety of nurses with different levels of training and responsibilities.

♦ Nurse's aides or hospital attendants complete a training program and may have many years of experience. They can give you direct hands-on care, but do not give medications.

♦ Licensed Vocational Nurses (LVNs) or Licensed Practical Nurses (LPNs) complete an educational program and can give medications and direct care. They work collaboratively with Registered Nurses (RNs).

♦ RNs receive their education from an associate degree program, a hospital training program or a Bachelor's degree program at a college or university. Many hospitals have different clinical levels of expertise and authority where RNs progress over time, based on merit and continuing education. An RN with cancer nursing experience can become an

Oncology Certified Nurse (OCN) by passing an exam that will certify her or his competency.

♦ Some nurses receive Master's degrees in cancer nursing. They practice as nurse practitioners, clinical nurse specialists, managers or researchers. Or they choose to continue to work as staff nurses at the bedside. In advanced clinical practice, these nurses teach and act as role models for other nurses, take part in advanced problem-solving, participate in clinical research trials and provide leadership.

The Ambulatory Care/Office Nurse You may not always receive your cancer treatment in a hospital. The preferred place of treatment in many places recently has shifted away from hospitals. You might, therefore, find yourself in a comprehensive cancer center, an out-patient clinic, an ambulatory care center or a private office.

One major reason for this shift is the tremendous costs of health care today. There is a great push to shorten hospital stays because out-patient care is more cost-effective for patients, insurance companies and health care plans. But more important, you benefit by going to an office or clinic, getting your treatment and then going home to recover in your own home and sleep in your own bed.

Antinausea treatments have become so sophisticated that many of the negative side effects that used to mean a long stay in the hospital for treatment have been eliminated. Of course, specialized or research cancer treatments still usually have to be given in the hospital so your condition can be closely supervised and monitored. But even then, you can spend more time outside the hospital than used to be the case.

Out-patient nursing includes giving all types of chemotherapy treatments ranging from a rapid injection to a five- to seven-hour infusion. Out-patient nurses learn the latest treatment protocols and investigational studies and can give you and your family important information about your disease, treatment, possible side effects and how to manage your medications. These nurses are experts at starting IVs or any of the surgically implanted catheters such as the Hickman, the Port-a-Cath and the Infusaid pump, to name a few. Their job may include mixing and preparing the chemotherapy drugs, syringes, IV bags or bottles.

NURSING IN THE HOME AND HOSPICE

For the same reasons that out-patient treatment has become more widespread, home care is becoming an important part of oncology care. There are now a variety of home care agencies that are staffed by oncology nurses. Many people choose this type of treatment simply because they prefer to get their chemotherapy in the privacy of their own homes with family and friends close by.

Care in the Home Nurses can spend anywhere from a few hours to 24 hours in your home. Chemotherapy is not the only treatment you can get at home. Under the direction of the oncologist, the oncology nurse can provide you with wound care, central venous (CV) line care and teaching, intravenous (IV) hydration, IV antibiotics and total IV nutrition.

Hospice Care Hospice can be an important alternative if your cancer becomes very advanced. In the terminal stage of cancer, hospice care gives you the choice of spending the final days not at a hospital but at home with loved ones by your side.

As with other oncology specialties, hospice nurses are closely involved with both you and your family. Under your doctor's guidance, the hospice nurse provides pain medication, including narcotics by many different routes.

They teach family and friends how to care for their loved ones and decrease their distress. The hospice nurse, together with social workers and clergy, also helps the family deal with the impending death and handle the bereavement period that follows. During that time, the hospice nurse spends many hours with the family and is available at all hours of the day or night.

SUPPORT FOR YOU AND YOUR FAMILY

The role of the oncology nurse varies depending on where and what kind of care is needed at any particular moment. But improving the quality of life for people with cancer is a primary goal of cancer nursing practice. To reach that goal, the oncology nurse is devoted to reducing your physical discomfort and providing emotional support to you and your family.

Managing Symptoms Cancer and the side effects of treatment may have symptoms that are distressing or affect your day-to-day life. Your health care team has to work together to identify and relieve these symptoms. There is now a great deal of nursing knowledge that lets the oncology nurse evaluate, advise and effectively take the edge off symptoms like nausea and vomiting, pain, constipation, diarrhea, mouth sores, shortness of breath, loss of appetite and emotional distress.

Support Groups and Other Resources It is important that whatever needs you have for emotional support be matched with the resources available in your community. These needs often change over the course of an illness and may depend on individual differences and the availability of family, friends and community support.

There are nurses, social workers, psy-chologists and psychiatrists in private practice who have a special interest in and experience with people who have cancer. Most oncology nurses and social workers will be able to give you information about support resources. Nurses are especially active in referrals for support services, particularly the cancer support groups that are widely available. These groups can be led or facilitated by social workers, psychologists or psychiatrists. Many are co-facilitated by nurses. There are many groups led by professionals who have themselves been diagnosed with cancer.

Not everyone with cancer wants or needs to take part in a structured support group. Many patients successfully use friends and family members as a source of strength. Some people choose individual psychotherapy, either along with or instead of a support group. Yet you should be aware that many people with cancer have credited their support groups with fostering hope and supporting their recovery.

A Special Relationship Many cancer nurses choose to specialize in oncology because they want to make a difference. They want to establish ongoing and meaningful relationships with people who have cancer and their loved ones. The oncology nurse truly touches many lives in many different ways. The nurses who specialize in oncology develop the technical skills needed for cancer care. They will support and inform you and your family throughout your illness. They will always be your advocate.

Simply stated, oncology nurses strive to treat you with kindness and caring, expertise and competence, warmth and good humor and, above all, dignity.

PART II:
SUPPORTIVE CARE

16
LIVING WITH CANCER

Ernest H. Rosenbaum, MD, Malin Dollinger, MD, Isadora Rosenbaum, MA, and Lenore Dollinger, RN, PhD

Cancer used to be thought of as a virtual death sentence. Yet more and more people have learned to view this disease in a very different light. Many now recognize that living with cancer means learning to live with a chronic disease. It means learning how to manage symptoms and treatments while returning to as many of the normal activities of daily living as possible.

It's important to have life go on as usual or at least as close to usual as you can make it. Maybe you won't be able to take a planned vacation. Maybe you won't be exercising or playing sports or making love as vigorously or as often as you used to. Then again, maybe you will. The point is that a cancer diagnosis doesn't have to be absolutely devastating—although it can be if you let it.

The key is to not feel as though you are a helpless victim of blind fate. Do that and you may easily lose the will to live. If you're going to be cured, go into remission or even just improve the quality of your life, *you have to take an aggressive stance.*

Fighting cancer is a joint effort, a shared responsibility between you and your medical team. This partnership is based on honesty, communication, education and a willingness to do your part. The medical team assumes responsibility for planning the most effective treatment and giving therapy and support. You have to assume responsibility for working on proper nutrition, proper physical exercise and the proper mental attitude.

Do your part and the result will be a much greater ability to cope, a strengthened will to live and a much more enjoyable life. Sometimes it may seem like a struggle, but you—just like many people before you—can learn to live with cancer.

TALKING TO FAMILY AND FRIENDS

Not too many decades ago, some illnesses were never discussed openly, even among family and friends. Tuberculosis was rarely mentioned in front of other people, for example. And any mention of cancer was made in hushed tones more suitable to talking about bubonic plague. *Cancer* gradually became the most feared word in the English language. It still is. Today, many people remain reluctant to talk about it, even though it is now a rather common disease and often a curable one.

How open you should be about the fact that you have cancer or about how your treatment is going is entirely up to you. There is no single "right" way to talk about it. There are no "right" words to use. Like everyone else, you will have to find your own comfort area and the words you're most comfortable using. If you would rather talk about your "malignancy" or "tumor" or "growth" or "lump" or "problem" than keep using the word "cancer" all the time, so be it.

Deciding Who to Tell Some people prefer to keep their cancer a very private matter, not telling anyone outside the family. One person in our experience has had cancer for 19 years and no one knows but her husband and her daughter, now age 21. The cancer started in 1971 with breast cancer metastatic to her liver and bones. Yet she works, she runs track and is active in the community. One of the reasons she has survived is because she is living with her cancer. For her, this approach is a very positive one. She wants to forget about it and get on with her life.

Others who need outside help pick one or two close friends who have indicated that they would be available emotionally to provide comfort and support when it is needed.

Deciding What to Say Although it can be hard, it makes sense to be open and direct with your family and close friends if you feel comfortable doing that.

Without candor and openness, concerned relatives and friends are left with their own darkest imaginings. They have their own fears and frustrations that will only grow into terrifying phantoms if they are left behind a veil of secrecy and ignorance of what you are really experiencing. The mutual confrontation of fears is a good way of keeping your own fears and the fears of others under control.

Being open doesn't mean that you have to start every conversation with the story of your latest aches and pains. Nor, if someone asks how you feel, do you necessarily have to answer with a long, detailed description. The litany of the person who wants sympathy or empathy—"I've got it bad. It hurts here and here. I've got to get this treatment"—makes a lot of people want to avoid you. People with cancer are often avoided because, by their own conversation, only bad things seem to happen to them.

Another person in our experience—a military man and pharmacist who had lymphocytic leukemia and, concurrently, colon cancer—was a very open, extroverted person. But if someone said to him, "How do you feel?" he always said, "I

never had it better in my life." For him, this was a great opener, ending any conversation about his cancer that he could have found depressing, demoralizing or inappropriate. It also made the association with others far less uncomfortable and much warmer because no one was made uneasy.

Short-circuiting painful conversations like this is one way of coping and getting on with your life. But, again, it is not the only way. What is right for you is your own decision. For you, it might not be helpful to just say "fine" if someone asks how you are doing. Such an automatic social response might be appropriate for friends, relatives or co-workers you are not particularly close with, but not if the person asking is someone close who is trying to be supportive.

The same caution applies the other way. When you are feeling low physically or mentally, many people will try to buck you up by telling you, "Don't worry, everything will be fine." This is a common, socially acceptable statement we are all taught to make to show support. But the true message seems to be, "Don't tell me that you don't feel good; tell me you're okay."

When you really aren't feeling so good, this kind of support obviously contradicts what you know to be true. At such times it is especially nice to have a close friend or relative who can say, "I'm sorry you're feeling down and I'm glad I'm here for you." For that special someone to be there for you, you have to be able to communicate truthfully how you really feel.

COPING WITH SPECIAL FAMILY PROBLEMS

Cancer is a personal disease, but everyone close to you suffers in some way. Cancer is especially hard on family members, particularly when you are in the hospital for an extended time. The period of separation can be traumatic.

Family caregivers are often very stressed. Everyone in the family wonders where you will be in a month or two months down the road—in the hospital, a nursing home, at home and needing nursing care? They are afraid you will have great discomfort or pain.

Very often, the family struggles with questions about how needs can be met and care arranged in such a way that insurance companies will pay for it. They wonder how other caregivers can become involved so they can get back to work. Relatives who live some distance away may have to make plans for taking care of their children so they can come and provide help for a few weeks or a month. Schedules may have to be rearranged, but people are often uncertain about when they should come.

And all members of the family have fears of losing someone who is an important part of the family's life, with meaning and value for love and companionship.

The Needs of Children When you are away in the hospital or when you are back home but feeling tired from treatment, it is not unusual for children to feel lost or neglected. You and other family members have to reassure them often that they are still loved. With younger children you may also have to quickly eliminate any notion that they somehow caused this illness.

Teenagers are especially vulnerable to stress. They have all the same worries that other members of the family have. They have the same needs for reassurance as younger children. And at the same time they may be burdened by having to take on adult responsibilities around the house. If all this becomes too much to bear, they can rebel by cutting the number of visits to the hospital, not doing their new chores at home or even taking alcohol or drugs.

Strained Relationships Not all families are supportive all the time. Realistically,

not everyone is able to be open, loving and intelligently supportive in a crisis. Families sometimes feel death before it even happens. Oncologists have seen patients take a turn for the worse, then have seen family members decide emotionally and psychologically that all is over and stop coming around to the hospital for visits. The family goes into mourning while the patient is still trying to get better and have hope. It's sad to say, but oncologists sometimes see family members fighting at the bedside over wills and codicils.

But even close families and stable relationships can be threatened by the pressures of a long-term illness. Emotional and physical exhaustion, frustration and constant worry and care can all take their toll. Anger and guilt can surface in sudden attacks, recriminations or indifferent or oversolicitous behavior. Other problems that may have been latent in a relationship for years can suddenly emerge.

All these possible strains just emphasize the need for everyone to look after his or her own needs. You have to do all that you can to look after yourself. Your family members have to be reminded that they need time for themselves. They need moments of rest and relief to keep themselves on an even keel emotionally and psychologically.

Both you and your family may be suffering from the same feelings of inadequacy, the same burdens of guilt, the same quiet anguish, the same sheer tedium of prolonged illness. Any or all of these can break the spirits of the most loving and courageous people.

No one can or should be blamed or criticized for the ways he or she responds to the crisis of cancer or the threat of change or loss. Some people and some relationships grow stronger. Some waver but hold fast. Some collapse. Some experience new heights of love, respect and understanding.

DEALING WITH NEGATIVE EMOTIONS

Nothing can undermine your will to live and your "battle-ready" posture so much as the negative emotions that are so often the response to a cancer diagnosis—anger, fear, loss of self-esteem and feelings of isolation. These emotions have to be resolved. If they aren't, helplessness, futility and resignation can easily take over.

Resolving Your Anger How you react to the cancer diagnosis depends on your personality and how you usually adapt to life's problems. If you are the sort of person who looks on adversity as one more problem to be attacked with determination or as simply something you have to make the best of, then your normal positive attitude will probably carry you through the initial shock of the diagnosis and the tough times ahead. But if you usually react to adversity by asking "why me?" you may spend most or all of your emotional energy being angry at the disease, the "gods" or other people for bringing this catastrophe down on your head.

Anger is a normal reaction. In some ways it can help you through the period of grieving that comes after the diagnosis. In fact, if you don't feel some anger and find some way of expressing it, you may be setting yourself up for a period of depression. But there is a time for anger and a time to put anger aside.

If anger stays unresolved, it takes away the energy that could be channeled into coping with the disease and living life as fruitfully as possible. The first step in resolving it is to recognize why you are angry. If you don't, you may find yourself taking out your anger on others, finding fault with friends or family, making a big deal about trivial matters or flying off the handle at the slightest provocation. The result may well be that you drive needed people away just when you need them most. But if you recognize your anger for what it is, you will be getting your mental attitude set to cope with it.

It's important to let your anger out. Talk about it. Scream. Punch a pillow or throw things around—anything to help release anger's hold on you. Then work to apply that energy in a positive and useful direction. Tell the world you just ain't ready to go, and put your anger to work to make sure you don't have to.

Coming to Terms with Fear Most people hear the word *cancer* and immediately think of suffering, prolonged disability or the phrase "nothing can be done." These responses may be okay for the movies, but except in unusual circumstances they don't have a lot to do with the reality of cancer treatment today. Something can almost always be done. Pain and other side effects of treatment can be controlled. Disability is not inevitable. Most people are surprised to learn that their ideas about cancer are much more pessimistic than the facts warrant.

But no one with cancer has any experience or training in how to deal with the sometimes scary events that happen day to day, week to week or month to month. Even if the surgeon "got it all out" or the radiation or chemotherapy seems to be working, there is always a fear that the cancer will come back.

Fear is a terrible master if you let it get a grip on your life. You can be literally "frightened to death." It is a documented phenomenon in modern medical practice that people who accept a cancer diagnosis as a death sentence can die quite quickly, long before the disease has progressed far enough to cause death by itself.

A diagnosis of cancer is not a death sentence. The first question people usually ask when they get the diagnosis is, "How long have I got?" Unfortunately, some doctors still answer with an unqualified "six months" or "a year" or "two years." Specific predictions like these are simply not valid. Such figures may be published averages for people with a specific type of cancer, but they are only averages. Obviously, some people did not live as long as the estimate, some lived longer.

No estimate of *individual* survival can be made until therapy has begun and the response to it has been established. Until then, predictions are, at best, guesswork and uncertainty that can only stifle hope and the will to live.

Knowledge and understanding are the keys to freeing yourself from unreasonable fear. If you want to know the truth about cancer, talk to oncologists and other members of your health care team. Don't listen to what friends, relatives or acquaintances tell you or take reports in the press as gospel. Fears can be resolved if you understand clearly the problems you face, if you understand the treatments and supportive measures that might be taken and if you have a reasonable and realistic estimate of the discomfort or inconvenience you can expect.

Dealing with the Fears of Others Even if your own fear is under control, well-meaning friends or family members can communicate their fears to you. Unless you are prepared for this, you might find your reserves of emotional energy drained and a depression coming on.

The only way out of this situation is to either hide the fact of your cancer or make sure your family and friends understand your disease and treatment. You may even want to include some of them in your consultations with your doctor so they can become part of your "informed" support team. This may also help your doctor, for, from the doctor's point of view, many of the problems in communication come from the family—the husband or wife, the sister or brother, the cousin or friend who has heard about a cure somewhere or about someone who's had better treatment. By making sure that all interested parties are kept informed, everyone can focus their ener-

gies and efforts in the most constructive channels.

Overcoming a Loss of Self-Esteem Your self-esteem can be threatened by the very idea of having cancer. Unfortunately, it's not unusual to feel that if you were somehow a better or more complete person you wouldn't have been stricken in the first place or that the cancer is some sort of divine punishment.

These are all superstitious beliefs that, sad to say, still cling to the word *cancer*. But having cancer doesn't mean that you are unworthy in any way or that you are guilty of some terrible wrongdoing. Cancer can happen to anyone. It will happen to one out of every four Americans.

Even if you don't fall victim to these superstitions, however, cancer can take away or change some of the things that have always given you a sense of self-esteem.

Your Body Image Changes to your body as a result of surgery, radiotherapy or chemotherapy can have a devastating effect on your self-esteem, especially if the changes are visible to other people. If you lose some part of your body, if you have scars or skin changes or if you lose your hair or a lot of weight, everyone can't help but notice. And you're bound to feel uncomfortable when they do, at least at first. If you have to have an ostomy you may feel humiliated by having to collect your body wastes in a bag. If you have surgery to your genitals, you may feel that you are no longer a "real man" or a "real woman."

But your body is not your self. Your true self is your spirit and your soul. It may be hard for you to accept this truth, but you can come to accept it with help and encouragement. Become involved with a support group and get to know other people who have had similar body changes. Just as you will be able to relate to them, other people will be able to relate to you just as you are. The volunteers who work with groups or other social agencies can help you adjust emotionally. You, in turn, may eventually be of value to others going through the same changes.

Loss of Independence and Control To some extent, these are inevitable for anyone with cancer. In the beginning, you will have to depend on the medical system for your very life. When you are in the hospital, other people may well determine when you eat, sleep, bathe, walk or even go to the bathroom. You may feel uncomfortable or humiliated by having to use a bedpan or having your body exposed to doctors, nurses and medical staff.

When you get home, you may have to depend on family, friends or social service agencies for help around the house, personal body care or meeting your financial obligations. You may start to feel "useless" or feel guilty about being a burden to people you care about.

You may have to simply accept your loss of independence for a while, but your sense of self-esteem can be improved if you take as much responsibility as you possibly can in the areas you *can* handle.
♦ Look after as many self-care tasks as you can.
♦ Be methodical and dedicated about eating the right foods and doing regular exercises to increase your strength and mobility.
♦ Keep charts of your progress to help you feel a sense of accomplishment.
♦ Carefully choose some little jobs you can do around the house, whether it's tending plants or caring for a pet or finding some other outlet for your ability to nurture.

Your self-esteem can also be improved if you get involved in a range of supportive programs such as special group counseling or patient support organizations. If there are no support groups in your area, talk to your local medical staff, social workers, clergy and other people with cancer and start one yourself.

Avoiding Isolation Our society likes to think that it is compassionate and willing to rehabilitate people who are disabled or suffering from chronic diseases. The reality is that disabled people are often shunted aside or even shunned. Employers and co-workers can keep their distance. Family and friends, attentive and sympathetic at first, can drift away over time as they deal with their own problems and live their own lives. Everyone can feel uncomfortable talking to someone who is seriously ill, not knowing quite how to relate or what to say. At times like these, it is easy to feel abandoned and lonely.

Even when you are surrounded by caring friends and family, you may feel cut off. Any life-threatening disease can put you in touch with the essential aloneness humans feel when contemplating their own mortality. Some people turn their attention and energies inward to such a degree that they lose contact with life and the rest of humanity.

Isolation and loneliness can often be self-inflicted. If you focus on grieving or feeling sorry for yourself or if you accept the diagnosis as a death sentence, you may snip your ties to the world and live as though you already belong to the dead. When that happens—just as when isolation comes from the outside and old connections are broken by others—you have to make new connections, building new bridges to people and activities that can renew your energy and zest for living.

You may be frightened or pessimistic about taking the first steps toward making a new life. But you *can* change direction. The benefits of doing so make the effort more than worthwhile.

SUPPORT GROUPS

Some people need special help to cope with their cancer, and their doctors can't always provide it. Doctors are as interested in their patients' emotional well-being as they are in their physical well-being, yet medical appointments are usually taken up with talks about treatment problems, side effects, precautions and complications.

Doctors do recognize the importance of dealing with emotional concerns and can often refer you to the many external support groups and systems available to you. These groups give all cancer patients the kind of help that only interested and dedicated people, often sufferers of the same disease, can provide.

At the Hospital Many local hospitals, especially those with cancer treatment centers, have support groups that are run by health professionals and often meet every week. These are groups designed just for individuals with cancer and for family members.

Some of these groups are specialized, dealing only with the common physical and emotional problems of people who have been treated for specific tumors. For example:
♦ People who have had ostomies—artificial openings created in the colon, intestine or bladder—have to learn what they can do to live as normal a life as possible.
♦ People who have had their larynx, or voice box, removed have to learn how to speak all over again.
♦ Women who have had a mastectomy have specific emotional problems. So do men with testicular cancer.

Outside the Hospital The American Cancer Society and other professional organizations have programs that help deal with physical, emotional and mental problems associated with having cancer. The Reach to Recovery program for women with breast cancer and the I Can Cope program of weekly seminars are two examples. Both include a comprehensive educational process for cancer patients and their families.

The Wellness Community is another example of an organization devoted to improving the quality of life of people with cancer. It features educational programs, seminars, discussion groups and the opportunity for everyone with cancer to relate to others with the same fears and worries. Many people find the approach of this rapidly expanding organization—which encourages you to become an active participant in your fight for recovery—extremely helpful (*see* Chapter 30).

Depending where you live, there also may be organizations designed to meet the needs of young adults who do not always feel comfortable in other support organizations. An organization called Vital Options, for example, meets these needs. This organization started in Los Angeles and is rapidly expanding nationally.

How the Groups Work There are great advantages to taking part in a group when you feel well enough to participate. A group of people in circumstances similar to yours can offer companionship and the chance to discuss many concerns and feelings.

How the support groups are designed and structured and what they cover vary. But they all have in common the gathering together of people with similar experiences. In these groups:
♦ You can tell your story, sharing your experience of cancer and its effect on your life.
♦ You can hear the stories of others, support their similar experiences and decrease their sense of isolation, fear and loneliness.
♦ You can share information and resources that will help you cope with specific problems.

Each group functions for better or worse, depending on the members and the leadership. *Not everyone is suited for a group.* Some people prefer and would do better not participating in a group. But many people with cancer have given credit to their support groups for helping them maintain hope and setting them on the road to recovery.

Where to Find the Right Group Local chapters of the American Cancer Society usually have a current listing of which groups are offered. Many cancer newsletters contain this information, and most oncology nurses and social workers can help you find support resources.

GETTING BACK TO WORK

Many people don't realize how much their feelings of self-worth depend on their being active, productive and capable of taking care of themselves and others. Then an illness strikes and it soon sinks in just how important all that is. Of course, a job is pretty much essential for financial well-being. But it can also be essential for psychological well-being.

This is especially true when you have cancer. The loss of self-esteem that often follows a cancer diagnosis or treatment can be magnified by sitting around doing nothing while you depend on family and friends for personal care, financial assistance and help around the house. So it is vital to your peace of mind to find ways of returning to productive work in some capacity. It might mean getting back to your old job. It might mean learning a new skill, studying or even simply doing work around the house. (*See* Chapter 28.)

Keeping a Positive Attitude Admittedly, getting back to work can sometimes be a problem. You may be disabled in such a way that you can no longer do the same job you had before treatment. And, you may have to confront some discrimination in the job market or prejudice in the workplace.

It's unfortunate, but there is still some stigma attached to having cancer. Employers and co-workers may react out of a vague fear or uneasiness about cancer in the abstract. Co-workers can stay at arm's length either because they just don't know what to say or because they have the irrational and completely mistaken notion that they'll catch something terrible if they go near you. Employers might be afraid of decreased production or financial losses because of the time you might need to take off for treatment. (*See* Chapter 31.)

A study by the American Cancer Society in the 1970s showed that cancer patients did face some discrimination in hiring, firing, job assignments, benefits and attitudes.

♦ Almost a quarter of the people who took part in the study reported either being rejected for jobs because of cancer treatment or being the target of negative attitudes.

♦ Slightly more than half described at least one illness-related problem.

But the good news was that 46 percent said they had *never* had problems at work because of their cancer. And over three-quarters said that after treatment they had earned salary increases because of promotions or increased responsibilities. Since that study was done many American states have passed legislation to outlaw discrimination because of medical conditions, including cancer.

What is absolutely essential is that you keep a positive attitude despite some rejection. Medical social workers, physical and occupational therapists and vocational counselors can all help ease the transition back into the workforce. They can help you match your skills with available jobs or help you get retraining if that is necessary. But learning to live with cancer is the key. Your positive attitude will strengthen your resolve and also just might rub off on employers and co-workers.

YOUR NEED FOR RECREATION

Recreation is an important part of living. We all need a break from the routine and stress of daily life to keep us steady even in the best of circumstances. Although it is sometimes hard to summon up the energy or the will, recreation is even more important when we are sick. Engaging in some kind of recreational activity helps relieve tensions and bring on a feeling of relaxation. It also contributes to feelings of self-worth and well-being.

When you are being treated for cancer, you may forget about recreation. Or you may think it's not important, inappropriate or just too hard to pursue. It is none of these. No matter what your limitations, you can start many activities while you are in the hospital and continue when you go home.

Being with a Group Working with a group or simply working on your own among other people engaged in the same activity has a lot of advantages. The companionship can give you the opportunity to talk about any problems or concerns you have. Better yet, it gives you the chance to talk about all kinds of things that have absolutely nothing to do with cancer. Either way, being with others can lift your spirits and calm your anxieties.

If you are up to it, you can arrange outings with one or more companions. You might want to do something as simple as take a walk in the park with an old friend or take in something entertaining like a movie or a play. If you are involved with craft work, go on an outing to a museum or library to pick up new information or broaden your appreciation of craft activities.

There are many outside resources you can contact, both for learning opportunities and companionship—the YMCA/YWCA, local clubs, schools, colleges and univer-sities, community centers, religious organizations. And keep looking in local newspapers and magazines for recreational activities that change from week to week.

Things to Do on Your Own If you feel more comfortable with solitary pursuits, check out the library in your neighborhood or at the hospital for suggestions. There are many games, crafts and other activities that you can become involved in no matter what your limitations in strength and energy. The list of possibilities is almost limitless, but you might:

♦ Start a scrapbook. Put all your loose photos and mementos into some pleasing arrangement. Divide them by subject or theme and write captions or amusing comments. Maybe you could devote part of the layout to tracing your family tree.

♦ Take up sketching, painting or some other artistic activity. If you have no experience with art, start with line drawings of still life. Once you've got the basic contours of the object on paper, fill in details and shadings and add color. Experiment with various materials. You might find you have talents you never dreamed you had.

♦ Listen to music. It not only "soothes the savage breast," it can raise your spirits, help you sleep, relieve pain and make mealtimes more pleasant and satisfying. Listening to music is not only enjoyable, it's downright therapeutic.

♦ Rent funny movies. If you have a VCR, watch as many comedies as you can. Whether your taste for humor is satisfied by Charlie Chaplin, the Marx Brothers, the Three Stooges or Monty Python, many comedies are available at your local videotape outlets.

♦ Watch comedians. Let Arsenio Hall, Jay Leno, George Carlin, Roseanne Arnold, Bill Cosby or anyone else you like tickle your funny bone. Laughter can change your whole outlook on life.

♦ Crochet or knit. Both activities can be very entertaining. And you can see the results of your labors quickly. Even if you've never done either before, you can easily learn to make simple afghans, scarves, shawls or hats for yourself or as gifts for others.

♦ Collect stamps, coins, figurines, recipes,

sports cards or anything else that catches your interest. Collecting gets your mind working on organizing, classifying and physically arranging your collection, as well as on what you need to make the collection more complete.

♦ Set up a golf putting course in your home or yard. A very simple arrangement is all that's needed. It will give you an opportunity to stay active and give you a challenge every day.

What kind of recreational activity you pursue is entirely up to you. But whatever you choose as a diversion should be just that—something enjoyable and fun that diverts your mind away from your illness. The relief from stress and the positive attitude fostered by enjoyment can be critically important to your recovery.

THE GOAL OF TOTAL REHABILITATION

Overcoming your anger and fears, developing the right attitude, getting your support system in place and arranging for productive work and recreation are just the start of your rehabilitation and recovery. All these "set the table" for all you have to do during the tough times ahead.

Once you have made the critical decision that you want to get well, you have to be willing to make sacrifices and believe that achieving the goal is worth the effort. You will have to pay attention to all kinds of things that are detailed in the next few chapters—coping with side effects, maintaining good nutrition, getting enough exercise, learning how to relax, becoming secure enough to express yourself sexually, and many more.

You will have to know your strengths and limitations and be able to set realistic goals. And you will have to be willing to compromise, to accept what cannot be changed and move on from there. Having cancer means that your life has to be restructured if you are going to get as full a rehabilitation as possible. This doesn't mean that you have to change the habits of a lifetime, even if you could. But it does mean you will have to make adjustments in your daily living patterns so that your time can be used in the most efficient and constructive ways.

If you pay attention to your mind and body and spirit, you will be well on your way not only to living with cancer but to achieving the highest level of success possible in the circumstances.

17
COPING WITH TREATMENT SIDE EFFECTS

Ernest H. Rosenbaum, MD, Malin Dollinger, MD,
Barbara F. Piper, RN, OCN, DNSc, and Isadora Rosenbaum, MA

————◇————

When you are ill, your overriding goal is to get well and return to an active life. If you are going to reach that goal, every part of your rehabilitation program is important—the psychological and social dimensions, nutrition, pain control and all the others. But unless the side effects of treatment are looked after, you might not have the energy nor even the desire to get back to a normal life. Side effects can be debilitating. They can sap your strength, weaken your resolve and generally just make life unpleasant.

With support from the medical team, family and friends, you can manage these side effects and eventually overcome them. It may take quite an effort on your part. But the benefits will be well worth that effort.

FATIGUE

Everyone gets tired. This is a universal sensation that is expected to occur at certain times of the day or after certain types of activities. Tiredness usually has an identifiable cause, is short-lived and is easily dissipated by a good night's sleep or rest. In contrast, the fatigue experienced by people with cancer is often described as an unusual or excessive whole-body tiredness that is unrelated or disproportionate to exertion and that is not easily dispelled by sleep or rest.

Fatigue may be short-term (acute), lasting less than one month. Or it may be more long-term (chronic), lasting any-where from one month to six months or longer. Whether acute or chronic, fatigue can have a profound negative impact on the quality of life. Fatigue interferes with the ability to perform the kinds of activities and roles that give meaning and value to life. So fewer activities are undertaken and those that are undertaken may require more effort and take longer to complete.

As fatigue begins to change what cancer patients can do for themselves, family members and other caregivers begin to assume many of the roles patients used to perform themselves. These increased demands can lead to fatigue in family members and to social isolation for both patients and their families.

What Causes Fatigue No one knows exactly why people with cancer and other chronic illnesses experience this unusual fatigue. Age, sex and genetic, socio-economic and environmental factors have been implicated in fatigue, but many other factors involved in both the disease and its treatment may also contribute.

♦ Changes in energy production and the availability of nutrients may cause fatigue. The tumor itself may make the body function in an overactive or "hypermetabolic" state, for example. Tumor cells compete for nutrients, often at the expense of normal cells' growth and metabolism. Weight loss, reduced appetite and fatigue are often the result.

HINTS ON HOW TO COMBAT FATIGUE

ASSESSMENT

♦Think about your personal energy stores as a "bank." Deposits and withdrawals have to be made over the course of the day or the week to ensure a balance between energy conservation, restoration and expenditure.

♦Keep a diary for one week to identify the time of day when you are either most fatigued or have the most energy. Note what you think may be the contributing factors.

♦Be alert to the warning signs of impending fatigue—tired eyes, tired legs, whole-body tiredness, stiff shoulders, decreased energy or a lack of energy, inability to concentrate, weakness or malaise, boredom or lack of motivation, sleepiness, increased irritability, nervousness, anxiety or impatience.

ACTIVITY AND EXERCISE PATTERNS

♦Identify which activities or situations make your fatigue worse or better and develop a plan to pace yourself. Schedule activities according to your fatigue and energy patterns, scheduling them ahead of time during the day and throughout the week to avoid becoming unusually tired.

♦Plan adequate rest and sleep periods so you can recover your energy before undertaking more activities.

♦Select the activities that are most important for you or that give you the most pleasure and do these activities first. Let the others go or delegate them to others.

♦Try to feel less guilty about restructuring your life to do what is most important for you and what gives you the most pleasure.

♦Reduce unnecessary energy expenditure by using special equipment or by placing equipment and supplies within easy reach. Physical therapy can help for bed and strengthening exercises using overhead trapezes, walkers and canes and with stair-climbing instruction.

♦Occupational therapy can help with equipment and energy-conserving activities. The American Cancer Society can help with transportation and supplies.

♦Begin to cultivate the fine art of delegating.

♦Stick to some form of individually tailored exercise program approved by your physician, nurse or physical therapist. Walking is an activity that most people can do at certain times during their illness.

♦Avoid exercising during the 24 hours immediately before and after your treatments. Also avoid exercise if you are running a fever, have low blood counts or if your bones are involved with disease. In such cases, consult your physician.

SYMPTOM PATTERNS

♦Monitor the effectiveness of medications and other strategies used to control other symptoms such as nausea, vomiting, pain and lack of sleep. Could these symptoms and/or their treatments be affecting your fatigue patterns?

NUTRITIONAL PATTERNS

♦Drink at least 8 to 10 glasses of liquids a day to maintain hydration and to eliminate the waste products of treatment that may be associated with fatigue.

♦Eat a balanced diet emphasizing complex carbohydrates (grains and vegetables) that give you a sustained source of energy supply.

♦Get dietary counseling, help with food preparation and shopping or Meals on Wheels to maximize and conserve your energy and to prevent your fatigue from becoming unusual, excessive or chronic.

DISTRACTION

♦Use distraction techniques to focus on things other than fatigue, disease or treatment. Listen to music, visit with friends, watch television or go for walks.

♦Focus on activities that can improve your emotional energy. These usually involve a change in routine to avoid boredom and doing things that catch your interest easily and are enjoyable or at least pleasurable. Try appreciating nature, doing something creative such as drawing, writing or pursuing a hobby or doing something socially with people you enjoy being with.

♦Contract with yourself to do these types of activities three times a week for at least 30 minutes at a time. Your mind, heart and spirit need exercising too!

PSYCHOLOGICAL PATTERNS

♦The negative effects of stress can be dissipated in many ways—exercise, progressive relaxation, visual imagery, meditation, prayer, talking with others and therapeutic counseling.

♦Social service agencies can help with referrals to support groups for yourself and family members.

REST AND SLEEP PATTERNS

♦Begin to direct your own activities.

♦Set limits on visitors if you need to or have someone else run interference for you when you need to rest and don't want to be disturbed.

♦Sit or lie down often. Short rest periods are better than longer ones.

♦Take naps as needed as long as they don't interfere with your normal sleep patterns.

♦Adhere to or re-establish bedtime rituals that help you fall asleep, stay asleep and enjoy a good quality of sleep.

♦Sleep-enhancing aids and sleep medications may be helpful at certain times during your illness and treament.

♦ Disease complications and/or treatment side effects such as anemia, infection and fever can create additional energy needs that your usual food intake cannot supply alone. Nutritional supplements and therapy may be needed.

♦ Also associated with fatigue are diagnostic tests, anesthesia, surgery, radiation therapy, chemotherapy, biotherapy and drugs used to control symptoms and side effects such as nausea, vomiting, pain and insomnia.

♦ Eighty to 96 percent of all chemotherapy patients experience fatigue, which is perceived to be more distressing and disabling than nausea and vomiting.

♦ Drugs such as vincristine and vinblastine may cause fatigue because of their toxic effects on nerves (neurotoxicity). With cisplatin, low magnesium levels, along with neuorotoxicity, may cause fatigue.

♦ Fatigue that increases over time (cumulative fatigue) occurs in radiotherapy patients regardless of treatment site. This usually improves within one month but may last up to three months after treatment stops.

♦ Fatigue may become so severe during biotherapy that treatment dosages may be limited.

♦ As cancer cells die in response to therapy, certain substances are released that may contribute to fatigue. More attention has recently been paid to the possible role of cytokines in the development of fatigue. Cytokines are natural cell products or proteins, such as the interferons and interleukins, that are normally released by white blood cells, lymphocytes and macrophages in response to infection. These cytokines carry messages that regulate other elements of the immune and neuroendocrine systems. In high amounts, these cytokines can be toxic and lead to persistent fatigue.

♦ Changes in the patterns of activity and rest can play significant roles in the prevention, cause and relief of fatigue. Unnecessary inactivity, prolonged bedrest and immobility contribute to loss of muscle strength and endurance. Muscle that is not exercised loses its ability to use oxygen, so more effort and more oxygen are required for the same amount of work performed by conditioned muscle. This is one of the reasons why aerobic endurance exercise—such as walking three or four times a week for 20 to 30 minutes—is often prescribed for patients and family members.

♦ Lack of restful or adequate sleep at night can lead to fatigue and increased sleepiness and napping during the day. Sleep disturbances such as insomnia, multiple awakenings and early waking are common symptoms of depression.

♦ Anxiety also can contribute to sleeplessness, increased energy demands and fatigue.

What Can Be Done The best way to combat fatigue is to treat the underlying cause. Unfortunately, it is not always easy to know what the exact cause is. Many factors may be involved and require treatment, particularly if the fatigue has become chronic. All possible causes must be thoroughly assessed.

If fatigue is related to anemia, for example, blood transfusions, supplemental oxygen and medications designed to increase red blood cell production may be prescribed. Other causes can be managed on an individual basis. This management may include physical therapy and strength training, nutritional assessment and support and psychological counseling.

NAUSEA AND VOMITING

Nausea is a feeling of stomach distress or wooziness accompanied by a strong urge to throw up. Nausea and vomiting are temporary side effects of both chemotherapy and radiotherapy. They can also be brought on by an obstruction in the intestine, irritation of the gastrointestinal tract (gastritis) or brain tumors.

Constant vomiting naturally makes it impossible for you to eat or take fluids, so whatever can be done to reduce nausea should be done *before* vomiting starts. Paying attention to nausea's psychological causes and using antinausea drugs will help control what can be disturbing events.

Nausea and Chemotherapy Drugs The goal of chemotherapy is to deliver a therapeutic amount of drugs with the least side effects. But each chemotherapy agent and each drug combination has a potential for causing nausea and vomiting. Getting three or four drugs at a time, which is often the case, can make the reaction even more severe. The dosage and the number of cycles to be given can also contribute to the reaction.

You, your family and even your friends should talk with your doctor about the type of chemotherapy you'll be getting. For each drug, a program should be established so that you feel you have some control over the situation. With psychological factors playing such a big part, it is very important that you be a participant in preventing nausea and vomiting.

Nausea Before and During Treatment It is estimated that up to half of all people receiving chemotherapy experience some nausea or vomiting not after they receive the drugs but *before* their treatment. This is known as anticipatory nausea and vomiting (ANV) and it usually makes the nausea and vomiting even more severe when the chemotherapy is actually given. This can eventually become such a set psychological pattern that it affects the amount of chemotherapy that can be given. And once the psychological pattern of ANV is established, it is much harder to control nausea and vomiting before and after treatment.

Anticipatory nausea is the result of a conditioned reflex. This means that if chemotherapy made you throw up once or twice, then you will will feel nauseated whenever you take the treatment or even when something triggers the very idea of treatment. This conditioned aversion often takes hold after two to four chemotherapy sessions and can last a long time. A standard joke among doctors is the one about the patient who met her oncologist on the street three years after therapy and threw up on the spot.

Your anxiety state, how you feel about yourself and your cancer and how you respond to stress and disease are all important factors in setting up this psychological pattern. And once the pattern is established, all kinds of stimuli can trigger feelings of nausea—the colors or odors in the room where the chemotherapy is given, the smell of alcohol used to prepare you for the IV needle, the sight of the nurse entering the room.

To deal with this problem, you will have to take steps both to relax before your chemotherapy and to not inadvertently set up situations that become associated with nausea.

♦ Try to relax in a quiet, darkened room before your treatment sessions.

♦ Use behavioral techniques to help you relax and control any triggering stimuli—hypnosis, relaxation therapy, imagery or listening to a tape of your favorite music or a relaxation tape (*see* Chapter 25).

♦ Perhaps try acupuncture or acupressure, which have been effective in controlling nausea or vomiting in some cases.

♦ The time of day when you get treatment can sometimes make a difference. If you have a problem with either the morning or the afternoon, try to change your appointment schedule.

♦ Avoid eating hot, spicy foods or other dishes that might upset your stomach or gastrointestinal tract.

♦ Eat slowly so you don't develop gas or heartburn.

CHEMOTHERAPY DRUGS AND THEIR POTENTIAL TO CAUSE NAUSEA

Highest Potential	Intermediate Potential	Least Potential
♦cisplatin	♦doxorubicin (Adriamycin)	♦bleomycin
♦dacarbazine	♦CCNU	♦5-fluorouracil (5-FU)
♦nitrogen mustard (Mustargen)	♦procarbazine (Matulane)	♦etoposide (VP-16)
♦dactinomycin	♦Cytosar (cytarabine)	♦methotrexate
♦Cytoxan	♦mitomycin-C	♦chlorambucil
♦streptozocin	♦ifosfamide	♦vincristine/vinblastine
♦BCNU	♦carboplatin	♦mercaptopurine
	♦Hexalen	♦melphalan (Alkeran)
		♦Taxol
		♦cytarabine
		♦hydroxyurea (Hydrea)
		♦mitoxantrone

♦ Try to avoid cooking odors that may bring on nausea by having friends or family prepare meals at their own homes and bring them over to you.

♦ Always avoid your favorite foods when you are getting chemotherapy. You might start to associate these foods with treatment, nausea and vomiting and develop a strong aversion to them.

Nausea After Treatment Nausea and vomiting are common side effects after chemotherapy (or after radiation therapy). They may begin one to three hours later or even as long as two to four days after treatment.

Like anticipatory nausea, post-therapy nausea and vomiting can have significant therapeutic implications. You may start to fear therapy, a fear that can gnaw at you and make you want to avoid treatment. It may also make problems such as pain control and maintaining an overall good quality of life much harder to deal with.

Fortunately, a wide variety of anti-nausea drugs has been developed and some combination tailored to your specific needs will usually do the trick to minimize or prevent the problem.

Antinausea Medications Two areas in the brain have been identified as being responsible for nausea and vomiting, and certain drugs and other methods can selectively block these areas. Your doctor can work out a program to combat your nausea, although if one drug or drug combination doesn't work as well as you would both like, you may have to experiment with different programs.

Generally, antivomiting drugs (antiemetics) should be taken 30 minutes before chemotherapy so that they have time to take effect.

♦ If vomiting has already started and you can't keep a pill down, antinausea suppositories such as Compazine or Tigan may help.

♦ Long-acting spansules such as Com-

pazine can be very helpful, since they work for 6 hours.

♦ Ativan and Decadron may help block the brain's vomiting center. It is also a very powerful combination to block anticipatory nausea and vomiting. Ativan can be taken under the tongue for rapid absorption during severe nausea.

♦ Ativan is also an antidepressant and sleeping tablet that can cause amnesia, which might take the edge off any memory of vomiting once the episode is over.

♦ Some forms of marijuana—the natural delta-9-tetrahydrocannabinol (THC) and the synthetic Marinol—may successfully control nausea and vomiting by working on the higher brain centers. But they can also cause drowsiness, dry mouth, dizziness, a rapid heartbeat and sweating.

♦ Ondansetron (Zofran) is the most significant drug used to control nausea and vomiting caused by intensive chemotherapy and radiotherapy. It may be needed when you are receiving "highest potential" chemotherapy drugs or when you cannot get relief with other antinausea agents. It is often given with Decadron IV. It suppresses vomiting in 60 to 80 percent of patients and is even more effective in combination with other antinausea drugs.

SORE MOUTH

The lining, or mucosa, of the gastrointestinal tract—which includes the inside of the mouth and throat—is one of the most sensitive areas of the body. Many chemotherapy drugs can inflame the lining, a condition called mucositis. Many drugs can also cause small ulcerations or sores to develop. Radiation delivered to the head and neck can irritate the lining and cause sores, too, and so can mouth or throat infections, especially fungus infections like monilia (thrush). All these can be very painful or at least uncomfortable.

If you are going to get over your mucositis, mouth care is very important. You will have to make sure your mouth stays clean and moist and that you eat the proper foods and get medication for any infections that develop.

Oral Hygiene A good oral hygienic program includes dental cleaning and scaling, followed by daily brushing and flossing to reduce plaque.

Any scaling, cleaning, tooth extractions or repair of cavities should be done before your cancer therapy begins. Extractions especially should be completed at least two weeks before therapy to give your mouth a chance to heal. Ill-fitting dentures should be fixed or replaced.

Before any dental work is to be performed, your blood counts should be checked to be sure that counts are adequate to take care of any possibility of infection or bleeding (low white cell counts can lead to infections and a low platelet count may lead to bleeding). So any periodontal or dental work has to be coordinated with your oncologist. If you have any mouth injury because of a dental procedure, antibiotics are certainly recommended.

The following daily steps will help your mouth stay in good shape:
♦ Use a soft-bristle toothbrush and soften it more by soaking it in warm water. You may also find that brushing with a paste of baking soda and water may be less irritating than commercial toothpaste.

♦ If brushing your teeth is painful, use either a cotton swab or commercial Toothettes, a sponge-tip stick impregnated with a dentifrice.
♦ Avoid commercial mouthwashes. Some of these have ingredients (especially alcohol) that can irritate your mouth even more. Lemon glycerin swabs may make your mouth feel clean but they are not recommended, because glycerin will make your mouth drier.
♦ A Water-Pik to cleanse your mouth is helpful.
♦ Peridex (oral rinse) will help gum inflammation and bleeding.

Dry Mouth Chemotherapy and radiation to the salivary glands can make your mouth very dry. This can make your mucositis or mouth sores more painful, so you should do everything you can to keep your mouth moist.
♦ Commercial preparations such as Moistir or MouthKot—an oral natural saliva substitute—may help.
♦ You can make your own mouthwash with liquid Xylocaine, baking soda and salt dissolved in 1 quart (1 L) of water.
♦ Sucking sour lemon hard candies or Tic Tacs can help. You can also suck on popsicles or flavored or plain ice cubes.
♦ Use lip balms or lipstick if your lips are dry.

COMMON ANTINAUSEA DRUGS

	Oral	IM	IV	Suppository
♦ Compazine (prochlorperazine)	X	X	X	X
♦ Ativan (lorazepam)	X	X	X	
♦ Reglan (metaclopramide)	X		X	
♦ Haldol (haloperidol)	X	X		
♦ Inapsine (droperidol)			X	
♦ Decadron (dexamethasone)	X	X	X	
♦ Benadryl (diphenhydramine)	X	X	X	
♦ Tigan (trimethobenzamide)	X	X		X
♦ THC (marijuana tablets)	X			
♦ Torecan (thiethylperazine)	X	X	X	X
♦ Zofran (ondansetron)	X		X	

Mouth Sores If the soreness in your mouth becomes severe, there are quite a few anesthetic agents you can use on a short-term basis. If your symptoms persist, you should have a complete dental hygienic evaluation.

♦ Benadryl elixir, lozenges and analgesics may help reduce mouth pain.

♦ Swishing and swallowing the anesthetic jelly viscous Xylocaine or Hurricane can also help you eat if you have pain in your mouth, pharynx or esophagus (a spray is also available).

♦ It may help to swish diluted milk of magnesia, Carafate slurry or Mylanta around your mouth.

♦ Orabase—with or without Kenalog—is a dental salve that covers mouth sores while they are healing. You may have to apply it several times a day.

Infections Mouth infections can be dangerous and have to be cared for. You should examine your mouth every day for any irritation or early fungus growth (white spots inside your mouth that don't wash off). Look under your tongue and at the sides of your mouth and report any changes to your doctor. If you do get an infection, it should be treated promptly.

♦ If you have a herpes virus—acute or recurrent—your doctor may prescribe oral Acyclovir.

♦ Monilia requires antifungal agents, including mycostatin oral suspension Nizoral tablets, Mycelex Troches or Mycostat Pastilles.

♦ You can freeze Nystatin Liquid in medicine cups in the refrigerator and let it melt in your mouth.

Nutrition A normal high-protein, high-calorie diet—with supplements as needed—will help your sore mouth or tongue heal faster. Drinking lots of fluids will also help the healing process as well as help make your mouth sores more comfortable.

A high-calorie, high-protein diet would include scrambled eggs, custards, milkshakes, malts, gelatins, creamy hot cereals, macaroni and cheese and blenderized or pureed foods. Commercial supplements such as Ensure, Sustacal or Carnation Breakfast Drink can also be helpful.

Until your mouth sores heal you should avoid:

♦ Very hot or very cold foods.

♦ Tomatoes and citrus fruits such as grapefruit, lemons and oranges, which can burn your mouth.

♦ Salty foods, which can cause a burning sensation.

♦ Hot, spicy, coarse or rough foods, including toast, dry crackers and chips.

♦ Alcoholic beverages and tobacco, both of which irritate the lining of the mouth.

♦ Any medications such as mouthwashes or cough syrups that contain alcohol.

LOSS OF APPETITE

Loss of appetite, called anorexia, is one of the most common side effects of chemotherapy. It can also result from radiation therapy, stress and anxiety, depression and the cancer itself.

For the sake of your health, your strength and your ability to fight cancer, you have to get enough nutrition. But it's hard to keep your appetite when your mouth and tongue are sore or you have trouble swallowing. Fortunately, these side effects are usually short-term, lasting only three to eight days. But even after they go away, you still might have trouble getting your normal appetite back.

You can talk to a dietitian, nurse or your doctor about ways to improve your appetite. If you don't seem to be making too much progress, you might also ask your doctor about medications that can stimulate your appetite, such as:

♦ Prednisone, a corticosteroid hormone, when given in small doses of 10 to 20 mg a day (there are side effects to consider).

♦ Megace (a progestin), 40 mg two to four times a day.

♦ Marinol, a legally available synthetic form of marijuana in capsule form. It is usually used as an antinausea drug, but stimulation of appetite is a positive side effect.

TASTE BLINDNESS

Many chemotherapy drugs can change your sense of taste and smell. What these changes are depends on the individual, but they are most common with foods that are either very sweet or very bitter. Oddly enough, sweet foods might taste sour and sour foods taste sweet. Chewed meat may have a bitter taste because of the release of proteins in your mouth. Sometimes there is a continuous metallic taste in your mouth after chemotherapy, which naturally enough can affect what you eat and how you eat.

Taste changes may not last long. But while you are experiencing them, you can do several things to lessen their effect.

♦ Brush your teeth several times a day and use mouth rinses such as diluted bicarbonate of soda.

♦ If foods and beverages taste bitter, add sweet fruits, honey or NutraSweet.

♦ If meat tastes bitter, substitute bland chicken or fish, eggs and mild cheeses or tofu. All of these might taste better if you use them in casseroles or stews.

♦ It will also help if you marinate meats, chicken or fish in pineapple juice, wine, Italian dressing, lemon juice, soy sauce or sweet-and-sour sauces.

♦ Add whatever flavorings you enjoy, but avoid spicy, highly seasoned foods.

♦ You might find that starchy foods such as bread, potatoes and rice have a more acceptable taste if you eat them without butter or margarine.

CONSTIPATION AND IMPACTION

Constipation means infrequent bowel movements. It also means a collection of dry, hard stools that get "stuck" in your rectum or colon. When you are constipated, you will often feel bloated and not have much of an appetite. If constipation persists, it may cause a stool "im-

---

Tips to Reduce Loss of Appetite

♦Plan your meals in advance and arrange for help in preparing them. You might also better tolerate meals prepared by friends or family, since cooking at home might produce offensive odors that will put you off food.

♦Make your mealtimes a pleasant experience.

♦Stimulate your appetite by exercising for 5 or 10 minutes about a half-hour before meals.

♦Have an aperitif such as a small glass of wine before meals. It will help you relax and stimulate your taste buds.

♦Relax for a few minutes before meals, using relaxation exercises.

♦Eat frequent, small meals and have snacks between meals that appeal to your senses.

♦Add extra protein to your diet. Fortify milk by adding 1 cup (250 mL) of non-fat dry milk to each quart (liter) of whole milk or milk recipe. Be creative with desserts. And use nutritional supplements.

paction"—a very large hard stool that you will have great difficulty passing.

It is important to try to prevent constipation and stool impaction, for both can cause great distress and pain. Patients with heart, respiratory or gastrointestinal diseases can be especially aggravated by the discomfort and pressure of an impaction.

Causes All kinds of things can make you constipated—lack of exercise, emotional stress, various drugs or simply a lack of high-fiber or bulk-forming foods in your diet.

Chemotherapy drugs such as vincristine and vinblastine are often constipating. So are narcotics such as morphine and codeine, gastrointestinal antispas-modics, antidepressants, diuretics, tranquilizers, sleeping pills and calcium- and aluminum-based antacids.

When prescribing these drugs, your doctor should anticipate the need for a stool softener and/or a mild laxative. Enemas or suppositories might also be needed.

Laxatives and Stool Softeners If you become constipated, talk to your doctor about a laxative program. It is essential that you take laxatives—and suppositories and enemas as well—only under your doctor's supervision. Don't try to diagnose and treat yourself since there may be more to the situation than you may realize. For example, diarrhea can occasionally develop at the same time as a stool

---

Hints to Prevent and Relieve Constipation

♦Eat foods that are high in fiber and bulk. These include fresh fruits and vegetables (raw or cooked with skins and peels on), dried fruit, whole-grain breads and cereals and bran. Avoid raw fruits and vegetables, including lettuce, when your white blood cell count is lower than 1,800.
Note: You should start a high-fiber diet before taking a chemotherapy drug that causes constipation.

♦Drink plenty of fluids—8 to 10 glasses a day. *Avoid dehydration.* Try to drink highly nutritional fluids (milkshakes, eggnogs and juices) rather than water, since liquids can be filling and may decrease your appetite.

♦Add bran to your diet gradually. Start with 2 tsp. (10 mL) per day and gradually work up to 4 to 6 tsp. (20 to 30 mL) per day. Sprinkle bran on cereal or add it to meatloaf, stews, pancakes, baked goods and other dishes. Dietary bran is helpful.

♦Avoid refined foods such as white bread, starchy desserts and candy. Also avoid chocolates, cheese and eggs, since these can be constipating.

♦To make your bowel movements more regular, take prunes or a glass of prune juice in the morning or at night before bed. Prunes contain a natural laxative as well as fiber. Warmed prune juice and stewed prunes will be the most effective.

♦Eat a large breakfast with some type of hot beverage, such as tea, hot lemon water or decaffeinated coffee.

♦Get enough rest and eat at regular times in a relaxed atmosphere.

♦Get some exercise to stimulate your intestinal reflexes and help restore normal elimination.

impaction, with the liquid stools moving around the impaction. If you decide to take antidiarrheal drugs, you can make the situation much worse.

There are many different ways to treat a wide variety of conditions, and your doctor may recommend several kinds of medications depending on your condition and other personal factors.

◆ *Stool softeners* help the stool retain water and so keep it soft. Stool softeners—Colace (DOSS, docusate sodium, 50 to 240 mg per day with a full glass of water) and Surfak, for example—should be used early, before the stools become hard, especially as it can be days before any effect is noticeable.

◆ *Mild laxatives* help promote bowel activity. Examples are milk of magnesia, Doxidan, cascara sagrada and mineral oil (a lubricant).

◆ *Stronger laxatives* include Phospha-soda (Fleet's), magnesium citrate and senna (Senokot).

◆ *Contact laxatives* such as castor oil or Dulcolax suppositories or tablets cause increased bowel activity.

◆ *Bulk laxatives* include dietary fiber, bran, methyl cellulose (Cellothyl) and psyllium (Metamucil).

◆ Laxatives with magnesium should be avoided if you have kidney disease. Laxatives with sodium should be avoided if you have a heart problem. (Laxatives that contain magnesium can also cause diarrhea.)

◆ If you are taking narcotics you should use stool softeners and mild laxatives rather than bulk-forming laxatives, because the combination can cause high colon constipation.

◆ Non-stimulating bulk softeners such as docusate (Colace) help to soften the stool and mineral oil or olive oil can be used to loosen the stool.

◆ Glycerin suppositories or Dulcolax suppositories may be used to stimulate bowel action as a contact laxative. (Dulcolax may cause cramping.)

◆ Bowel stimulants such as Reglan may be useful.

◆ Lactulose (chronulac) is an acidifier that softens the stool and increases the number of bowel movements.

All laxatives should be used with care. If you use them continually, you might develop a gastrointestinal irritation that can make it difficult to regain your normal bowel habits once you stop taking them. Increasing doses can also make your colon and rectum insensitive to the normal reflexes that stimulate a bowel movement.

Treating Stool Impaction A stool impaction develops when all of a stool doesn't pass through the colon or rectum. The stool gradually gets harder and harder as water is absorbed by the bowel. Then the stool gets larger and larger. If you can't pass it, it may partially obstruct the bowel or cause irritation of the rectum or anus. If you do pass it, it may cause small tears or fissures in the anus.

The primary treatment is to get fluids into the bowel to soften the stool so it can be passed or removed. Using enemas—either oil-retention, tap water or phosphate (Fleet's)—may help accomplish this goal. Sometimes it might be necessary for a health professional to use a gloved finger in the rectum to break up a large bulky mass or to extract the stool.

DIARRHEA

Diarrhea is a condition marked by abnormally frequent bowel movements that are more fluid than usual. It is sometimes accompanied by cramps.

You may get diarrhea because of chemotherapy, radiation therapy to the lower abdomen, malabsorption because of surgery to the bowel or sometimes a bowel inflammation or infection. Some antibiotics, especially "broad spectrum" antibiotics, can cause diarrhea, and it might develop because of an intolerance to milk.

Treating Diarrhea Effective treatment depends on finding the cause. A good general approach is to limit your diet solely to fluids to allow the bowel to rest. Drink plenty of mild liquids, such as fruit drinks (Kool-Aid and Gatorade), ginger ale, peach or apricot nectar, water and weak tea. Hot and cold liquids and foods tend to increase intestinal muscle contractions and make the diarrhea worse, so they should be warm or at room temperature. Allow carbonated beverages to lose their fizz—stir with a spoon—before you drink them.

When you are feeling better, gradually add foods low in roughage and bulk—steamed rice, cream of rice, bananas, applesauce, mashed potatoes, dry toast and crackers—eaten warm or at room temperature.

As your diarrhea decreases, you may move on to a low-residue diet. Frequent small meals will be easier on your digestive tract. Low-residue nutritional supplements such as Precision Low Residue, Vivonex, Flexocal or Citoein can also help.

Foods to Avoid Many types of foods are likely to aggravate your diarrhea and should be avoided. These include:
♦ fatty, greasy and spicy foods;
♦ coffee, regular (non-herbal) teas and carbonated beverages containing caffeine;
♦ citrus fruits such as oranges and grapefruit;
♦ foods high in bulk and fiber, such as bran, whole-grain cereals and breads, popcorn, nuts and raw vegetables and fruits (except apples); and
♦ beverages and foods generally that are served too hot or too cold.

Replacing What Is Lost Diarrhea can cause dehydration, so you will have to drink plenty of fluids. To replace the fluid, sugar and salt you will lose, a good general formula is: 1 quart (1 L) boiled water, 1 tsp. (5 mL) salt, 1 tsp. (5 mL) baking soda, 4 tsp. (20 mL) sugar and flavor to your taste. As with any specially prepared concoction, however, you should check with your dietitian or doctor to make sure you can tolerate the particular ingredients.

Potassium is also lost in diarrhea. It is a necessary mineral, and it must be replaced. Foods high in potassium include bananas, apricot and peach nectars, tomatoes, potatoes, broccoli, halibut, aspara-

---

Diarrhea Medications

♦**Kaopectate**. Take 2 to 4 tablespoons (25 to 50 mL) after each loose bowel movement.

♦**Lomotil**. One to two tablets every four hours as needed. You can take Lomotil with Kaopectate or Imodium. Maximum eight Lomotil tablets per day.

♦**Imodium.** Two capsules initially, then one to two capsules every two to four hours. Maximum 16 capsules per day.

♦**Paregoric**. Take 1 tsp. (5 mL) four times a day. It may be used with Lomotil.

♦**Cholestryamine**. A bile-salt sequestering agent. One packet after each meal and at bedtime.

♦**Donnatal or Robinul**. Anticholinergic, antispasmodic agents for bowel cramping. One to two tablets every four hours as needed.

♦When all else fails, try Metamucil plus Kaopectate.

gus, citrus juices, Coca-Cola and milk. Supplementary potassium tablets sometimes have to be taken.

Milk Intolerance Some people are born with lactose intolerance and some develop it as they grow older. The intolerance results from a deficiency of lactase, an enzyme that digests milk sugar (lactose) in the intestine, and is marked by cramping and diarrhea.

A lactase deficiency can sometimes develop after intestinal surgery, radiation therapy to the lower abdomen or chemotherapy. Because you can no longer digest milk sugar properly, you feel bloated and experience cramping and diarrhea.

♦ If your diarrhea is caused by milk intolerance, you should avoid milk and milk products such as ice cream, cottage cheese and cheese. Depending on how sensitive you are to milk, you may also have to avoid butter, cream and sour cream.

♦ If you are very sensitive, look for lactose-free, non-fat milk solids. You can even make your own lactose-free milk by adding Lactaid—a tablet containing lactase—to your milk and keeping it in the refrigerator for 24 hours before using it.

♦ You can use buttermilk or yogurt because the lactose in them has already been processed and is digested. You might also tolerate some processed cheeses.

♦ You might try Mocha-mix, Dairy Rich and other soy products, or some lactose substitutes like Imo (an imitation sour cream), Cool Whip or Party Whip.

SWOLLEN LIMBS (LYMPHEDEMA)

Lymphedema—the medical term for swelling caused by the buildup of fluid (lymph) in the soft tissues—develops because of some blockage of the lymphatic system. Most lymphedema in cancer patients results from scarring after the surgical removal of lymph nodes or after radiation therapy. It usually involves areas next to large collections of lymph nodes in the armpit (axilla), pelvic region and inguinal (groin) areas. The lymphatics are obstructed and swelling in the arms or legs is the result.

In its early phase, the swelling of the limb will "pit" with finger pressure. Elevating the arm or leg or using an elastic support arm glove or stocking will help reduce the swelling and improve the lymphatic flow.

Acute and Chronic Lymphedema Acute lymphedema may be a temporary condition. It can happen after a radical surgical procedure with lymph node dissection or after an acute inflammation such as an infection in the limb. More often seen in cancer patients is chronic lymphedema. Sometimes it results in only minor swelling and discomfort. But occasionally it can lead to grave disability and disfigurement.

Chronic lymphedema is more difficult to reverse than the acute variety because the more the limb swells the harder it is to drain the fluid adequately. People with chronic lymphedema are also more susceptible to infections or local injuries, which results in more scarring and additional lymphedema. Infections of the limb—known as cellulitis—often develop after even minor cuts or abrasions and they can often only be controlled with long-term antibiotics.

Occasionally lymphedema becomes prolonged and severe. It can be aggravated by poor protein intake that may result from loss of appetite or nausea and vomiting from chemotherapy. It can also be aggravated by a decrease of the protein in the blood called albumin. The decrease results in leakage of water into the tissues, which leads to additional arm or leg swelling.

Who Gets It A small number of people with cancer develop lymphedema. It is not unusual after treatment for several common cancers.

♦ Breast cancer. Primary radiotherapy to the breast is rarely associated with lymphedema. It is more common if you are treated with radiotherapy after surgery to the regional lymph node areas.

♦ Malignant melanomas with lymph node dissection and/or radiation involving an extremity.

♦ Prostate cancer or gynecologic cancers after surgery, with or without radiation.

♦ Testicular cancer with lymph node dissection, with or without radiation.

♦ Patients who have had several courses of radiotherapy to the axilla, shoulder or groin, especially if surgery has also been performed there to treat recurrent cancer.

Hints for Preventing and Controlling Lymphedema

1. Whenever possible, keep the swollen arm or leg elevated, preferably above the level of the heart. When you are sitting, put your leg on a chair or stool.

2. Clean and lubricate your skin every day with oil or skin cream.

3. Do everything you can to avoid injuries and infection in the affected limb:
♦use an electric razor to shave the limb to avoid skin cuts
♦wear gloves when gardening or doing housework and wear thimbles when sewing
♦suntan gradually, if at all, and use a sunscreen
♦avoid walking barefoot, particularly on the beach or wading in water
♦use insect repellants and wear protective clothing to avoid insect bites
♦clean any breaks in your skin with mild soap and water, then apply an antibacterial ointment
♦use gauze wrapping instead of adhesive tape on any skin wounds
♦if you develop a rash, consult your doctor
♦try to minimize all the "invasive" procedures for drawing blood and giving medications—injections, finger pricks and IVs—on the affected arm or leg
♦take good care of your nails and don't cut the cuticles
♦cut your toenails straight across
♦see a podiatrist for any foot care problems
♦keep your feet clean and dry and wear cotton socks
♦avoid extreme hot or cold—ice packs and heating pads, for example—on the swollen limb.

4. Avoid constrictive pressure on your arm or leg:
♦ don't cross your legs while sitting
♦ wear loose jewelry and clothes with no constricting bands
♦ carry handbags on the non-swollen arm
♦ don't use blood pressure cuffs on the swollen limb
♦ wear only elastic bandages or stockings without constrictive bands
♦ don't sit longer than 30 minutes without changing position.

5. Check the limb daily for signs of change. Especially watch for signs of infection—redness, pain, heat, swelling or fever—and call your doctor immediately if any signs appear. Be sure to report any sensation of swelling or sudden increase in fluid.

6. Practice your drainage-promoting exercises faithfully.

7. After the limb has healed, *gradually* return to your normal activity. But always practice protective procedures—edema can come back if you get an injury.

Preventing Lymphedema If you have had any of the above procedures, you will have to take extra special care of the limb that might be affected. You should treat your arm or leg with the same care and attention you give to your face.

You can do a lot to prevent lymphedema—good nutrition with a high-protein diet, active physical exercise to help your muscles pump the lymphatic fluid, control of obesity. You should also try hard to avoid infections from small cuts you might get working around the house or by doing physical work that might damage or injure the skin on the affected arm or leg.

Even if you follow a prevention program faithfully, lymphedema can occasionally develop years after surgery. This often happens after a local infection, although sometimes it happens for no apparent reason at all. If you develop any evidence of inflammation or infection (cellulitis) with redness or increased swelling, report it to your doctor. He or she can evaluate your condition and prescribe any necessary antibiotics. You may have to stay on antibiotics for several weeks or even months.

Milking Your Muscles Exercising your muscles is vital if you want to prevent lymphedema. It is just as vital if you want to control it. The compression of your muscles helps to milk the fluid in the lymphatics back toward your heart.

Physical therapists can recommend the most appropriate exercises for you. Many people are often encouraged to walk or ride a bicycle to help improve the lymphatic flow. Breast cancer patients are usually instructed to go through a series of hand and arm exercises after surgery. A similar program is used by patients with melanomas involving the limbs. Therapists can instruct you in the use of lymphedema milking pumps that can reduce your swelling, which can be an effective approach for chronic lymphedema.

HAIR LOSS

Losing your hair (alopecia) can be quite an emotional experience. As the most visible side effect of cancer treatment, it is often the most upsetting. In fact, you may find it helpful to have your mate or a close friend or relative with you when you talk to your doctor about the potential for hair loss.

Why You Might Lose Your Hair Chemotherapy drugs circulate throughout your body and they aren't selective about which cells they affect. They change normal as well as malignant cells and have an especially destructive effect on rapidly growing cells like your hair and the cells lining your mouth and gastrointestinal tract. So hair loss is a common side effect of chemotherapy, especially with drugs such as Cytoxan, Adriamycin and vincristine. Your chances of losing your hair are increased if you are getting combination therapy.

When You Lose Your Hair You may not lose all your hair. It may just become thin or patchy. The loss might also be sudden or gradual. It usually happens within the first cycle (usually around Week 3), but it may not happen until the second cycle. And, whether the loss is partial or complete, you may develop some scalp irritation, dermatitis or scaling that will need medical attention.

The hair almost always comes back. It may take three to six months or it might come back while you are still on chemotherapy. When it does come back it might have a slightly different texture or color or curl.

Hair Loss and Radiation You might lose some hair after radiation therapy to the skull or brain. This may be total and permanent, but if lower doses are used the hair sometimes comes back within two to three months.

Preparing for Hair Loss This is one side effect you can plan for well in advance.

There are several things you can do before you begin treatment that will make losing your hair not quite as upsetting.

♦ Get a short haircut so that the hair loss won't be as noticeable either to others or to you when you look in the mirror.

♦ Treat your hair and your scalp gently by avoiding hairsprays, perms and dyes.

♦ Select hair covers that you'll need during the period of hair loss—turbans, scarves, hats, wigs and scarves with hair fringes that look like your own hair. Many insurance companies will pay for a hair piece or wig since they are a "part" of treatment, so ask your doctor for a prescription. To get the best possible match, buy a wig before you lose your hair.

Tourniquets and Ice Caps Scalp tourniquets and ice caps can be used to prevent or reduce hair loss. But they are not very useful when the chemotherapy drugs tend to stay in the bloodstream for several hours or if the drugs are taken orally, which leads to the same time effect. Even so, using caps and tourniquets during therapy might make you feel better by reducing anxiety.

Tourniquets and ice caps are *not* recommended if you are being treated for cancers that are likely to have hidden scalp metastases—melanoma, kidney cancer, leukemia, lymphomas and tumors that spread in the bloodstream.

18
MAINTAINING GOOD NUTRITION

Ernest H. Rosenbaum, MD, Malin Dollinger, MD, Lawrence Margolis, MD, and Isadora Rosenbaum, MA

◇

Good nutrition is vital to all of us all the time. It is impossible to stay in good health without consuming the right foods in the right amounts. Good nutrition gives us the energy and the building blocks our bodies need to function properly and stay in good repair.

Good nutrition is even more necessary when you have cancer. Your body is fighting disease and food is a critical weapon in the fight. You will need even more nutrients than usual—a metabolic need about 20 percent higher than a healthy person who engages in moderate activity. The extra nutrients will help your body fend off weakness, repair damaged tissues, help boost your immune system and create a feeling of general well-being.

COMMON PROBLEMS

Many people with cancer have a hard time maintaining good nutrition since the cancer itself and the therapies that fight it can make it hard to eat enough food. (*See* Chapter 17.) There are several major common problems.

♦ *Loss of appetite* This is the most serious problem. Pain, nausea, vomiting, diarrhea, constipation or a sore or dry mouth can easily make you lose interest in food. You may also tend to eat less because of fear, anxiety or depression about having cancer.

♦ *Malabsorption* For a number of reasons, nutrients may not be absorbed normally into the bloodstream from the intestines. Cancer of the pancreas can cause a decrease in the digestive juices that regulate absorption. Abnormal connections between surgically created loops in the intestine may divert food past the parts of the intestine where nutrients are usually absorbed. The intestines may become less able to absorb nutrients if your normal food intake is reduced for a lengthy time.

♦ *Physical problems* Tumors in the mouth and neck area, as well as radiation therapy directed to those areas, can make it hard to swallow or cause pain in the mouth or throat. Radiation directed to the abdomen or the removal of part of the stomach or intestinal tract can cause diarrhea, cramps or decreased absorption.

♦ *Changes in smell and taste* Chemotherapy or radiation to the neck and mouth can distort the perception of smell and taste, and the loss of taste tends to be greater if the tumor is more advanced. Some foods can start to taste bitter or rancid, especially meat, which might taste bitter and metallic. It is common to develop strong aversions to foods such as meat, eggs, fried foods or tomatoes. All these changes make your appetite worse, making it even more difficult for you to avoid weight loss.

♦ *Early filling* The feeling of being full after taking only a few bites of food is a common problem and will lead to weight loss if you try to stick to the usual three meals a day.

Because of all these problems, many people with cancer become malnourished almost to the point of starvation. And malnutrition can have very serious effects.

THE DANGERS OF WEIGHT LOSS AND MALNUTRITION

Malnutrition affects your whole body, making you steadily weaker. It can also decrease your immunity and make you more susceptible to infections. It can promote tissue breakdown that can lead to "fistulas"—leakage from the natural gastrointestinal tract—and poor healing of any surgical wounds. Malnutrition can also worsen any problem of malabsorption of food you may have as a side effect of treatment, resulting in cramping, bloating and diarrhea.

But the worst effect of malnutrition is the excessive weight loss so often seen in cancer patients. Losing a great deal of weight unfortunately sets up a vicious cycle. A decreased appetite and weight loss lead to fatigue and depression. Depression and progressive weakness lead to reduced activity and an even smaller appetite. More weight loss and weakness lead to a lower resistance to disease and a decrease in immunity. Lower resistance may limit the amount of chemotherapy, radiation therapy or surgery that can be delivered, leading to a poorer prognosis.

Anyone with cancer who is potentially curable may fail to be cured because of poor nutritional management.

Planning for Improved Nutrition The key to keeping this cycle at bay is to do everything in your power to prevent malnutrition from occurring in the first place. Once weight loss begins, it is hard to reverse. The time to start thinking and planning for proper nutrition is not when you have already lost a lot of weight but when the diagnosis is made or your treatment gets under way.

If you lose more than 5 percent of your usual weight, you and your doctor should consider the loss significant. Losing 10 percent of your normal weight is a danger signal. A 15 percent weight loss may result in a further decrease in your

---

HOW MANY CALORIES AND HOW MUCH PROTEIN DO YOU NEED?

Your normal weight   _____pounds

Your desirable weight   _____pounds

♦ Your *minimum* daily protein requirement =   _____grams
desirable weight (pounds) x 0.5

♦ Your *minimum* daily calorie requirement =   _____calories
desirable weight (pounds) x 18 (men)
desirable weight (pounds) x 16 (women)

♦ Keep a daily record of your weight
(and your protein and calorie intake).

If you are losing weight, increase your protein and calorie intake to:

protein grams = desirable weight x 0.7 =   _____grams

calories: desirable weight x 20 (men) =   _____calories

calories: desirable weight x 18 (women) =   _____calories

---

appetite, depression, fatigue and progressive weakness that will limit your chance of recovery.

Good nutritional management and careful food selection may also be necessary to avoid *gaining* a substantial amount of weight. Some patients, especially those receiving chemotherapy, tend to use eating as a way of managing nausea. Some of the hormones used to manage breast cancer can also stimulate the appetite.

THE BEST APPROACH TO EATING

What you will need is a totally different approach to eating. Forget the signals that have always told you when to start eating and when to stop. They will no longer be a reliable guide. You will have to approach eating as a necessary part of your therapy and learn to eat even if you don't feel like it.

Nutritional support is usually best directed by your physician and dietitian, preferably at the start of therapy. But the hospital nutritionist can plan an individualized program for you after two or three days of observation and analysis of any deficits in your intake of calories, protein or fat. You and your family can be instructed in basic nutritional requirements, such as the four basic food groups—protein, milk, vegetable-fruit and bread-cereal.

The nutritionist can also explain how you can deal with the special dietary problems associated with cancer and cancer therapy, such as anorexia, bloating, heartburn, constipation, diarrhea, nausea, vomiting, sore or dry mouth, indigestion and taste blindness.

Special Diets Your nutritional needs may change during therapy. After surgery, for example, you may need to go on a liquid diet and work your way up through a soft diet before getting back to your regular foods. You may need a lactose-restricted diet, a high-fiber diet and/or a high-protein diet. You might also need special food supplements, either with or between meals, to increase your daily intake of nutrients.

These might include lactose-free high-calorie, high-protein drinks such as Ensure, Resource, Sustacal and Nutren.

Some chemotherapy drugs can prevent absorption or cause the depletion of certain vitamins and minerals. Your doctor or dietitian may advise you to take oral supplements to counter the depletion of magnesium caused by cisplatin. 5-fluorouracil may cause a loss of potassium, which can be replaced with medication and/or a diet rich in apricots, bananas, oranges and potatoes.

There are diets to prevent kidney stones from forming and diets to prevent diarrhea, constipation, nausea and vomiting. There are diets to help improve taste and appetite. All of these preventive and palliative techniques, including occupational therapy to improve your ability to swallow, can be used along with other supportive programs to control depression, relieve any pain and promote physical activity.

Fad diets may be very tempting and appear to follow sound medical principles, but they can be dangerous. They may not supply the macro- and micronutrients you need during this special time. Macrobiotic diets are not recommended.

A Team Effort With guidance from your doctor, the nutritionist and a few good pamphlets and brochures, you and your family should be able to handle most nutritional problems at home.

And remember that good nutrition is a team effort. It requires not only the expertise of nutritionists and the medical team but the tact and concerned attention of family and friends. Your support team should know that you will be more likely to respond to enjoyable company and gen-

Guidelines for Overcoming Weight Loss

♦ Help ease the problem of early filling by eating smaller portions of food more frequently throughout the day and by drinking fluids between meals instead of with food.

♦ Eat by the clock at regularly scheduled times. Your appetite signal may not be intact.

♦ Snack between meals with high-protein diet supplements, milkshakes, eggnogs and puddings.

♦ Add extra calories to your diet by adding cream or butter to soups, cooked cereals and vegetables and by using gravies and sauces with vegetables, meat, poultry and fish.

♦ Add extra protein to your diet by using fortified milk, peanut butter, cheese and chopped hard-boiled eggs.

♦ Taste blindness makes it critical that you do everything you can to enhance the smell, appearance and texture of food. So cook dishes that appeal to your sense of smell and be especially creative with desserts.

♦ Choose foods that you like, within any dietary restrictions your doctor or nutritionist tell you about.

♦ Exercise about half an hour before meals to stimulate your appetite.

♦ Make mealtimes pleasant by doing relaxation exercises beforehand to reduce stress, by setting an attractive and colorful table and by eating with family or friends.

♦ Plan daily menus in advance. If possible, prepare many portions of food and have them frozen and ready to heat and serve.

tle encouragement than to harassment and manipulation. The preparation, serving and sharing of food expresses the concern of care givers, family and friends. And that concern can have a direct effect on your sense of well-being.

Also remember that planning for good nutrition early in your disease not only may result in your being able to take more intensive therapy but can also make the difference between survival and death.

So eat often and well. You will feel better mentally and physically. You will heal faster after surgery and have fewer unpleasant side effects from radiation or chemotherapy. You may be able to tolerate more chemotherapy. Your radiotherapy will not have to be interrupted as often. Your immune system will be better

able to resist infection. And, not least, you will be able to lead a more active and enjoyable life.

TUBE AND INTRA-VENOUS FEEDINGS—ORAL SUPPLEMENTS

The *ideal* way to get enough food is by eating normally—put the food in your mouth, chew it well and swallow. The food is absorbed naturally, using a functional gastrointestinal tract to meet nutritional needs. This is also the least expensive method of nutritional support.

But there are times when normal eating just isn't practical. You may not be able to swallow. You might be suffering through a bout of nausea, vomiting or diarrhea.

Your mouth, throat, esophagus or stomach might be so inflamed that you can neither chew nor swallow. You might also have some obstruction or irritation in the gastrointestinal tract.

These kinds of problems are not unusual after surgery, chemotherapy or radiotherapy. And it is when you have these kinds of problems that the possibility of malnutrition becomes a critical concern. Your body must somehow get enough nutrients.

Enteral Nutrition As long as your stomach and bowel are still working properly, enteral—or tube—feedings can be a practical and low-cost way of providing good nutrition.

Feeding tubes can be placed:
♦ through your mouth (orogastric);
♦ through your nose (nasogastric); or
♦ directly into your stomach through the abdominal wall (gastrostomy) or the small bowel (jejunostomy). This can be done during or after surgery, when the need for high-calorie and high-protein nutrition is most critical. There is also a technique called percutaneous gastrostomy (PEG) that allows a stomach tube to be placed through the skin into the stomach without the need for surgery.

Oral and Enteral Formulas Obviously, solid food can't be delivered to your stomach or jejunum through a tube. So you will need enteral feeding formulas, which can be prepared by pureeing food, or you can buy any of the nutritionally complete formulas your physician or nutritionist might prescribe. Which formula to use depends on your individual situation. There are special formulas for lactose intolerance (lactose-free) and for high-calorie, high-protein intake. Or you may need a low-residue and/or chemically defined liquid diet.
♦ Ensure, Resource, Sustacal and Meritine are soy-based, lactose-free, low-residue, high-calorie, high-protein supplements in beverage form.
♦ Lactose-free (unflavored) supplements used mainly for tube feeding diets include Nutren, Isocal, Osmolite and Jevity. All except Jevity are also low residue.
♦ Vital-HN, Vivonex-TEN and Peptamen are low-residue, lactose-free chemically defined diets with hydrolyzed protein and crystalline amino acids and/or dipeptides. These are useful when you have malabsorption problems or an inflammatory disease like gastroenteritis.
♦ Glucerna and Vitaneed are special supplements used for tube feedings for diabetics.
♦ Nepro (high protein) and Suplena (low protein) are specific electrolyte-controlled supplements used in cases of renal deficiency. Glucerna, Nepro and Suplena can also be taken by mouth.

Side Effects of Enteral Feeding Though effective in delivering enough nutrition, feedings through nasogastric tubes can produce some side effects.
♦ You may suffer some throat irritation, nausea or vomiting.
♦ Some formulas, including cold or concentrated formulas, may cause diarrhea. The formula may have to be changed to lactose-free isotonic solutions at room temperature.
♦ Impaction and constipation can occasionally develop, possibly leading to an obstruction in the intestine.

Parenteral Nutrition When neither oral nor enteral nutrition methods are appropriate, you can still get all the nutrients you need through a process called total parenteral nutrition (TPN), formerly called hyperalimentation. What it means is that you get all the proteins, carbohydrates, fats, vitamins and minerals you need intravenously.

While you are receiving TPN, you may also eat solids and drink fluids, although TPN sometimes decreases the appetite.

SPECIAL PROBLEMS OF RADIATION PATIENTS

Radiation oncologists try to select the most effective dose of radiation to destroy a tumor while still protecting normal tissues. Nonetheless, there are often acute effects during treatment, mainly on rapidly growing tissues that are in the radiation field such as the skin, the mucous membranes (mucosa) in the esophagus, the bladder, small intestine and rectum. These tissues usually heal within a few weeks after radiation. There may also be late chronic effects that can result in the formation of scar tissue, ulcerations or damage to an organ.

Depending on which part of the body is irradiated, you may develop special problems that will affect your ability to get enough nutrition. But many of these problems can be prevented or eased by careful planning and treatment. Your close cooperation with your radiation oncologist and dietitian will let you complete your treatment with as few side effects as possible.

Mouth Problems Radiation to the mouth and throat may result in painful sores on membranes (mucositis), dry mouth, dental problems and taste changes or the loss of taste.

♦ *Dental problems* If you are getting radiation to the oral cavity or pharynx, a complete dental evaluation is essential before treatment. Your teeth should be x-rayed and any decayed teeth either repaired or removed. If you have to have a tooth extracted, the site must be completely healed before treatment to avoid late and irreversible bone damage. Radiation treatment should generally not start until about 14 days after any extraction. Your other teeth should be treated daily with a topical fluoride to help prevent cavities.

♦ *Mucositis* Radiation mucositis fre-quently occurs after radiation to the head and neck. If the membranes lining your mouth and throat are inflamed, you will need a nourishing soft diet. Sharp-edged or salty foods, such as pretzels and potato chips, should be avoided. So should extremely hot or cold, acidic or spicy foods that may irritate the membranes even more. You should also stop drinking alcoholic beverages and smoking or chewing all forms of tobacco immediately, since they can irritate the mouth and throat.

When you have mucositis, good oral hygiene is crucial. Frequent use of a gentle mouthwash can help reduce discomfort or pain, especially if you use a solution of baking soda and salt dissolved in warm water instead of commercial mouthwashes that might irritate the mucosa.

If the mucositis is severe and interferes with eating or drinking, you can use a topical anesthetic such as viscous Xylocaine, gargling 1 tsp. (5 mL) before meals. A slurry of sucralfate (Carafate)—prepared by dissolving sucralfate in water and sorbitol, which is available at most drug stores—can also coat the oral membranes and soothe any discomfort.

Your radiation oncologist will have to check your mucositis carefully and often to rule out monilia (fungus) infection. These infections can be treated locally or systemically with mycostatin (Nystatin) oral suspension or tablets, ketoconazole (Nizoral) or Diflucan.

♦ *Dry mouth* Xerostomia, or dry mouth, isn't unusual after radiation to the mouth or pharynx, since you can't produce as much saliva after irradiation of the salivary glands. This may be a temporary condition, though if the total dose exceeds 4,000 cGy, you may have some degree of permanent mouth dryness. You can minimize symptoms by using an artificial saliva such as Salivart, moisturizing gels such as Oral Balance and a special dry-mouth toothpaste such as Biotene. It will also help if you increase your intake of fluids, particularly with meals, and if you use creams, gravies and sauces to moisten dry, hard food.

♦ *Loss of taste* Irradiation of the taste buds can make you lose your sense of taste. The decrease in, or the thickening of, saliva from irradiation of the salivary glands can contribute to the problem too. Taste will usually come back within two months after radiation treatment is completed.

Problems in the Esophagus Radiation is frequently delivered to the upper chest (thorax) to treat lung cancer, esophageal cancer and lymphoma. And the esophagus usually has to be within the radiation port. If you get doses over 3,000 cGy in three weeks, the lining of your esophagus may

---

ENTERITIS: Hints on Food Tolerance

Foods to Avoid

♦ Whole-grain or high-bran breads and cereals.

♦ Nuts, seeds, coconut, beans and legumes.

♦ Fried, greasy or fatty foods, which may be hard to digest.

♦ Fresh and dried fruit and some fruit juices (such as prune juice).

♦ Raw vegetables.

♦ Rich pastries.

♦ Popcorn, potato chips and pretzels.

♦ Strong spices and herbs.

♦ Chocolate, coffee, tea and soft drinks containing caffeine.

♦ Alcohol and tobacco.

♦ Milk and milk products. Exceptions are buttermilk and yogurt, which are often tolerated because lactose is altered in the presence of lactobacillus. You might be able to tolerate processed cheese, because the lactose has been removed. You may use milkshake supplements such as Ensure, which are lactose-free.

Foods to Enjoy

♦ Fish, poultry and meat (preferably broiled or roasted).

♦ Bananas, apple juice, peeled apples, apple and grape juices.

♦ White bread and toast.

♦ Macaroni and noodles.

♦ Baked, boiled or mashed potatoes.

♦ Cooked vegetables that are mild, such as asparagus tips, green and wax beans, carrots, spinach and squash.

♦ Mild processed cheese, eggs, smooth peanut butter, buttermilk and yogurt.

Helpful Hints

♦ Eat foods at room temperature.

♦ Drink 12 glasses of fluids per day. Let soft drinks and other carbonated beverages go flat before you drink them. You can help the process along by stirring the drink until the bubbles disappear.

♦ Add nutmeg to food. This will help to increase mobility of the gastrointestinal tract.

♦ Start a low residue diet on Day 1 of radiation therapy.

---

react, causing some pain when you swallow. The reaction will go away gradually. But it is possible that the daily dose can be reduced or your treatment interrupted for a short period to allow rapid healing.

In the meantime, a soft, bland diet, antacids and a topical anesthetic such as a viscous Xylocaine (lidocaine) solution will often minimize the symptoms. A slurry of sucralfate will coat the esophagus and soothe the discomfort as it does in the mouth. If symptoms persist, you may have a candida infection, which can be effectively treated with ketoconazole (Nizoral) or mycostatin (Nystatin).

Problems in the Bowel (Radiation Enteritis) With their rapidly dividing cells, the membranes lining the large and small bowel and the rectum are quite sensitive to even low doses of radiation. So any radiation delivered to the upper abdomen or pelvis can cause an irritation of the bowel known as radiation enteritis.

Only 5 to 15 percent of people treated with radiation to the abdomen will develop chronic problems, and the severity of the symptoms will depend on several factors—how much of the abdomen or pelvis is irradiated, the daily dose, the total dosage required and the possible use of chemotherapy at the same time. People with a history of abdominal surgery, pelvic inflammatory disease, atherosclerosis, diabetes or hypertension are also more likely to suffer radiation injury.

Symptoms If you are getting radiation to the upper abdomen, you may experience bouts of nausea and vomiting. Pelvic irradiation is more likely to cause irritation in the rectum, frequent bowel movements or watery diarrhea. These disturbances to the intestinal mucosa may change the way your gastrointestinal tract absorbs nutrients from the food you eat. It may become much more difficult to absorb fat, bile salts and vitamin B_{12}, for example.

Your doctor will evaluate the extent of the enteritis by assessing how often you have diarrhea, the character of the stools, whether you have any rectal bleeding and whether your abdomen is enlarged (distended). He or she will also watch for possible dehydration or an electrolyte mineral imbalance in your blood resulting from diarrhea and/or malabsorption.

Managing Enteritis The medical management of radiation enteritis includes dietary changes, medication and, in severe cases, an interruption of radiation treatment. If you are getting abdominal or pelvic radiation you should start on a low-fat, low-fiber, low-residue diet right from the beginning of treatment.

Medications If radiation enteritis persists despite changes in your diet, it may be necessary to reduce the daily dose of radiation to the abdomen and pelvis. You may also have to use medications such as:

◆ Kaopectate (2 to 4 tablespoons/25 to 50 mL after each loose bowel movement).

◆ Lomotil (one to two tablets every four to six hours as needed to a maximum of eight tablets a day). Most patients find they need only two or three tablets per day after the diarrhea has been controlled.

◆ Imodium (two capsules initially, followed by one capsule after each loose stool, the total dosage not to exceed 16 capsules per day). Imodium is also available in a liquid form (half-dose strength) that does not require a prescription.

◆ Donnatal or Robinul (one or two tablets every four hours for abdominal cramping).

◆ Paregoric (1 tsp./5 mL orally every four hours for diarrhea).

◆ Compazine (10 mg every four hours), Ativan (1 mg every two to four hours) or Reglan tablets or liquid (10 mg four times daily, 30 minutes before each meal and at bedtime) can usually control nausea.

19
CONTROLLING PAIN

Eliot S. Krames, MD, FACPM, Ernest H. Rosenbaum, MD, and Malin Dollinger, MD

"Pain is an even more terrible lord of mankind than even death itself."
— *Albert Schweitzer*

—————◇—————

Fear of pain is a large part of any patient's fear of cancer. Sixty to 90 percent of people with advanced cancer develop pain severe enough that they need some type of pain-relieving therapy, so this is a realistic concern. But not all cancers produce pain equally, and some cancers, even when advanced, may not cause pain at all. Cancers involving bone, either directly or through spread, or the abdomen are usually associated with pain when advanced. Cancers of the blood system such as leukemias or lymphomas may not be.

Pain can have a terrible effect on the way you live. It can lead to depression, loss of appetite, irritability, withdrawal from social interaction, anger, loss of sleep and an inability to cope. If uncontrolled, pain can destroy the very fabric of your life and your will to live.

Fortunately, pain *can* be controlled. What is needed is an understanding by your caregivers of the nature of the pain, of what causes it and of the appropriate treatments for the type of pain involved, as well as a commitment to relieving it. Your doctor and/or pain specialist are well equipped to handle your pain.

SOURCES OF PAIN

Pain is a complex phenomenon. It certainly has physical causes, but has emotional and psychologic components too. How each individual responds to pain is also complex. The extent of disease and the type of pain contribute to the painful experience. But pain is also modified by remembrances of past painful experiences, the special meaning of pain to each individual, the expectations of family and friends, religious upbringing, racial background and personal coping skills and strategies.

Cultural background and beliefs also play a part. Certain cultures teach tolerance of pain or that the outward expression of pain is inappropriate. People from these cultures bear their pain without complaining or even expressing their needs. They appear to have a higher threshold or tolerance to pain. Other cultures readily and outwardly express painful experiences and appear to have a low threshold or tolerance.

Types of Pain Not all pains are the same. There are two kinds of physical pain, and recognizing their differences is the key to selecting appropriate treatment plans. Patients generally use different words to describe these two types of pain. One type is called somatic pain and is often described as sharp, dull, throbbing or aching. A second type, neuropathic pain, is often described as sharp, shooting, electrical or lightning-like.

Most pains we experience in our daily lives—the pains from cuts and bruises or pains from broken bones or surgery—are usually somatic pain. Some pains from bone cancer or cancer of abdominal organs such as the stomach or colon may also be somatic. These somatic pains usually respond to narcotic therapies and are well suited to treatment according to guidelines for cancer pain management developed by the World Health Organization (WHO).

Neuropathic pain is totally different. This type of pain is caused either by damage to the peripheral or central nervous system or by the abnormal processing of painful information in the central nervous system caused by such damage. Examples might include pain due to nerves being damaged by chemotherapy drugs, surgery or radiation, to a tumor pressing on nerves or to the direct invasion of cancers into nervous tissue. Neuropathic pain is often resistant to or unresponsive to narcotic therapies. The dosages of narcotics needed to control this type of pain may be greater than the dosages used to control somatic pain. Sometimes, caregivers may have to choose other forms of medications or other pain treatments to relieve neuropathic pain.

Unfortunately, not everyone has purely somatic or neuropathic pain. Some people may have both, and choosing a treatment to fit the pain type in patients who have mixed somatic and neuropathic pain can be difficult.

Physical Sources Cancer pain can be caused by the cancer itself, the drugs used to control or cure cancer, surgical treatments or radiation therapy. People with cancer can also have all the pains that people without cancer have—back pain from a "slipped disk," a broken bone from a skiing accident or daily headaches from stress. In other words, the onset of pain or the development of a new pain does not necessarily come from the cancer or mean that the disease has spread.

♦ Somatic pain from the cancer itself may come from a bone that breaks because the tumor has weakened the bone structure or from an obstruction in the intestine or urinary tract.

♦ Neuropathic pains may come from the spread of the tumor directly into nerves, such as the spread of colon cancer into the pelvis where the nerves to the legs or pelvic structures reside. Neuropathic pain may also result from pressure on the nerves, as in spinal tumors pressing on or pinching nerves to the arms or legs.

♦ Surgery may cause both somatic and neuropathic pain. Pain from the surgery itself is somatic and usually responds to narcotic medications, but surgical damage to nerves may cause burning, shooting pains that do not respond to narcotics.

♦ Chemotherapeutic drugs act like poisons to tumors and may act the same way on some vulnerable nerves. Drugs such as antiviral agents or vincristine can cause peripheral neuropathy, which is often felt as a burning in the hands and feet. This may respond to narcotics, but may also require drugs specific for neuropathic pain or some other intervention for relief. The sore mouth (mucositis) that is sometimes a side effect of these drugs is one example of somatic pain from chemotherapy.

♦ With radiotherapy, pain may be due to skin reactions to the radiation, breakdown of mucous membranes or even scarring of the nerves (fibrosis), which can produce a neuropathic pain.

Emotional Sources Pain is made worse by worry and fear—fear of death, suffering, deformity, financial disability or isolation. The onset of pain or a new pain may trigger fears about the spread of the disease or of impending death. All these fears can be magnified when a kind of pain in the spirit comes on. This might be triggered by surroundings, low levels of emotional support or feelings of loneliness and desperation. How you approach the problems of life makes a big difference to how you perceive pain. And that makes a big difference to whether your pain is controlled.

THE TREATMENT PLAN

Treating and controlling pain is a primary concern for all members of the health care team, including your doctors, nurses and any consultants, such as pain care specialists, involved in your care. Ongoing assessment of the types of pain that develop and change during the course of the cancer is essential to prescribing appropriate pain treatments.

Your doctor will assess your pain before administering therapy. He or she will ask you about the nature of the pain, to describe it, locate it and describe any changes in its nature over time. Questions about successful or unsuccessful therapies in treating your pain are also important. The goal of pain therapy is complete and total pain relief and comfort, but sometimes this goal may not be obtainable. Reasonable expectations should be discussed with your caregivers early and often during therapy. Your support group—friends and family and others—should be in on these discussions.

The Pain Control Ladder According to the WHO committee on cancer pain, 90 to 95 percent of all cancer pain can be well controlled using a set of guidelines called the Pain Control Ladder. These guidelines separate pain into levels of intensity and suggest tailoring the strength and potency of prescribed pain-relieving medications to the intensity. Not all cancer pain requires strong narcotics. But *strong* pain requires *strong* medications.

The guidelines suggest that:
♦ mild pain be treated with non-narcotic medications such as aspirin, acetaminophen (Tylenol) or other aspirin-like drugs called non-steroidal anti-inflammatory drugs (NSAIDs);
♦ moderate pain be treated with a combination of NSAIDs and weak narcotics such as codeine (Tylenol with codeine), hydrocodone (Vicodin or Lortab), Percocet, Percodan or propoxyphene (Darvon); and
♦ severe pain be treated with strong opioids such as morphine, Demerol, Dilaudid, fentanyl or methadone in combination with an NSAID.

The guidelines also suggest adding an adjuvant medication to these narcotic and non-narcotic medications, where appro-

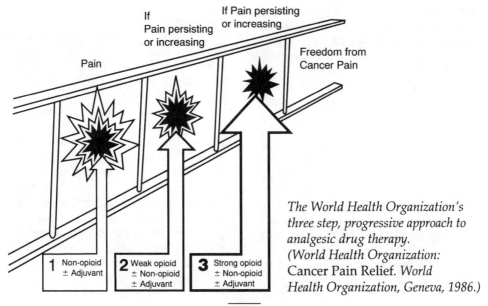

The World Health Organization's three step, progressive approach to analgesic drug therapy. (World Health Organization: Cancer Pain Relief. World Health Organization, Geneva, 1986.)

priate. These medications—which include steroids, antidepressant and anticonvulsant medications, antihistamines and sedatives—are often useful in treating opioid-resistant pain. For whatever reason, they do relieve pain although they are not usually labeled as pain relievers.

Simple measures such as aspirin or Tylenol, with or without codeine, or ibuprofen may do the job well enough. But when pain is severe, the dosage has to be increased or the drug has to be taken more frequently. If these simple measures don't help, then you have to step up the ladder, increasing the strength or potency of the medication. Sometimes, just the addition of an adjuvant medication is all that is needed.

Side Effects Not all people tolerate all drugs equally. Some people are allergic to various medications. Some develop side effects from medications that others taking the same drugs do not share. Some people tolerate one specific drug in a class of drugs, but do not tolerate others in the same class. Some do not tolerate any drugs in a particular class. Everyone is an individual.

WHO guidelines suggest that doctors try a given drug in a class to see if the patient will tolerate it. The dosage is increased until the patient gets either pain relief or intolerable side effects. Side effects that may occur with narcotic medications include nausea, vomiting, constipation, sedation, difficulty in urinating or hallucinations.

Medication is tailored not only to your needs but according to your tolerances. If you cannot tolerate one drug (too many side effects), another drug is tried before abandoning that class of drugs. The guidelines also suggest that if side effects occur, they be managed with side-effect treatments—drugs for nausea, constipation, loss of appetite or sedation and so on—before abandoning the therapy.

Treatment Options Why do some patients fail to respond to these guidelines? Some pains don't respond to narcotics at all and some may require extremely high doses for pain control. Some patients may achieve pain control with a given dose of narcotic when they are lying quietly in bed, but their pain increases as soon as they are moved. This type of narcotic-resistant pain is called incident pain.

Besides physical reasons for not responding to the narcotic ladder approach, there are other reasons why patients do not get good pain control. Just as beliefs and experiences color the experience of pain, the beliefs and knowledge of caregivers, patients and their families influence whether patients receive appropriate pain care. Doctors may be uncertain about the role of narcotic therapy for patients with early pain or treatment-related pain. They may under-treat the pain because of a lack of knowledge of narcotic therapy, failure to assess the type of pain adequately or because they overestimate the risks of addiction. Your own and your family's beliefs about narcotic treatment, fears of addiction and under-reporting of pain may also lead to poor pain control.

If 90 to 95 percent of patients receive adequate pain control using the narcotic ladder, what about the 5 to 10 percent who do not have their pain controlled by these guidelines? Certain direct interventions by specialists can modify or block pain information from reaching the central nervous system. These interventions include "nerve blocks," alternative delivery systems—such as administering narcotics under the skin (subcutaneous) or into the spine—spinal local anesthetics or therapies that destroy nerves causing the pain. These invasive, interventional therapies may require the expertise and skills of a pain specialist to whom your doctor may refer you if needed.

MYTHS ABOUT NARCOTICS AND CANCER PAIN

A lot of cancer patients want to avoid taking narcotics. Many have fears that they will become addicted to these medications and some feel that narcotics should be used only as a last resort for fear that they will not be effective when they are "really needed." Doctors may also share some of the "myths" about narcotic medications. These myths form barriers to good and effective relief of cancer pain. These myths need to be understood and addressed by patients and their caregivers.

Myth 1. *People given narcotics for pain control are always doing worse or are near death.*

Just because a person is placed on a narcotic does *not* mean that he or she is gravely ill. Narcotics are highly effective medications that can be used at any stage in the disease when severe pain requires strong medication.

Myth 2. *All patients getting morphine or other narcotics will become addicts.*

Addiction is a psychologic need for a drug and rarely, if ever, develops in people using narcotics for pain control. Physical dependence, however, always occurs in patients taking narcotics for a long time. Physical dependence is a problem only when a patient is suddenly taken off the drug. If this happens, a physical reaction, called withdrawal syndrome, takes place. If your disease becomes cured during therapy and you no longer need narcotic medications, they can be withdrawn slowly so that the withdrawal syndrome does not develop. The bottom line is that *physical dependence does not equal addiction.*

Myth 3. *Patients who take narcotic medications develop tolerance and always need more and more medicine.*

There are many reasons behind the need for increased doses of a narcotic. One is spreading disease or a change in the type of pain, such as a new neuropathic pain problem developing with tumor spread.

Another reason is tolerance, which is defined as an increasing dose of a drug needed to achieve a desired result. Tolerance, if it develops at all, does not develop suddenly, and doctors can respond to its development by increasing the dose you are taking. Remember, narcotic medications do not have a "dose ceiling." If you no longer get pain relief at one dose level, the dose can be increased again and again. The sky is the limit.

Myth 4. *Narcotics are dangerous because they can make breathing harder for a terminally ill patient.*

Morphine and other narcotic drugs are not dangerous respiratory depressants in patients with cancer and pain. Doses are gradually increased and tolerance to the respiratory-depressant effects of these drugs usually develops before tolerance to their pain-relieving effects.

Myth 5. *People taking narcotics always have to get shots since narcotics are poorly absorbed by mouth.*

Most narcotics are absorbed very well when taken orally. A fair amount of the dose taken by mouth is "lost" to non-target body tissues and therefore wasted, however, so larger dosages of the drug are required than the doses needed for shots. The pain equivalency between oral and intramuscular (shots) morphine is 3 to 1 when taken over time, meaning that 30 mg of oral morphine is equivalent to 10 mg of morphine by shot.

USING MORPHINE AND OTHER NARCOTICS

Morphine remains the gold standard of medical practice. Morphine and other narcotics can be taken in a variety of ways. All methods control pain very effectively.

♦ Intravenous or direct IV morphine can be used when you are in the hospital or even at home. This route delivers the drug directly into the bloodstream. A single IV dose rapidly relieves pain, but has a short duration of action. Continuous infusion can be given this way.

♦ Morphine, Demerol, hydromorphone (Dilaudid), methadone and oxycodone (Percodan and Percocet or Tylox) are available in pills or oral solution. Morphine and methadone are available as long-acting pills (8 to 12 hours) and morphine, Demerol, hydromorphone and oxycodone are available in short-acting pills or solution.

♦ Most narcotics are available in rectal suppository form.

♦ Narcotics can be given by injection into muscles or under the skin.

♦ Most narcotics, but most often morphine and hydromorphone (Dilaudid), can be given through a portable infusion pump with a small butterfly needle inserted under the skin or as a slow intravenous infusion.

♦ Fentanyl, a very potent narcotic, can be given through a patch worn on the skin. These patches come in various strengths and can provide pain relief for up to three days.

♦ Most narcotics can be given intraspinally. All narcotics relieve pain by binding to narcotic receptors in the spinal cord and brain much like a lock and key, so narcotics given by this route are very effective at very low doses. While the pain equivalence between oral and intramuscular morphine is 3 to 1, the equivalence between intraspinal and oral morphine is 300 to 1. This very large ratio usually means a much smaller dose is needed, which means far fewer side effects. Patients unable to tolerate narcotics when given by mouth, shots or intravenously might tolerate drugs given intraspinally.

Supportive Techniques It is important to look after the emotional and psychological components of pain too. Psychological counseling can help in many ways—finding sources of emotional support, reducing any sense of loneliness and isolation, coming to terms with your situation or planning for the future. Talking with clergy or other trusted spiritual advisers might also reduce anxieties and fears that contribute to your pain.

Basically, anything that helps you relax can help your efforts at pain control. Relaxation exercises, massage, transcutaneous nerve stimulation, biofeedback, acupuncture and acupressure may all be of help.

Perhaps surprisingly, one very effective pain control device may be as close as your stereo. Music has been rated to have an analgesic effect twice that of a plain background sound. So listen to your favorite musical works and artists. Music can help you relax, raise your spirits, give you great joy *and* help you control your pain.

20
GUARDING AGAINST INFECTIONS

Margaret Poscher, MD, Lawrence Mintz, MD, W. Lawrence Drew, MD, PhD,
Ernest H. Rosenbaum, MD, and Malin Dollinger, MD

◇

Everyone with cancer runs a high risk of catching some sort of infection. This is so because the cancer and the methods used to fight it affect the immune system defenses that normally keep infections at bay.

Our first line of defense against infection is the outer and inner linings of the body—the skin and the mucous membranes. Both these barriers are punctured by the invasive procedures necessary to diagnose or treat cancer problems. Chemotherapy and radiation are particularly damaging to mucous membranes. And the needle in the arm to draw blood for testing, the IV lines, the catheters and pumps all create potential ports of entry for infectious organisms.

Once an infection does get into our bodies, one of the most important defenses—the white blood cell—usually goes into action. But the number of these cells is dramatically reduced by chemotherapy, radiation therapy, leukemia and bone marrow transplants. Low white blood cell counts are common in cancer patients, and as the count decreases the risk of infection increases.

Another defense mechanism is known as cellular immunity, in which specialized white blood cells called T lymphocytes attack invading organisms. But some cancers such as Hodgkin's disease can cause defects in cellular immunity, and so can chemotherapy, radiation and drugs that suppress the immune system.

Another part of the immune defense system is known as humoral immunity. Here other specialized white blood cells called B lymphocytes produce proteins—antibodies—to fight infections. This part of the system can be damaged in cases of multiple myeloma and chronic lymphocytic leukemia or when treatment requires the removal of the spleen.

We all have "resident" bacteria (called normal flora) that are usually harmless but can cause serious infection when our defenses are down. We can try to prevent infections, but nevertheless they do occur.

THE DIFFERENT TYPES OF INFECTIONS

Infections are defined by the type of organism involved and the location in the body. The most common organisms fall into three broad categories.

Bacterial Infections A major source of these infections is bacteria normally found in our own gut (gastrointestinal tract). In a phenomenon known as sepsis, these organisms find their way into the bloodstream and can "seed" various organs.

Bacteria on the skin can get into the bloodstream if an IV line is in place, resulting in sepsis or a local infection called cellulitis. A urinary catheter to drain the bladder can sometimes lead to a urinary tract infection. You may also have a greater chance of catching infections through social contact with people who already have an infection. A depressed immune system will make you more likely to acquire an infection in this way.

Once any area of your body is infected with bacteria, the opportunity exists for bacteria to get into the bloodstream, spread and cause sepsis.

Viral Infections When your cellular immunity is decreased, new viruses can take up residence in your body and old viral infections can be reactivated. Cold sores, for example, are caused by the herpes simplex virus. This is a virus that stays with you, although it can have long quiescent periods. When your cellular immunity is damaged, the virus can flare up and give you quite severe cold sores. Another herpes virus—the same one that causes chicken pox—can reactivate and cause shingles (herpes zoster) that can become widespread and quite severe.

Fungal Infections These are common when white blood cell counts are profoundly low and IV lines are in place.

SIGNS AND SYMPTOMS

There are several common signs and symptoms of infection. Some might be caused by something other than an infection, but you should consult your doctor as soon as any of them appear.

♦ Fever. This is a very reliable sign of infection and has to be attended to immediately, especially if your white blood cell count is low.

♦ Shaking chills.

♦ Severe night sweats.

♦ Nausea and vomiting, especially if accompanied by fever.

♦ Diarrhea, especially with a fever or with blood in the stool.

♦ Burning or pain when urinating, which could indicate a bladder infection.

♦ Coughing, shortness of breath or chest pain, all of which may be the first signs of pneumonia or bronchitis.

♦ Sore throat.

♦ A sore IV site from a permanent catheter for chemotherapy such as a Hickman or Port-a-Cath.

♦ Headache or neck stiffness with fever. This could indicate meningitis, a very serious infection of the nervous system that should be treated immediately.

DIAGNOSIS

Once you notice any of these signs and symptoms, your doctor will start searching for the origin of the infection. He or she will follow the usual steps in the diagnostic procedure, first asking you about your medical history, which may provide some clues about where the infection comes from. Shaking chills and fever are clues that sepsis may be present, which will prompt your doctor to order blood cultures. A cough might indicate pneumonia, which can be confirmed by a chest x-ray. Soreness and pains will lead the search to specific areas of your body.

The physical exam can confirm the leads given by the symptoms and may lead to the discovery of abnormalities you may not be aware of. Your abdomen will be examined for signs of enlargement or tenderness in organs that may be involved with infection. Your skin will be checked for signs of redness or tenderness. Even if there are no symptoms, pneumonia might be detected simply by listening to your chest. A careful neurologic exam will be done and sophisticated tests can be ordered if the exam reveals any abnormalities.

Once the history and physical exam are completed, your blood, sputum and urine will be analyzed. Stools, spinal fluid and skin lesions might be tested too. Depending on the results of the complete blood count and serum chemistry panel, you may undergo other diagnostic studies—x-rays, CT or MRI scans or nuclear medicine studies such as gallium or indium scans.

All the information from the history, exams, tests and studies will be used to plan the most appropriate therapy.

TREATMENT

There is a huge array of antibiotic, antifungal, antiviral and immune modulating therapies available to fight infections. Which to use depends on the organism involved and the site of infection. Someone with multiple myeloma, as well as some other patients, might benefit from the boost to the immune system provided by intravenous immune globulin. Someone with a herpes virus might need an antiviral drug like acyclovir. Someone with a serious fungal infection might be give an antifungal drug like amphotericin B or Fluconazole.

In an ideal world, the infecting organism would be identified quickly and the most effective drug against it would immediately be given. But cultures and lab test results may take 24 to 48 hours to get. While the offending organism still isn't known, what is called "empirical" therapy will begin, meaning that broad spectrum drugs will be directed against the most likely culprit. Someone with leukemia, for example, with a fever and a low white blood cell count would be given a combination of broad spectrum antibiotics effective in treating the kinds of bacteria known to infect this type of patient.

Once the organism is identified, treatment can be modified, if necessary. The broad spectrum drugs may be replaced by a specific antibiotic most effective against the bacteria or may be continued if tests show they are likely to be effective. If the fever and low white cell count continue after a week or 10 days of antibiotic therapy, an antifungal drug might be added.

Length of Treatment When to stop antibiotic treatment depends on the situation. If you've had fever and a low white cell count but neither the organism nor the site of infection could be identified, then antibiotics will usually be continued until the fever is gone and your white cell count is returning to normal.

If the site of infection is known—as in pneumonia, for example—and your temperature and white blood cell count is normal, antibiotics will be continued for one to two weeks.

If blood tests have isolated the organism, your fever is gone and the white count is back to normal, antibiotics will usually be stopped five to seven days after the fever disappears.

WHAT YOU AND YOUR DOCTOR CAN DO TO AVOID INFECTIONS

There will be certain times during the course of your illness when you will be more susceptible to infections, particularly when your white blood cell count is at its lowest. This point is called the nadir. Infections are most likely when the nadir is down to 1,000 cells per cubic millimeter or less. You should do everything you can to avoid possible sources of infection at all times. But be especially vigilant when your susceptibility is greatest.

How Your Doctor Can Help It has become standard practice in many chemotherapy programs to raise white blood cell counts by giving colony-stimulating factors such as G-CSF (Neupogen) or GM-CSF (Leukine). These are synthetic forms of substances the body naturally secretes to stimulate bone marrow to produce white blood cells.

♦ CSFs are very effective and are used with chemotherapy to shorten the time when the white blood cell count is extremely low. Raising the count decreases significantly the risk of serious infections.

♦ Much has been learned from the AIDS epidemic about giving antibiotics to people at risk before any infection has developed. Prophylactic antibiotics have many benefits. Ciprofloxicin, for example, can decrease bacterial infections when the white blood cell count is low.

♦ During the time when people receiving bone marrow transplants are profoundly immunosuppressed, the prophylactic use of gancyclovir can prevent cytomegalovirus infections and oral Fluconazole can prevent fungal infections.

♦ Getting a shot of influenza vaccine every autumn can help you avoid flu during an epidemic.

What You Can Do The best single preventive measure you can take against infection is to wash your hands often and well. Also keep the following guidelines in mind:

♦ Stay away from people with colds or the flu.

♦ Avoid intimate contact with people who have open sores such as cold sores or other viral infections.

♦ Avoid enclosed public areas where there is little ventilation, such as airplanes, theaters and shopping malls.

♦ Cut your nails carefully to avoid small nicks.

♦ Shave with an electric razor rather than a blade.

♦ Use gloves for protection when doing physical work that might damage the skin.

♦ Avoid dental work or cleaning if you are taking chemotherapy or if your white cell or platelet counts are low (less than 3,000 WBC or less than 100,000 platelets).

♦ Avoid raw vegetables and fruit that can't be peeled by someone else.

♦ Avoid lettuce completely when the white cell count is very low.

♦ Don't eat undercooked meat and poultry.

♦ Avoid constipation, using a stool softener if necessary. The act of straining can cause small tears in the anus and the lining of the intestine. This is dangerous when the white blood cell count is low.

♦ Avoid rectal thermometers and any other manipulation of the anus or rectum.

♦ Don't clean cat litter boxes or bird cages. Avoid all contact with animal stool and urine.

♦ Don't garden. It doesn't make sense to "play in the dirt." For this reason, plants (except plastic or silk ones) are usually kept out of patients' hospital rooms when the white cell count is very low.

21
LIVING WITH AN OSTOMY

Kerry Anne McGinn, RN, BSN, MA

—————◇—————

Some of my good friends just happen to have ostomies.

Like Virginia. She's the one stretching her four-foot 10-inch self so that her head shows above the podium for the speech she's giving. After 10 years with a colostomy—10 years of energetic work as an organizer, publicity person and grandmother—she says, "My colostomy's just part of me."

Like Joe. "My urostomy is a positive asset. When we go camping and everyone has a little beer, I'm the only one who doesn't have to get up in the middle of the night to trudge to the Porta-toilet."

Like Carol. She may be hard to find, between her trips to Australia and Finland, her teaching and her writing contracts. She says, "My ostomy is a minor nuisance. I barely remember it most of the time. Actually, I did have to be a little extra-cautious when I ran the marathon in Helsinki."

These three are a few of the hundreds of thousands of people who have had a passageway constructed through the abdominal wall as an exit for feces or urine. This change becomes necessary if the normal outlet cannot be used because of disease, trauma or birth defect.

Without their ostomy surgeries, none of these people would be alive. With their ostomies, each is happily, comfortably, normally alive.

A FEW DEFINITIONS

There are various kinds of ostomy—the surgical creation of an "opening into" some organ to connect it with the skin. A tracheostomy can be performed to improve breathing, for example. Most ostomies are performed to allow the elimination of body wastes through the abdominal wall.

"Ostomy" is the word for the total change the surgeon makes. "Ostomate" is one common term for a person who undergoes this change in personal plumbing. The new opening that can be seen on the abdomen is called a stoma.

There are three general categories of these abdominal exit ostomies:

♦ *Colostomy* is the rerouting of the colon, or large intestine. This change may be permanent or temporary.

♦ *Ileostomy* is such a detour in the ileum, the last section of the small intestine.

♦ *Urostomy*, or urinary diversion, covers a number of surgical procedures that redirect urine to the outside of the body when the bladder or another part of the urinary tract has to be bypassed or removed.

COLOSTOMIES

A colostomy is the most common ostomy. Surgeons perform colostomies for colorectal cancer, for other cancers of the abdomen or pelvis that press on or invade the large intestine and for conditions that have nothing to do with cancer.

In this surgical procedure, part of the colon is removed or disconnected and all or part of the rectum may be removed too. The end of the remaining colon is brought to the surface through the skin of the

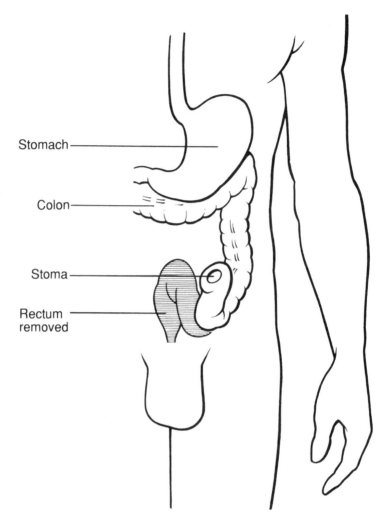

Stomach

Colon

Stoma

Rectum removed

Sigmoid colostomy after abdominal-perineal resection for rectal cancer.

abdomen, folded back like a turtleneck and stitched in place to form the stoma.

Adjusting to the Ostomy How does your body change when you have a colostomy? What stays the same?

Everything we eat, from apple pie to zucchini, must be broken down into tiny particles and changed to simpler chemical substances that can be absorbed into the bloodstream. The resulting nutrients make their way to cells throughout the body,

providing constant fuel and materials for energy, growth and rebuilding. This complex process of digestion takes place in the long—28 ft. (8 m) or longer in an adult—twisting channel that starts at the mouth and ends at the anus.

By the time food reaches the colon—the last 6 ft. (2 m) of the channel—most of the nourishment has been absorbed. Here the major tasks are absorbing water and some mineral salts in the first portion of the colon, then transporting and storing the indigestible remains of the food in the rest of the colon and the rectum. At the far end is the anus, a ring-like sphincter muscle that opens to release feces.

The body adjusts quite nicely to a shortened digestive tract. If your ostomy occurs near the end of the colon, as it does in many colostomies, you've lost only a storage area and a sphincter to release feces. If your ostomy is higher up in the digestive tract, you may lose part of the ability to absorb water so the discharge will tend to be less formed, more liquid. (This is much more of a problem for the person with an ileostomy, who has no colon and may have a problem absorbing mineral salts also. But ileostomy surgery is rare for cancer.) The remaining intestine eventually takes over some of the water-absorbing function. The kidneys, the major regulators of water and mineral salts, handle the rest of the adjustment.

Temporary and Permanent Colostomies With new surgical techniques available, surgeons are performing fewer "permanent" colostomies—in which the rectum and anus are removed—than they did several years ago.

But if a cancer occurs near the very end of the digestive tract, this may be the best way to remove all the cancer and save a life. An abdominal-perineal (A-P) resection is the usual surgery, with the surgeon making incisions in both the abdomen and the perineal area around the anus to remove the cancer and construct the colostomy.

Often, a surgeon constructs a "temporary" colostomy, which can sometimes last for years. This operation involves bypassing, but not removing, the rectum and anus. For instance, a surgeon might cut out a colon cancer but want the area to heal without feces passing over it. Or a large tumor that can't be removed causes pain because it's blocking the passage of stool. Using one of several techniques, the surgeon can form a colostomy using the colon

ahead of the affected section, leaving the problem area alone. Stool then can pass out of the body, but through a new exit. Later, the colostomy can be reversed so that stool moves through the anus again.

How the Stoma Functions The stoma that results from a colostomy could be described as a soft valve. Since it is made from the digestive tract that winds from the mouth to the anus, it is the same red-pink color as the mouth, and is lined with essentially the same kind of soft velvety mucous membranes. It stretches to permit waste to be expelled. During inactive periods, the tissue pulls together rather like puckered lips (stoma, in fact, means mouth). Although it expands and contracts, the stoma does not have the firm muscle control of the anal sphincter. So voluntary control of a bowel movement must be replaced by something else.

For many people with colostomies, that "something else" is a pouch (also called an appliance or bag). This is made of thin flexible plastic or rubber, which adheres to the skin over the stoma to hold feces until a convenient time for disposal. These are comfortable, odor-proof and secure.

An alternative for many colostomates with fairly solid stool is "irrigation," a kind of enema through the stoma done every day or two. This permits them to empty the bowel at a convenient regular time. They wear only a tiny pouch or a soft pad over the stoma the rest of the time.

URINARY DIVERSIONS

Urinary diversions or urostomies are often performed for cancer in the urinary tract.

Normally, once the kidneys have filtered wastes out of the blood, they flush excess fluid and wastes as urine through narrow tubes to an expandable storage area—the bladder—and then out of the body. At least some kidney function is essential for life, but any other part of the urinary tract can be removed or bypassed. Because reasons for urostomies vary from birth defects to bladder cancer, the age range of urostomates is wide and many different surgical techniques are used.

Making the Conduit To treat bladder cancer, surgeons may create an ileal conduit (also called an ileal loop or Bricker loop). The surgeon removes the bladder or sometimes just bypasses it. A section a few inches long is cut away from the last part of the small intestine (the ileum), keeping the blood and nerve supply intact. This section is closed at one end, the narrow tubes from the kidney are attached to it and the open end is brought through the abdominal wall to form a stoma.

The remaining ends of the intestine are reconnected and resume their function of moving feces out of the body. If the surgeon prefers to use a section of colon rather than ileum, the ostomy is called a colonic conduit.

The conduit is not an artificial bladder. It doesn't store urine. It is simply a passageway, and urine continues to drip out of the stoma all the time. This means that if you have this kind of urinary ostomy you wear a pouch at all times and drain it into the toilet as needed.

TAKING CARE OF YOUR STOMA

Although the stoma usually shrinks somewhat in diameter as postoperative swelling subsides and you resume your normal diet and exercise, the red-pink color remains.

Unlike an incision, a stoma requires little healing. A urostomy stoma starts to expel urine immediately, even before the new urostomate has left the operating room. Colostomies start discharging feces in a few days, usually with a lot of gas and watery stool until the bowel settles down after surgery.

Stomas come in many shapes and sizes, depending on the kind of ostomy and the person who owns it. Since it is made from the large intestine, a colostomy will be wider than an ileal conduit urostomy made from the small intestine. Some "temporary" stomas may be quite large and have two openings in one stoma or two stomas near each other. Most stomas should protrude from the skin enough so that feces or urine discharge away from the skin rather than pooling around the stoma.

At first, it's a temptation to feel overprotective about a stoma. You might feel that it is so fragile it might be damaged by a breeze or a bump. While reasonable protection is essential, the stoma is surprisingly tough. It is not harmed by water, by contact during sex or even by gentle bumps against furniture. But it does bleed easily, even from as little cause as an overzealous wipe with a washcloth, because many tiny blood vessels are very close to the surface of the stoma. A pouch or a soft pad will protect it from the friction of clothes.

GETTING SUPPORT

When you have an ostomy you can eat, work and play normally. But there are new skills to learn. Fortunately, there are many resources to help and give you moral support.

♦ An enterostomal therapist (ET nurse) is a registered nurse with special training in the care of ostomies and ostomates. ET nurses work in hospitals or have private practices. With their information and caring, they are a godsend for both new and long-time ostomates. Ask your doctor for the name of the ET nurse in your hospital or community.

♦ The United Ostomy Association (UOA) is an organization of more than 50,000 people with ostomies. The association holds local meetings and provides ostomy visitors—volunteers matched for sex, age and type of ostomy—for the new ostomate. Some people come to the meetings for information, some for moral support, some for the social contact. Some people come because they are having problems, others because they have solved problems and are happy to pass on their experience.

Some are desperate, discouraged, depressed. Many of them find answers and all of them find support and a place where they can talk freely about what concerns them. Local chapters of UOA may be listed in the phone book or can be located through the American Cancer Society. The national organization publishes a quarterly journal and holds regional and national conferences.

Keeping a Positive Attitude Hearing that you have cancer and need an ostomy is a double jolt for anyone. It takes time, information and support to adjust. But it's not the end. Definitely not.

I'll never forget Roger. A year before I met him, the doctor in his small town had diagnosed rectal cancer and had recommended colostomy surgery. "No way," stormed Roger. "You're not going to see me with one of those awful bags."

Despite his doctor's urging, Roger refused surgery. He underwent radiation and chemotherapy, but the tumor spread. When Roger came to our big-city hospital and, by some administrative quirk, to my orthopedics floor, he was deathly ill. But he was still adamantly opposed to "those damned bags."

I was scarcely an ostomy expert at the time, but I knew someone with a colostomy—my mother. I knew people could be happy with a colostomy, bleak as Roger's chances seemed to be. So Roger and I talked. Just quiet talk. I passed on what information I had and my own confidence that ostomy surgery might make him feel much better. Meanwhile, his bowel became totally blocked, his pain became agonizing and his temperature soared. The bowel had burst and infection had set in. Too ill to protest much, Roger agreed

to surgery. The doctors did minimal surgery, creating a "temporary" colostomy so that stool would no longer spill into his abdomen.

To our astonishment, Roger survived both the surgery and a very rocky postoperative course. As he grew stronger, we started teaching him about caring for his ostomy, created in haste and none too neat. Remembering my mother's experiences with the United Ostomy Association, I asked the doctor's permission to call UOA for an ostomy visitor to see Roger, a real boost indeed. Eventually, still with his "temporary" colostomy, Roger was well enough to go home to his hometown hundreds of miles away, where we alerted the UOA chapter to expect him.

After he left, I wondered how he was, what had happened to him, whether he was still alive. His chief pleasure at home, besides his family, had been riding his horse, but I rather doubted that he'd ever be able to do that again.

Nine months later he returned to our hospital and was again admitted to our floor.

"Roger! What's the matter?"

"You'll never believe it, Kerry," he said, with a fine combination of sheepishness and pride. "I was at the rodeo."

"Hey, that's great! You've been getting out of the house some. Have you been able to ride at all?"

"Sure, that's what I was doing, roping cattle at the rodeo."

I took a deep breath. "But Roger, what about your colostomy?"

"No problem. The pouches you gave me stick on fine. You know, I just wish I'd known back then how easy a colostomy is. If only I'd known."

"Why are you here?"

"Well. . . I took a tumble from the horse and broke my ankle."

22
THE LOOK GOOD... FEEL BETTER®
COSMETIC PROGRAM

The Cosmetic, Toiletry, and Fragrance Association Foundation

◇

Just about anyone's quality of life is seriously diminished during cancer treatment. Fatigue and changes in daily routine, in physical appearance, personal emotions and reactions from family, friends and colleagues can all weigh heavily on cancer patients.

If you are a woman getting cancer treatment, you may find that physical changes are especially hard to bear. Your personal appearance directly affects your self-image and your psychological well-being. And if you are experiencing some of the common side effects of radiation or chemotherapy, you may start to believe that you're in worse medical shape than you really are. The face you see in the mirror each morning is a harsh reminder of your disease. Every day you can't escape your loss of hair, eyelashes and eyebrows or the changes in your skin tone and texture.

Looking in that mirror, you may start thinking that you couldn't possibly lead a "normal" life. But in today's world, leading a normal life—with all the family relationships, work and social demands normal life involves—is essential while you are getting cancer treatments. What you need to get back to a good quality of life is help to overcome the changes in appearance that cancer treatments bring.

Fortunately, to help you do just that, Look Good. . . Feel Better® (LGFB) is a free national public service program designed to teach women with cancer—through practical hands-on experience—the beauty techniques that help restore their appearance during chemotherapy and radiation treatments.

So while your medical treatment helps heal the inside of your body, the Look Good. . . Feel Better program helps you renew your self-esteem by enhancing your "outside" appearance. It encourages you to pay attention to yourself during a time of dramatic physical changes.

HOW THE "LOOK GOOD... FEEL BETTER" PROGRAM WORKS

Until recently, the kind of service offered by LGFB was largely unavailable. The program began in 1989, when three national organizations pooled their resources to develop the service and make it available to women across the country. The program was founded and developed by The Cosmetic, Toiletry, and Fragrance Association (CTFA) Foundation —a charitable organization supported by the members of the cosmetic industry's trade association—in partnership with the American Cancer Society (ACS) and the National Cosmetology Association (NCA). The NCA is a national organization that represents hairstylists, wig experts, estheticians, makeup artists and nail technicians, among others.

These three organizations provide:
♦ Patient education—through group or individual sessions—by volunteer cosmetologists and beauty advisers.
♦ Complimentary makeup kits for every-

one participating in a group program. (Look Good. . . Feel Better is "product neutral" and does not promote any specific cosmetic product line or manufacturer.)
♦ Free program materials such as videos and patient information pamphlets.

The Look Good. . . Feel Better program is administered nationwide by the ACS and is designed to meet the needs of local communities. The NCA organizes volunteer cosmetologists who can evaluate your skin and hair needs and who will teach you the appropriate beauty techniques to deal with the appearance-related side effects of cancer treatments. The CTFA Foundation provides the makeup, materials and financial support for the program.

All volunteers for Look Good. . . Feel Better are trained and certified for participation by the ACS and the NCA at local, statewide and national workshops. The purpose of this training is not only to discuss important hygienic guidelines and helpful cosmetic tips, but also to promote sensitivity and understanding about what a cancer patient goes through during treatment. This is a necessary step for each volunteer.

Group Sessions Each group session usually consists of eight to ten women led through a one-and-a-half to two-hour program by beauty professionals. Through practical hands-on experience, the women learn a 12-step makeup program and are shown beauty tips about hair, wigs, turbans and scarves. To ensure that every participant gets the same working tools, each woman in a group program receives a complimentary bag of makeup containing 12 items, which match the 12-step program.

THE TWELVE-STEP MAKEUP PROGRAM

1. Cleanser	**7.** Eyeliner
2. Moisturizer	**8.** Eyeshadow
3. Concealer	**9.** Eyebrows
4. Foundation	**10.** Mascara
5. Powder	**11.** Lipliner
6. Blush	**12.** Lipstick

Look Good. . . Feel Better group programs are located in comprehensive cancer centers, hospitals, ACS offices, and community centers.

Personal Consultation A free one-time consultation in a participating salon may also be available, depending where you live. A list of all salons willing to provide this service has been compiled by the NCA and has been distributed to all ACS divisions as well as to a toll-free number you can call for information (1-800-395-LOOK).

Program Materials There are several materials available free of charge from the ACS. These include a patient brochure, a 14-minute inspirational video and a 33-minute video, which includes a detailed demonstration of the 12-step program and alternatives to looking bald.

HOW AND WHERE TO FIND PROGRAMS IN YOUR COMMUNITY

Many doctors, nurses, social workers and

other medical professionals recognize how important outward appearance is to their patients. And with their help, Look Good. . . Feel Better is now reaching out to tens of thousands of women across the United States.

The growth of the program has been remarkably rapid and widespread. Two pilot programs were successfully operated at the Memorial Sloan-Kettering Cancer Center in New York City and the Vincent T. Lombardi Cancer Research Center at Georgetown University Hospital in Washington, DC, in the fall of 1988. By March 1989, the program was off and running. Since then, Look Good. . . Feel Better has been implemented in all 50 states and the District of Columbia and 22 of the 28 National Cancer Institute-designated comprehensive cancer centers. Group programs served 24,000 women with cancer in 1993. LGFB materials are also available in Spanish.

For more information, or to find out about programs in your area, call your local unit or state division of the American Cancer Society, or call toll-free 1-800-395-LOOK.

23
BECOMING SEXUALLY ACTIVE AGAIN

David G. Bullard, PhD, Ernest H. Rosenbaum, MD, Malin Dollinger, MD,
Jean M. Stoklosa, RN, MS, and Isadora R. Rosenbaum, MA

◇

Cancer affects all aspects of your life. So it's not surprising that it can affect your sexual feelings and the ways you express those feelings. You and your spouse or partner remain sexual beings and may have much the same needs and desires as you had before the illness struck.

Sexuality can be expressed in many ways—in how we dress and how we move and speak, as well as by kissing, touching, masturbation and intercourse. Changes in body image, tolerance for activity and anxieties about survival, family or finances can strain the expression of sexuality and can create concerns about sexual desirability. But if you were comfortable with and enjoyed your sexuality before your illness, the chances are excellent that you will be able to keep or regain a good sexual self-image despite any changes brought about by cancer.

Many people, healthy or dealing with an illness, find that being sexually active is not important to them. This can be a healthy, normal choice for any individual or couple. But if sexual intimacy has been a comfort to you, you may want to continue being sexually active once your cancer has been diagnosed and treated.

This may require some adaptation of your normal sexual patterns, and it might be a challenge to change them. Support groups with the right orientation can give understanding and encouragement, and open, comfortable communication with your partner is essential. You may also need specific information and guidance from your doctor. But the subject of sexual health for people with chronic illnesses—especially cancer—has been neglected for far too long. Members of your medical team may find it hard to initiate discussions about sexual problems. But don't make the mistake of trying to be a "good" patient by not complaining and simply suffering in silence. Sexuality is a legitimate area of concern. Take the initiative and ask your doctor any questions you have about your sexuality. You can overcome many problems, reduce tensions and get much more sexual satisfaction.

THE PHASES OF SEXUALITY

Understanding the phases of sexuality and how cancer can affect one or more of them can help you increase your satisfaction with sex.

♦ *Desire* This varies from person to person, ranging from an uninterested, indifferent attitude to a very active desire for sex. Desire can often be increased by physical, visual or fantasy stimulation.

♦ *Excitement* The body reacts to stimulation with increased blood flow in the sex organs and increased heart rate and blood pressure. Sexual interest and stimulation are characterized by an erection in men and increased vaginal lubrication in women, although a person may feel desire without those physiological responses.

Sexual problems often occur during the excitement phase. This can lead to considerable anxiety and distress. Men may lose the ability to get or keep an erection. Women may not have enough vaginal lubrication for comfortable penetration, making intercourse difficult or painful.

♦ *Orgasm* This is a peak of pleasurable expression followed by a gratifying relaxation. It is both a physical release and an emotional high.

Some men might ejaculate only after prolonged stimulation. Sometimes nothing happens despite prolonged effort. Or the ejaculate might be reversed into the bladder (retrograde) rather than going forward and out the penis. The feeling of orgasm still occurs, but there is no semen or liquid.

For women, the painful intercourse (dyspareunia) that sometimes follows cancer treatment can inhibit orgasm.

♦ *Resolution* Many people feel relaxed and satisfied after sex regardless of whether or not they reach orgasm. For others, who have had problems in the desire, excitement or orgasm phases, the satisfying resolution may be replaced by sexual tension, discomfort in the pelvis or emotional frustration.

THE SEXUAL PROBLEMS OF SPECIFIC CANCERS

Treatment for some cancers may have little effect on sexuality beyond the effects of fatigue, pain, weakness or other temporary side effects. Younger men who receive extensive chemotherapy, however, might consider sperm banking before treatment in case the sperm count does not return to normal. But the treatment of several kinds of cancer may directly affect how well you function sexually.

Bladder Cancer Surgical therapy for bladder cancer can lead to decreased desire, a reduced ability for men to get an erection,

retrograde ejaculation and orgasm problems including a lower intensity. About half the women who have this therapy end up with a shorter and narrower vagina, making penetration more difficult. Communication with her partner will become especially important, as will the use of lubricants such as K-Y jelly or Crème de la Femme.

Breast Cancer Psychological counseling is helpful for all women treated for breast cancer given the symbolic sexual significance of the female breast. Even 10 percent of women who have a *benign* biopsy may want to discuss sexual concerns. And 30 to 40 percent of women who have a modified radical mastectomy experience sexual dysfunction. Fewer sexual problems are reported if a lumpectomy is done, which results in less change to body image. Treatment with low doses of testosterone can help women regain desire and sexual enjoyment.

Colon Cancer There is twice the amount of sexual dysfunction after surgery for colon cancer than there is after surgery for benign causes such as an ilieostomy for ulcerative colitis. People with ostomies may have embarrassment or worry about their partner's reaction that might interfere with their sexual responsiveness. Direct communication with and reassurance from a partner can be very helpful.

Gynecological Tumors A woman having gynecological surgery may have a premature loss of estrogen. This in effect is a premature menopause with hot flashes, mood swings, sleeping problems, anxiety and depression. Sexual partners often have a hard time coping with these changes. All this can reduce a couple's ability to have sex or their inclination to even think about it. With the feelings of abandonment and rejection that often follow, the relationship can definitely suffer. But the right kind of help and counseling can assist the couple in talking about and coping with these problems. Hormonal replacement therapy may also resolve some of these issues.

Hysterectomy and radiation treatment to the female genitals may lead to problems in the excitement phase. The surgery might also affect orgasm, and painful intercourse can result from radiation. The frequency of intercourse might be reduced. Women who have had hysterectomies for benign disease have similar problems—a decrease in sexual desire especially in the first six months after the operation, with desire usually returning to normal after a year.

Radical surgery to the vagina and vulva can so change the physical aspects of the genitalia that sexual activity can become very difficult both physically and psychologically because of the fear of pain or bleeding during intercourse. Plastic surgery to reconstruct the organs, along with sex counseling, can be very helpful to some, while others may learn to enjoy love-making without intercourse.

Hodgkin's Disease About 20 percent of men and women with this type of cancer lose energy and interest in sex. Hodgkin's disease doesn't usually affect the ability to get an erection, but problems with ovaries may lead to painful intercourse for women. Lengthy treatments and impaired fertility may cause marital stress unless both partners are encouraged to communicate their feelings.

Cancer of the Penis and Testicles Men who lose part of their penis may still be capable of getting erections, having orgasms and ejaculating. Removal of the whole penis naturally can cause very severe sexual difficulties. But orgasm may still be possible with stimulation of the bones, pubis, perineum and scrotum and ejaculation through a urethrostomy.

With testis cancer, the sexual problems depend on the type of tumor. With non-seminoma, removal of a testicle and the lymph nodes in the area usually result in a decrease in fertility and sexual activity. Some men with seminoma who have had a testicle removed plus radiation therapy report low or no sexual activity, decreased desire, problems with erections and orgasms, and decreased volume of semen.

Prostate The diagnostic biopsy might result in less seminal fluid in the ejaculation. Surgical removal of the prostate can cause similar problems and, with hormonal therapy, the ability to get an erection and ejaculate may be lost altogether.

Radiation produces problems too, but only half as many as the surgical approach. When the pelvic lymph nodes are removed and a radiation implant is used for localized tumors, 15 to 25 percent of men have difficulties with erections and about 30 percent have a retrograde ejaculation. New surgical approaches and new chemotherapy treatments may help reduce erection and ejaculation problems.

Drugs That Affect Sexual Activity Most cancers occur in people over 50, many of whom are usually already experiencing some decrease in sexual activity. This decrease can be accelerated by the very fact of having cancer and by the drugs that are often taken for other diseases such as high blood pressure, diabetes, alcoholism or psychological problems. A great many drugs can affect sexual activity and can lead to sexual dysfunction:

♦ alcohol
♦ anticancer drugs and hormones
♦ antihypertensive drugs, including beta blockers
♦ pain medications
♦ antidepressants
♦ sleeping medications
♦ codeine or other narcotics
♦ psychedelic and hallucinogenic drugs

EXPRESSING YOURSELF SEXUALLY AFTER TREATMENT

With all the possible effects of cancer treatment, the prospect of having a normal sex life may seem out of reach. But whatever your cancer, there are steps you can take that will help you increase your sexual enjoyment.

If You've Had an Ostomy People with ostomies and their partners have to learn about ostomy appearance, care and control. Women may be comfortable wearing special undergarments that cover a pouch while still permitting sexual stimulation. Specially designed and esthetically attractive pouches are available.

If You've Had a Laryngectomy Laryngectomy patients should be acquainted with how to deal with sounds and odors escaping from their stomas. Wearing a stoma shield or T-shirt will muffle the sound of breathing and will minimize your partner's feeling the air that is pushed through the stoma.

If You've Had a Mastectomy After a mastectomy, you may be worried about how you look. Undressing in front of your partner or sleeping in the nude may feel awkward and uncomfortable. That's natural, especially in light of the overemphasis our culture places on the sexual significance of breasts. Grieving over what you have lost is important. But with time and patience, most women overcome their self-consciousness and feel secure and comfortable with their bodies again.

♦ Some women have found it helpful to explore and touch their bodies, including the area of the scar, while nude in front of a mirror. You may want to try this alone at first and then with a spouse, lover or close friend. Share your feelings about your new body.

♦ Be aware that your partner may not know what to say. Your spouse or lover may not know how or when to bring up the topic of sexuality and so wait for you to do it. Your partner may be afraid of hurting or embarrassing you and want to protect your feelings. Sometimes this "protection" may feel like rejection. Although you might feel that it's risky to break the ice and approach the topic yourself, most people feel relieved once they've done it.

♦ You both may also worry about pain. If your incision or muscles are tender, minimize the pressure on your chest area. If you lie on your unaffected side, you can have more control over your movements and reduce any irritation to the incision. If your partner is on top, you may protect the affected area by putting your hand under your chin and your arm against your chest.

♦ If you feel any pain, stop. And let your partner know why you are stopping. If he knows that you'll tell him what is painful, he will feel more relaxed and will be less inhibited in exploring and experimenting with you. Taking a rest or changing position may help you relax, and relaxing will usually decrease any pain. You can also apply extra lubrication. With communication and cooperation, you can work together to find positions and activities that give you the most pleasure.

♦ Experimentation and time seem to be the keys to finding satisfactory ways of adapting to the loss of such a symbolically important part of the body as the breast. Talking with other women who have had mastectomies—women from the American Cancer Society's Reach to Recovery program, for example—can provide support and encouragement as well as suggestions about clothes and prostheses.

♦ Some women find breast reconstruction important for their emotional well-being.

♦ Treatment with testosterone may also be beneficial.

If You've Had Treatment to the Genitals or Reproductive Organs Even the prospect of surgery or radiation treatments for these cancers can make you intensely concerned about your body image. But it is usually impossible to predict the effects of treatment for any one person. Treatment can affect some people's ability to get erections, ejaculate or have intercourse. The same treatment for someone else might result in little or no change in sexual functioning.

Anxiety Sexual problems that seem to be the physical results of treatment may actually be due to anxiety. You can reduce your worry by discussing potential problems and possible solutions with your doctor or other members of the health care team *before* treatment. This discussion will also reassure you that if problems do come up there are ways of handling them. Since in most situations physical and emotional causes of sexual problems interact, your exploration and experimentation about what you can do is very important. Your diagnosis does not dictate what is possible for you sexually.

Painful Intercourse If you find that intercourse is painful after treatment for genital cancer, have a gynecological examination to find the cause. The problem may be related to surgery, radiation or chemotherapy. Then again, it may result from a simple problem like an infection.
♦ If the cause is not enough lubrication, natural lubrication such as saliva or products such as water-soluble lubricants can reduce friction. Artificial lubricants such as K-Y jelly, Jergen's Lotion and other creams may make coitus possible where the lack of circulating estrogens has caused dryness. A new way to get adequate lubrication for sexual arousal and intercourse is Replens, a vaginal gel applied three times a week. In some cases, small amounts (one-third to one-half a tube) of a poorly absorbed estrogen like

Dienestrol may help restore lubrication and atrophy of the vagina. But if breast cancer has been diagnosed, use of estrogens may be unwise.
♦ Surgery or radiation therapy can cause shortening of the vagina or make the vagina less elastic. Either situation may make intercourse difficult. Your doctor may recommend dilators to exercise and stretch the vagina. Getting back to intercourse soon after treatment can also help prevent these problems. Different positions during intercourse, especially sitting or lying on top of your partner, may let you move in pleasurable ways.

Communication Again, the most important thing to remember is to stop when you first feel pain. And tell your partner ahead of time that you will let him know immediately about any pain. Stopping to rest, slowing your movements, breathing deeply and sharing your feelings will help you relax. By exploring together, you and your partner will eventually discover the kinds of sexual activity that suit you best.

If You Have Trouble Reaching Orgasm The natural interruption in the ability to experience sexual pleasure after an illness may make having orgasms more difficult for some women. If this is a problem for you, learning to re-explore pleasurable body sensations may be helpful.

It is important to do this when you can be alone and not distracted by having to please or perform for your partner. So find a comfortable place where you can be alone—your bedroom or bathroom—and a time when you won't be interrupted. Undress slowly and gently stroke your whole body. Then focus on the most sensitive areas—your neck, breasts, thighs, genitals or any other area that feels good to you.

Use different kinds of touch, soft and light, firm and strong. Try moistening your hands with oil, lotion or soap. Pay attention to the sensations you feel and discover which ones are most pleasurable.

Learning which kinds of touch feel best will help you heighten your sensation and will give you information to share with your partner.

If You're Having Trouble with Erections
Since some drugs can temporarily interfere with the ability to have erections, you may want to ask your physician about possible side effects of your treatment.

Physical and Emotional Causes If you can get an erection by masturbating or you wake up with an erection in the night or morning, it is most likely that anxiety or "trying too hard" is the cause, and it's not a physical problem. If you are not sure of the cause, ask your doctor to refer you to a urologist or sex therapist for evaluation and treatment.

Taking the Pressure Off The more options you have for sexual expression, the less pressure there is on having erections. This in turn makes it more likely that they will happen. Many couples report that they have learned to have very pleasurable sexual experiences without erections or intercourse. Many kinds of sexual expression and stimulation do not require an erect penis. It may be reassuring to know that to have an orgasm many women need or prefer direct stimulation by hand or mouth on or around the clitoris. This is stimulation that even an erect penis in a vagina can't provide.

If you explore other kinds of sexual touching and expression for a while, you may discover that erections will return with time or that the increased variety of sexual options satisfies both you and your partner. Patience, communication and time are critical factors in developing pleasurable sexual experiences.

Counseling If erections don't come back and intercourse is important to you and your partner, ask your doctor to refer you to a sex therapist for counseling.

Counseling will help you with relaxation techniques, with planning time for proper stimulation and with methods for using visual stimulation and fantasy. Group counseling with cancer survivors who have had the same problem can also help.

If you are still not getting erections, the counselor may refer you to a urologist. Together with you and your counselor, the urologist can explore options such as a penile implant, injections or use of a vacuum pump.

GENERAL GUIDELINES FOR RESUMING SEXUAL ACTIVITY

Whenever you are sick, your usual sense of control over your body may be shaken. You may feel inadequate and helpless. An illness can change the way you experience your body or it might actually change the way you look because of surgery, amputation, scarring, or weight loss.

These changes can create painful anxiety. You wonder whether you'll be able to function in your usual social, sexual and career roles. You wonder what people will think of you. This anxiety—and the depression and fatigue that often go along with it—understandably make sexuality seem less important. But once the immediate crisis has passed, sexual feelings and how to express them may become important again.

Feeling anxious about resuming sexual activity is normal and natural. It is easy to "get out of practice." You may have questions about whether sexual activity will hurt you in some way. You may wonder how you will be able to experience sexual pleasure and your partner may share the same worries. He or she may be especially concerned about tiring you out or hurting you somehow.

But once you resume sexual relations, your comfort and confidence should gradually increase. If not, sexual counseling may help you discover ways to deal with whatever problems you are having. For many people, a "new start"—by themselves or through counseling—is refreshing. It might even create opportunities for greater intimacy and sharing than ever before.

What to Do When You Are in the Hospital Your cancer treatment might involve long stays in the hospital and long separations from those you love. Hospitals or convalescent facilities don't usually provide much privacy, so there may be little opportunity for sexual expression unless you speak up.

Although health care facilities are rarely designed to ensure patients' privacy, there is no reason why you and your partner can't have time for intimate physical contact in the hospital. With a little friendly intervention doctors might be able to arrange for a special room where you and a loved one can spend some time alone. Or you can always make a sign reading "Do Not Disturb Until __ o'clock" or "Please knock" and hang it on the door to your room. The nurses will respect your wishes.

If this sounds important to you, ask your doctor to speak to the hospital staff and help foster a caring and respectful attitude toward your need to express your sexuality with guaranteed privacy. It takes some education and maybe a change in the "way things are always done around here," but it's well worth the effort.

Developing Helpful Attitudes and Practices Whenever you are ready to become sexually active again, there are a few things you should keep in mind.

♦ *You are loved for who you are, not just for your appearance.* If you were considered lovable or sexually desirable before you got cancer, chances are that you will be afterward too. Your partner, your family and your friends will still love you and value you, as long as you let them.

♦ *We are all sexual beings.* Whether we are sexually active or not, sexuality is

part of who we are. It is not defined just by what we do or how often we do it.

♦ *Survival overshadows sexuality.* If you've lost your good health, it is normal and natural for stress, depression, worry and fatigue to lower your interest in sex. Just coping with basic everyday decisions can seem like a burden. But take one day at a time and be patient. Sexual interest and feelings will probably come back when the immediate crisis has passed.

♦ *Share your feelings.* Making relationships work is a task we all face, but it can be made more difficult by worries about our worth and attractiveness. Whether you are looking for a new relationship or already have a regular partner, you may find yourself in the position of having to share your sexual feelings with someone, perhaps for the first time.

This sharing may feel awkward at first. Learning how and when to talk about sexual issues may not come easily. You may feel shy or nervous about exploring new and different ways of finding sexual pleasure. You may wait for your partner to make the first move while your partner is waiting for you to make the advances. This familiar waiting game is often misunderstood as rejection by both people. It may be frightening to think of breaking the silence yourself. Yet a good move is to make the first move. Try sharing some of the myths or expectations you grew up with about sexuality. Often this is humorous and may break the ice in starting a frank discussion about your sexual needs and concerns. Try not to make broad, generalized statements. Talk about what is important to *you* and about how *you* feel. The payoff is greater understanding of each other's needs and concerns, and that is worth the effort.

♦ *Expect the unexpected.* The first time you have sex after treatment, physical limitations or fears about your performance, appearance or rejection may keep you from focusing on the sheer pleasure of physical contact. On the other hand, you may be surprised by unfamiliar pleasurable sensations. If you expect some changes as part of the natural recovery process, they will be less likely to distract you from sexual pleasure if they do happen.

♦ *Give yourself time.* You and your partner may be frightened of, or even repulsed by, scars, unfamiliar appliances or other physical changes. That's natural too. But such feelings are usually temporary. Talking about them is often the first step to mutual support and acceptance. Don't pressure yourself about having to "work on sex." A satisfactory and enjoyable sex life will happen one step at a time. You may want to spend some time by yourself exploring your body, becoming familiar with changes and rediscovering your unique body texture and sensations. Once you feel relaxed doing this, move on to mutual body exploration with a partner.

♦ *Take the pressure off intercourse.* Almost all of us were brought up to believe that intercourse is the only real or appropriate way of expressing ourselves sexually. Yet sexual expression can encompass many forms of touching and pleasuring that are satisfying psychologically and physically.

When you resume sexual activity, try spending some time in pleasurable activities—touching, fondling, kissing and being close—without having intercourse. Re-experience the pleasure of playing, of holding and of being held without having to worry about erections and orgasms. When you feel comfortable, proceed at your own pace to other ways of being sexual, including intercourse if you like.

Experiment and explore to discover what feels best and what is acceptable. If radiation therapy, for example, has made intercourse painful, try oral or manual stimulation to orgasm, or intercourse between thighs or breasts. If you are exhausted by the disease or movement is painful, just cuddling or lying quietly next to your partner might be a satisfying form of intimacy.

♦ *Don't let your diagnosis dictate what you can do sexually.* Your sexuality cannot be "diagnosed." You will never know what pleasures you are capable of experiencing if you don't explore. Try new positions, new touches and above all new attitudes. Your brain is your best and most important sex organ. And its ability to experience sensation is virtually limitless.

♦ *Plan sex around your changing energy levels.* Life with cancer can be exhausting. Fatigue, depression and just feeling sick are almost normal for cancer patients at certain times. The amount of energy you have for all kinds of activities, including sex, can vary from day to day or week to week. So plan sexual activities to coincide with the times when you think you will feel best.

♦ *Ask for help if you need it.* Don't hesitate to seek counseling or information if you have problems. Help is available from a wide range of sources. If you want to discuss any problems, bring them up with your health care providers. Ask them to recommend competent sex counselors or therapists in your area. There may also be other resources available nearby, such as people who have had both cancer and experience in talking about sexual concerns.

♦ *Be patient.* The important thing is to be patient, with both yourself and your partner. You won't adjust overnight. Give yourself time to explore and share your feelings about your body changes and time to again see yourself as a desirable sexual being. When *you* can accept the way your body looks and recognize your potential for sexual pleasure, it will be easier to imagine someone else doing the same.

The satisfaction and good feelings—emotional and physical—that can come from a sexual relationship require patience, communication, respect, cooperation and a willingness to remember that in some respects the relationship must be learned all over again, physically if not emotionally.

Everything may not work properly at first. Everything may not be enjoyable at first. But have the courage and confidence to keep trying.

24
STAYING PHYSICALLY FIT

Ernest H. Rosenbaum, MD, Malin Dollinger, MD, and Francine Manuel, RPT

◇

If you were involved with an exercise program before you became ill, you will probably be open to the idea of getting involved in an active program all through your recovery. But if you have never been involved in an organized exercise routine you may need some encouragement. Welcome this encouragement if you get it. If you don't get it, seek it out, because getting and staying physically fit should be one of your most important goals.

WHY YOU SHOULD EXERCISE

Physical fitness is healthy for everyone, of course. But it is essential for all cancer patients. Even though it's hard to find the energy to exercise when you are sick, the benefits of keeping your body in an active state are too great to ignore. When you participate in a daily exercise program:

1. You will improve your prognosis If you are in good physical condition, you may tolerate therapy better. This, in turn, may allow you to have more aggressive treatments and so stand a better chance of remission or cure. It is well known that successful treatment and an improved prognosis depend directly on physical status. The simple truth is that if you are physically fit, you may live longer and enjoy a more active life.

2. You will stop your muscles from wasting away When we are healthy, we all usually exercise our muscles one way or another—by walking up and down stairs, doing housework, going shopping, taking part in athletic activities like golf and tennis or simply by walking as we go about our business. Even a low level of activity helps to maintain muscle tone and strength. But during an acute or chronic illness, prolonged bedrest is often necessary. Muscles shrink in size and strength when they're not used for a long time. An exercise program will make sure that doesn't happen to you.

3. You will recover faster If you do not exercise after surgery or while you're undergoing radiotherapy or chemotherapy, your muscles will get weaker and weaker. The tissues that may be broken down by therapy will not be repaired as quickly as they should be. By exercising, you can help your tissues rebound and you can minimize any deterioration in your joints. You might also help prevent complications such as bone softening, blood clots and bedsores. And, not least, you'll get some relief from the boredom and depression that often come with being confined to bed.

WHEN TO START

Become physically active as soon as possible after treatment. It is now the general practice within one day of surgery to get out of bed and at least sit in a chair. Even this minimal activity helps reduce the loss of muscle mass and increase strength.

True, pain can limit physical exercise

after a mastectomy, bowel surgery or some other major operation. And you may be depressed by a change in your body image and not feel like doing anything. You may need help to get going. But with appropriate timing, you should turn your attention to rehabilitation.

In the Hospital At least a gentle exercise program should begin while you are still in the hospital. This may involve simple muscle tightening while you lie in bed or passive muscle exercises. As your strength returns, different forms of physical activity—isometric and isotonic exercises and rhythmic repeated movements for various muscles—will help get you on the path to improved fitness. Massage therapy can complement these activities, helping you relax your mind and body and improving your circulation.

You might think all this will involve too much of an effort while you're still in the hospital. But you will feel much more confident when you do go home if you have already started to regain your strength. You will also be less prone to falls or other accidents that might result from a weakened condition.

PLANNING A PROGRAM

Before you leave the hospital, physical therapists can assess your physical condition and come up with an appropriate set of exercises. Everyone has different wants and needs, so programs are usually customized. They will also be flexible, taking your energy level into account. The staff of the Physical Therapy Department can also instruct you, your family and other caregivers on how to proceed with your program at home. Their recommendations on an appropriate program may be essential to your recovery.

Safety Rules When you begin exercising, keep in mind a few simple rules for safety:
♦ Ask your doctor if you're ready to exer-

cise. Let him or her set limits to your activity.
♦ Have someone join you. This will make the exercise more enjoyable and safer, especially when you are just getting out of bed and may feel dizzy.
♦ Stop and rest if you feel tired or if your muscles are sore.
♦ Leave out any exercises that seem too difficult and try them another day when you feel stronger.
♦ Try to repeat each exercise three to five times at first, then gradually increase the repetitions to ten or twenty.
♦ Try to exercise at least twice a day, more often if you feel up to it.

The most important rule is to start out gradually. Don't overdo it. Muscles that haven't been used for days or weeks will strain very easily. Light warmup exercises several times a day will be useful, both as a starting point for your program and as a daily prelude to more vigorous exercises later on.

When you start your exercise program, you might experience some fatigue, dizziness or even nausea. Discuss any problems with your doctor or physical therapist. But these side effects usually pass fairly quickly.

Working Through the Stages A graduated program may take you through three stages:
♦ *Stage 1—Beginning to Move Exercises.* These are simple exercises that help you maintain and increase your range of motion. They don't require much exertion and can be done while you are lying in bed.
♦ *Stage 2—Increased Activity Exercises.* A small weight (up to 2 lb./1 kg) is used to increase resistance. These exercises can be done when you are spending part of the day out of bed sitting in a chair.
♦ *Stage 3—Up and About Exercises.* These exercises will build up your strength when you are able to stand, walk and spend the whole day out of bed. (For more detailed information, consult

Rehabilitation Exercises for the Cancer Patient, by Ernest Rosenbaum, Francine Manuel, Judith Bray, Isadora Rosenbaum and Arthur Cerf, available from Bull Publishing, PO Box 208, Palo Alto, California 94302.)

Setting a Regular Routine Once you are back on your feet and approaching your normal level of activity, you can establish a set routine, naturally within any limitations or restrictions identified by your doctor. A very enjoyable workout program can be created.

♦ Aerobic programs are very helpful. You take your pulse before beginning, then take it again halfway through and at the end of the routine. The aim is to roughly double your heart rate, although your physician may set a specific rate that you should not exceed.

There are a great number of aerobic programs to choose from. You may even alternate programs to avoid boredom. A variety of TV shows can take you through an aerobic workout every day, although aerobic programs need only be done for twenty minutes three times a week to achieve maximum benefits. If you have a VCR, Jane Fonda or other celebrities can take you step by step through a program with their videos. These videos are widely available and offer an ideal way to work up to a full routine. Some of the videos show a slower group on one side and a more athletic group on the other. You can also stop the tape or limit the number of repetitions.

♦ If aerobics are not for you, there are all kinds of machines—stationary bikes, stair climbers, treadmills, rowing or skiing machines and so on—that use weights or hydraulics to build all your muscles. Home equipment is worthwhile if you have a busy schedule and want to work out at your own pace at your own convenience. Some of these units are expensive, but some can be purchased cheaply, especially during special sales.

♦ You can go to a health club if you want a variety of equipment to choose from and to be with people who are also working out.

♦ If you don't feel comfortable with any formal program, there is always stair climbing and brisk walking. You can go up and down your stairs at home for 15 to 20 minutes every other day or take a long walk, perhaps during your lunch hour, every other day.

Whatever your routine, staying active will build up your body's reserves so that if you do need a temporary period of bedrest your energy stores won't be depleted.

While you should think of your program as being as much a part of your recovery as visits to the doctor, try to enjoy yourself. Exercising can be a lot of fun. And it can be very stimulating.

If you have days when depression and boredom get you down and exercising seems like too much of a burden, just remind yourself of all the benefits of exercising regularly. Your program will improve your energy level and stamina, improve your appetite, help you relax and help you sleep at night.

The more you exercise, the better you will feel.

25
RELAXATION AND CANCER RECOVERY

Lenore Dollinger, RN, PhD

We are all beginning to recognize that health is a balance of many factors—physical and environmental, emotional and mental, lifestyle habits and spiritual beliefs.

Stress plays a key role in this balance. Stress is well known as a contributing factor in a broad range of disorders. In fact, it's estimated that 50 to 80 percent of illnesses have some stress component. Stress is recognized as a risk factor in addictions, obesity, high blood pressure, peptic ulcer, colitis, asthma, insomnia, migraine headaches, lower back pain and many psychological disorders.

Whether stress is also a risk factor in the development of cancer is unknown. Some people believe it plays a part, others do not.

POSITIVE AND NEGATIVE STRESS

Stress is not always negative. Positive stress allows us to act, think, move and respond to situations with purpose. We wouldn't function without it. The stress I am talking about in relationship to your need for relaxation is what I call *negative* stress.

People with cancer suffer a lot of negative stress. There are many sources:
♦ fear of dying
♦ loss of ability to work, which may lead to financial insecurity
♦ pain
♦ changes in appearance
♦ changes in relationships
♦ mental confusion
♦ "life-and-death" decisions that have to be made
♦ less energy
♦ less mobility
♦ severe physical symptoms
♦ feelings of aloneness
♦ anxiety about medical or surgical procedures
♦ anxiety and nausea before and during chemotherapy

Negative stress is the stress that increases your fears. It makes you feel helpless and unable to function. This is the kind of stress you can't seem to cope with. It is known that negative stress will make it especially hard for you to cooperate and assist in your therapy. It may also weaken your immune system.

You want to do all that you can to manage this stress.

RELAXING TO REDUCE NEGATIVE STRESS

Relaxation is an excellent way to manage stress. Many people believe that relaxation techniques alone can reduce all levels of stress. This is generally true for people who are *not* in crisis. But people in crisis—and people with cancer often are—have to take practical steps toward stress reduction before a healing relaxation can occur.

Reducing Pain It is pretty well impossible to relax if you are suffering acute or chronic physical and emotional pain. So the most important practical step you can take to reduce stress is to reduce your physical pain. You may have to take pain medication or antianxiety medication at first. But you will notice that as you follow through on a stress-reduction and relaxation program, you will become less and less dependent on these medications. Once the mental and emotional struggle and severe pain have been attended to, then you can get down to the business of deep relaxation.

Enjoying Yourself You can take many other practical steps to reduce stress. Make up your own list, perhaps starting with these suggestions:
♦ exercise appropriate for your condition
♦ listening to music
♦ support groups
♦ sharing feelings with friends and family
♦ adopting a pet
♦ professional counseling
♦ watching funny movies
♦ reading comic or comical books
♦ getting a massage
♦ showing gratitude
♦ helping someone else

You reduce stress by doing those things you need to do—getting second opinions, counseling, controlling your symptoms and sharing your feelings. You also reduce stress by doing the things you enjoy doing—listening to music, going to movies, enjoying your favorite hobby or finding a new hobby or attending religious services.

Successful methods for stress reduction are different for everyone. One person might meditate quietly, another might run a few miles. Most people find music relaxing, but one person might listen to rock 'n' roll while another listens to Mozart. There is no right way or wrong way.

DEEP RELAXATION TECHNIQUES

The relaxation techniques described here do more than just reduce stress. They bring you into what is called an alpha state. Alpha describes a brainwave pattern that represents a deeply relaxed and meditative state. In this alpha state, stress is reduced enough to increase your sense of well-being, improve your ability to function, improve your immune system and make it easier for you to participate in your own recovery.

Before you can relax enough to be in the alpha state, you must decrease the negative stress you are experiencing. Then you can use several relaxation methods known to produce alpha states—acupressure, meditation and visual imagery.

Getting in the Mood Before using any of these methods, put yourself in a calm and quiet mood. One way to do this is to sit in a chair or lie down. Make sure you are comfortable. Make sure your surroundings are quiet or at least without distraction.

Then start taking very deep breaths. Breathe into your abdomen. You can check this out by resting your hand on your abdomen and feeling your hand go up and down. This is deep abdominal breathing. It's also called hara breathing, a healing kind of breathing that is very relaxing. Do this a number of times slowly and deeply until you feel relaxed.

You might also use a relaxation tape. There are many different tapes and many different ways of relaxing. Sources for these tapes are listed at the end of this chapter. Each tape will give you instructions.

Whatever method you use, once you're in a relaxed state you can go on to actively use one or more of the following techniques:

Acupressure This involves the application

of finger pressure on points where it is believed that our life force or energy comes to the surface of the body. These points are the same ones used in acupuncture.

One acupressure technique you can use

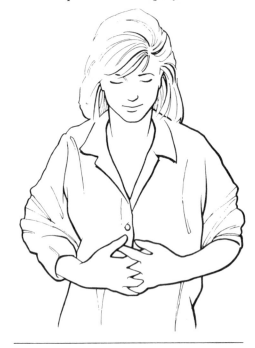

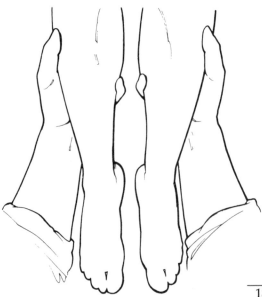

to create deep relaxation is to interweave your fingers and place them over your solar plexus, which is found in the center of your body just below the breastbone. Then sit back and quietly relax. Experience the feeling that you have—a sense of calm or sedation. You will soon be in a very relaxed state.

You might ask a friend or family member to sit at your feet. Have them put a hand under each calf, spreading their fingers. Have them sit there with their hands under your calves for about 15 minutes. This too will put you in a deeply relaxed state.

Meditation This is the act of focusing the thoughts in your mind. Another way of describing it is "engaging in contemplation or reflection." You can do this in many ways. A common way of putting yourself in a meditative state is to focus your attention on a single object. It could be a piece of fruit or the flame of a candle.

Another method is to repeat a sound. A common sound you may be familiar with is "om," which many people use in meditation. You can use any sound you are comfortable with.

Meditation takes practice. When you put yourself in a relaxed state and then meditate, you will notice that your mind tends to be very busy. You will have trouble staying focused. When your mind does start to wander, take a deep, slow breath and let the object or sound you are repeating come into rhythm with your breathing. Then continue.

Visual Imagery Again, put yourself into a relaxed state through deep breathing or a relaxation tape. Then visualize a scene or a color you find very, very relaxing. A peaceful, pleasurable setting might be a warm beach or a lush green meadow or a cool, refreshing mountain lake. It could be an image of floating on a soft white cloud.

Something else that might be relaxing

for you is the color blue (or pink or white). Take this color and visualize yourself being flooded by it and relaxing. There is no right or wrong here. Whatever relaxes you when you visualize it is right for you.

Acupressure, meditation and visual imagery are methods that are known to induce deep relaxation and to create a fertile environment for recovery. You can use all of them or just one. And remember that stress reduction and deep relaxation are two separate actions but can be performed simultaneously.

Using these techniques can help you control pain, improve your immune system and increase your sense of well-being. They can also increase your ability to tolerate therapy and improve the quality of your life.

These techniques cannot be overused. You can use them for as long as you are comfortable. But don't struggle to keep doing them. Remember, your goal is to relax; you will notice that the more you do them, the longer you will be comfortable doing them. And once again, remember that there is no right or wrong way. Just "your way."

WHERE TO FIND STRESS MANAGEMENT TAPES

Audiotapes that help you reduce or manage stress have become so popular that many are now available in drugstores and health food stores as well as bookstores and libraries.

You can also order tapes or ask for catalogs by contacting:

The Enterprises Store
1200 N. Lake Avenue
Pasadena, California 91104
(818) 798-7893 or 1-800-826-0364

Gateways Institute
PO Box 1778
Ojai, California 93023
(805) 646-8148

**Jin Shin Do Foundation
for Bodymind Acupressure**
PO Box 1097
Felton, California 95018
(408) 338-9454

Potentials Unlimited, Inc.
4808-H Broadmoor SE
Grand Rapids, Michigan 49508
1-800-221-6121

SelfCare Catalog
PO Box 130
Mandeville, Louisiana 70470-0130
(504) 893-1195

Whole Person Press
PO Box 3151
Duluth, Minnesota 55803
(218) 728-4077

26
HOME CARE

Ernest H. Rosenbaum, MD, Malin Dollinger, MD, Isadora Rosenbaum, MA,
Pamela Lemkin, RN, BSN, and Stephen Lemkin, MD

◇

Most people feel much more comfortable in the warm, familiar surroundings of home than they do in a hospital or convalescent home. Medical facilities naturally seem strange. They are antiseptic, regulated and sometimes forbidding. Yet many cancer patients prolong their hospital stay. Why? Because they—or their families—are afraid they won't get proper treatment at home or be able to cope with home care problems.

These fears are understandable, but they can be overcome. Medical and non-medical crises can be anticipated. And they can often be avoided by training in the elements of home care—for patients and families alike—before discharge from the hospital.

Is Home Care for You? Home care can play a vital part in your rehabilitation. But it isn't for everyone. There are times when going home is just not practical. Not only your physical needs but also the ability of you and your family to cope with the psychological stress of a home care situation have to be assessed.

It is often hard for someone with cancer to endure the indignities that daily dependence on family members can bring. And the stress of having a chronically ill person at home may be too much for a family already stressed by other responsibilities. You may well be better off in a nursing facility.

Home care is a cooperative effort. You, your family and your medical team are all

involved and the decision to go home has to be made by all concerned—the attending physician, discharge planners, family members and you.

PLANNING TO GO HOME

The key to successful home care is planning. Problems have to be anticipated. Changes might have to be made in the way your home is organized. You might have to buy or rent special equipment and work out the routines necessary for proper care. All this may seem like a lot of work, maybe even too much of a burden. Yet a comfortable and workable home care environment can be devised. And it can be a helpful step to recovery.

Discharge Planning Once you, your doctor and others make the decision to go home, you should be able to call on the services of a discharge planner. This planner—who may be a medical social worker, public health nurse or discharge coordinator—will help define your needs and match them with the resources available in your community.

Training Depending on the hospital, you, your family and any other potential caregivers might be able to enroll in the home care training programs now provided by many hospitals. These programs are usually taught by nurses and home care planners and vary in length.

The first part of the program may be

devoted to making sure that home care really is practical and appropriate for you and your family. The rest of the program may combine personal and/or videotape instruction with teaching in the hospital, followed by your practicing the skills to be used at home. The home health nurse will be able to reinforce or complete the training you receive in the hospital.

Assessing Your Resources Since the objective of home care is to keep your home life as normal as possible while still providing you with quality medical care, the first step to effective home care is taking a good look both at the support available to you and at the physical layout of your home.

Home care requires a willingness of family and friends to accept the responsibility of helping you on a sustained basis. Some key questions have to be answered.
♦ How much time can your family and friends spare?
♦ How will they balance providing support to you with their work and other responsibilities?
♦ If more than one family member will be providing care, can a rotation schedule be worked out?
♦ Will infants or growing children make other demands that will have to be met?
♦ Can each caregiver have enough free time to maintain his or her own physical and emotional well-being?

In the home, you and the home care planner should look closely at the physical setup. You'll have to pay special attention to the bathroom and bedroom, the location of stairs and the space available for extra equipment. You might have to get rid of scatter rugs or small objects on the floors. Railings might have to be installed and rubber strips attached to the tub and shower to prevent slipping.

Equipment The planner will also help you decide what equipment you will need. Commonly needed aids include:
♦ Hospital beds—manual, semi-electric

or electric; safety side-rails; overhead trapeze bars; overbed tables
♦ Wheelchairs—standard folding or powered chairs
♦ Walking aids—canes, crutches, walkers and folding walkers
♦ Bathroom safety equipment—bath benches, grab bars, shower attachments, elevated toilet seats and toilet assist frames
♦ Patient aids—commode chair, flotation pads, sheepskin pads, transfer lifts and respiratory equipment
♦ Patient care items—foam cushion rings, bedpans, urinals, heel and elbow protectors, sitz baths and incontinence pads and pants.

Most of this equipment should be available through local supply companies. And most medical insurance policies will cover the cost of rental or purchase.

Other Resources The planner can also put you in touch with the home health agencies in your community and direct you to other community resources. The local chapter of the American Cancer Society can also provide information on support groups and organizations devoted to specific problems, such as the United Ostomy Care Association or the Reach to Recovery Program.

GETTING TREATMENT AT HOME

One reason some cancer patients put off going home is that they're worried they'll have to be always going back and forth over long distances for their therapy sessions. This was a legitimate concern not many years ago, but things have changed.

In a way, things have come full-circle. In the first half of this century, medicine had much less to offer in the way of specific therapies than it does now. Before the age of antibiotics, modern diagnostic tools and effective treatment for many now curable diseases, doctors sent their patients to the hospital only when they were extremely ill. Medical care was given primarily in the home or in the doctor's office. But as medical advances and technological developments gradually led to superb diagnostic and treatment methods, hospitals became the primary centers for medical care. People were admitted for complex diagnostic studies and for the initiation of therapy, especially for serious diseases like cancer.

But the pendulum has been swinging away from the hospital as the focus of medical care and back to the home and the doctor's office. Both can be just as effective places for treatment as hospitals are. And both are a lot more convenient.

Doctors have realized for some time that they could deliver the same chemotherapy program they gave in hospitals in the comfort of their own offices where efficient and experienced oncology nurses, lounge chairs and television distraction were available. Patients also found this far more acceptable and desirable than a stay in the hospital, especially for treatment that lasted only four to six hours. After a few years of observation that this office procedure was effective, safe and satisfactory, it was not a radical step to perform the same procedure in a person's home.

Now hospitals are again used mainly for serious, life-threatening medical problems or complications, major surgery or beginning complex therapies that require sophisticated equipment or observation that can't be obtained elsewhere.

The New Home Care Services Home and office care offer significant advantages—lower cost, the avoidance of a strange and unfamiliar environment and especially the ability of a family to offer direct, supportive care.

Home care services are expanding in many areas. Where these services are available, a variety of important treatment procedures—including chemotherapy,

antibiotics, total parenteral nutrition and pain management—can be given in the home by an oncology nurse working under the supervision of an oncologist. The ability to give home chemotherapy safely has been greatly improved by the use of implanted venous access devices such as the Hickman, Broviac or Groshong catheters or Infusaport devices.

If you need these services, the nurse can remain with you for as many hours as necessary and your family members can be taught to give other medications to control symptoms and side effects.

Insurance companies and other third party payers are rapidly agreeing to pay for home care in many instances, especially when the cost of performing the service at home is shown to be a lot less than it is at a hospital. Medicare and Medicaid will pay for professional nursing visits, physiotherapy, occupational therapy and a medical social worker, provided your physician believes it is a necessary part of your treatment program.

CARING FOR YOUR BODY

Like most people with cancer, you are probably going to have a number of problems in body care. But these too can be anticipated and dealt with before discharge from the hospital. You and your family should be instructed in specific care techniques.

Bowel and Bladder Care You should be given a practical approach to bowel and bladder care. Special attention will be given to the problems of constipation, diarrhea and incontinence. You and your family should have a basic knowledge of laxatives, enemas, catheters and dietary management. (For more detailed information, *see* Chapter 17.)

There are two main problems with the bowels, both uncomfortable but both preventable in many cases:

Constipation Irregular or infrequent bowel movements can be caused by many things—chemotherapy drugs, pain-controlling narcotics, changes in diet or environment or lack of activity.

It can be prevented by adding foods high in fiber and bulk to your diet, such as fruits, vegetables, whole-grain breads and cereals and bran. You should also drink plenty of fluids and be as active as possible. Stool softeners, stimulating laxatives and suppositories can help. More severe constipation can be relieved by enemas (either commercially prepared or a home mixture of 1 tsp./5 mL of table salt and 1 pint/500 mL of tap water). If your white blood cell count or platelet count is severely depressed, talk to your doctor about what to do for constipation.

Diarrhea Unusually frequent and liquid bowel movements can result from chemotherapy, radiotherapy, emotional stress or sensitivity to certain foods. Your doctor can help find the cause and advise you if you need medication.

To relieve the discomfort, restrict yourself to warm fluids so your bowel can rest. Then gradually add foods low in roughage—dry toast, crackers, mashed potatoes, applesauce and rice. As you slowly return to your normal diet, drink plenty of liquids to replace the fluids lost in the diarrhea.

Incontinence If you have a problem controlling urination, two kinds of catheter can be used. Men can use a condom type that fits snugly on the shaft of the penis and is attached to a gravity drainage bag. The other type is a Foley catheter that is inserted directly into the bladder and attached to a bag that is changed regularly.

With either type, it is important to keep the skin clean and dry. With the Foley catheter, special care has to be taken to keep the connections and drainage port free of contamination. A nurse can show you and your family the procedures to follow before you leave the hospital.

Skin Care If you have to remain in bed for long periods, you'll have to pay special attention to the condition of your skin. When some part of the body lies against a surface like a mattress for a long period, nutrients and oxygen can't reach the skin cells. The area breaks down and the skin cells die. This creates pressure sores or bedsores.

Your tailbone, hips, spine, elbows, heels, ankles and shoulder blades are particularly susceptible to these sores. It is especially important to prevent your skin from being damaged by this kind of chafing because the sores can become infected. And weight loss and the side effects of radiation or chemotherapy can lower resistance to infection.

Proper skin care, along with adequate nutrition, helps prevent pressure sores and will also keep you feeling refreshed. A nurse or physical therapist can instruct you and your family in the basic techniques of skin care, such as:

♦ frequent position changes (most important)
♦ dry, wrinkle-free linen
♦ heat
♦ gentle massage
♦ good hygiene
♦ the use of talcum and skin lotions
♦ the use of a foam rubber ("egg crate") mattress or a foam or sheepskin pad to cushion your body and provide better air circulation.

Mouth Care Daily care of your mouth and teeth is always necessary, but cancer treatment can create special problems. Radiotherapy affects the mouth when it is given directly to the area and mouth sores may be a side effect of chemotherapy given for tumors in any part of the body.

You should brush your teeth daily with a soft-bristled brush. You might also floss daily to clean between the teeth, although it could be too irritating to your gums.

Your mouth should also be kept moist, both for oral health and for comfort. If a dry mouth is a problem, your doctor can prescribe an artificial saliva or a saliva stimulant. Rinsing your mouth frequently with water, chewing sugarless gum or sucking on ice chips or sugarless candies can also help keep the mouth moist.

PAIN CONTROL

Patients about to go home from the hospital are often worried about how they will deal with pain. If they've been getting medication from nurses and doctors to relieve pain, they often wonder, "Who will give me the medicine at home?" "What if I run out of medicine?" "Suppose I need an injection?" "What if I'm alone and the pain gets worse?"

The important point to remember is that most pain can be relieved. There are many medications available and one or more of them will certainly help. (For detailed information, *see* Chapter 19.)

Also remember that pain is a complex experience that is not only physical. Psychological and emotional factors play a major role in anyone's response to pain. Chronic pain that is relieved for a while and then returns can be very tiring. That fatigue in turn can make the pain worse. Acute or sudden pain can set off anxieties and fears.

The key to overcoming pain is to feel that you are the expert and you *can* do something about it. Having control over pain helps you relax. Relaxation means less anxiety, and less anxiety means less pain.

Keeping Track of Your Pain The first step in your gaining control over pain will be taken in the hospital when your doctor recommends the type and frequency of medication. You and/or your family should then keep a record of how the medication affects you.

Monitor where the pain is, what it feels like—sharp, dull, intermittent or stab-bing—how long it takes the medication to start working, how long the relief lasts and whether there are any side effects. Grade your pain on a scale of 0 to 10, with 0 being non-existent and 10 being severe. All this information will help your doctor make minor changes in dosage or prescribe other, possibly more effective medication. Keeping track of the effects while you are still in hospital will also prepare you to be self-reliant in pain control once you get home.

Injections You might be prescribed medication in the form of pills, liquids, rectal suppositories or injections. Pills, liquids and suppositories are familiar and usually easy to take. But many people are afraid to give themselves injections.

These fears can be overcome with help and a little training in the proper techniques from hospital staff. After all, many diabetics give themselves injections every day. A nurse can show you and your family how to measure the medication and draw it into the syringe, how to prepare the skin and how to inject the needle. A little practice will be needed before you feel able to give a shot safely and comfortably. But once you know you can do it you will have more confidence that you can control your pain.

Where to Give the Injection The doctor or nurse will also advise you about where to give the injection. Generally, medications that are either irritating to the skin or designed to act quickly are injected deep into the muscle tissue (intramuscular). Non-irritating medications are often injected just below the skin (subcutaneous).

The three common places for intramuscular injections are the upper outer portion of the buttocks, the thigh midway between the hip and the knee, and the upper arm about a third of the way down from the shoulder to the elbow. Subcutaneous injections can be given at many places, the most common being the fleshy part of the upper arm.

Infusions Continuous infusions of pain medicine, either through an IV catheter such as a Hickman, or subcutaneously through a small plastic needle, may be used for severe pain or pain not relieved by a variety of oral or injected medicines. Small pumps, approximately 8 oz. (225 g) in weight, are used so you can remain mobile and be as active as your condition allows.

A home health nurse will instruct you and your caregiver about the operation of the pump and will be available by phone 24 hours a day.

Side Effects Pain medications can produce side effects such as nausea or constipation, but both can be treated. It's very important, however, that you tell your doctor about the side effects and let him or her recommend what to do about them. Treating them yourself can cause complications. If you take certain types of bulk laxatives at the same time as narcotic pain medication, for example, the laxative can actually *cause* rather than relieve severe constipation.

EMOTIONAL SUPPORT FOR YOUR FAMILY

When you get home from the hospital, you may be a little frightened. But you'll probably be eager to get back to sleeping in your own bed and returning to your normal routines. Your family will be happy you're coming home, but they'll be worried too. They will wonder about providing you with proper care. They will have to deal with new routines, changing roles, new expectations. Not least, they will have to deal with the many changes of mood and behavior you'll go through as you cope with your illness.

Home care is a major undertaking for family members. They give not only their physical services but also their empathy and compassion. Many people with cancer, because of the intensity of their illness, are often able to give little emotional support in return.

So family members may need special emotional support. They may feel left out of critical decisions, burdened with responsibilities, afraid of what the future will bring. They may feel angry about the disruption of their own lives and guilty for any number of reasons. Family members must be especially helped to not feel guilty for considering their own needs as well as yours and for taking time for their own social and recreational activities. It is also important to include children in discussions appropriate to their age and level of understanding.

The Importance of Communication The emotional needs of everyone can best be met by planning and open communication. If more than one family member is involved in care, a schedule to rotate responsibilities should be arranged. If one person is the main caregiver, he or she has to be allotted some free time for mental and physical well-being. Resentments and fears should be discussed as freely as possible so that frustrations don't simmer and rise to the boiling point. Shared feelings are always easier to handle.

Psychological counseling or support groups made up of families of other cancer patients can also give family members a forum for emotional release. Your doctor, medical social worker or local medical organizations can put family members in touch with appropriate groups.

And if your home situation grows tense or emotionally exhausting, you might consider a temporary stay in a nursing home. Giving family members some respite from the rigors of home care—even for a few days—might let everybody come back to the home care setting in a refreshed and more relaxed frame of mind.

IF THERE'S AN EMERGENCY

One of the biggest fears you and your family may have when planning to go home is what will happen if there's an emergency. Your doctor, home care planner or medical social worker can help you and family members prepare for emergencies. They will go over with you what situations might come up and the procedures for getting help quickly. They can also instruct family members in appropriate first aid procedures.

For your own peace of mind, you should follow a few procedures as soon as you get home:

♦ Prepare a card listing the telephone numbers of your doctor, pharmacy, ambulance service, fire department, police and a close relative or friend. Keep the card by the telephone.

♦ Prepare a self-care card recording important facts about your condition and medications. You may not always be able to reach your own doctor and if you or your family have to explain things to another doctor on call, you may get confused or lose valuable time if vital information isn't at your fingertips. The self-care card should include your name, diagnosis, the treatment you've been getting, which chemotherapy drugs you've been on, any other medications you are taking, any allergies you may have, the names of other doctors involved in your care and your blood type, if available.

What to Do If an emergency does arise, you or your family members should follow three basic principles:

1. Stay calm. Remember that help is always available and will usually arrive within minutes of an emergency call.

2. Determine the problem and call for help. Check the pulse rate to see if it is fast, slow or irregular. Check for breathing problems, changes in mental state, new pain or sudden increases in pain, nausea or vomiting, or injuries from a fall or other accident. If the symptoms seem to require immediate attention, call the doctor or appropriate emergency service at once.

3. Take appropriate action while waiting for help to arrive. The most common emergencies are heart-related problems, breathing problems, bleeding, broken bones and falls.

Though hospital staff can give family members some training in dealing with these emergencies, the best preparation is the first aid courses offered by the Red Cross or other organizations in the community. These courses will teach family members the technique of cardiopulmonary resuscitation (CPR), the Heimlich maneuver to deal with choking, how to operate oxygen equipment rented for use at home, how to stop serious bleeding and what to do to keep someone comfortable when bones are broken.

The most important thing for family members to keep in mind is, *when in doubt, call for help*. It is far better for a doctor or paramedic to find the situation not as serious as originally thought than to risk the life of a loved one.

27
PALLIATIVE CARE

Margaret I. Fitch, RN, PhD, and Leslee J. Thompson, RN, MScN

◇

For some people with cancer, a cure will not be possible. The most appropriate route in such cases is treatment and care that are directed toward palliation.

Palliative care is a form of comfort-giving care that fully recognizes that cure or long-term control is not possible. The primary concern of palliative care is quality of life. Palliative care is provided so that people who are dying can be helped to maintain the best possible level of physical, emotional, mental, spiritual, vocational and social life during their remaining time, no matter how much limitation may be imposed by their advancing disease.

It is so important to understand that the phrase "there is nothing more we can do" usually means to the doctor that the disease cannot be cured. It does not mean that we have run out of ways to help. There are still many things that can be done to promote comfort and ease distress.

The Range of Services Providing palliative care requires special skill and expertise from a variety of health care professionals and includes close attention to controlling symptoms and providing psychosocial and spiritual support. Both patient and family are involved in palliative care to ensure that the patient can live as fully as possible in the face of impending death and the most satisfactory quality of time together can be achieved. Family members benefit from such support during the illness and, later, during their time of grieving.

Another term sometimes used is *hospice* care. First used in England, hospice refers to a place where palliative care is given and also to the concept that palliative care, after active treatment is no longer appropriate, is especially important and worthy. It now also applies to *any* palliative care, whether in an institution (hospice) or in the home ("hospice care").

Palliative care/hospice care is, then, a set of ideas or beliefs about what is important when people are dying and how they can be helped. The ideas have been used to develop special programs or ways of offering help to patients and families. In some hospitals, palliative care teams of nurses, doctors, social workers and others will visit a patient in the hospital. In some communities, palliative care experts and health professional teams will visit a person at home. There are also volunteer hospice organizations across the country that can provide support and assistance for people at home. The exact type of service available from place to place is apt to vary. Not all communities will offer the same services, and what is available may not be widely publicized. Patients and families may have to ask about which services are available in their community.

The health care professionals and volunteer visitors involved in this work are trained in helping the person who is dying feel supported and cared for. However, not everyone has the same comfort level in talking about death and dying. Patients and families who want palliative care may have to request it or turn to other health care professionals than those they have known to find the support they need.

There is sometimes a feeling that a palliative care unit is a "place to go to die." What is important to know is that the focus in such a unit is on *living* until death. The emphasis is on achieving comfort (freedom from pain) and maintaining as much activity as possible. Often the regulations and atmosphere in a palliative care unit are more relaxed than in a typical hospital setting. In many instances arrangements can be made for family gatherings or visits with pets. A palliative care unit can become "a home away from home."

THE ROLE OF PALLIATIVE CARE

Hospice or palliative care focuses on life. Hospice recognizes that death is a part of life and dying is a normal process. We are human beings and death will come to each of us.

For most of us the idea of our own death or the death of someone we love is inconceivable. In North America, thoughts of death are pushed aside. We are a death-denying society. So, when faced with the inevitability of death—our own or that of one whom we love—most of us feel ill prepared. Many of us feel overwhelmed by the situation and are not certain where to turn for help. Sometimes we are not sure what kind of help we need.

Hospice or palliative care services exist in the hope and belief that through receiving appropriate care, people who are dying and their family members might be free to discover a satisfactory degree of mental and spiritual preparation for death.

The route to appropriate care is through working in partnership—patient, family and health care team members working together—with a clear focus on issues of patient autonomy and patient and family preferences.

MAIN GOALS OF PALLIATIVE CARE

The main goals of palliative care are:
♦ to provide relief from pain and other distressing symptoms;
♦ to provide psychological and spiritual care; and
♦ to provide support for the family during the illness and the grieving period that follows.

Pain and Symptom Relief (*See* Chapter 19) Individuals with advancing disease can experience a variety of symptoms, depending on the specific type of disease. The most common symptoms include pain, loss of appetite, fatigue, weakness, weight loss, constipation, difficulty breathing, confusion, nausea, vomiting, cough, and dry or sore mouth.

The nurses and doctors may try several approaches to find the most appropriate way to achieve comfort. It is important that both patient and family members keep a close eye on the symptoms a person is experiencing, and note whether a particular approach is helpful. If the approach is not effective, another should be tried quickly and the search continued until comfort is achieved.

One of the most commonly experienced symptoms, pain, no matter how chronic or severe, can almost always be controlled without harmful side effects. By using a variety of medications, nurses and doctors work to discover the "tailor-made" plan to relieve pain. Several different approaches may need to be tried. Each patient may have pain for different reasons and respond to pain differently.

The most important medications used to relieve pain and prevent side effects are called analgesics. When milder analgesics such as aspirin or codeine are no longer effective, there should be no hesitation in using stronger analgesics (called narcotics) such as morphine. The dose of the narcotic is exactly matched to the level of pain the person is experiencing and adjusted whenever the pain changes. In some situations, patients remain alert despite large doses of medication. The patient does not become "accustomed" to the drug or require increasingly higher doses to control the pain; nor does he or she become addicted.

Medications may be given by mouth (liquid or pill), by suppository, by injection into a vein, by continuous infusion with a "pain pump" or in a "patch" on the skin.

For chronic pain, medication must be given regularly. It is inappropriate to wait until the patient is in pain again before the next dose is given. Sometimes, taking regular doses means the patient will need to be awakened from sleep, especially at night. But it is important to maintain the schedule to prevent the pain from reappearing or "breaking through." Use of the pain pump is becoming more common. The pump is designed to give a continuous dose of medication 24 hours a day through a small portable, computerized device so that patients can remain independent and out of hospital.

Each of the other symptoms (constipation, cough, difficulty breathing, diarrhea, confusion, etc.) requires the same close attention that pain requires if patients are to be comfortable. It is important that patients and families discuss any symptom with the nurse or doctor and state any preferences they may have for managing it. If patients are involved in planning how to treat or relieve symptoms, they are more likely to feel in control of their symptoms. This sharing process will also help patients understand the physical changes occurring to their body.

One of the changes that can occur for cancer patients as their disease advances is loss of weight and wasting of body tissues. This can be accompanied by changes in skin color and loss of appetite. Watching these changes can be difficult both for the patient and for family members. The changes are part of the normal course of the advancing disease. As death draws closer, all bodily functions slow. Weakness and fatigue can be profound, and there may be periods of confusion. Finding the energy to talk is often difficult.

As the time for death draws nearer, many people have questions about what their death might be like. Some have heard about others' experiences with dying and wonder if their experiences will be the same. In most instances, nurses and doctors can anticipate how an individual will die based on the type of disease and the symptoms. Patients and family members feel better prepared if they talk with the nurse or doctor about what bodily changes to expect and how things might feel.

Psychosocial and Spiritual Care To be faced with one's own death releases a range of emotions. Each person will react in his or her own way. There can be shock and disbelief that this could be happening, anger that it is happening at this time in one's life, or acceptance that one's appointed time has come. A range of worries will usually emerge as a person begins to imagine the ending of life and what will happen to the people he or she loves. There may be financial concerns, legal issues and worries about how one's family will manage. As bodily changes occur and the need to depend on others for help increases, many people have concerns about not contributing to the family in their usual way and worry about being a burden.

This can also be a time when people question what their lives have truly meant and experience a range of spiritual questions. Regrets about things one did as well as things left undone can create a sense of guilt and remorse. Sometimes people feel that they are very alone, that no one could possibly understand what they are going through. This can also be a time for inner growth and reaching a sense of profound peace. As individuals review their lives, they may gain insight about themselves and an understanding about some of the events and relationships they experienced.

Not everyone will experience all of these feelings, but they are all natural and it is helpful to talk about them. Various professionals—nurses, social workers, chaplains and psychologists—can be of assistance in listening, helping you with choices and assisting you in organizing any additional help you might wish. Some people find it helpful to talk with their close friends or family. Some will turn to their rabbi, minister or priest.

As difficult as these feelings are to face and to talk about, they do not go away if they are ignored. Finding a comfortable way to acknowledge and express them will be helpful. While some people will talk to another person, others will write in a diary, paint a picture, write a poem or compose a song. Others may find solace in listening to music, reading or meditation. Feelings can be expressed in many ways. What is useful to one person may not be helpful to another. Each of us needs to find the way that works best for us.

Support for the Family Family and friends also experience a range of emotions. They too share the shock and disbelief, the feelings of unfairness and anger and the overwhelming sense of helplessness to change the course of events. In some instances, there may also be a sense of relief that the suffering and struggle is nearly over or relief that death brings an end to a troubled relationship. In turn, some feel guilt for holding those feelings of wanting things to be over quickly.

Loved ones will experience their own concerns about the future. There is a sense of their world suddenly being changed so that it will never be the same again, and a fear about how they will face the challenge of managing alone. The world without their spouse or parent or child is impossible to imagine. There is an over-

whelming sense of dread and despair, an emerging sense of profound loss. It is difficult to concentrate or focus. Suddenly all one's priorities have shifted and the world seems turned upside down.

For some people, the time they have together can strengthen their relationship and create lasting memories. There is time to share, in a deep and profound way, what their lives together have meant. There is time to talk about the past and to make plans together. Such discussion could cover plans and dreams for children's futures, what to do about the house, what to do with finances, what the funeral should be like or what should happen to the body. Not all people will be able to discuss these topics easily and may need assistance in doing so. Nurses, social workers, chaplains, psychologists and palliative care volunteers may be called upon for help.

It is helpful to remember to focus on life and living until death comes. People need to live until they die. Celebrations and life pleasures are still there to be enjoyed, to be shared. Birthdays, anniversaries, graduations and achievements offer time for families to gather and to affirm life.

On the other hand, it is important to discuss with the person who is dying what would be helpful for him or her. The presence of too many people all at the same time could be overwhelming and tiring. Perhaps the more appropriate plan would be for visitors to come in small numbers and be able to sit and talk quietly. Sometimes, too, it is the little things that can make such a difference—a trip to the countryside, listening to a favorite record, sitting in the garden, feeling the sun on one's face, hearing children's laughter, seeing a sunset. Family and friends can play an important role in making these things happen.

Reactions to a family member's impending death will differ from family member to family member. Not everyone will feel exactly the same way at the same time. There is no "right way" to cope, and no "appropriate" time schedule for feelings. One person may feel strong at a time when another feels most vulnerable. One may cry easily while another does not feel able to cry. One may bury himself or herself in work while another is unable to concentrate. Talking to people who are not aware of the upheavals can create added tension for some people. What is important is that a family can understand these differences and find ways to draw on one another's strengths. Talking with one another, or with someone else, about one's feelings can be helpful.

Young children are part of the family and it is important that, when appropriate, they be included and involved in conversations about what is happening. It is very easy for a child to think he or she has caused the death if no other explanation is provided. There are many helpful books about talking with children about death.

Making funeral arrangements and preparing a will are two activities that, if completed before death, can make the time of death and period of mourning less stressful. Most funeral homes provide a "prearrangement" service for families; many of the details for visitation and the funeral ceremony can be made ahead of time. This approach can also enable the individual to be involved in planning for the funeral and the disposition of his or her body. Writing a will provides a vehicle for a person to plan with certainty how his or her possessions will be dispersed.

The choice between dying in a palliative care unit or in a hospital and dying at home can be difficult for both patients and families. Both settings have benefits and drawbacks. In a unit there is 24-hour nurse support, while in the community the nurse may visit only once or twice a day; in a unit the patient is more separated from family and familiar environment, whereas at home he or she could be the center of the household; in a unit the family can visit and provide help in some ways, while at home the family carries the major burden of caregiving.

Before making a choice about which approach to take, the patient and family should talk over the details and explore the benefits and drawbacks with the nurse or doctor. In some instances arrangements can be made to take advantage of both settings at different stages of the illness.

PART III:
QUALITY OF LIFE

28
THE DECISION TO LIVE

Ernest H. Rosenbaum, MD, and Isadora Rosenbaum, MA

"Choose life—only that and always, and at whatever risk.
To let life leak out, to let it wear away by the mere passage of time,
to withhold giving it and spreading it, is to choose nothing."

—Sister Helen Kelley

◇

As medical professionals, we have always been fascinated with the power of the will to live, with the way some of our patients cope with chronic disease even under the threat of death. We've observed how they refuse to let physical discomfort affect their enjoyment of family and friends or prevent them from going to work or pursuing outside interests.

Inspired by their fortitude, we asked some of them how they were able to transcend their problems. As we listened to their stories, we realized that however diverse they are in ethnic or cultural background, age, educational level or type of illness, they have all gone through a similar process of psychological recovery. They all consciously made a "decision to live." After an initial period of feeling devastated, they simply decided to assess their new reality and make the most of each day.

If these people were to give one piece of advice to anyone who has been diagnosed with cancer, it would be, "It's up to you. You can learn to live with it, live around it, live in spite of it. You don't know what you can do until you try."

Elsewhere in this book authors have referred to the gamut of emotions you experience when the unthinkable—a diagnosis of cancer—occurs. You feel terrified, angry, depressed, sorry for yourself and dehumanized by medical procedures. Everything you took for granted yesterday, even the things you complained about, suddenly belong to another life that you'd give anything to recapture.

You'd also like to recapture the image of yourself as a healthy person—independent, jovial, outgoing or competitive. Unfortunately, you've probably accepted the historical (but no longer true) image of a cancer patient as a helpless victim. And you naturally assume that's how everyone is secretly going to label you.

You probably can't even find reassurance in the words of family members and friends. Sure, they care, but how can they really know how you feel? It isn't happening to them. It's happening to *you—now!*

FACING REALITY

Your feelings are normal, particularly your anger and self-pity. Experiencing these emotions is part of being human. But at some point you will probably begin to seek ways of regaining control and living as normal a life as possible.

The first step in this process is to become well informed. This book is a beginning, providing you with basic information about the many different diseases we call cancer, how they affect our bodies and what the treatment options are. In these pages you'll also learn the valuable art of asking questions of your medical team and discover other types of support, from relaxation techniques to cancer support groups to ways of handling relationships.

To fight your disease, you also need goals. You're probably beginning to re-examine your most deeply held values and priorities. A threat to our existence has that effect, and it is an effect not easily forgotten. You can't help but appraise the kind of person you are, what's really important to you, how you want to live the rest of your life and what you want to accomplish.

As you make the transition from help-less victim to activist, one of the most important realizations is that *you* have everything to do with how others perceive you and treat you. If you can accept your condition and hold self-pity at bay, they won't feel sorry for you. If you can discuss your disease and medical therapy in a matter-of-fact manner, they'll respond in kind without fear or awkwardness.

In brief, you are in charge.

You can subtly and gently put your family, friends and co-workers at ease by being frank about what you want to talk about or not talk about and by being explicit about whether and when you want their help.

COMPROMISE: THE ART OF LIVING

You can live with your cancer, but you'll probably have to make compromises, as you've done all your life. When you have a major physical problem, compromise involves adaptation to any physical limitations. It may mean you have to give up a rigorous physical regimen and seek a less strenuous form of exercise. It may mean a change in job or hobbies. It will certainly require experimentation with alternative ways of doing things.

But whatever compromises you must make in your daily activities, remember one thing: your intellectual and emotional potential have not diminished. On the contrary, they have probably been enhanced by your illness. You may even find that you're willing to take risks you were too timid to take in the past. You may open your mind to new ideas, go places you've never been and do things you've never done.

Perhaps the hardest compromise most people have to make is to ask for or accept help. But the help of others may be necessary at times. Moreover, your family and friends *want* to be told what they can do for you. People feel good when they can be of service.

Besides, you can give to them in other ways. You can listen to them. As one patient said, "I feel I'm still in the ball game if a friend comes to me with a big problem and upsets me or if he comes to me with a great happiness and makes me feel glad. Either way, it means I have a sincere friend who wants to share a real part of his experience, whether it's tears or laughter."

REACHING OUT TO OTHERS

You have something extra to give your friends because of what you are going through. You've developed sensitivities that enable you to reach out to others, especially those who are just beginning to wage their own battle—to make their own decision to live.

To relieve another person's loneliness, to give hope that there's something to live for, is, we believe, what life is all about. It frees people from their own problems. That is perhaps the most valuable lesson we have learned from our patients: that happiness comes from the satisfaction of sharing with and helping others.

But before you can help others, you have to take responsibility for yourself and see that your needs are met. It requires tapping that reserve of spiritual strength you didn't know you had and using the power that is yours: to learn all you can about your illness, to reject out-moded attitudes toward cancer "victims," to determine by your own behavior how others will treat you, to make compromises where necessary, to take risks, to share tears or laughter with family and friends.

As our patients would say, "It's up to you."

29
LIVING WITH MORTALITY: LIFE GOES ON

Malin Dollinger, MD, and Bernard Dubrow, MS

We revel in life's beginning, wrestle with its challenges and take pride in our achievements. We know deep down that we are mortal and that our life will end some time in the future—the distant future, we hope—but we are not consciously aware of our mortality from day to day.

The media bombard us with flashes of death in stories and graphic pictures of car accidents, plane crashes, murders and wars, but we block them out in our minds. We feel protected and safe. We can accept the deaths of war heroes and old people, but reject the idea of its happening to us. We focus on guarding and enjoying our life and intuitively distance ourselves from thoughts of our mortality.

But what happens when we are jolted by the diagnosis of a possibly fatal chronic illness such as cancer? After recoiling from the shocking news and accepting its reality, how can we cope with this new state of uncertainty? How can we adjust our lifelong attitudes and renew our trust in life? For the first time, we find ourselves in the strange and disruptive situation of having to cope with living and dying at the same time. How can we do it?

The threat of serious illness unleashes a wide range of moods and emotions. We swing back and forth between fear and hope, nostalgia and yearning, sadness and joy, self-affirmation and self-doubt, confidence that modern medicine offers the prospect of fighting the disease and concern that treatments can fail. Religious people sense God's closeness at times and at other times feel abandoned.

Searching for Answers To avoid confusion and despair, these and other contradictory feelings have to be sorted out, faced squarely and dealt with.

New social and economic questions also arise. Should you keep trying to fulfill your ambitions, to build and compete? Will telling your friends and co-workers that you have cancer adversely affect your prospects for success? How should you protect your family from financial disaster? How do you emerge from the loneliness that seems to accompany illness and find meaning within your silent universe?

Denial of your illness lessens your capacity to find answers to these and other vital questions. But if you retain control of the illness as much as possible, you will be able to look directly at your own mortality and deal with it.

THE STAGES OF LIVING WITH MORTALITY

The process of living with mortality begins when you are first told the diagnosis. A new cancer "victim" develops fear, despair, hope, depression, anxiety and determination to find answers. It doesn't matter if there is a 50 percent chance of a cure or 80 percent or 95 percent. As long as there is even a 5 percent chance that the cancer is *incurable*, the emotional turmoil persists and the need to learn how to go on living in a purposeful way, despite the fear and worry, remains.

Many people diagnosed as having a chronic potentially fatal disease react, think and behave in similar ways, following a similar pattern. Not everyone will go through all the stages described below. Some will skip one or two or even come back to an earlier stage if a new symptom or other significant event occurs. But it is useful to become aware of these common reactions, whether or not you experience all of them yourself. Understanding these experiences will help you face your own uncertainties and fears and help you put in perspective some of the decisions you will have to make.

When faced with the threat of death or dying, many patients and their families turn for understanding and guidance to the highly regarded work of Dr. Elisabeth Kübler-Ross. She illustrates five stages— denial and isolation, anger, bargaining, depression and acceptance—that occur during a terminal illness. But the Kübler-Ross model applies to death in the near future of weeks or months. These circumstances do not apply to cancer patients who have been told they have a *potentially* fatal illness and that they might die of it, but cannot know when, and, then again, may not die of it but may not know that for years to come.

Living with a chronic potentially fatal illness associated with a lifespan measured in years involves responses that differ in many important ways from those described by Dr. Kübler-Ross.

Understanding the patterns of reaction to a prolonged illness with perhaps years of remission and a significant chance of being cured will help you put your emotional survival in focus while your doctor tries to take care of your physical survival. You will also realize that whatever stage you may be in, you are not alone. Your loved ones will be able to help you go on living. You will renew your confidence

and zest in life, deal with fear and worry, discover new value and meaning in your life, achieve gratification and even attain peace of mind.

DISBELIEF

When the diagnosis of cancer is made, many people first go through a stage of disbelief.

You will likely be unprepared for this sudden insult to your normal physical and emotional existence. There may be some denial involved. You may think, "The diagnosis is wrong . . . it will go away . . . it can't happen to me." You wish you could make a poor prognosis go away by picking up the phone and saying, "Hello, Heaven, please hold."

But you can hope—and with good justification—that you have significant time left, whether you are cured or not. The opportunity remains for you to enjoy life's pleasures.

Eventually, you are able to accept the idea, "The cancer victim is really me." At that point, you can proceed to the next stage.

DISCOVERY

Now you need to know all about the kind of cancer you have. You need some details about its stage and prognosis. You have to find out, to whatever extent is personally meaningful, all that is important to know about the illness. What tests do you need? What treatments are available? Are there alternative treatments? What are the advantages, disadvantages and risks of each? Where should you go for treatment? Is a second opinion important? What questions should you ask your doctor? You need to do whatever you have to do to be satisfied you're getting the best possible treatment.

One of the main purposes of this book is to help you with this discovery stage. Another pathway to discovery is through a connection with a key physician, sometimes your own physician and sometimes a specialist, with whom you can develop a relationship of confidence and trust. This physician will advise and guide you through the journey ahead.

Besides discovering technical information, you also have to discover your own strengths and weaknesses, your spiritual beliefs, how others can be of help and who your friends really are. Do your relationships with others need clarification?

When you have gathered this essential information and gained understanding of your situation, you are able to redefine and take charge of your life. A new phase of dealing with life begins.

REDIRECTION

You need to continue, adapt or invent a lifestyle and an attitude that let you function physically and emotionally. This is an opportunity to redirect your life in fresh, productive ways.

The method of redirection is an individual choice and depends to a significant extent on how you have dealt with major life problems in the past. Some people need logical, sensible, step-by-step discussions and explanations, with lists of ideas and choices. Others need only minimal consultations with their physicians. Some feel protected and supported by their religious beliefs and make trust in God a major part of their redirection. Some are helped by their relationships with their family, friends and support groups. There is no single right answer to how we should approach life.

Balancing Worry and Hope The powerful emotions of fear, hope, despair, anger and guilt released by a serious illness fade with recovery, but anxieties accumulate with a chronic possibly fatal disease. Tensions rise and fall and moods swing in cycles of highs and lows.

You may worry so much that you lose sight of the possibility of optimism. You may also become so hopeful and confident that you lose sight of reality. Your main challenge is how to balance your worry and your hope, integrating both into your day-to-day life without losing sight of either. As you ride this roller coaster of emotion, you should persist in finding the reality of each situation. The struggle is difficult, but great is the reward of finding peace of mind.

Controlling Negative Emotions It's just human nature to believe that if things are going well for us we must be doing something right. We also tend to believe the opposite: if things aren't going well and some misfortune occurs, we have *not* been doing the right things.

If a construction site collapses or a power plant erupts, we feel the need to mount a thorough investigation to find out why it happened and especially to find and punish whoever was responsible for the disaster. It is not surprising that we sometimes assume personal responsibility for our own illness and single ourselves out as deserving punishment. Explaining illness as a kind of punishment for a tragedy stemming from doing something wrong is, of course, a psychological reaction, a distortion of reality arising from the destructive emotion of guilt.

There is also a reaction called "survivors guilt." By remaining alive when others have died, some survivors dare not feel too confident or reassured for fear of somehow being punished for enjoying good fortune. They may feel that they have survived at the expense of others, although obviously they have not!

The redirection stage can be a time to learn how to lessen the destructive impact of emotional issues. Some people gain support and insight from spouses, family members or close friends. Sometimes professional help is useful, including clergy, psychologists, psychiatrists, social workers and counselors. For some, attending group meetings where feelings can be shared in a comfortable setting can relieve many psychological stresses. This will not abolish all anxiety, but will give expression to the deep emotions—fear, anger and guilt—that arise during a prolonged life-threatening illness. The first step toward control of negative emotions is recognizing them during this stage of living with mortality.

Affirmation During this stage, some people approach life with renewed enthusiasm, especially if a battle plan has been formulated to conquer the cancer.

You need to find ways to reaffirm your interest in life, in pleasurable activities, in your profession or your hobbies. The role of loved ones and friends is especially important. They have to give you "permission" to share your worries and fears. They can do this by encouraging you to tell them about your problems rather than turning off communication by trying to simply cheer you up. Giving blanket reassurance by saying "everything will be okay" sends the message that they want to hear only good things. They have to affirm that they are truly interested in you as an individual going through perhaps the most critical time of your life.

This stage—which, one hopes, can last a long time—also includes key medical judgments such as the affirmation that the correct physician is in charge of your care and is making the correct decisions about treatment. Sometimes a relapse, a setback or even an uncertain lab test or x-ray report may disrupt the redirection process. You may suddenly find yourself back in a stage of disbelief or discovery, but you will be better prepared to settle on and handle the course of action required to resolve new questions or problems.

During this stage you will also usually be forced by circumstances to deal with physical, emotional, financial and social effects, whether your illness is considered to be cured, is in remission or requires continued treatment. You must master the techniques of how to get on with your life and enjoy yourself despite problems such as denial of health insurance claims, prejudice in the workplace and trying to find people with whom you can share your problems.

You have to learn to retain your independence and to keep the anxieties of illness from suffocating you. Redirection helps shape your life and makes it more productive.

RESOLUTION

Finally, the stage of resolution is reached. This may occur if your cancer is cured and you are able to accept this fact and put the experience behind you. It may also occur when you realize that cure is not possible.

If your cancer cannot be cured, this stage is not necessarily associated with a sudden dismal change in attitude or depression, although certainly your spirits and emotions may be at a low ebb.

Having known for months or years that some day this time might come, someone who has been dealing productively with his or her illness will have spent time getting renewed enjoyment from life in whatever way possible, perfecting relationships with significant people and sorting through the things in life that are important.

You may have discovered the meaning of life in general and of your life in particular. In some cases, there may even be relief that the long-awaited catastrophe need no longer be feared in the abstract but can be dealt with directly.

You have worked through the complex and progressive emotions that the illness created in you as well as in the lives of those you love. You know that everything possible has been done and are comforted by the fact that you have gained additional time and meaning. You know that if there is to be a brief period of ending that it will be made as comfortable and as free of suffering as possible. This may mean aggressive medical treatment to relieve symptoms, hospice care when appropriate or the cessation of active anticancer treatment if that is appropriate.

If the previous three stages have successfully dealt with problems and needs, the final stage of resolution represents the attainment of peace of mind. It can become a validation that your struggle has been worthwhile and of value to you, your loved ones and your close friends.

If your cancer is gone, many months or, more often, several years after apparently successful treatment—which can often be complex, difficult and lengthy—your mind finally allows you to believe that you are cured. You can then reach the stage of resolution by regaining your belief once more that you are a normal person. You finally accept that the hoped-for goal has been achieved. You have a new awareness of the value of life and what in life holds special meaning for you.

EMERGING VICTORIOUS

The miracles of modern medicine have created a new dilemma for millions of people with chronic illnesses such as cancer, heart disease and stroke. Prolonged illness, especially if potentially fatal, generates anxiety, tension and worry that may be more troublesome than the illness itself.

Those who have cancer are labeled "cancer patient" and often agree somehow to accept this new identity. Loved ones and friends treat you differently, not to mention employers, insurance companies and everyone else who hears the news that you have cancer.

You want to get on with your life. You want to feel and look normal. Your doctor has told you that you are okay now. But that's hard to believe when every trip to the doctor's office, even for a checkup, reawakens old fears. Anxiety will not disappear completely, but a way of thinking about and understanding the emotional stages cancer patients face will help you cope with the awareness of mortality that cancer evokes.

In our society, the prospect of dying makes most people shrink and hide from a significant part of life. But you have to think positively. You have to recognize the potential within each of us even during prolonged illness.

For some of us, the threat of death increases our creative energies. Friends and family ties can draw closer and long-standing conflicts can be resolved. In spite of, or perhaps because of, the prospect of suffering, life intensifies and takes on added importance. Time is telescoped, and greater sensitivity to the wonders of the world is often gained.

It is unfortunate that our society shuns the thought of dying and turns away from the large segment of the population marked with the stigma of a chronic potentially fatal illness like cancer. We deny the self-worth of millions of capable and active people.

We have to learn to recognize that medical technology has greatly extended life by offering effective treatments to people who are seriously ill. Such people are living full lives and deserve full acceptance by society. When a chronic and potentially fatal illness is not dealt with effectively by patients, family or friends, emotional problems will inevitably mount and social fears will continue to fester.

But if the threat to life by disease is accepted, understood and dealt with, life, not death, will be the winner.

30

WELLNESS: PARTICIPATING IN YOUR FIGHT FOR RECOVERY ON THE PSYCHOSOCIAL FRONT

Harold H. Benjamin, PhD

———◇———

People with cancer now have a choice. They can choose to be *Patients Active*, a part of the team fighting for their recovery, or they can choose to be *Patients Passive*, handing over responsibility for their recovery to their health care team.

Thirty or 40 years ago, most cancer patients didn't know they had any options. They were Patients Passive and their role was well defined. It included following their physician's instructions, accepting his or her ministrations and, if the patient was so inclined, praying for divine intervention. That was the only role they thought they could play.

But there's a new field of scientific study—an additional method of fighting for recovery—evolving. It's called psychoneuroimmunology, or PNI for short. It is broadly defined as the study of the effect that mental and emotional activity have on physical well-being. It has taught us that patients can play a much larger role in their recovery—a role that may actually affect the outcome of the illness, may prolong life *and will probably improve the quality of life.* Further along in this chapter you will find studies that support that concept.

This chapter is about that choice. First, it suggests activities you can do and attitudes you can develop that will help you become a Patient Active. These activities and attitudes have been learned by working with thousands of cancer patients at The Wellness Community.

Second, it explains why someone with cancer who takes specific, conscious, purposeful actions to fight for recovery *will* improve the quality of his or her life and *may* enhance the possibility of recovery.

There are three important points to consider when thinking about the possibility of recovery:
♦ The stronger the immune system, the more likely the recovery.
♦ The immune system may be enhanced by pleasant emotions.
♦ The immune system may be weakened by long-term, unremitting, unpleasant emotions.

If you understand these statements, everything that follows will be much more meaningful.

The assumptions on which this chapter is based should be emphasized.

First, treatment by a competent medical team is the primary method of fighting to recover from cancer. The psychosocial methods described here are supportive of, and adjunctive to, medical treatment. They are not alternatives.

Second, there really is a choice. But there is no right or wrong choice. There is no choice that is good or bad, brave or cowardly. Every decision you make is the right decision for you. Choose the passive role or the active role. Both will be right. In these matters, you know better than anyone else what is good for you. If you decide to try all or none of the following suggestions, that is the right decision for you. You cannot make a wrong decision.

Another fact that's important for you to know is that if you decide to try any or all of these suggestions and they don't seem to be working, that doesn't mean that you aren't doing them right or that you're not trying hard enough or that you're inadequate in some other way. Be assured that you are doing whatever is to be done as well as "it" can be done.

ATTITUDES AND ACTIVITIES TO HELP YOUR FIGHT

Before reviewing the following suggestions, understand that not all of them apply to everyone with cancer. Nor are they easy to accomplish. They are listed here because we want you to know what methods are available so you can choose what is best for you in your own unique circumstances.

Also keep in mind that although the main purpose of each suggestion is to try to direct the course of your illness toward health by strengthening your immune system, our experience is that a most important benefit to the people who use these suggestions is an improvement in the quality of their lives. And that's reason enough to give them serious consideration.

1. Make plans for the future.
People don't plan for the future if they believe there is no future in their future. If you are not making plans you may be unconsciously giving up. So you may find it helpful to come up with a list of short-term goals and long-range plans. Making plans in itself is a pleasant and positive experience. Why not enjoy yourself while giving yourself hope for the future?

2. Fight unwanted aloneness.
This is easier said than done. People with cancer know that many of their friends and family act differently toward them after the diagnosis. If you find yourself in this situation, then communicate, communicate, communicate. Tell your friends and family what you want and expect of them. When this is discussed openly, some—maybe not all, but some—of them will change. You might also become part of a support group in your area. It may be very important to fight the unwanted aloneness that can be so depressing.

3. Make sure you are not acting like a recluse.
Many people with cancer find it difficult to be with their friends and family in the way they were before the diagnosis. If you are having similar feelings, decide whether that's what you really want. If not, remember that although cancer has brought about physical and emotional changes that may make it more difficult to communicate, you are basically the same person you were before you developed cancer. Revitalizing old relationships is probably easier than you think. Do what you can to renew relationships and not be alone more than you want to be. Tell your friends what you are feeling and ask them to help you not be reclusive. Communicate, communicate, communicate.

4. Regain and maintain as much control over your life as is reasonable.
Most cancer patients have to give up some control over their lives to health professionals, family and friends. So will you, probably. But don't give up more than you need or want to. Make a list of the control you've lost and make a conscious decision about what is reasonable for you to take back. Feeling that you're not in control is a very unpleasant emotion.

5. Use some method to evoke the relaxation response.
The relaxation response is the name used to describe a physical state arrived at by several methods, including acupressure, meditation and directed visualization (*see* Chapter 25). The relaxation response is

important to people with cancer because when that state is achieved, the immune system is enhanced for a while. And that may have a beneficial effect on the course of your illness. It is easy to do, takes very little time, has no unpleasant side effects and almost always leaves you feeling more peaceful and relaxed.

We suggest that you choose some method of meditation or directed visualization that suits you and use it regularly. There are those who believe that learning to trigger the relaxation response is the most important part of being a Patient Active.

6. Be careful of the words you use about your illness.

To describe yourself as a victim afflicted with a catastrophic or fatal disease leaves little room for anything but despair—a very unpleasant emotion. So why not use less dramatic and less ominous words? If you persuade yourself by the words you use that you are doomed, you may unconsciously give up. Try to describe your illness and your battle with it with words that are as hopeful as you can make them.

7. Pursue happiness and avoid stress.

This is easy to say but sometimes difficult to do. Remember, pleasant emotions may enhance and unpleasant emotions may suppress the power of the immune system. So do as much as you can to bring about those pleasant emotions and avoid unpleasant ones.

"Not so fast," you say. "That's not so easy. You may not know it, but I'm not feeling great. I have a lot to worry about." And of course you're right. But leaving aside any effects on the immune system, here you have a suggestion that is almost sure to at least improve the quality of your life. It may not be so easy, but isn't an improved quality of life worth the effort?

Trying to increase pleasant emotions

and decrease unpleasant ones is probably what we all should be thinking about all of our lives. But now, if you have cancer, it is particularly important to be *consciously* aware of how and where you spend your time and whether or not you are enjoying yourself as much as possible. The pursuit of happiness is a reasonable part of your fight for recovery.

8. Become partners with your physician.

Some patients want to hear nothing but instructions. Others want to have every bit of information they can get and be involved in the decision-making process. Most physicians are now flexible enough to act in any capacity that is in the best interests of their patients, including acting more as your partner in achieving better health. So decide with your physician what you both want the relationship to be. Communicate, communicate, communicate. A strained relationship with this very important person in your life can bring on unpleasant emotions for both of you.

9. Be with other people who have cancer.

Many people with cancer say that only someone else with the disease truly knows what having cancer feels like and understands the struggle. Being with people who do understand forms an esprit—a camaraderie—that is a most pleasant emotion. It also relieves tension because you can't frighten them as you do your friends and family. You don't have to be constantly on your guard.

If there is no cancer support group in your area, you can find other cancer patients by asking your physician, your local cancer society or other organizations that provide services to people with cancer.

10. Do what you can to keep up hope.

Hopelessness is one of the most unpleasant emotions known to humankind. But when the diagnosis is cancer, many of us believe that there is no hope. That's just not true. There are millions of people in the world today for whom cancer is just a memory. There is no type of cancer that does not have some recovery rate. Forty to 50 percent of all people who develop cancer in the United States will eventually conquer the illness. Others will live long lives controlling the cancer as they would some other chronic disease. Hope is not only desirable but emotionally *reasonable.*

11. It is not necessary to give up intimacy and affection.
If you and your intimate partner want to maintain some type of physical affection after the diagnosis, adjustments can almost always be made to accommodate that desire despite psychological and physical problems. Once again, the solution is communication. Perhaps it won't be easy, but if intimacy has been reduced or eliminated and it's important to you to regain it, make the effort.

WHY YOU SHOULD BECOME A "PATIENT ACTIVE"

To understand fully the implications of these suggestions, it is best to review a few basic facts about cancer.

Cancer cells are not necessarily powerful, dominant engines of destruction. They may be thought of as weak, confused, abnormal cells, which appear in all of our bodies from time to time. Their primary abnormality is that they continue to divide and subdivide long after a normal cell would have stopped. If they continue unchecked, they form a continuously growing clump of cells called a tumor, which, when it becomes large enough, will interfere with the performance of nearby organs.

If these abnormal cells are of the type that can grow only at the place of origin, they form a benign (non-cancerous) tumor that can usually be surgically removed. If they are of the type that can travel and spread to other parts of the body, the ill-ness is categorized as one of the more than 200 illnesses called cancer.

One theory holds that although cancer cells may appear in everyone's body from time to time, all of us do not develop cancer because our immune systems are strong enough to destroy the cancer cells as they appear. That's what the immune system is for. According to this theory, then, for cancer to develop the cancer cell must appear and the immune system must be weak enough not to be able to handle it.

Recovery and the Immune System But how important is the immune system to someone who already has cancer? What part can it play in the fight for recovery? Until recently, the conventional wisdom was that the immune system had no part to play in the fight. That wisdom said that the only way to fight cancer was to try to remove the cancer cells from the body surgically or to kill them with chemicals or radiation.

Then along came immunologists who hypothesized that if the immune system were strengthened by various methods—including the introduction into the body of chemicals such as interleukin-2 and interferon—the system could destroy the cancer cells from within. This investigation continues worldwide with varying degrees of success.

PNI Studies The scientists of particular interest here are those involved in psychoneuroimmunology (PNI). They also believe that if the immune system is strengthened, recovery following conventional medical treatment will be more likely. But they are looking for ways to strengthen the power of the immune system not chemically but by psychological and social (psychosocial) means as an adjunct to conventional medical treatment.

As noted, PNI studies have suggested that long-term, unremitting, unpleasant emotions weaken the immune system while pleasant emotions strengthen its power. This information led the scientists to hypothesize that people with cancer can consciously take action to enhance the power of their immune systems, which *may* make the possibility of recovery more likely. In other words, if you increase the number of pleasant emotions and decrease the number of unpleasant emotions, it may help redirect the course of the illness toward health.

Although there is as yet no statistical evidence that enhancing the immune system increases the likelihood of recovery, four current studies have had interesting results. The most recent was a 1992 Australian/New Zealand study of over 300 women with metastatic breast cancer done by Alan Coates, to determine the efficacy of various ways of measuring the quality of life of women with that illness. Although they were not looking to see if quality of life was a predictor of longevity, they found that women with a higher quality of life at the outset of their illness lived longer than those who were less happy at that time.

Dr. David Spiegel of Stanford University, in the early 1980s, studied women with metastatic breast cancer to determine what effect group support had on their quality of life. The immediate result of the study was the finding that "support groups can clearly improve the quality of life (for women with metastatic breast cancer)." In a 10-year follow-up, they found that the women who had participated in the one-year group support lived twice as long as the women in the control group who did not receive group support.

In the late 1980s, Dr. Fawzy I. Fawzy at UCLA studied the effect of group support on melanoma patients. That study found, in a six-month follow-up, that the patients who participated in the support groups "showed significantly lower depression, fatigue, confusion . . . as well as higher vigor" than patients who did not. The study also found that there were encouraging immune system consequences of being in the group.

A 1988 study conducted by Lee Berk at Loma Linda Hospital investigated the effect

laughter had on the immune system and found that "laughter may be an antagonist to the classical stress response." What that means is that laughter may actually strengthen the immune system, a fact commented upon extensively by Norman Cousins.

KNOWING THAT YOUR CANCER IS NOT YOUR FAULT

If you have cancer, it is important for you to know that no matter what anyone says, you cannot be blamed for the onset of the illness. You may find that hard to believe, especially since there are many so-called experts who, for reasons of their own, try to persuade cancer patients that they developed cancer because they subconsciously wanted to or were in some way negligent or inept in the decisions they made.

Certainly, from all of the foregoing information, it's clear that there is the possibility that lifestyle—such as being under too much stress—just might play a part in the evolution of cancer. But unless you smoked after the Surgeon General's report came out and then developed lung cancer or exposed yourself to too much sun after being warned that it might cause skin cancer or melanoma, *there is no possibility that you can be at fault.*

It is true is that there are many actions people with cancer can take that may have a beneficial effect on the fight for recovery. Unhappily, there is no guarantee that such actions will have the desired result.

Fight for recovery with all your might, if that's what you want. Do everything in your power to make your body the world's most inhospitable place for a cancer cell to live. And if the illness does not seem to be abating, don't let anybody tell you that you aren't doing "it" well enough or that you are not trying hard enough. That's nonsense. Whatever you are doing is right and proper for you. You are doing "it" as well as "it" can be done.

You are the very best "you" that ever was or ever could be.

31
SURVIVORSHIP: OBSTACLES AND OPPORTUNITIES

Susan Nessim and Diane Shader Smith

—◇—

When treatment was over and I had to go back to the real world, the world outside the hospital, I thought my life would be the same. I went about doing things the way I'd always done them, but nothing worked. You're not the same person. You can never go back.—Anita, 38-year-old breast cancer survivor.

The concept of cancer survivorship is quite new but is finally being recognized. The 8 million cancer survivors in this country are a living testament to the fact that cancer is not always a death sentence. Thanks to medical advances in diagnosis and treatment, we can confidently look beyond the disease process to life after cancer. By the year 2000, the number of survivors will top 10 million.

Clearly, a physical cure does not mark the end of the healing process. And only by examining the impact that a cancer illness has on a person's life can strategies be devised to ease the difficult transition from a state of illness to one of well-being.

Survivors often liken their cancer experience and their efforts to resume a normal life to that of returning war veterans. Their sense of balance is lost. The immediate crisis of fighting for life itself is over. Then comes the time to lick their wounds and assess the damage. The post-treatment period brings with it myriad emotions. It is not unusual to feel a strange mixture of elation and anxiety. The disease has been eradicated, but there is still a "second war" to be fought, a struggle with less tangible but still threatening physical, psychological and social ramifications.

ASKING THE HARD QUESTIONS

Society values those who can assimilate quickly, who can bounce back from tragedy without skipping a beat. The message survivors receive from all sides is, "You're so lucky to be alive. Now get on with your life."

That's great in theory, but the reality is that once cancer has touched your life, nothing will ever be the same. Relationships are tested, employment issues surface and priorities are re-evaluated. Perhaps the most important factor is that a survivor has faced mortality and emerged transformed, keenly aware of how fragile life is.

Survivors and those close to them must acknowledge all that has happened. Only then can they move forward. Only then can they derive meaning from their experience. This is the challenge facing all survivors.

The obstacles you may encounter when you finish treatment are totally unexpected but can be overcome. Denying that you have changed or that you feel differently about every aspect of your life will only delay the recovery process. It's important to stay in touch with your feelings and to ask yourself some hard questions.

You probably won't be able to answer

these questions right away, but asking them is a good place to start your new life as a survivor.

♦ Who am I now that I've had cancer?
♦ Will I get it again?
♦ Can I survive another bout with cancer?
♦ What is the best way to spend my time?
♦ Does my career really make me happy?
♦ Do my relationships work?
♦ Am I contributing to society?
♦ Will I ever feel secure in my future?

RENEGOTIATING RELATIONSHIPS WITH FAMILY AND FRIENDS

Once I was given a clean bill of health, the doctor told me, "You're out of the jungle but you're in the woods." I went home and I was cured and nobody wanted to hear about cancer anymore. I wasn't supposed to say the word or even think about it. I pretended along with everyone else that I never had cancer and that way everything was okay.—Derek, 29-year-old Hodgkin's disease survivor.

It is common for family members and friends to react with uncertainty to your new status as a survivor. They may have pulled away from you as a self-protective mechanism during your diagnosis and treatment. Those close to you probably prepared themselves emotionally for the possibility of your death. This process of distancing—therapists call it anticipatory grief—is understandable. But once you recover, loved ones realize an incorrect assumption has been made, so expectations have to be adjusted. This reaction is called the Lazarus syndrome, named for the biblical figure who rose from the dead.

Once you are past the acute stage of the illness, family members and friends may feel it is safe to allow their suppressed emotions to surface. Guilt, resentment, anger, denial and fear are often by-products of the crisis brought about by cancer. As a survivor, you have to encourage hon-

est and open expression so that bonds can be re-established.

Keep in mind that how a family has dealt with a crisis in the past is a good indicator of how that family will deal with a cancer illness. Also bear in mind that cancer is a family event, that cancer changes *all* relationships and, especially, that change can be positive.

The following suggestions will help you mend any ties that might have been damaged.

For the Family
♦ Share your feelings with family members, by talking or in writing.
♦ Reach out to other survivors through support groups.
♦ Go for individual counseling.
♦ Give yourself and those close to you time to sort through feelings.

With Friends
♦ Let go of negative emotions.
♦ Embrace friends who support your recovery.
♦ Take the initiative with those who have been uncomfortable with your illness.
♦ Allow friends to re-enter your life.
♦ Sever friendships that don't work anymore.
♦ Mourn your losses.

WORKPLACE DISCRIMINATION

I was laid off right after I was diagnosed with cancer. After I finished treatment, I tried to get a job but nobody would hire me. I felt like I was a displaced person. I had the education, the experience, the talent, but because I had the big "C" I couldn't get a job anywhere.—Chris, 54-year-old prostate cancer survivor.

For centuries, fear of cancer has caused those with the disease to be stigmatized. By the nineteenth century, the public had developed a horrible phobia about cancer. People viewed the disease as sinister, relentless and possibly contagious. Cancer was considered so shameful that people had trouble even speaking the word. Until the middle of this century, doctors were as helpless in treating cancer as they were in explaining what caused it. Even they regarded it with fear and fatalism, just as their patients did.

The Cancer Stigma in the Workplace: Common Myths Ignorance about cancer is what gave rise to the myths, misconceptions and prejudices that still prevail today. Unfortunately, these often influence the way employers and co-workers regard those who have survived the disease. Among the myths and misconceptions are:

♦ *Cancer is a death sentence.* Many people incorrectly believe that those with cancer will die prematurely. Employers can be reluctant to make an investment in someone they believe won't be with them over the long term. This attitude is not based on fact. The National Cancer Institute reports that more than half of all people diagnosed with cancer today will survive their illness.

♦ *Cancer is contagious.* It has been proven time and time again that cancer is no more contagious than heart disease or arthritis. Yet surprisingly, some people still cling to this antiquated notion. Superstition is the basis for this myth, which can result in a survivor's unnecessary isolation from peers at work.

♦ *Cancer makes workers unproductive.* Perhaps the most widespread belief, this myth assumes that once you've had cancer, you won't be able to contribute fully to your job. Despite employers' concerns, turnover and absentee rates are not higher for cancer survivors. According to a study by MetLife Insurance and Bell Telephone, survivors showed no difference in any aspect of job performance than non-survivors. On the contrary, survivors often work harder to prove that they are still able to compete in the workplace.

Questions to Ask Yourself When You Are Back at Work When you do get back to work, you may notice many changes in the way your employer and co-workers treat you. Some of these changes may be subtle, some may be blatant. Ask yourself:
♦ Have your responsibilities been reduced?
♦ Have you been transferred without prior consent?
♦ Have you been overlooked for a promotion?
♦ Are co-workers or superiors treating you differently?
♦ Have you been required to take a medical exam that is unrelated to your job duties?
♦ Have you been asked to provide detailed medical information?
♦ Have your insurance benefits been cut?

Actions You Can Take If you feel that your position in the workplace has changed, there are things you can do to improve or at least come to terms with the situation.
♦ Try not to read too much into someone else's actions.
♦ Remember that your return to work will require adjustment on everyone's part.
♦ If your health is being questioned, get a note from your doctor to confirm that you are able to perform your job duties.
♦ If you feel you are being treated unfairly, request an informal meeting with your office mates.
♦ Keep copious notes if you feel discriminated against in any way.
♦ If all else fails, you might consider filing a complaint with the management of your company or taking legal action.
♦ If you are unable to keep your job because of a cancer-related disability or discrimination, vocational training is available through your state-run Vocational Rehabilitation Administration.

Legal Protection The Americans with

Disabilities Act of 1990 is sweeping legislation that makes it illegal to discriminate against any qualified applicant who is disabled, has a history of disability or is perceived as having a disability. This bill enables survivors to have recourse if they have a legitimate case. For more information, please write to the Equal Employment Opportunity Connection, 1801 L St. NW, Washington, DC 20507.

WHERE TO GO FOR HELP

Cancervive was founded in 1985 to assist cancer survivors by helping them make sense of their cancer experience and work through any lingering emotions. What makes this organization unique is that it deals exclusively with *post-treatment* issues.

Cancervive provides individual and group therapy, a quarterly newsletter and public education about survivorship.

If there is no Cancervive chapter in your community, you can start one yourself with the help of the Cancervive national office in Los Angeles. The address is 6500 Wilshire Blvd., Los Angeles, CA 90048. You can also contact your local hospital to find out if there is a hospital-sponsored survivorship program in your area.

Suggested Readings for Survivors
♦ *At the Will of the Body* by Arthur Frank (Houghton Mifflin).
♦ *Cancer and Hope: Charting a Survival Course* by Judith Garrett Garrison, MEd, LSW, and Scott Sheperd, PhD.
♦ *Cancer Stories* by Esther Dreiff-Kattan (The Analytic Press).
♦ *Cancervive: The Challenge of Life After Cancer* by Susan Nessim and Judith Ellis (Houghton Mifflin).
♦ *Charting the Journey* by Dr. Fitzhugh Mullan and Barbara Hoffman, JD (Consumer Reports Books).
♦ *Upfront: Sex & the Post-Mastectomy Woman* by Linda Dackman (Viking Press).
♦ *Where the Buffaloes Roam* by Bob Stone and Jenny Stone Humphries (Lapidum Press).
♦ *Witness to Illness* by Karen E. Horowitz and Douglas M. Lanes, MD (Addison Wesley).

32
PAYING FOR CANCER CARE

Joseph S. Bailes, MD, Barbara Quinn and Malin Dollinger, MD

◇

Newly diagnosed cancer patients are suddenly confronted with critical questions about their insurance coverage. Paying for medical care is complicated. There is a vocabulary of words and initials that is confusing even to health care workers.

The insurance industry—both public and private—has its own policies, guidelines and methods of payment specific to cancer care. Each company's rules may be different. It is important for you to know and understand how your insurance company's payment system works so you will get the care you need at a cost you should be able to pay. It is especially important to know your policy restrictions.

As a cancer patient, you are probably uncertain and unclear about the scope of your coverage as well as how you can obtain the benefits you are entitled to under your insurance contract. Not being fully informed can put you at great financial risk. You may end up paying for services that should have been covered by your insurance.

TYPES OF HEALTH CARE COVERAGE

There are many types of payment plans, insurance plans and medical groups.

Medicare This is a government-sponsored health insurance program for people age 65 and older. It also covers people who are permanently disabled and who have received Social Security benefits for at least two years.

Medicare is divided into two parts:

♦ *Part A. Hospital Insurance.* This covers your inpatient hospital stay, limited skilled nursing care, part-time home health care and hospice for those who are eligible. It is available without payment of a premium, although some services require a deductible or co-insurance. Medicare Part A is administered by the Health Care Financing Administration (HCFA) through insurers called intermediaries.

♦ *Part B. Medical Insurance.* This covers physician services and hospital outpatient care, such as blood transfusions, x-rays and lab tests. There is limited coverage for medical equipment such as wheelchairs and walkers. Enrollment is optional and the payment of a premium is required. Medicare Part B covers 80 percent of allowed charges. You are responsible for the other 20 percent of allowed charges, called co-insurance. You must also meet a yearly deductible (currently $100) before Medicare Part B coverage applies.

Medicare Part B is directed by the federal government through the HCFA and is funded through a monthly premium, which comes out of your Social Security check. It is administered through contracts with a number of insurers (called carriers) throughout the United States. If you need additional information, as well as a free handbook describing the Medicare program, contact your local Social Security office.

Medigap This insurance is sold by private carriers and traditionally covers the 20 percent Medicare co-insurance you are responsible for. Federal law requires that there are 10, and only 10, standard types of Medigap policies available. These policies vary widely in the scope of their coverage. You should thoroughly familiarize yourself with the particular Medigap policy you are considering purchasing so that you have the coverage appropriate for your situation.

Medicaid This is a joint federal- and state-funded program for low-income individuals. It provides coverage for inpatient care, outpatient services, diagnostic testing, drugs, skilled nursing facility care and home health care. Each state has different rules about eligibility for the Medicaid program. Your local social service or welfare department is the best place to obtain information about Medicaid.

QMBE This is a program in which the state pays co-insurance and premiums for certain low-income Part B beneficiaries even if they don't qualify for Medicaid.

Traditional Indemnity Insurance Sometimes called "Major Medical Coverage," this is insurance sold by numerous private insurance companies. It is the most common type of insurance coverage for people not covered by Medicare or Medicaid. This insurance typically pays the usual fee for service each time you see your doctor.

There is usually a deductible or co-payment associated with traditional indemnity insurance. This means, for example, that you might pay the first $250 or $500 in charges each year or perhaps might pay 10 percent or 20 percent of the fees. There may be limits in the policy, such as hospital room and nursing costs, treatment for psychological problems, a maximum dollar amount that will be paid or limitations of a physician's fees to the "usual and customary."

An employer will often have a plan for general insurance coverage for each employee.

Managed Care Plans Managed care is usually thought of as a situation where an individual pays either a fixed fee for a certain set of services or sees a physician who has agreed to discount his or her fees for particular services.

There are many variations of Managed Care plans:

♦ *HMO (Health Maintenance Organizations).* These are prepaid health plans that require you to use a specific network or group of provider physicians, hospitals and labs. For a fixed fee each month, HMOs provide care specified by your contract. This care may or may not be all-inclusive, so it is important to read and understand the contract of your particular HMO. For instance, some HMOs have no outpatient prescription drug benefit. In an HMO, you are usually required to select one physician as your primary or family doctor. This individual coordinates your care.

Examples of HMOs include Kaiser Permanente, Cigna Health Plans and Blue Cross HMO plans.

HMO members over 65 years of age should remember that the HMO plan replaces Medicare coverage and you must stay within your HMO plan for your claims to be paid by Medicare.

♦ *PPO (Preferred Provider Organization), EPO (Exclusive Provider Organization) or IPA (Independent Practice Association).* Traditionally, these are groups of physicians and other participating providers who have agreed to offer a discount from their usual fees in order to participate in a particular group. These function as "old-fashioned private practice" in that the physician or other provider receives a fee each time a service is performed or each time you see the physician. You do have a choice of using providers or physicians who are not in the plan, but if you do, you will have to pay a larger portion of the cost.

WHAT DOES YOUR PLAN COVER?

Your health benefits manual, insurance representative or the health plan manager at your place of employment should be able to answer the following questions.

♦ What is the effective date of the policy? In other words, when does your coverage begin?

♦ What is your deductible? This is the amount you need to pay before your insurance plan starts paying the rest. Only medical care received as a benefit under your policy is calculated against your deductible. Non-covered benefits that you pay yourself do not count.

♦ Do you have a stop loss? This is the amount you must pay out of your own pocket before your insurance pays at 100 percent.

♦ What percentage of billed charges is paid by your insurance? Some policies pay 80 percent or 90 percent of some costs. Others might be paid only at 50 percent. Look carefully at your policy booklet.

♦ Do you have coverage for home care, nursing visits at home, private duty nursing (24-hour care) and care at a skilled nursing facility or convalescent hospital? Most insurance companies cover only skilled care. Custodial care—such as housekeeping, bathing, laundry, assistance to the bathroom or other activities—is not usually a covered benefit.

♦ Does your plan cover hospice care?

♦ Does your insurance provide coverage only if you go to contracted providers?

♦ Is authorization required for doctor's visits, hospital admissions or outpatient testing?

♦ Are there any waivers that would preclude payment for treatment for your condition? This might include prior treatment (within one year for, example) for the same or a similar condition.

♦ What is your lifetime maximum? This is the maximum benefit your insurance will pay in your lifetime. It can be $25,000 or up to $1 million or more.

♦ How do you get care after hours or in an emergency?

♦ If you have group coverage through your employer, does coverage end if you are fired or laid off? If so, is there a way to continue coverage?

WHY CLAIMS MAY BE DENIED

Even though your policy may appear comprehensive, denials for medical care claims are common. Sometimes this only reflects missing information or incorrect documentation. Sometimes the policy does not cover certain types of care. This is often a matter of interpretation of your specific care needs. If this is the case, you will need to go to bat along with your doctor or other health care provider to establish that your care should be covered even though the insurance company's agent interprets the policy as appearing to exclude it.

Pre-Existing Condition Your claim may be denied if your medical condition existed before you became eligible for or bought your policy.

Non-Covered Benefit This is usually explained in the section of your policy that lists illnesses or services excluded from coverage. Because of the possibility of non-covered benefits, it is a good idea to check your insurance plan before any treatment or tests are ordered. Some treatments are covered only when given or administered in the hospital, for example. In such cases, you or your physician's office may be able to make specific arrangements for outpatient coverage in lieu of hospitalization. Services may actually be cheaper that way.

Not an Authorized Provider Many insurance plans require that you use providers in their network. Specialists usually require a referral for a consultation and all subsequent treatment. Failure to go to contracted providers with a written referral can result in a complete denial of all treatment provided.

Investigational Treatment Many insurers will deny claims deemed to be investigational (experimental), unnecessary or inappropriate. Bone marrow transplants and certain other new treatments often fall into this category. While there is no guaranteed way to prevent denial of such a claim, make sure you attempt to receive pre-approval for the treatment from your insurance carrier in writing. To do this, you should have a letter of medical necessity from your physician documenting that the proposed treatment is medically appropriate, along with supporting clinical literature and a full description of the procedure or services to be provided. The anticipated cost and duration of the treatment should also be included.

Off-Label Treatment Your insurer may deny a claim if the drug your doctor has prescribed is used for other than its labeled indication or the use listed on the drug company's "package insert." The claim may also be denied if the drug is used in a new dosage, according to a new schedule, given by a different route or combined with other drugs.

You should be aware that fully half of all uses of cancer drugs are *not* those listed on the official package insert or label. Such use reflects advances in cancer treatment that occurred after the drug was released onto the market and are in fact the ordinary, proper and *accepted* uses of such drugs. *Not* to use certain drugs for established "off-label" uses may be inappropriate.

When there is a denial of payment for a claim because the use of the drug was "off-label," it is very important that this be appealed to the insurance carrier. These denials are usually reversed, especially if the use of the drug is standard in the community and is a medically necessary and effective treatment for your illness. Most pharmaceutical companies will provide clinical literature if needed to help support your claim. In fact, they often provide reimbursement "hotlines" to provide assistance. Your oncologist's insurance office is usually familiar with ways to help you with this problem should denial occur. In many states, cancer physicians have formed organizations to advise insurance companies about effective new treatments for cancer, especially the uses of established drugs in off-label use.

Non-Payment of Premiums It is very difficult to obtain an insurance policy once you have a pre-existing condition. Make sure that premiums are kept up to date to ensure that your insurance policy is not canceled.

SUBMITTING CLAIMS

You must bring proper insurance plan identification on your first visit to your oncologist's office. Your insurance provider—whether it is Medicare, Medicaid, a PPO, HMO or Private Indemnity plan—should give you an identification card. This card will have your subscriber identification number (often your social security number), group number, office co-pay amount and the address where you have to submit your insurance claims. If your insurance also requires a claim form to be submitted, also bring a fully completed and signed claim form to the office.

Inform your physician's office of any changes in your address, phone number, employment or insurance information. Notifying the office immediately will prevent a lot of unnecessary delays in claim submission and the need for re-submission, as well as possible denials of payment. It will also result in quicker payment of claims.

Most oncology offices have an insurance or finance department. Their patient representatives will explain the billing procedures to you before you begin treatment. They should also inform you whether they will submit your claim or if you are to submit the claim yourself. Always request a copy of your charges, which should include an itemization of all services and the diagnosis and code for your visit.

COMMON TERMS AND ABBREVIATIONS

To better understand the claim submission and processing procedure, you should understand the terms and abbreviations used by most insurance carriers. The most common are:

♦ ICD-9 CODE (International Classification of Diseases, 9th Edition). This is the coding system used to identify your illness. All claims submitted to your insurance carrier will require the correct code. Carriers will not pay your claim if this code is not provided.

♦ CPT CODE (Current Procedural Terminology). This is the coding system used to identify medical, surgical and diagnostic services rendered by your physician. It is used by most insurance carriers to identify what services were performed. Claims are paid using these codes.

♦ Deductible. This is the amount you have to pay before your insurance starts paying the rest. Only medical care received as a benefit under your policy is calculated against your deductible. Non-covered benefits that you pay yourself do not count against your deductible.

♦ Co-payment. This refers to the amount of your bill that you are responsible for. The co-payment is usually a specific dollar amount rather than a percentage of the bill. Prescription drug programs, for example, often have a co-payment, usually a fixed dollar amount per prescription.

♦ Co-Insurance. This is the percentage of the bill you are responsible for after you have met your deductible. If your policy has a $100 deductible and a 20 percent co-insurance, for example, you would pay your $100 deductible and 20 percent of all covered expenses. You are also responsible for all services not covered by your policy.

♦ E.O.B. (Explanation of Benefits). This is the statement you will receive from your insurance carrier when your claim has been paid. It will show the provider of services, the place of service and how the benefits were paid. If you have a deductible or co-insurance, this will also be stated on your E.O.B. If you have a secondary insurance carrier, that company will need a copy of your E.O.B. in order to pay its portion.

♦ Assignment of Benefits. This is required by most physicians' offices. It means that you want your insurance company to send payments directly to the provider of services. Assignment of Benefits is usually signed in the physician's office on an office form. There is also a place for your signature on your claim form.

♦ Medicare Assignment. Any physician can accept the fee schedule set by Medicare in an individual case. A participating provider in the Medicare program has agreed to always take the set fee schedule ("assignment").

If your physician takes Medicare assignment (fees), you are then responsible only for non-covered services, your deductible and your co-insurance. If the physician is not a participating provider in the Medicare program, you can be responsible for more than the 20 percent co-insurance. If the physician's charge is more than the Medicare allowable charge, for instance, the physician would receive 80 percent of the Medicare allowable while you would be responsible for the rest of the bill.

Make sure you ask ahead of time if

your physician participates in the Medicare program and will accept assignment of benefits for your care.

♦ E.O.M.B. (Explanation of Medicare Benefits). This is sent to you as soon as your claim has been paid. It will state the provider of any service, the amount allowed under the Medicare fee schedule, the amount paid and what charges were applied toward your deductible. If your physician is a Medicare provider, the check will be sent directly to his or her office. You will need this explanation of Medicare benefits in order for your secondary insurance company to pay your claim.

♦ UCR (Usual, Customary and Reasonable). This is the fee determined by your insurance carrier to be the usual fee charged for the same service by the average provider with similar training in your geographic area. This may be different than the fee your physician charges.

♦ Pre-Authorization. This is a requirement by your insurance carrier that certain services be authorized before the services are rendered. If your insurance contains this requirement, make sure your physician's office is aware of it.

♦ Superbill. This is a standard itemized "checklist of services" in widespread use. It will contain all the required codes (CPT and ICD-9) that will enable you to submit your claim.

♦ C.O.B. (Coordination of Benefits). When you are enrolled in two separate insurance plans, those plans will coordinate their benefits so that your claim is paid at no more than 100 percent of the covered benefits. If you have more than one insurance plan, make sure you notify your physician's office so the office can submit both claims for you.

NEW WAYS OF PAYING FOR MEDICAL CARE

Our society is engaged in a great effort to reform the health care payment system.

There used to be only two "players" in the system: the doctor and the patient. Now there are several others: the health insurance industry, various federal and state regulatory agencies, employers (who often provide employee health care plans) and the federal government. New rules and regulations are being proposed and implemented that will change the basic concepts and practices of health care.

The patient's need for skillful, dedicated and considerate care by the physician has never changed. From the viewpoint of the physician—now called a health care provider—what has changed is that there needs to be interaction with other parties and agencies that have taken over some of the decision making that used to belong to the physician alone. Many decisions now need outside approval. These include the decision to hospitalize, where to hospitalize, which consultants may be called, what types of treatment may be used and, especially, how health care resources are to be allocated and provided. Authorization required to order tests and x-rays is just one example. Many doctors' offices now have more people handling insurance than they have nurses. Physicians will need to be increasingly accountable to outside agencies.

"Managed care" is one common expression for a coordinated effort by physicians, hospitals and insurance payers to work together to create an optimum balance between incredibly sophisticated medical technology and our inability as a society to afford paying for every possible test and treatment while looking for every possible diagnosis for each person in every situation. The "practice guidelines" now being developed will probably become increasingly important in how services are provided and covered.

Because the patterns of delivering and monitoring health care are complex and changing and new payment systems are being created, it is absolutely essential that you completely understand the provisions of your health insurance plan. With increasingly expensive tests and treatments, and more and more controls over payment for medical care, your best insurance is to completely understand your insurance.

In this rapidly changing medical world there will have to be a greater effort and understanding by all the participants in medical care—patient, physician, the health care team and the governmental/insurance payers—to provide cost-effective state-of-the-art health care.

33
PLANNING FOR THE FUTURE

Ernest H. Rosenbaum, MD, and Malin Dollinger, MD

"The best way to get something done is to begin."
—*Elmo A. Petterle*

———————◇———————

The chances for living a long and healthy life are now greater than ever before. Age is just a number that measures time. As George Burns said, "You're not old until the candles on your birthday cake cost more than the cake."

Today, we have better nutrition, better physical fitness, improved living conditions, new drugs, new advances in medical science such as transplants, bypasses and other life-prolonging discoveries. More and more cancers are becoming curable when they are diagnosed at an early stage. Cancer treatment techniques are constantly being developed and new therapies like immunology and genetic engineering are holding out the prospect of curing more cancers in the future.

Yet living with cancer remains a fearful, anxious time despite all the promise of medical advances. No matter how well informed you are about your cancer or all the therapies that might be used to treat it, you still feel some loss of control over your fate. You put your life in the hands of specialists and live in uncertainty, hopeful one day, gloomy the next.

Although living with uncertainty may seem uncomfortable, it does allow room for hope and positive thoughts. You may discover that life can be more meaningful. Little pleasures can become very important. You may even begin to "stop and smell the roses." Once any anger or bitterness about having cancer is put aside, you will find there is still tremendous room for enjoyment.

And, if you are like many other people faced with uncertainty, you may get your life in focus with more clarity than you have known before. Thinking about their own mortality, perhaps for the first time, many people decide to make plans for the future if the best happens or if the worst happens. In either case, the act of making plans wonderfully concentrates the mind. If you make that decision yourself, the act of planning will let you face the uncertain future with clarity, simplicity and the comforting knowledge that your affairs are in order and that as few things as possible are left undone.

YOUR LEGACY OF LOVE

We all know that at some time death will take us. And each of us makes—or should make—some plans for when the time comes. Most of us buy life insurance to provide financially for the people we love. We make wills so that when death occurs there is a clear plan for the distribution of our earthly possessions.

But beyond these basics, few of us take the time to prepare in detail for the time when we are no longer around. Making such preparations isn't pleasant. In some ways it may be very difficult. It is something that we often put off, partly because we all consider ourselves immortal or too young to worry about death and all its implications.

But avoiding discussing or thinking about it only puts off the kind of planning that really should be done. The burden just passes on to our survivors. More than 90 percent of survivors in America are unprepared to handle the responsibilities and immediate needs when a loved one dies.

Making Your Medical Choices You should discuss with your physician any concerns you have about how your medical care should be delivered, especially during a medical crisis. In the event of a sudden drastic complication, such as a heart stoppage or cessation of breathing, hospitals are often legally required to "call a code," to resuscitate you with cardiopulmonary resuscitation (CPR). This is sometimes called a Code Blue. Many health care givers also believe they are morally and professionally obligated to call such a code.

Code status varies, however, and it is important to consider how far *you* want your physician to go to attempt resuscitation should a crisis occur.

♦ Full Code means that treatment and support will be very aggressive, with the use of cardiac resuscitation, breathing tubes and machines.

♦ A "Chemical Code" calls for a less aggressive plan. Drugs and intravenous treatments will be used to save or prolong life, but if breathing or the heartbeat stop, no attempt will be made to restart them.

♦ If you agree to a No Code status, no extreme measures will be used for life support and resuscitation.

The decisions about what life support measures should be taken should be made by you in advance of a hospitalization or major illness. Then make your wishes known. This can take the form of an Advance Directive, a paper you fill out in advance with your instructions in case you have a serious illness and are not able to speak for yourself. There are also documents called Living Wills and Durable Power of Attorney. (These decisions can

be reversed at any time.) This will protect you as a patient even if you are unable to convey the information at the appropriate time. It will also protect your family from the stress of making sudden medical decisions for you.

The best way to define the code status you wish and ensure that your wishes are followed is through written documents.

♦ A Living Will should include your decision on the extent of treatment in the event you become so seriously ill you might die. You may amplify the Living Will with a codicil or statement of your wishes for additional pain and comfort care if the end is near and the primary goal is keeping you comfortable under all circumstances. You can include a written request for adequate doses of morphine or sedatives, for example.

♦ Durable Powers of Attorney should include a summary of your wishes on limits to preserving or extending life. Those responsible for monitoring and delivering your health care can then act in accordance with your wishes should you become physically or mentally unable to make your own medical decisions.

This information should be in the medical file kept by your doctor and in your hospital record. Always carry in your wallet a medical emergency information card containing all vital information about codes, diagnoses and any medications you take. In some states, the code status request can be included on the driver's license organ donor card.

Planning Tools A book by Elmo A. Petterle called *Getting Your Affairs in Order (Legacy of Love)* (Petterle Publications, 3 Greenside Way, San Rafael, CA 94901) is a practical guide on how you can make life easier for the people you leave behind. Its objective is to approach the problem of potential death with compassion and sensitivity. The book was designed for everyone—young, old, rich, poor, married, single, healthy and ill.

It was not written to scare you into thinking that your time is running out because of age or any other reason. It is simply a strategic planning tool, a workbook you fill in yourself. It deals with realities in a very practical and organized way so that your survivors know what they need to know and are properly instructed and prepared for what has to be done.

♦ The book introduces you to the material you will be working on, including how to start planning for your beneficiaries. It gives advice on will preparations, on what you have to do, what the first priorities are and what is not important.

♦ It covers the details on how you wish to be cared for if you become very seriously ill, including a Living Will and Durable Powers of Attorney.

♦ It gives advice and a place to fill out your instructions about your choice of a cemetery or other resting place, mortuary and funeral arrangements, memorial or other types of services, newspaper information and advice on death benefits that are available in the United States.

♦ It provides survivors with a list of immediate after-death contacts and phone numbers in order of importance. This is convenient at a most awkward time. In their grief, people often don't think clearly and may make errors such as being sold costly funeral services that might directly contradict your wishes, which should be honored.

♦ It also lists the proper contacts to be made within the first 10 days—such as instructions for the post office or motor vehicles departments—and what contacts should be made within the first month—telephone, gas and electric, water companies, waste disposal, newspapers, credit cards, clubs and organizations, cable TV and other organizations that deserve to be listed.

♦ It provides guidance and planning space to be filled out on financial plans, any investments you've made, property and casualty insurance, as well as information about home and personal property

insurance. It is amazing how ill informed many people are about life insurance policies, social security benefits, medical insurance, pensions, profit-sharing plans, IRAs and Keogh provisions that have often been made years before. Working through this section may give you a few surprises.

♦ It lets you catalog vital information on banks, savings accounts, loans, safety deposit boxes and so on so that this information is available when it should be.

♦ It gives advice on how to deal with bureaucracies that are often insensitive to the needs of people at such personal times.

♦ It provides necessary information about medical history that may be important to the family, as well as about family history and where personal letters can be found.

There are other tools that can assist you in your planning. One especially helpful book is *The Diagnosis is Cancer*, by Edward J. Larschan, JD, PhD, and Richard Larschan, PhD (Bull Publishing, PO Box 208, Palo Alto, California 94302). This book covers some of the same ground as *Legacy of Love*, but from a different perspective, dealing primarily with the legal arrangements necessary for survivors.

Many people unfortunately procrastinate, but books like *Legacy of Love* and *The Diagnosis is Cancer* give all thoughtful people an opportunity to lessen the pain and suffering of their survivors, simply because they love them.

HOPE AND THE WILL TO LIVE

Like every creature in the animal world, human beings have a fierce instinct for survival. The will to live—that instinct to fight when our lives are threatened by illness or some other crisis—is a natural impulse in all of us.

Yet some people are easily destroyed by the mental and physical effects of disease while others call on inner resources to sustain them through the experience. Why do some people respond positively to suffering while others cannot endure? Maybe the survivors have learned to be resilient by coming through earlier crises, becoming strong, tough and confident in the process. Maybe the small flame of gritty determination that makes us keep struggling at even the lowest ebb just burns brighter in some than in others. But the most important reason may be hope.

Many doctors have seen how two patients of similar ages, with the same diagnosis and degree of illness and the same treatment program experience vastly different results. And the only noticeable difference between the two was that one person was pessimistic and the other was optimistic.

Hope, courage, effort, determination, endurance, love and faith all nurture the will to live. And the greatest of these is hope. There may be times when you feel exhausted and overwhelmed by never-ending problems, when you feel ready to give up the struggle to survive. Yet if you have hope you can carry on.

As long as there is even a remote chance for survival, as long as there are even minor improvements, hope can be kindled and nurtured. As long as your family, friends and support team keep a positive attitude, hope can see you through any crises or times of reversal.

But hope has to come mainly from within. You can have hope if you are willing to fight for your life and if you are ready to do everything you can to improve your health. Just as soldiers have a revival of mood and spirit as they march home singing from an exhausting day, so you can find new energies and new strength.

Even at the roughest times, you probably have untapped reserves of physical and emotional strength at your command. Call on them and use them to survive another day. These resources are the foundation and the source of your recovery.

PART IV:
NEW ADVANCES IN RESEARCH, RISK ASSESSMENT, DIAGNOSIS AND TREATMENT

34
THE FUTURE OF SCIENTIFIC RESEARCH AND TREATMENT

Vincent T. DeVita, Jr., MD

———————◇———————

Think of a world without cancer. It is a difficult concept to even begin to comprehend. Those of us living today have never known such a world. Cancer is embedded in our literature and our culture. Years ago we did not talk much about cancer, and the news that any relatives had it was kept under wraps, as if having cancer was some sort of disgrace.

Yet many diseases that have dominated our lives and culture, such as tuberculosis, polio and smallpox, have either diminished as major health problems or disappeared, like smallpox. It has happened before and it can happen again, although it has sometimes taken centuries to accomplish.

It took two hundred years, from the first effort to vaccinate against it, to eradicate smallpox from the face of the earth, but eradicated it is. Paralytic polio is virtually gone as well. Although tuberculosis has re-emerged as a serious health threat, it is nowhere near the killer it was in the nineteenth and early twentieth centuries, when it killed more than 2,000 out of every 100,000 people in the Western world. Cancer was not much of a problem in those days because people died of these other scourges before getting cancer.

The pace of the current revolution in biology and medicine is really quite astonishing and should reduce the time it takes to make sweeping changes in medicine. It will not and should not take centuries to markedly reduce the impact of today's major killers, including cancer.

The major roadblock to reaping the benefits of this research may well be the ability of our medical system to absorb and translate advances into medical practice, a difficult problem for our cumbersome and economically besieged health care system. Given these complexities of the war on cancer, we should also especially be on guard for the negative influence of the self-fulfilling prophecy. If we believe that cancer can never be eradicated, then it never will be.

MONITORING PROGRESS IN THE WAR AGAINST CANCER

Given this background, the public needs a way to continuously monitor how cancer is being controlled. Unfortunately, there is no systematic way to get progress reports on cancer research that the general public can understand, even though their tax dollars paid for much of it. We are mostly deluged with bad news. If anyone wants to get a high profile for an environmental cause of any kind they just say it causes cancer.

But there is a national system to monitor progress in the control of cancer. It is called the SEER Program (Surveillance, Epidemiology and End Results), which studies a sample of 12 percent of the U.S. population for cancer incidence, survival and mortality. This is a marvelous program, and 12 percent is a huge sample size as these things go, so these data are truly reliable. Statistics are always out of date, however, because it takes so long to collect and publish the information, and statistics are, and always will be, confusing to doctors and lay people alike. Statistics are also subject to manipulation by anyone who wants to create suspicion by quoting information out of context.

Here is one example of how statistics can confuse. Even if we are successful in reaching the goal set by the National Cancer Institute of reducing mortality from cancer by 50 percent by the year 2000, cancer will move from the number two killer in the United States, behind heart disease, to number one. This is because mortality from heart disease is declining much faster than cancer mortality. Think of the confusing stories this will generate in the press. The National Cancer Program will take its bow for achieving what would be a singular success, and the critics will shout, "Despite billions spent on the war on cancer, cancer moves to number one killer in the U.S.!"

Another example of the possibility for confusion relates to breast cancer. The dominant news in the past year has been about the "epidemic of breast cancer." This is an epidemic that does not exist. The apparent recent increase in breast cancer incidence is actually a success story because the evidence suggests it is due to successful screening programs that have detected cancers today that would have become a problem later.

The number of women screened in the U.S. today has increased substantially to about 70 percent of women who should be screened, from a dismal handful in 1984. When the National Cancer Institute detailed its "Goals for the Year 2000," it made the point that to capitalize on the known beneficial effects of screening mammography, we needed to reach the current rate of screening by 1990 to see the 30 percent reduction in mortality from breast cancer we know we can get from mammography screening by the year

2000. And we did it. The newly diagnosed cases that constitute "the epidemic" are really "money in the bank." Because of the early diagnosis, most of these women will not die of their cancer, but the decline in mortality will not be detectable in national statistics until the year 2000. Nonetheless, the rising incidence is being used—and in most cases by well-meaning people—as bad news to drum up support for research in breast cancer and women's health issues in general. These are good causes, to be sure, but this support comes at the price of public confusion and ultimate loss of credibility, which in the end usually results in a decrease in support.

WHAT HAS BEEN ACHIEVED

Before looking at the future of cancer research and treatment, let us take a quick glance at the past. A mere 20 years ago the cancer cell was a black box. We could look at it, describe it, measure it, weigh it, but we could only guess at what was going on inside. We approached the treatment of cancer, and still do, by finding it as early as possible, before it had a chance to spread, outlining its extent (staging), and either removing it or treating it with an x-ray beam. If neither was possible, it was called an advanced cancer and it was, in those days, considered incurable.

By the 1950s it became apparent that those patients who failed this kind of treatment had recurrences because the tumors had metastasized. Some of their tumor cells had sneaked away from the primary lump and developed secondary growths elsewhere. This accounted for the recurrence of cancer even when surgeons thought they had removed it all. Cells that escaped and circulated in the blood needed something that was also put into the blood to chase and destroy them; this was developed first in the form of chemotherapy, chemicals that can get anywhere and kill circulating tumor cells, and now in the form of biologic therapy, chemical substances that either mimic a natural material found in the body or a purified form of a natural substance in the blood.

What most people do not realize is that when patients die of cancer, they do not die from the effects of the cancer where it started. They die of metastases, because these secondary growths eventually crowd out normal organs, usually the liver, the lung or the brain.

It was in the mid- to late 1960s when we first were able to cure some forms of advanced cancer with drugs and attack the problem of metastases directly. The treatment of cancer is the treatment of metastases we can see on x-rays and other tests or metastases we can presume are present because of a known high risk of recurrence with a localized form of treatment. Treatment with chemotherapy or biologic therapy because of a presumed risk of recurrence—adjuvant therapy—is applicable to a larger number of patients and was successfully introduced in about 1970 only after we could show that we could cure more advanced cancers. It is now known to work for many common cancers, like breast and colon cancer, although not well enough.

Using these approaches, we can now cure about half of all patients with serious cancers in the U.S. By serious cancers we mean those that would lead to rapid death if not treated effectively. We exclude about 500,000 easily curable and rarely lethal skin cancers, so strictly speaking our ability to cure all cancers is much higher, about 58 percent. The problem is that 50 percent of patients with serious cancers are still dying, and since we now freely discuss cancer, they are more visible to us than in the past. Patients who are cured are less visible because they largely go about enjoying life and look and act like the rest of us.

New Understanding The major investment of the war on cancer was in basic laboratory research. Because of the advances made in the laboratory, the lid of the black box has been pried open and the black box has become a blueprint. Using powerful new tools that probe our very genes, we can literally see inside the cancer cells and watch the wheels go round. We have, in the process, uncovered the most amazing array of signaling systems that normal cells use to talk to each other. They mostly involve the cancer genes, called oncogenes.

When these systems, or genes, are damaged, by an accident of nature, deficiencies in our diet, cigarette smoke or environmental agents, the cells can still talk to each other but they often cannot hear. The result is that the programs once used to carefully control growth and development of an egg to a fetus or a child to an adult have no brakes, and the wild and destructive growth that emerges is cancer. One of the reasons why understanding the cancer process well is so important is that it is the very stuff of life itself. Understanding this process has important implications for human development and particularly the aging process, the last frontier of medicine.

In medicine we make progress by a process of trial and error even when we do not understand what we are doing. But we make much more progress when we understand things, and we are now at a level of understanding of the cancer process that was unforeseen by even the most optimistic of scientists in 1971, when the U.S. Congress passed the National Cancer Act that poured billions of dollars into cancer research. Yet the fruits of this investment in basic understanding of cancer are just now reaching the level of clinical application and are hardly measurable yet in national statistics.

Improved Techniques We also continue to use and improve the old ways—surgery, radiotherapy, chemotherapy and biotherapy. These older ways have been aptly described by the author Lewis Thomas as "halfway technologies." When the Cancer Act was passed, a concerted effort was made to improve these technologies especially in testing ways to use them together, rather than separately, to improve results and give the investment in basic research time to bear fruit. It was not considered appropriate to allow a generation of cancer patients to suffer unnecessarily if their lot could be improved by tinkering with current tools. This investment has also paid off, first in cancers in the young and now in common cancers such as breast cancer and colon cancer. Like recent laboratory advances, the most dramatic advances in breast and colon cancer treatment are still too recent for their effects to be measured until about the year 2000.

When the Cancer Act was passed, the national survival rates were 38 percent for all cancers combined (again excluding skin cancers). The improvement in the use of technology is responsible for the increase up to 50 percent in the last figures reported in 1989, and the substantial decline in national mortality from cancer in all people all the way up to age 65.

The more effective use of technology has led to another dramatic change in cancer treatment that is often overlooked. Treatment has become far less difficult to take. To be sure, it is still not considered easy but, compared with 20 years ago— when patients regularly bled to death or became infected and died, even when their cancers were responding to treatment, for the want of good supportive care—the availability of ways to prevent bone marrow toxicity has much improved. Even nausea and vomiting, never a lethal side effect, but the bane of existence for cancer patients receiving radiotherapy or chemotherapy, has, in only the past few years, become almost totally under control.

Prevention What about preventing can-

cer? As a profession, we are often criticized for not paying enough attention to cancer prevention. Before 1971, however, we knew little about how to prevent cancer besides urging people not to smoke. Even with smoking, we did not then have the information about the harmful effect of second-hand smoke that has recently given the anti-smoking drive so much steam. We knew much more about how to treat cancer than prevent it until a large investment in a research area called epidemiology, which did not start in earnest until around 1978, gave us the necessary leads to pursue in cancer prevention. We now know we should be able to prevent most cancers.

We also have new techniques to identify people who are at risk and methods to explore to prevent common cancers. In fact, it may soon be possible to test cord blood from a newborn infant and determine his or her risk of getting cancer as an adult. As exciting as it may be, this process will present scary ethical dilemmas if our ability to prevent cancer does not keep pace with our ability to detect those at risk. Chemicals are already in hand that are known to interrupt the wild signaling process of a cancer cell that can prevent cancer cells in culture from maintaining the malignant state. The National Cancer Institute is supporting more than 50 clinical trials around the world that attempt to prevent cancer, and there have already been some glimmerings of success.

OVERCOMING LIMITATIONS

So what are the cancer treatments of the future? They center around overcoming the major limitations we have been dealing with in the past. These are also now possible to overcome with newly developed technology.

A major limitation has been our inability to know what we are doing to the cancer cell with treatment on a moment-to-moment basis. After a treatment is administered we need to know whether most of the cells are dead or dying to know when, or whether, to administer more and what type of treatment. There are two new techniques available in some institutions to do this. One is nuclear magnetic resonance spectroscopy, a variant of MRI scanning. The other is positron emission tomography (PET scanning). Both are highly sophisticated physical tools that can measure the ability of cancer cells to grow while they reside in the body.

Another major limitation is the inability to tell if a cancer cell has developed the ability to metastasize. Since patients die of metastases, it is extremely important to know when metastases are present even when they cannot be seen with the naked eye or a microscope. We now know that the process of metastases is a modification of a process normal cells use to travel to the proper place to form our various organs when we are embryos. Since all these processes are controlled by genes, the abnormal counterparts of these genes in cancer cells can be probed to determine if a cell has executed this program. If cancer cells cannot travel, then we can deal with a cancer at its primary site in the breast, lung, colon and so on by local means alone, such as refined and limited surgery or even laser surgery. There is also computer-driven radiotherapy that shapes the beam precisely to the tumor and avoids the normal tissue (referred to as conformal radiotherapy) now available in a few places in the U.S. If it is known that the cell has already developed the capacity to metastasize, then we need to do more regardless of how favorable the cancer looks to the doctor.

We have also been severely hampered by our inability to determine after surgery, radiotherapy or chemotherapy if we got all the cells. Older techniques could measure only one cancer cell in a hundred normal cells. Smaller numbers were missed and treatment was stopped

or a necessary treatment not given because the patient appeared free of cancer. Now we have the ability to measure one cancer cell in a million normal cells with newer techniques of molecular biology. We are using these techniques wherever the opportunity presents itself to monitor treatment so we give enough treatment of the right dose, but no more.

Another limitation that affects the use of chemotherapy is the ability of cancer cells to exclude cancer drugs from the inside of the cell, where they do the most damage. Cancer cells can be quite clever. We humans grow up in a world surrounded by all kinds of natural chemicals. Many of them are found in plants or are made by bacteria in soil for the purpose of protecting plants from insects and birds or protecting bacteria from other bacteria. We get our best antibiotics and anticancer drugs from these sources. It should come as no surprise, then, that cells of normal humans, and other species, have developed ways to prevent these chemicals from entering our normal cells in order to avoid being poisoned. The cancer cell regularly usurps these mechanisms to defeat cancer treatment, and we have only recently begun to understand them well enough to develop methods to overcome what we refer to as "drug resistance." Now we are testing elegant tools to do this.

Finally, the whole field of biologics—the use of natural products—to treat cancer is new. Before the 1970s we could get biologic materials only in very small amounts. With gene cloning now a routine technique, we can turn bacteria and yeast into factories and make virtually unlimited supplies of these materials to test as ways of controlling cancer. This includes, for the first time, making pure vaccines to test against cancers that appear to respond better to immune manipulation than chemotherapy, such as malignant melanoma.

The above are scientific limitations. The

socioeconomic limitation we face is making the transfer of technology fast and efficient. This is a real problem in our medical system, and a major responsibility of the National Cancer Institute's network of comprehensive cancer centers.

The architects of the National Cancer Act should be proud of what has been accomplished. It has been a long and arduous trip to this point, and although there is still a lot of work ahead of us, it is becoming increasingly apparent that the cancer cell is a vulnerable target and there is much room for optimism.

It is possible to begin to think of a world without cancer.

35
CANCER PREVENTION, SCREENING AND RISK ASSESSMENT

David S. Alberts, MD, Mary Klein Buller, MA, Ernest Rosenbaum, MD, Malin Dollinger, MD, and Guy Newell, MD

◇

Most of our lives have been, or will be, touched by cancer. But there are positive measures we can take to prevent or survive this disease. More than one million new cases of cancer are diagnosed in the U.S. annually. As the second leading cause of death after heart disease, cancer claims the lives of more than half a million Americans each year.

Although that translates into one death from cancer every minute, there is reason for optimism. Significant advances in the prevention, early detection and treatment of several cancers have enabled half of all patients with cancer to survive. More than 8 million Americans alive today with a history of cancer can attest to recent successes.

The medical community is credited with increasing the cancer survival rate from less than 20 percent in the 1930s to nearly 50 percent today. Their efforts continue and hold promise for the future. New research approaches may hold the keys to reducing the number of cancer deaths or someday even curing the disease. New clinical and screening procedures may be developed to detect even more cancers in their early and treatable stages. Genetic research may discover what turns a cancer cell on and find a way to turn it off. Biologic research could lead to an antitumor vaccine much like vaccines for measles and other diseases. But these research results may be many years away.

Prevention and Early Detection The real strides that can be made against cancer right now are in the areas of prevention and early detection. These victories will be won not only by the medical community but also by individuals who realize that a fuller, healthier future is within their reach.

♦ Cancer prevention is trying to keep cancer from developing by reducing risk.

♦ Early detection is finding cancer in its earliest, most curable stage, often before symptoms appear.

The benefits to be gained by prevention and early detection are especially desirable. Although the risk of cancer increases with age, cancer can strike anyone at any time. It can change your life drastically. It can be debilitating, painful, costly to treat and fatal in half of all cases. Why take that chance when you can do something about it?

Lifestyle, environment and heredity, alone or in combination, help determine cancer risk. The way you live your life, such as choosing to smoke or not eating a healthy diet, can have the greatest impact on your risk. More than 70 percent of all cancers may be related to personal behaviors and habits.

Since you have the ability to change and control your behavior, you also have the ability to reduce your risk for cancer. Both outright prevention and early detection require that you assume greater responsibility for your health and that you work actively in partnership with health care professionals to make personal

TABLE 1

HEALTHY PEOPLE 2000 OBJECTIVES FOR THE PREVENTION AND EARLY DETECTION OF CANCER

	From Baseline Of	To Goal Of At Least
Smoking Cessation:		
Reduce cigarette smoking among people aged 20 and older.	29%	15%
Reduce the number of youth who become regular cigarette smokers by age 20.	30%	15%
Increase smoking cessation by pregnant women.	39%	60%
Reduce the proportion of children who are exposed to tobacco smoke at home.	39%	20%
Reduce smokeless tobacco use by males aged 12 through 24.	6.6% (12-17 yrs) 8.9% (18-24 yrs)	4% 4%
Diet:		
Reduce dietary fat intake among people aged 2 and older.	35% of calories	30% of calories
Reduce average saturated fat intake among people aged 2 and older.	13% of calories	10% of calories
Increase adults' consumption of fruits and vegetables.	2.5 servings/day	5 or more servings/day
Increase adults' consumption of grain products.	3 servings/day	6 or more servings/day
Sun Exposure:		
Increase the proportion of people of all ages who limit sun exposure, use sunscreens and protective clothing, and avoid artificial sources of ultraviolet light.	n/a	60%
Breast Cancer Screening:		
Increase the proportion of women aged 40 and older who have ever received a clinical breast examination and mammogram.	36%	60%
Increase the proportion of women aged 50 and older who have received a clinical breast examination and mammogram within the preceding 1 to 2 years.	25%	60%
Cervical Cancer Screening:		
Increase the proportion of women aged 18 and older who have ever received a Pap test.	88%	95%

Increase the proportion of women aged 18 and older who have received a Pap test within the last 1 to 3 years.	75%	85%
Colon Cancer Screening:		
Increase the proportion of men and women aged 50 and older who have received fecal occult blood testing within the last 1 to 2 years.	27%	50%
Increase the proportion of women and men aged 50 and older visiting a primary care physician in the last year who have received a digital rectal examination.	27%	40%
Increase the proportion of women and men aged 50 and older who have ever received a proctosigmoidoscopy examination.	25%	40%
Oral Cancer Screening:		
Increase the proportion of women and men aged 50 and older visiting a primary care physician in the preceding year who have received an oral examination.	n/a	40%
Skin Cancer Screening:		
Increase the proportion of women and men aged 50 and older visiting a primary care physician in the preceding year who have received a skin examination.	n/a	40%
Physician Counseling:		
Increase the proportion of primary care providers who routinely counsel patients about cancer screening recommendations.	52%	75%

Source: Public Health Service. *Healthy People 2000: National health promotion and disease prevention objectives.* Washington, DC: US Government Printing Office, 1991. DHHS Publication No. (PHS) 91-50212.

choices and decisions that may positively influence your destiny.

Cancer prevention and early detection can be extremely successful. Nearly all cancers of the lung, bladder, mouth and skin could be avoided by eliminating tobacco use, heavy alcohol consumption and unprotected exposure to sunlight. It is estimated that cigarette smoking alone is responsible for 30 percent or more of all cancer deaths. Food can be both a friend and foe when it comes to cancer. Risk may be reduced by increasing consumption of foods rich in beta-carotene and fiber that may have the ability to prevent certain cancers, while limiting high-fat foods that may promote some cancers.

Early detection can save lives because treatment can begin promptly at a more curable stage. Many types of cancer, including cancer of the breast, colon, cervix, skin, prostate, testes and mouth, can be detected early through routine screening procedures and self-examinations. It is up to you to follow the recommended guidelines for cancer screening and report any suspicious symptoms to your physician.

National Objectives The U.S. Surgeon General and the Department of Health and Human Services have proposed a goal-oriented public health program known as the *Healthy People 2000 Objectives*. The program's objective for cancer is to reduce cancer deaths by 50 percent by the turn of the century, saving around 230,000 lives each year. Whether we achieve this goal will be determined in large part by our own behaviors over the rest of the decade.

The plan focuses on state-of-the-art treatments, early detection, screening and prevention. In the short term, it's expected that increased use of state-of-the-art treatments will bring about the greatest reduction in the number of deaths. But earlier and more effective screening and prevention eventually should save more lives by reducing the incidence of cancer.

The success of the Year 2000 Objectives for cancer hinge on two things that are within your power:
♦ Your eagerness to increase your understanding of the causes of cancer and the risk factors associated with it.
♦ Your willingness to act upon that information to reduce your chances of developing cancer and enhance the quality of your life.

RISK FACTORS AND RISK REDUCTION

As outlined in Chapter 1, the transformation of normal cells into cancerous tumors may be caused by insults or "hits" to the cell's genetic structure. These hits—a combination of genetics, environmental factors and especially lifestyle habits—interact and accumulate over time.

There are hits that initiate cancer—tobacco smoke, x-rays, certain hormones and drugs, sunlight, industrial chemicals and some sexually transmitted viruses.

And there are promoters such as alcohol and stress. It takes at least one or two hits to damage a cell and affect the DNA. As the hits accumulate, a breaking point is eventually reached and a normal cell mutates, changing into a cell that grows uncontrollably—a cancer cell.

We can do nothing about some risk factors. But most are a matter of choice.

Heredity When there is a family predisposition to cancer, heredity may be the first event that promotes the growth of cancer. A cell may then be changed into a cancer cell by a single hit of a carcinogen. Although a tendency or susceptibility to developing cancer can be inherited under certain conditions, probably less than 2 percent of malignancies are caused directly by heredity. The vast majority of family histories of cancer result from a complex interaction of genes, environment and lifestyle.

Geographic Area People living in areas where there are vitamin or mineral deficiencies such as selenium deficiency may run a higher risk of cancer. The biggest influence of geographic area, however, is on diet, which may also be influenced by cultural habits.

Many studies have been carried out on cancer rates among migrant workers. Two studies looked at Japanese migrants who moved to Hawaii and whose next generation moved to California. The incidence of breast cancer was found to be very low in Japan, probably because of dietary factors. When the same hereditary population moved to Hawaii and adopted some American customs, the incidence of breast cancer rose. When the same genetic population then moved to California and adopted the American-style diet, the cancer rate increased to the same level found in native-born Americans.

Diet Obesity, defined as being 40 percent or more overweight, may increase your risk for several types of cancer. High levels of fats in the diet—both saturated (hard, mostly animal) and unsaturated (liquid, mostly vegetable oil)—appear to play a role in causing cancers of the colon, rectum, prostate, testes, breast, uterus and gall bladder. Even lean people, if they eat high-fat and low-fiber diets, run increased risks of developing these tumors.

Low fiber consumption may contribute to the rise in colon and rectal cancers. Grains have always been one of humanity's basic foods. In days past, we would eat grains, and foods made from them, in their simplest form—whole and unrefined. Paleolithic people ate five to ten times more fiber than we do now. About 150 years ago, a new milling process tempted our tastebuds with refined white flour. But when the husk was removed from the grain, so was the fiber. Fiber has the power to dilute cancer-causing toxins, such as dietary fat, and move them through the bowel quickly so they have less time to cause harm. Some studies suggest that people who eat a high-fiber diet may reduce their risk for colon cancer by up to 40 percent.

Adequate intake of some vitamins and minerals (found in fruits, vegetables and other foods) may protect against certain cancers. Low levels of vitamins A and C increase the risk for cancers of the larynx, esophagus, stomach, colon, rectum, prostate, bladder and lung. Low levels of selenium also may increase the risk of skin and other cancers.

Eating preserved foods, especially smoked or nitrate-cured meats, increases the risk for cancers of the esophagus and stomach.

Even the way food is cooked may increase cancer risk. Cancer-causing substances may be formed when meat, poultry and fish are cooked at very high temperatures.

Exposure to Environmental Carcinogens
Exposure in the workplace to cancer-caus-ing chemicals such as coal-tar-based products, benzene, cadmium, uranium, asbestos or nickel can greatly increase the risk of developing cancer. Carcinogens are also showing up in the air, water and soil. Excessive exposure to radon in homes and other buildings with poor ventilation may increase the risk of lung cancer, especially in smokers.

Exposure to Sunlight On sunny and even cloudy days, intense amounts of ultraviolet rays may affect your skin. With the thinning of the protective ozone layer, these rays are becoming even more intense and more dangerous. Excessive exposure to sunshine can cause sunburn, wrinkles, premature skin aging and leathery or rough skin. Cumulative sun exposure can also produce skin cancers such as basal and squamous cell carcinomas.

Some evidence suggests that intermittent intense sun exposure (severe or frequent sunburning), especially during childhood and adolescence, may increase risk of developing dangerous malignant melanoma later in life.

Exposure to the radiation in artificial sources of sunlight, namely sun lamps and tanning booths, may also increase the risk of developing skin cancer. Unfortunately, sun damage from ultraviolet light is cumulative over a lifetime. Once exposed, you can never reverse the exposure. But you can limit further exposure and more severe skin damage by starting today to stay out of the sunshine.

During the last 20 years all types of skin cancer have increased dramatically throughout the United States and especially in the Southwest. Southern Arizona, for example, has the second highest rate of skin cancer in the world behind Queensland, Australia. Skin cancer is the most common malignancy in the U.S. The national goal is to increase to 60 percent by the year 2000 the proportion of all people who limit sun exposure, use sunscreen, wear protective clothing when outdoors and avoid artificial tanning devices. Public health education programs, the media and the cosmetics and pharmaceutical industries that manufacture sunscreens have helped bring the magnitude of the skin cancer problem into national focus.

Sexual Practices Sexual history and habits influence the chance of developing cancer. They can either protect you or promote the growth of tumors. Childbearing reduces the risk of cancers of the ovary, uterus and breast. And women who give birth before age 30 are less likely to develop breast cancer in later life.

The more sex partners you have, the more likely you are to be exposed to sexually transmitted viruses. Some of these can cause cancers of the head and neck, cervix, penis and anus, as well as AIDS and AIDS-related cancers.

Alcohol In about 7 percent of males and 3 percent of females—about 4 percent of people overall—alcohol can lead to cancers in the head and neck, the larynx and possibly the liver and pancreas. Alcohol consumption also has a strong relationship with smoking, a combination that greatly increases the risk for cancers of the mouth, throat and esophagus.

Tobacco Smoke Despite the claims of the tobacco industry, there is no longer any question about the causal relationship between smoking and cancer. The link has been established statistically since 1950, though it was apparent long before that.

In the early years of the century lung cancer was a rare disease. There were probably not more than 400 or 500 cases each year. Some professors of medicine were advising their students as late as 1920 that they might see only one case of lung cancer in their professional careers. But when inhalable Burley Turkish tobaccos (which didn't cause excessive coughing) came on the market in 1912, smoking became much more popular.

By 1950, when the first report relating smoking and lung cancer was published in the *Journal of the American Medical Association,* there were 18,000 lung cancer deaths per year in the U.S. By 1982, there were 111,000. In 1993, there were an estimated 149,000 deaths. This tragically high death rate has started to decrease in men but is still increasing in women. As late as the 1950s the disease was relatively uncommon in women, but by the late 1980s lung cancer replaced breast cancer as the number one cause of cancer deaths in women.

In response to recent research evidence, environmental tobacco smoke has been classified as a Class A carcinogen by the Environmental Protection Agency. Nonsmokers who are exposed to the toxic tobacco smoke of others are at greatly increased risk for heart disease, lung cancer and other health hazards.

Habitual use of smokeless tobacco is also threatening the lives of several million people in the U.S., especially young males. Without a doubt, chewing tobacco and dipping snuff can lead to the development of cancers of the mouth.

GUIDELINES FOR PREVENTION

Studies are confirming what doctors and many others knew 25 years ago—lifestyle does make a difference in the risk of developing cancer. With 30 to 35 percent of cancers associated with diet, 30 to 32 percent caused by smoking, 4 percent related to alcohol and 3 percent related to sun exposure, more than 70 percent of cancers are likely the direct result of the lifestyle choices we make.

Two-thirds of cancer cases, then, can be prevented if enough people make different choices. Reducing the number of smokers in the U.S. by 50 percent would save more than 75,000 lives each year by 2015. Dietary improvements would save at least 20,000 lives annually. But although many people have become aware of cancer risk factors, few seem willing to change their habits.

What You Can Do to Reduce Your Risk of Cancer

Diet No diet can guarantee that you won't develop cancer. But a diet low in fat and rich in a wide variety of fruits, vegetables and whole grain products may reduce your risk for cancer.

1. Reduce your intake of dietary fats—both saturated and unsaturated—from the current estimated level of 36 percent of total calories to less than 30 percent, and increase your consumption of fiber from 8 to 12 grams to 20 to 30 grams per day (about 1 to 2 cups [250 to 500 mL] of wheat bran cereal, for example).

2. Increase your consumption of fruits and vegetables to at least 5 servings per day (a serving being equal to an apple or a 6 oz. [175 mL] glass of orange juice). Fruits and vegetables contain vitamin A, vitamin C, vitamin E, the minerals zinc and selenium, and fiber.

3. Eat cruciferous vegetables—cabbage, cauliflower, broccoli, brussels sprouts, rutabagas and turnips. These are good sources of the indoles (natural cancer-prevention substances) and fiber that help reduce the risk of several cancers, especially colon cancer.

4. Reduce your consumption of smoked or charcoal-broiled foods. Before you begin cooking on the barbecue, first microwave meat for a few minutes and pour off the accumulated juices. This will decrease carcinogen exposure.

5. Drink moderate amounts of alcoholic beverages if you drink any at all. Ideally, you should have less than one drink or 4 oz. (125 mL) of wine per day.

6. Reduce your consumption of red meats, animal fats and tropical oils such as palm and coconut.

7. Keep physically trim and fit to avoid being overweight. This helps prevent cancer by reducing excesses of hormones that may promote cancer growth. It is as important to exercise as it is to maintain good nutrition. Even moderate exercise, such as brisk walking, helps to burn fat, make muscles firm and reduce fat bulges. Of course, exercise is also good for the heart!

Lifestyle
1. Don't smoke. If you do smoke, stop.
2. Limit your alcohol intake to one drink a day or less.
3. Don't drink and smoke at the same time. This combination increases the chance for head and neck cancers by about 50 times.
4. Reduce stress or practice stress-management techniques.
5. Protect yourself from sexually transmitted viruses by using latex condoms when appropriate. There is an increased incidence of cancer in patients with homosexual practices and an increased incidence of cervical and penile cancers in women and men who have multiple sex partners.
6. Follow the recommended guidelines for cancer screening and advocate public policies to make early detection affordable and available to everyone.

Environment
1. Avoid excessive unprotected exposure to the sun's ultraviolet radiation (UVA and UVB). UVB (sunburning rays) and UVA, which penetrates deeper into the skin, may lead to premature aging of the skin, wrinkling, sunburn, permanent skin damage and skin cancer.

Avoid midday outdoor activities, wear protective clothing and hats and use sunscreen with a Sun Protection Factor (SPF) of 15 or more to reduce sunlight's damage to your skin. The higher the SPF number, the longer you will be protected, but all sunscreen should be reapplied periodically, especially after swimming or perspiring heavily. Several broad-spectrum sunscreens that absorb both UVB and UVA are now available. Lighter complexioned, blue-eyed, red-headed, blond or freckled people will need to be especially vigilant because they lack built-in sun protection from melanin pigment in the skin.

2. People in areas with high levels of radon can decrease the risk of lung cancer by providing adequate ventilation in homes and other buildings. Radon is an odorless radioactive gas that is emitted naturally from the ground and can become trapped in buildings with poor ventilation. Some buildings have more radon than others. Commercial tests are available to measure radon levels.

3. Reduce or control any exposure to known chemical carcinogens such as benzene and industrial asbestos by using protective techniques. Preferably, avoid contact altogether.

4. Help in any way you can to enact legislation that will establish clean air and water standards.

THE MOST EFFECTIVE PREVENTIVE MEASURE: DON'T SMOKE

About 2.5 million people worldwide, including 400,000 Americans, die each year because of smoking. Smoking causes death from cardiovascular disease, lung diseases such as emphysema, bronchitis and pneumonia, stroke and several types of cancer. Not surprisingly, these are the leading causes of death in our society.

Cancer rates have not increased significantly over the past half century, except for lung cancer. Smoking is responsible for 85 percent of lung cancer cases. It is the leading cause of cancers of the larynx and mouth and plays a role in causing cancers of the stomach, bladder, kidney, pancreas and cervix.

Cancer cure rates have improved steadily from 20 percent to 50 percent, except for lung cancer. No effective treatment for advanced lung cancer exists. Yet 46 million Americans continue to smoke.

Cigarettes are cancer factories. Cigarette tar contains toxic cancer-causing chemicals and many other carcinogens enter cigarettes during production—pesticides and fertilizers in the field and chemicals during processing and manufacturing.

A burning cigarette gives off almost 7,000 chemicals such as carbon monoxide, argon, nitrosamines, benzpyrene, radioactive polonium 210, cadmium, methane, benzene, formaldehyde, vinyl chloride, arsenic and hydrogen cyanide. More than 4,000 of these chemicals are toxic and 43 are known to cause cancer. The same carcinogens are also found in the tobacco used in pipes and cigars.

A non-smoker sitting in the same room as a smoker cannot escape the toxic compounds released in tobacco smoke. In fact, second-hand smoke has significantly higher concentrations of the carcinogenic compounds found in mainstream smoke. Because "involuntary" smoking leads to the deaths of an estimated 53,000 people in the U.S. each year, including 4,000 from lung cancer, second-hand smoke has been granted status as a known human carcinogen by the Environmental Protection Agency.

When the Surgeon General first advised about the dangers of smoking in 1964, 52 percent of Americans smoked. The percentage is now down to 27 percent, thanks largely to warnings, smoking cessation programs, restrictive indoor air policies, education, social pressures and the availability of the transdermal nicotine patch. These have helped turn the tide against the clout of the tobacco industry.

The *Healthy People 2000* goal is to reduce cigarette smoking to no more than 15 percent of adults, reduce the initiation of smoking by children so that no more than 15 percent have become regular smokers by age 20 and increase the number of women who quit smoking during pregnancy to at least 60 percent.

Because it is a matter of choice and

takes so many lives, smoking is the most preventable cause of death in America. Smoking is an addiction, perhaps the most deadly form of drug dependence, and is a difficult habit to break. But quitting is possible, as over 44 million ex-smokers in the U.S. can confirm.

EARLY DETECTION

Despite all the advances in treatment, early detection can probably prevent more cancer deaths than any other approach. If tumors could always be detected and removed when they are tiny, no one would ever have to worry about metastatic disease.

Early detection depends on recognizing cancer's warning signals and receiving prompt medical attention when symptoms appear. But what helps early detection immeasurably is self-examination and simple screening tests performed as part of an annual medical examination.

Self-Examination A simple way to help detect breast cancer early is breast self-examination. This is a low-risk, non-invasive evaluation that does not involve any radiation exposure or any cost. It's estimated that 90 percent of cancerous tumors can be detected by monthly breast self-examination. Training programs that teach women how to perform a full examination have had great success.

Men should also practice self-examination, feeling each testicle every four months to detect any lumps. Although testis cancer is uncommon, it is one of the most common cancers in men aged 20 to 35 and is curable, especially when detected early.

With some training and experience, men and women could examine their skin and moles, mouth, thyroid gland, genitals, rectal area and lymph nodes for any suspicious changes, lumps or patches.

Clinical Examinations and Screening Tests During your yearly physical examination, your physician should examine various cancer-prone organs such as the skin, oral cavity, prostate, lymph nodes, thyroid, testes, rectum, breasts and ovaries. More involved procedures such as mammography, Pap smears and pelvic examinations should be performed for women. Stool blood tests and flexible sigmoidoscopy are recommended for both women and men. These screening tests are recommended at varying intervals depending on your age, since cancer risk increases with age. Periodic chest x-rays may be warranted for people at high risk for lung cancer.

Research studies are still collecting evidence on the benefits of some cancer screening tests, but other procedures have been proven effective at reducing cancer incidence and death.

♦ The regular use of mammography and clinical breast examination may reduce deaths from breast cancer by 30 percent among women aged 50 and older. Younger women may benefit to a lesser degree.

♦ Since the Pap test became widely used, the incidence of cervical cancer has fallen dramatically around the world as more precancerous lesions and early carcinomas have been found. In the U.S., the rate has been cut in half.

There are a few newcomers to the cancer-screening arsenal.

♦ A blood test for prostate specific antigen (PSA) has proven useful in the early detection of prostate cancer.

♦ Prostatic (transrectal) ultrasound, a rectal probe that emits ultrasonic waves to make an image of the prostate, is being investigated as another strategy for detecting malignancy early, often in combination with the PSA test. The specificity and sensitivity of transrectal ultrasound are higher than for a digital rectal examination, the current screening recommendation. The combination of digital rectal examination, PSA and transrectal ultrasound may work best to detect prostate

TABLE 2
AMERICAN CANCER SOCIETY RECOMMENDATIONS FOR THE EARLY DETECTION
OF CANCER IN PERSONS WITH NO SYMPTOMS AND AVERAGE RISK

CLINICAL EXAMINATIONS FOR WOMEN

PROCEDURE	CANCER SITE	AGE	FREQUENCY
General Exam	Thyroid, Ovaries, Lymph Nodes, Skin and Mouth	40 and older	Every year
Pelvic Exam	Ovaries and Uterus	Women who are 18 or older or sexually active	Every year or every 1-3 years after 3 normal yearly exams
Pap Test	Cervix	Women who are 18 or older or sexually active	Every year or every 1-3 years after 3 normal yearly exams
Endometrial Tissue Sample	Endometrium (uterine lining)	At menopause for high-risk women	At menopause
Clinical Breast Exam	Breast	20-39 years old 40 and older	Every 3 years Every year
Mammography	Breast	35-39 years old 40-49 years old 50 and older	Baseline Every 1-2 years Every year
Digital Rectal Exam	Rectum	40 and older	Every year
Stool Blood Test	Colon and Rectum	50 and older	Every year
Sigmoidoscopy	Colon and Rectum	50 and older	Every 3-5 years after 2 normal yearly exams

SELF-EXAMINATIONS FOR WOMEN

SELF-EXAM	CANCER SITE	AGE	FREQUENCY
Breast	Breast	20 and older	Every month
Skin	Skin and Moles	All ages	Every month
Oral	Mouth	All ages—smokers	Every month

CLINICAL EXAMINATIONS FOR MEN

PROCEDURE	CANCER SITE	AGE	FREQUENCY
General Exam	Thyroid, Testes, Prostate, Lymph Nodes, Skin, and Mouth	40 and older	Every year

Digital Rectal Exam	Rectum and Prostate	40 and older	Every year
Stool Blood Test	Colon and Rectum	50 and older	Every year
Prostate Specific Antigen (PSA)	Prostate	50 and older	Every year
Transrectal Ultrasound	Prostate	Not specified	If PSA and DRE are abnormal
Sigmoidoscopy	Colon and Rectum	50 and older	Every 3-5 years after 2 normal yearly exams

SELF-EXAMINATIONS FOR MEN

SELF-EXAM	CANCER SITE	AGE	FREQUENCY
Testicular	Testes	15 and older	Every month
Skin	Skin and Moles	All ages	Every month
Oral	Mouth	All ages—smokers	Every month

Source: American Cancer Society. *Guidelines for the cancer-related checkup (1991), Recommendations and rationale*. In *American Cancer Society Textbook of Clinical Oncology*. Atlanta: American Cancer Society. ACS Publication No. 91-50M-No.3347-PE.

cancer. In 1993, the American Cancer Society revised its national recommendations to include a PSA every year for men aged 50 and older, and transrectal ultrasound if digital rectal examination and PSA are abnormal.

◆ Women may benefit from advances in vaginal ultrasound technology. The Pap test, though extremely useful for discovering cervical cancer in its early stages, is marginally effective for the early detection of endometrial cancer and not effective for ovarian cancer. Studies are under way to evaluate vaginal ultrasound plus a common blood test, CA-125, for the early detection of ovarian cancer.

Preventive screenings are particularly important if you come from a family with a history of cancer or if you have ever had cancer yourself. If you have had one cancer you are more likely to get another one, so you should have periodic checkups and evaluations as advised by your physician.

The American Cancer Society and National Cancer Institute, as well as other professional groups such as the American College of Physicians, American College of Surgeons and American College of Obstetricians and Gynecologists, have proposed various recommendations for cancer screening that, although not exactly the same, are very similar.

People without a history of cancer and with no symptoms should follow these established guidelines for the early detection of cancer.

RISK ASSESSMENT AND SCREENING

Screening someone with a specific complaint such as a breast mass or a digestive problem will obviously lead to more diagnoses of breast or colon cancer than screening apparently normal, healthy people.

But screening apparently healthy people with no specific complaints to see if a cancer might be discovered has become a significant and popular field of activity. These screening programs could lead to earlier treatment and much higher chances for cure. There are two ways of approaching cancer screening: whole populations can be screened or individual risk assessments can be conducted.

Risk Assessment Some people may be at greater risk to develop cancer. This may be because of their genetic makeup, their exposure to some environmental cancer-causing substance or their having close (first-degree) relatives who have had cancer.

To identify such people, cancer risk assessment programs have been developed at many medical centers. In these programs, the "client" fills out a questionnaire detailing his or her life history, family history, medical history, work history and lifestyle habits. The questionnaire data is fed into a computer and analyzed. A report containing a comprehensive and detailed analysis of the risk of cancer in that particular individual is then produced and given to the "client" and/or a designated physician.

These programs often suggest preventive measures that might be taken, including some medical treatment or lifestyle changes. A history of heavy cigarette smoking, for example, would lead the program to recommend regular chest x-rays and physical examinations, as well as a recommendation to quit smoking. A family history of colon cancer would lead to a recommendation that family members be screened by sigmoidoscopy or colonoscopy at regular intervals and that stools be examined yearly for bleeding.

Quite a few cancer risk assessment programs are available for use by the general population. But it is important to understand that the programs are designed solely to give information about the increased risks for developing specific types of cancer.

Completing a risk assessment questionnaire is not a medical procedure and such programs do not constitute the practice of medicine. No physician-patient relationship exists. There is no physical examination, no blood tests or x-rays. Nor is any information provided beyond an estimate of the relative risks of certain types of cancers and general ways in which those risks could be reduced or specific cancers detected.

Widespread Screening There *is* a medical relationship with a physician when apparently healthy people have specific tests done to detect cancer in its early stages.

During these examinations, the doctor's attention is directed to specific sites that may harbor cancer. Which sites depend on the patient's case history. The larynx might be examined with a mirror, the lungs by chest x-ray, the bowel by endoscopy or x-rays and the pelvis by x-ray, ultrasound and physical examination.

Although there has been a great deal of information published on the usefulness of extensive screening of healthy people, the practice has not yet been widely accepted by the medical community nor, especially, by insurance companies and other third-party payers, because of costs.

On an individual basis, each person certainly merits screening. Anything that creates an earlier diagnosis is to be encouraged. But questions inevitably have been raised about the expense, complexity and cost-effectiveness of screening programs for large groups of people. It has been especially difficult for some insurance companies to justify spending the substantial sums needed to diagnose a small number of cases.

There has been some acceptance of the concept, though. Many health maintenance organizations and some small and large insurance companies have begun to promote and cover preventive screening services. In 1988, Medicare approved payment for routine mammograms because it has become increasingly clear that for certain age groups this simple procedure can detect breast cancers earlier and in a potentially more curable stage. A mammogram can provide a diagnosis about one year before a tumor could be detected otherwise.

JOINING THE NATIONAL FIGHT AGAINST CANCER

Following the guidelines for cancer prevention and screening means that you are willing to take responsibility for your own health. In so doing, you will be playing a part in achieving the national goals to reduce cancer incidence and death. But there are also other ways that you can become involved in the fight against cancer.

Community-Based Cancer Prevention and Control Initiatives Several national health and voluntary organizations—such as the National Cancer Institute, Centers for Disease Control and Prevention and the American Cancer Society—have launched large cancer prevention and control research initiatives. These community-based research studies and educational programs are designed to advance our understanding of ways to prevent, detect and control cancer.

They offer the public a tangible opportunity to participate in cancer prevention research. Predominant cancer sites such as the breast, lung, prostate and colon are targeted by these initiatives.

♦ With the passing of the Breast and Cervical Cancer Mortality Act, an anticipated 30 states will receive funds to coordinate comprehensive programs for the early detection of breast and cervical cancer in underserved women.

♦ The National Institutes of Health and the Department of Health and Human Services recently initiated several important cancer prevention and screening studies. Nationwide, 150,000 women age 50 to 79 will join the Women's Health Initiative to evaluate the benefits and risks of hormone replacement therapy, a low-fat diet and calcium/vitamin D supplementation on cancer, heart disease and osteoporosis.

♦ The Breast Cancer Prevention Trial, the first of its kind, is designed to determine whether tamoxifen, an anti-estrogen drug used to treat breast cancer, will prevent cancer, heart attacks and bone fractures in postmenopausal women and premenopausal women at high risk for cancer. Up to 16,000 women will participate in this 10-year study.

♦ The Prostate Cancer Prevention Study will assess the value of finasteride (Proscar) for preventing prostate cancer. Eighteen thousand healthy men age 55 and older will be recruited into this study.

♦ The Prostate, Lung, Colorectal and Ovarian Trial (PLCO) will evaluate the effectiveness of cancer-screening techniques. The study will randomly divide 74,000 men and 74,000 women into either intervention (screening) or control (no screening) groups for four years of screening and ten years of monitoring. Screening procedures to be tested include the digital rectal examination, prostate specific antigen test (PSA), chest x-ray, flexible sigmoidoscopy, pelvic examination, serum CA-125 blood test and vaginal ultrasound.

♦ The American Stop Smoking Intervention Study (ASSIST) is designed to reduce the prevalence of smoking in 17 states to less than 15 percent of adults by the year 2000. The study is expected to reach 18 million smokers.

♦ The National Cancer Institute has joined forces with the produce and food retail industries to launch a diet and cancer prevention program called "5 A Day For Better Health." This program will combine supermarket promotions, media messages and programs in the workplace, school and community to motivate individuals to eat five or more servings of fruits and vegetables every day.

Cancer Control Advocacy Along with AIDS (acquired immune deficiency syndrome), Americans list cancer as the most important health problem facing the nation today. According to a recent Gallup poll, we want cancer to be placed higher on the national health care agenda. Legislative action and public policy can complement research and education to reduce cancer incidence and mortality.

What is needed is for people not just to answer polling questions, but to speak out and demand action from Congress and from state and municipal bodies. Much has already been achieved by such public advocacy. To improve quality standards for mammography, U.S. mammography facilities are now required to be accredited and inspected. Smoke-free public buildings and worksites are commonplace. The government budget for breast cancer research has increased. And Medicare reimburses for screening mammography.

Additional public advocacy is warranted in areas such as prohibiting the sale of tobacco products to youth, increasing access to cancer screening, cancer survivors' rights, clean indoor air policies, funding for cancer research and insurance coverage of screening procedures.

36
INVESTIGATIONAL ANTICANCER DRUGS

Franco M. Muggia, MD

————————◇————————

The field of chemotherapy is very active. The National Cancer Institute (NCI) and the pharmaceutical industry are always searching for promising new chemotherapies.

Six to ten new drugs are introduced each year. Most are modifications of previously known drugs (analogues) or new formulations of old drugs. A number of new compounds also enter trial each year, but many are found early in their development to have problems or to share mechanisms of action or resistance with older compounds without possessing any obvious advantages.

Before being approved by the Federal Drug Administration (FDA) for the treatment of cancer, a chemotherapeutic drug is tested by patient volunteers in clinical trials (*see also* Chapter 4). Government and industry at national and international levels have shown a fair degree of cooperation in testing new drugs over the years.

PHASES OF INVESTIGATION

Current cancer drugs were discovered through drug-screening programs that measured the drugs' effects on prolonging the survival of leukemic mice.

More recently, the NCI has sought to improve specificity and reduce costs by first developing a profile measuring how actively a drug kills tumor cells of a particular type growing in laboratory cultures. This profile is compared to the pro-file of established drugs. If the new drug seems promising, its effects against tumors in animals are studied, including human cancers transplanted into mice.

Many of the new generation of compounds are designed by computers to attack certain biochemical targets known to be more common in cancer cells than in normal cells. But most compounds continue to be introduced because of knowledge acquired through the study of older drugs already proven effective against some cancers and through the application of new concepts.

Preclinical Testing Drugs of interest undergo preclinical testing. At this stage, they are characterized according to their stability and purity and their toxicity in animals. This testing ends with the development of a pure and stable preparation for administration to humans.

Phase I This is when clinical study begins. A starting dose level (based on the drug's effects on mice) is given to groups of patients who volunteer for a clinical trial because their standard treatments have not been effective. This dose is then increased in groups of similar patients by increments initially of 10 times the dose previously shown to be safe, and by lesser increments as toxicity is noted.

Sometimes noteworthy toxic events occur. These are very carefully documented and promptly treated. The increases in the dosage are interrupted and further study at the highest safe level is conducted. Researchers also study what happens to the drug in the body (drug metabolism and pharmacology).

What provides the "green light" to proceed to Phase II is the discovery of a dose level that causes only mild or manageable toxicities but also produces drug concentrations in the blood that are in the range for antitumor effects found in preclinical experiments. It is even more encouraging if patients are seen to benefit even when some received doses later found to be too low or when most have tumors that resist treatment.

Phase II For a more accurate assessment of potential, the drug in this phase is tested for effectiveness in patients who meet very specific requirements. Taxol, for example—which was in short supply— was advanced to three Phase II studies involving women with ovarian cancers that resisted the established drug cisplatin. This was done to confirm the substantial improvements seen in patients with this disease during the initial testing.

Phase III This begins when a drug has proved to be effective in Phase II. A randomized study is usually necessary to make the drug part of the standard treatment strategy. In a randomized study, half the patients receive the best standard therapy and the other half the new therapy.

In the case of taxol, Phase III studies of women with ovarian cancer after surgery compared taxol + cisplatin to the standard treatment of cisplatin + cyclophosphamide. Even before these studies were fully analyzed, the FDA approved taxol for treating women who had not responded to cisplatin. The approval was based on taxol's consistent effects and the unusual circumstance that many well-studied drugs had failed to show such activity.

Other Trials Drug combinations—particularly with a new compound such as taxol—are the subject of many investigational studies, often called pilot studies, that are based on experimental or early clinical observations. Patients enrolled in these trials often benefit from the drug programs. The risk of unexpected toxicities is minimized by the studies being performed in facilities with both experienced physician-investigators and the tools for accurate data collection.

Groups of patients also often receive certain investigational drugs from the NCI when the drug has been found useful but, for a variety of reasons, cannot be made commercially available.

APPROVED USES FOR DRUGS

The FDA approves chemotherapeutic drugs for one or more specific kinds of cancer. For example, taxol was first approved only for treating ovarian cancers that resist cisplatin or carboplatin. In time, however, drugs tend to be used to treat patients with other types of cancer. The FDA does not restrict the use of a drug for non-approved situations. Many such uses, based on literature reports or the personal experiences of oncologists, have become common and appropriate practice.

When a drug is first released, insurance companies in particular tend to regard non-approved uses as "experimental." But distinctions between "established" and "investigational" or "experimental" uses are often blurred. Drugs under investigation have often become therapeutic alternatives for patients who have failed standard treatments or have cancers with no known life-prolonging therapies.

Patients with metastatic breast or ovarian cancers, for example, will have failed standard combination chemotherapy programs before being treated with an investigational drug. An investigational treatment may appropriately be considered by someone with metastatic cancer whose primary site cannot be determined because, in such a case, no "tailor-made" drug therapy has been found to be superior.

TYPES OF NEW DRUGS

The drugs detailed here are at various stages of study. Some that have recently become commercially available are still being investigated against tumor types not included in the FDA-approved indication. The drugs are classified according to definitions introduced by the Cancer Therapy Evaluation Program of the NCI in the late 1970s:

♦ Group A drugs are at the earliest stage of development (Phase I).

♦ Group B drugs are in widespread testing by cancer centers and cooperative groups or by industry.

♦ Group C drugs are in routine use by qualified oncologists before commercialization.

♦ Drugs in the miscellaneous category are given together with chemotherapy, either to protect against toxicity or to enhance antitumor activity.

GROUP A DRUGS

Many compounds entering Phase I trials encounter unforeseen obstacles during their development, so individual drugs will not be detailed. Several classes of drugs are in active development.

One group is made up of new Topoisomerase I inhibitors. Topoisomerase is a DNA-modifying enzyme. These drugs are derivatives of the drug camptothecin, originally tested in 1970.

Another promising new set of drugs are antifolate compounds. These counteract some of the actions of the vitamin folic acid derivatives that act as co-factors in vital enzyme reactions. Except for edatrexate (*see* "Group C Drugs"), these new compounds have different enzyme targets than the original antifolate, methotrexate. Iometrexol is in Phase I trial, whereas ZD1694 has advanced to Phase III trials in colon cancer.

GROUP B DRUGS

These drugs are undergoing study because a suitable dose and schedule has been found in Phase I trials. Phase II studies are trying to establish the drugs' effectiveness, usually in a wide range of tumor types. Several drugs already show promise against certain types of cancer, but this information is very preliminary.

Gemcitabine (difluorodeoxycytidine) is an antimetabolite introduced by Lilly Laboratories. It has shown encouraging activity—20 percent or more responses—in lung, ovarian and breast cancers. Some patients with pancreatic cancer have also shown improvement, although objective responses will likely not exceed 10 percent of patients even when they have been given no treatment before.

The toxicity profile is quite favorable. The drug has mild effects on the bone marrow. Short-term skin rashes and flu-like symptoms are the most commonly observed side effects.

Mitoguazone (Methyl-GAG, MGBG) is an old investigational drug. It had shown activity against malignant lymphomas and Hodgkin's disease, as well as some squamous cancers, but with considerable toxic effects to many organ systems. Its unique mechanism of action and the likelihood that new schedules or drug combinations will prove useful have piqued interest in re-assessing its role.

Oxaliplatin is a platinum derivative that has had all its initial studies in France. It has no toxic effects on the kidney and causes minimal bone marrow depression. The only troublesome toxicity has been numbness and tingling in the extremities, but these feelings are diminished by timing the infusions to be given in the afternoon and are relieved by discontinuing the drug. Its activity against colorectal cancer when combined with 5-fluorouracil is generating a lot of interest. Trials are awaited in the United States.

Oxanthrazole derivatives are drugs bearing some chemical resemblance to the standard agents doxorubicin and mitoxantrone. One of the three derivatives under study has shown considerable activity (60 percent) in breast cancer. This derivative has been selected for widespread study.

PALA is an antimetabolite that proved too toxic when given by itself, but has shown some promising activity at low doses when combined with 5-fluorouracil for treating colorectal cancer.

Suramin is an old drug used to treat the parasite responsible for sleeping sickness. Interest in it as an anticancer compound followed a description of how it interferes with growth pathways in tumor cells. Activity has been noted against prostate cancer. Additional studies have awaited details of its pharmacology in relation to toxicities and antitumor effects. Life-threatening side effects have occurred in many organ systems, but these should become uncommon with greater experience of its complex metabolism.

Tumor necrosis factor is a biologic response modifier. It is also labeled a cytokine because of its effect on other cells. It is normally produced by the "clean-up" cells called macrophages and, with recombinant DNA technology, can be produced in the laboratory. It has remarkable actions on the coagulation pathways but has shown few antitumor effects even at dosage levels that are quite intolerable, causing weight loss, fever and low blood pressure. A number of experimental observations, however, has meant that interest persists in studying it in combination with chemotherapy.

GROUP C DRUGS

These drugs have shown definite antitumor activity but are still classified as investigational for a variety of reasons.

♦ The trials seeking FDA approval may be incomplete or currently inconclusive.

♦ A drug sponsor has not been identified or is under negotiation.

♦ The circumstances in which the drug has been shown to be useful do not easily lend themselves to the drug approval process, so approval is no longer being sought.

For oncologists registered in good standing as clinical investigators, drugs in the last two categories are often obtainable through the National Cancer Institute. Drugs are also available—rarely—from industry sponsors for "compassionate" use. In other instances, a referral to an ongoing clinical trial will allow entry into a randomized study, generally with a 50-50 chance of receiving the experimental treatment.

Amsacrine is distributed by the NCI for the treatment of resistant acute leukemias. It is chemically related to drugs such as doxorubicin. It has a generally favorable toxicity profile but less activity against all other tumors. It is still being tested in various combinations against malignant lymphomas.

Azacitidine is also an antileukemic agent distributed by the NCI for some resistant leukemias.

Edatrexate is related to the standard agent methotrexate and is under study by Ciba-Geigy. It may have a wider spectrum of activity and be more suitable for combinations that the older compound. Major disease targets are lung cancer, head and neck cancers and gynecologic cancer. Combinations with cisplatin, and with leucovorin rescue (*see* "Miscellaneous Drugs"), appear promising.

Epirubicin is one of several second-generation doxorubicin derivatives and is more closely related to it than the other derivatives. It is commercially available in Europe and Canada. The drug is identical to doxorubicin in its actions but differs both in its pharmacology and its potency. A possible advantage for epirubicin is that it reportedly has better tolerance in drug combinations, particularly against breast cancer.

Irinotecan (CPT-11) is a Japanese drug that shows activity against a large number of tumor types, with or without exposure to other drugs. It is in the family of camptothecin derivatives. Toxicities include decreased white blood cell and platelet counts, diarrhea, hair loss, anemia, nausea and vomiting. There have been responses in patients with lung cancer, colon and other gastrointestinal cancers, gynecologic cancers and lymphomas and leukemias. Very active combinations are also being reported. Wide testing of these leads, sponsored by the NCI, is expected in the United States.

Navelbine (Vinorelbine) is under study by Burroughs Wellcome as a mitotic inhibitor of the vinca alkaloid family. Compared with vinblastine given for adult solid tumors, it shows greater activity with less toxicity. It is also active when taken orally. It has shown promise against drug-resistant breast cancer and has also shown antitumor effects against lung cancer, for which drug approval has just been obtained.

Taxotere is a more potent and water soluble derivative of taxol. It has been under study by Rhone Poulenc in Europe and very recently in the U.S. As with taxol, antitumor responses have been noted in ovarian, breast and lung cancers. The drug has an advantage over taxol in that it requires less premedication and is easily administered as a one-hour infusion. On the other hand, skin toxicity, edemas and pleural effusions have complicated its administration. Patients who did not respond to taxol would not be expected to benefit from taxotere, but this point has not been extensively studied.

Topotecan is a semisynthetic, water-soluble derivative of camptothecin, a plant product first tested in 1970. It is of great interest since it does not share the unpredictable toxicities of the parent compound and is active against a number of cancers in animals that are resistant to standard chemotheraputic agents. It is currently undergoing early clinical trials in humans in a number of dosage schedules. Activity has been reported for a number of solid tumors.

Toremifene is an antiestrogen related to tamoxifen. It has some differences, however, that may make it useful against desmoid tumors and useful as a drug to reverse multi-drug resistance. It may also exert an effect on estrogen receptor negative cells along with the usual effects through estrogen receptor binding.

Tretinoin (all-*trans* retinoic acid) is undergoing widespread testing after it was clearly demonstrated that it induces remissions in the rare acute promyelocytic leukemia. It has become the prototype of this chemical class of vitamin A derivatives to be studied for striking antitumor actions. These actions are possibly related to inducing a malignant cell to differentiate toward a more mature and no longer dividing cell. In this way, a cancer cell may apparently change into a normal cell.

Another form of the drug is commercially available for the treatment of acne. Both drugs are generally well tolerated by mouth at lower doses. The first signs of toxicity are dry skin and sores at the corners of the mouth, followed by short-term liver malfunction. Very high doses lead to high calcium levels, headaches and increased pressure within the skull.

Many trials of the drug, either alone or in combination with other drugs such as interferon-alpha, are expected in the future. The biological actions of retinoids are just beginning to be understood and are quite striking.

Uracil-Ftorafur (UFT) is an oral preparation from Japan's Taiho Pharmaceutical Company that can result in consistent 5-fluorouracil blood levels. It is widely used in Japan for treating gastrointestinal and breast cancers. Studies are ongoing in the U.S. in combination with leucovorin.

Vindesine is a vinca alkaloid available through Lilly Laboratories outside the U.S. Studies are no longer being performed in the United States. It is midway between vincristine and vinblastine both in potency and in causing neuritis and low white blood cell counts. Studies had suggested some advantage over these other compounds when treating leukemia, lung cancer and breast cancer.

MISCELLANEOUS DRUGS

Knowledge about how anticancer drugs work has stimulated the search for drugs that counteract toxicities (protectors) or enhance their effectiveness (potentiators).

♦ Protectors include the thiol amifostine, other thiols including glutathione, dexrazoxane and the colony-stimulating factors.

♦ Potentiators—also named modulators—include buthionine sulfoximine (BSO), L-leucovorin, dipyridamole and drugs such as cyclosporin and its derivatives that reverse multi-drug resistance.

Amifostine (Ethyol, WR2721) is under study by US Bioscience as a protector against the bone marrow toxicity of cisplatin and cyclophosphamide and possibly as a protector against some other toxic effects of cisplatin, such as those on the nerves and kidney. Antitumor effects

appear to be unchanged. Vomiting and low blood pressure are its principal side effects.

Dexrazoxane (ICRF-187, ADR 529) protects against the toxic effects on the heart of anthracyclines such as doxorubicin. The FDA withheld approval, however, because of doubts about the slight protection of antitumor effects as well. The drug may play a role in preventing cardiotoxicity in children, the effects of which show up later in adolescence. Its use also has to be considered in adjuvant programs that include doxorubicin where a long life expectancy might be affected by cardiac events.

Buthionine sulfoximine (BSO) is under investigation as a drug to deplete glutathione and make alkylating drugs such as melphalan or platinum derivatives more effective.

L-leucovorin and *dipyridamole* (persantine) are used to enhance the actions of 5-fluorouracil. Leucovorin's role as an enhancer is somewhat paradoxical, since it was initially introduced as a rescue agent for methotrexate.

Cyclosporin A analogues that do not suppress the immune system will undergo testing to reverse multi-drug resistance. We have improved our ability to identify tumors that have become resistant by expression of the gene named MDR. Many drugs of various kinds are being tested to counteract this resistance, but the restoration of drug effectiveness has yet to be shown convincingly.

OTHER INVESTIGATIONAL STUDIES

There are many other investigational studies being carried out beyond those specifically directed at finding new chemotherapeutic drugs.

♦ Some involve biological therapy. These include the study of new cytokines, tumor vaccines and monoclonal antibodies, some with programmed "warheads" that deliver anticancer drugs directly to tumors.

♦ Special formulations of existing drugs are also under investigation, including orally active preparations of intravenous drugs and intravenous preparations of orally available drugs such as hydroxyurea.

♦ Liposomal preparations are under testing. In these studies, the active drug is attached to very tiny fat particles. Liposomes with very prolonged circulation in the blood and with preferential tumor distribution may help make drugs such as doxorubicin more effective and less toxic. Special kinds of liposomes containing cytarabine are being tested for administration into the central nervous system.

37
ADVANCES IN CANCER GENETICS

Christopher Benz, MD, Ernest H. Rosenbaum, MD, and Malin Dollinger, MD

Each cell in our bodies contains all of our genetic information in 46 chromosomes, 23 inherited from each parent. Each chromosome contains many thousands of genes, small subdivisions of the material that is the blueprint of life, DNA.

Genes are the carriers of genetic knowledge. A gene is capable of transmitting a single characteristic such as eye color from parent to offspring. There are an estimated 50,000 to 100,000 genes within a human cell. Only about 100 of them are known to regulate cell growth and division.

First proposed about 80 years ago, it is now well proven that one of the causes of cancer is changes or defects in our chromosomes. But only recently have new techniques in molecular biology made it possible to see abnormalities in the chromosomes and their genes, including small mutations in DNA. These new methods, along with other research initiatives, have led to discoveries that have profound implications for the diagnosis, prognosis and treatment of cancer.

TUMOR-CAUSING AND TUMOR-SUPPRESSING GENES

The DNA abnormalities that lead to the development of cancer may occur in either of two types of genes—those that promote cell growth or those that suppress cell growth.

Both types function normally and in a coordinated way during human growth and development. But genetic changes can cause the normally well regulated growth-promoting mechanisms within a cell to become uncontrolled.

Oncogenes One of the more exciting discoveries in the past decade is that some of our normal genes may be activated in various ways and transformed into genes capable of changing a normal cell into a cancer cell. These activated and cancer-causing genes are called oncogenes.

We all carry unactivated or normal forms of oncogenes in our chromosomes. In the unaltered state, these genes are referred to as proto-oncogenes. They stay dormant or perform useful functions throughout our lives unless they are stimulated, mutated or otherwise activated to become oncogenes. Once activated, they can work with other genes to transform a normal cell into a cancer cell. This is believed to be a multistep process in which the DNA undergoes an initial change, then more decisive changes complete the process of malignant transformation.

A proto-oncogene is activated to an oncogene by a metabolic defect that occurs inside the cell. This defect may spontaneously arise with aging or by exposure to a physical or chemical agent (a carcinogen) that can damage chromosomes or DNA. Radiation in the form of sunlight or x-rays, chemicals and other environmental factors such as cigarette smoke or asbestos, for example, are all carcinogens that are known to cause cancers with excessive exposure, probably by producing one or more oncogenes.

Some defects can be repaired, but the cell's ability to repair DNA damage weakens with age. It is also thought that the genetic machinery of aging cells becomes more error-prone by accumulating unrepaired defects. The unrepaired persistence of the activated oncogene will predispose a person to develop cancer in the tissue containing that gene.

While there are several theories about the cancer-causing mechanisms of these genetic changes—such as a virus inserting its own DNA into a normal cell's chromosome, a virus acting as a random mutating agent or a single carcinogenic bullet that knocks out or rearranges a critical gene—the most commonly accepted theory suggests that multiple genetic insults, or accumulated hits, are necessary to cause cancer (*see* Chapter 1). A single gene loss can be inherited and lead to family histories of cancer. Other genetic hits may accumulate because of a combination of aging, environmental carcinogens or lifestyle indiscretions such as smoking or overeating.

There are more than 60 known oncogenes. They are often named for the types of cancer they induce in animals, such as *ras* for rat sarcoma. Oncogenes may stimulate other genes by producing increased amounts of special proteins. Some may produce abnormal amounts of growth factors or cellular receptors for growth factors. There is usually more than one oncogene activated in any given tumor and these may coordinate with each other or with the loss of tumor suppressors to produce cancer. Exactly how most oncogenes and their protein products cause cancer to develop is still not understood.

Tumor-Suppressor Genes As their name implies, tumor-suppressor genes are normally protective, acting to prevent the unregulated growth that is characteristic of a cancer cell. They can also prevent the cancer-predisposing effect of an activated oncogene. If one of these genes is absent or its protein product is unable to work

properly, the cancer-producing action of an undetected oncogene may not be completely suppressed and a tumor may develop.

Many tumor-suppressor genes have been identified recently. Some are referred to by their protein size—p53, for example—while others are named for the cancer in which they were first discovered, as in WT (Wilms' tumor) and RB (retinoblastoma).

Tumor-suppressor genes are most commonly discovered in inherited cancers, since abnormal forms of these genes are passed to offspring by either egg or sperm. But they also play important roles in non-inherited cancers. Almost all cancers show a defect in one or more tumor-suppressor genes. A typical colon cancer, for example, may have at least four inactivated tumor-suppressor genes (p53, DCC, APC and MCC).

The RB gene was the first tumor-suppressor gene to be discovered and characterized, and retinoblastoma remains the model of a cancer caused by the loss of a tumor-suppressor gene product. Retinoblastoma is a rare and often fatal eye cancer occurring in children. It may be inherited or arise spontaneously.

♦ In the inherited form, one RB gene derived from one parent is non-functional. Sometime during childhood, the normal RB gene from the other parent becomes lost or mutated, predisposing cells in the retina to form a retinoblastoma.

Children with the inherited form often develop tumors in both eyes and may develop other malignancies later in life, such as sarcomas, leukemia or melanoma.

♦ In children with the spontaneous form, the tumor cells also have defects involving both RB genes, but these defects have not been inherited. These children usually have only one tumor and are not predisposed to develop other cancers.

If detected early, both inherited and spontaneous forms of retinoblastoma are curable with radiotherapy, and vision can

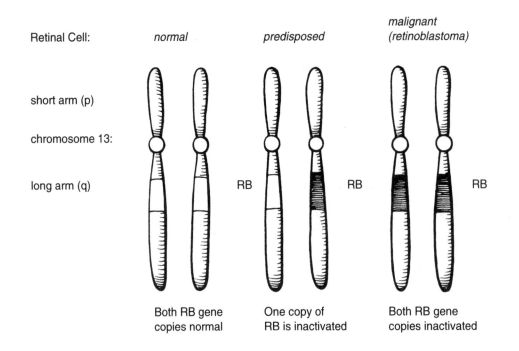

Retinoblastoma occurs when a retinal cell has lost the tumor-suppressing function of both RB genes on chromosome 13. With the inherited form, retinal cells are predisposed at birth since an inactivating mutation was transmitted by either sperm or egg. In the sporadic form, both genetic defects occur in the retinal cell during development but are not passed on to offspring.

be preserved. Genetic probes can detect the abnormal RB gene, identifying children at risk. These children need careful clinical monitoring and frequent eye examinations.

GENETIC SCREENING, DIAGNOSIS AND TREATMENT PLANNING

Single and multiple genetic defects associated with tumors are now being identified in clinical and laboratory research programs.

It is now possible to identify in any individual whether a specific oncogene has become activated or whether a tumor-suppressor gene is defective or absent. It is likely that within a few years these genetic factors will be used routinely to

determine both the diagnosis and the prognosis of people with cancer.

Since the presence of certain genetic defects may predispose some cancers to spread, genetic tests can enable physicians to identify individuals who are at higher risk for developing metastases. In these cases, more intensive clinical follow-up can then be offered or more effective adjuvant therapy can be given to improve the chance for cure.

The routine use of specific genetic tests has already begun and the new knowledge about and understanding of cancer genetics is also having an influence on cancer therapy.

Screening Techniques that test for genetic defects including activated oncogenes and abnormal tumor-suppressor genes are becoming available for use in selected situations such as detecting familial polyposis of the colon, a benign condition caused by inactivation of the APC tumor-suppressor gene that predisposes some people toward developing colon cancer.

Prenatal and postnatal tests can detect abnormalities involving any of the known tumor-suppressor genes like RB that are associated with inherited forms of cancer, thereby identifying infants or children who are at risk for developing malignant disease later in life.

Diagnosis FDA approval of the first DNA probe-based diagnostic test for chronic myelogenous leukemia launched the now rapidly expanding field of molecular diagnosis as it relates to cancer.

The Philadelphia chromosome (Ph1), a specific abnormality in this type of leukemia, was the first well-described chromosomal marker related to a gene rearrangement in cancer. The changes that result in this chromosome transforming a normal cell into a leukemic cell are now known. A proto-oncogene called c-*abl* normally resides on chromosome 9. It is activated—in other words, becomes an oncogene—when it travels to a critical point on chromosome 22. The exchange of genetic material between chromosomes 9 and 22 results in a shortened chromosome 22, the Philadelphia chromosome. It is believed that the activated c-*abl* oncogene produces an increased amount of an enzyme known as a protein tyrosine kinase that sends stimulative signals to the cell's nucleus. The result of this persistent signaling in a blood cell is development of a leukemic cell.

The importance of this genetic mechanism from a diagnostic point of view is that a DNA probe is now available that confirms the diagnosis of chronic myelogenous leukemia.

Similar DNA probes are being developed as aids in the diagnosis of different types of leukemia, lymphomas and other cancers. They appear to be able to recognize gene rearrangements and mutations in a high number of breast, ovary and bladder cancers, as well as in other malignancies such as retinoblastomas, renal tumors, brain tumors and sarcomas. They are also being used to help pathologists distinguish between malignant, premalignant and benign forms of disease.

Although much research is still needed to improve our understanding and expand the application of DNA probes, genetic techniques such as these will likely be used on a more routine basis in the future to accurately diagnose and classify all malignant diseases.

Treatment Planning Different types of genetic abnormalities may cause the growth-promoting mechanisms within a cell to become uncontrolled. An oncogene may become "amplified," meaning that there is more than one DNA copy of the oncogene, which increases its effect on the cell. Alternatively, a different genetic process can lead to the mutation of a single DNA component, resulting in the loss of a normally functioning growth-suppressor gene.

Such abnormalities in both oncogenes and suppressor genes can lead to uncontrolled cellular growth and are believed to occur in a large percentage of if not virtually all human cancers. Since these genetic abnormalities seem to have a bearing on prognosis, their identification can be helpful in planning treatment.

Gene Amplification Some breast cancers are associated with DNA amplification and overexpression of the proto-oncogene called HER-2/*neu* (also c-*erb*B-2). About 25 percent of breast cancers have multiple DNA copies of this oncogene. Detecting its amplification or the overproduction of its protein product (a growth factor receptor on the cell surface) may be useful clinically. It may help in determining patient prognosis and in deciding, for example, if adjuvant therapy should be given after surgery.

Since many breast cancers recur even though they have apparently good risk factors—such as small tumor size, positive estrogen receptors or negative lymph node involvement—it is hoped that new tests such as those for the HER-2/*neu* oncogene will be able to identify women at an exceptionally high risk for recurrence and for whom additional therapy might increase their chances for cure or prolonged survival.

The HER-2/*neu* oncogene has also been found to be amplified or overexpressed in ovarian, gastric and non–small cell lung cancers. In these cases, there also appears to be a correlation between this abnormality and poor prognosis with increased mortality.

Genetic Losses Recent studies have suggested that one tumor-suppressor gene—p53, found on chromosome 17—is defective or missing in many cases of cancer, including those arising in the breast, colon and bladder. Missing segments of other chromosomes have also been identified, suggesting that other tumor-suppressor genes are abnormal in these three common cancers. Losses on chromosomes 9, 11 and 17 occur in bladder cancers, for example, and losses on chromosomes 3, 6 and 11 occur in ovarian cancer.

These findings support the theory that multiple genetic losses and not just a single gene defect lead to cancer progression.

ONCOGENE THERAPIES

With the diagnostic and monitoring potential of cancer genetics already being realized, researchers are now trying to develop therapies to inactivate the oncogenes that turn on tumor cells and to correct defective suppressor genes. Several approaches are being investigated.

Gene Therapy The approach that theoretically could lead to the most specific and curative form of treatment is commonly called gene therapy. This involves replacing a defective oncogene or tumor-suppressor gene with its normal counterpart.

Since retinoblastomas, Wilms' tumors and lung, breast and colon cancers are known to be caused by genetically inactivated tumor-suppressor genes, these cancers might be obvious targets for gene therapy designed to replace abnormal tumor-suppressing genes.

Gene therapy can also take the form of inserting newly designed or foreign (recombinant) genes into bone marrow, blood, skin or other cells removed from a patient. When returned to the patient, these new genes can make therapeutic proteins.

The first attempts at gene therapy for humans were undertaken by medical investigators at the National Cancer Institute in the early 1990s. Now, investigations across the country have ongoing genetic protocols for certain cancer patients as well as non-cancer patients.

There are, however, at least three major technical obstacles that must be overcome before gene therapy will be routinely available for the treatment of human cancers:

♦ Tumor cells tend to reject foreign genes even after they are transferred into the cell.
♦ It is not yet possible to get the corrective genes into all the cancer cells in a patient's body.
♦ The amount of protein currently produced in cells bearing a newly transferred gene is often too low to expect complete correction of the tumor-causing defect.

Other Approaches Researchers are investigating anticancer vaccines and antibodies directed against oncoproteins such as HER-2/*neu* and EGFR (epidermal growth factor receptor). The therapeutic use of antibodies—alone or as carriers of powerful drugs, cell toxins or radionuclides—has already been shown to interfere with the tumor-causing action of oncoproteins. Such antibodies can selectively inhibit cell growth in cell cultures and in cancer patients and will likely be the most easily realized anti-oncogene therapy.

A different approach involves new drugs that can inactivate oncoproteins such as *ras* or associated enzymes such as protein tyrosine kinases. Yet another approach focuses on DNA- or RNA-binding drugs that recognize specific gene sequences such as antisense oligomers directed against the c-*myc* and c-*myb* transcripts that can inhibit intracellular expression of specific oncogenes.

These approaches all attempt to develop cancer treatments that target specific genetic defects. In theory, such treatments will be able to reduce the uncomfortable and life-threatening side effects now associated with chemotherapy.

Most important, some form of oncogene therapy could potentially be used to prevent tumors in people who are at a higher than normal risk for cancer because of their family history or environmental exposure.

38

ACCESS TO CANCER INFORMATION: THE NATIONAL CANCER INSTITUTE'S PDQ (PHYSICIAN DATA QUERY) SYSTEM

Susan Molloy Hubbard, BS, RN, MPA, and Vincent T. DeVita, Jr., MD

◇

Successful cancer treatment is often closely linked to care from knowledgeable doctors with experience in the delivery of the best available cancer therapies. Current statistics on cancer mortality suggest that wider use of effective, state-of-the-art cancer treatments could sharply reduce cancer deaths throughout the country over the next decade.

To make information on effective treatments more widely known, the National Cancer Institute (NCI), the major source of federal funding for cancer research, has developed a computerized information system called PDQ (Physician Data Query). The PDQ system provides doctors with the most current information on the treatment of cancer, the management of complications of cancer and its treatment and the early detection and prevention of the disease. It also contains up-to-date information on clinical trials designed to test new cancer detection, treatment and prevention approaches, a directory of doctors who treat cancer and a directory of facilities that have accredited early detection and/or cancer care programs.

How PDQ Is Organized The PDQ system is composed of information that is organized in interconnected computer files that are stored in electronic form and make up a database.

The information is organized and stored in electronic files for several reasons. First, computerized data files can be transmitted from one location to another over standard telephone line. Second, the files can be updated frequently with new treatment information; the PDQ files are updated every month. Third, the data files can be interlinked in such a way that users can retrieve information from different files concurrently with a simple command.

CANCER TREATMENT AND DETECTION INFORMATION

The PDQ Cancer Information File contains information on:
♦ prognosis (chance of recovery)
♦ staging (the extent of spread)
♦ histopathology (tumor cell type)
♦ state-of-the-art (effective or standard) treatment options
♦ promising clinical research
♦ supportive care (the management of complications)
♦ screening (early detection).

The treatment information in PDQ is written by cancer specialists with input from experts around the country. Treatment guidelines are provided for all major types of cancer—more than 80 different types—and information on a growing number of rare cancers is being added.

The files also contain information from important articles published in the medical literature that document the effectiveness of the therapies recommended in PDQ's statements. Short summaries of these articles can be displayed on request for review.

Because treatment for a patient with a cancer that has not spread from its site of origin is often quite different from the treatment for a patient whose tumor has spread to other organs (metastasized), PDQ generally recommends treatments by the stage of disease. In certain cancers, other factors such as the location of the tumor or the type of cells that have become cancerous can be more important in the selection of treatment. In such situations, PDQ recommends treatment options by those factors. When there is no effective standard therapy, the PDQ recommendation is for doctors and their patients to consider clinical trials that are evaluating new approaches to treatment (*see* "The PDQ Protocol File" below).

Format The treatment information in PDQ is provided in two formats:
◆ state-of-the-art statements written for health care professionals using detailed medical terminology; and
◆ patient information summaries that health professionals can share with patients when discussing the prognosis and treatment options. These summaries are written in simpler language and contain references to additional printed materials written for cancer patients. The summaries are designed to complement discussion with a doctor rather than serve as a primary source of treatment advice. A doctor will know facts about an individual patient's condition that may affect the selection of treatment.

The diagnosis of cancer and subsequent decisions about therapy can be overwhelming, and patients are often confused and upset. It is important for patients to discuss treatment options with medical experts and with family or close friends. Doctors and patients (and their families) can use the material in the PDQ patient information summaries as an educational resource to promote understanding of the diagnosis and treatment options. The treatment recommendations in this book have been written for patients and their families based on the treatment information provided in PDQ.

Information on how to provide supportive care to ease the side effects of cancer or its treatment—such as pain, digestive problems, nausea and vomiting, fever, itching, sleep disorders and fatigue—is also provided in PDQ.

Information on the early detection of cancers of the breast, cervix, ovary, colon and rectum, stomach, mouth, prostate, skin and testes is summarized. Each summary provides information on the effectiveness of screening both in detecting early cancer in people without symptoms and in reducing mortality.

Information on promising approaches to cancer prevention and new drugs to treat cancer is included in the database.

The state-of-the-art statements, patient information summaries, supportive care statements and information on the design of clinical trials have been translated into Spanish to facilitate access to current treatment information by Hispanic health professionals and patients.

Keeping PDQ's Files Current The treatment information file is updated monthly based on the recommendations of two Editorial Boards composed of about 30 doctors and nurses with expertise in treating cancer patients. One board reviews cancers that occur in adults; the other reviews information on childhood cancers. These boards meet once a month to review and discuss new treatment information and to update treatment recommendations. A group of associate editors—over 60 specialists from across the

United States and representing all aspects of cancer treatment—complements and extends the expertise of these two core Editorial Boards.

Information on early detection, the effects and management of side effects and promising new investigational drugs is regularly updated by separate editorial boards composed of experts in their respective fields. Each of these boards also has a group of associate editors. In total, more than 150 specialists review and update information for PDQ.

THE PDQ PROTOCOL FILE

New methods of cancer detection, prevention and treatment must prove safe and effective before they can be made widely available. The PDQ protocol file contains summaries of treatments being given to cancer patients in organized clinical research programs called clinical trials. The file contains two summaries on the design of clinical trials, one for health professionals and one for patients and families. The summaries describe what clinical trials are, what their objectives are and how they are performed, and also discuss biomedical, ethical and other concerns.

There are many kinds of clinical trials. They range from studies of new methods to prevent, detect, diagnose, control and treat cancer to studies of the psychological impact of the disease and of new ways to improve a patient's comfort and quality of life. More than 1,500 clinical trials open to patient participation are summarized in PDQ's protocol file. Each clinical trial in PDQ is designed to answer specific research questions and to find new and better ways to help cancer patients.

All of the clinical trials supported by NCI are listed in the PDQ protocol file. Clinical trials being performed with other sources of support can be voluntarily submitted by the doctors performing them and are listed in PDQ following approval by the cancer specialists on the PDQ Editorial Board. The NCI invites doctors to submit their cancer treatment protocols to PDQ.

Finding an Appropriate Clinical Trial
New treatments often use surgery, radiation, chemotherapy and biological therapy alone or in combination with one another. The clinical trials in PDQ are classified by:
♦ the research goal (prevention, detection, treatment or management of complications);
♦ the primary tumor type (colon or breast cancer, for example);
♦ the "modality" or type of treatment (surgery, radiotherapy, chemotherapy, biological therapy, early detection, chemoprevention, supportive care);
♦ accrual status (open, closed, approved but not yet active, standard, investigational);
♦ the study phase (Phase I, II, III or adjuvant trial); and/or
♦ specific drugs or biologic substances.

Protocol summaries give detailed information on the objectives of the study, the patient entry criteria (medical requirements) and details about the treatment regimen, including drug dosages and schedules. Each protocol also provides the names, addresses and phone numbers of the doctors performing the study. Information on protocols is updated monthly.

Searching the PDQ Protocol File Doctors may easily search the PDQ protocol file to identify clinical trials for patients with a specific type and stage of cancer, as well as trials being performed in a particular place (one or more cities, states, and/or Zip codes). The protocol file gives a doctor the latest information on clinical trials being offered anywhere in the United States and includes information on studies being conducted in Canada and several European countries.

With this information, doctors can help

patients who want to participate in a clinical trial to become enrolled in one that is suitable for them. The descriptions of the clinical trial and the medical requirements of patients who fit into the study are very technical, so a doctor who is familiar with the patient's case should make the contact with the doctors listed in PDQ as being directly responsible for the protocol.

The Phases of Clinical Trials Clinical trials show doctors which therapies are more effective. For example, some compare the best-known surgical treatment with a newer operation to see if one produces more cures and causes fewer side effects than the other. Many standard treatments were first shown to be effective in clinical trials. The state-of-the-art therapies recommended in PDQ should be considered a foundation for building new and better treatments. Treatment protocols are designed to take advantage of what has worked in the past and to improve on this foundation.

Clinical trials are carried out in distinct steps, or phases. Each phase is designed to discover certain types of information. Each phase depends on, and builds on, information from an earlier phase. Patients may be eligible for studies in different phases, depending on their general condition and the type and stage of their cancer.

♦ *Phase I* The purpose of a Phase I study is to find the best way to give a new treatment and how much of it can be given safely. The new treatment is given to a small number of patients, and doctors watch carefully for any harmful side effects. The treatment has already been well tested in laboratory and animal studies, but the side effects in humans are not completely predictable. For this reason, Phase I studies may involve significant risks and are offered only to patients whose cancer has spread and who would not be helped by known treatments.

Side effects are carefully assessed and recorded. Patients are also observed closely for anticancer effects by repeated measurement of the cancer sites present at the beginning of the trial. If those sites shrink appreciably, the patient is said to have responded to the treatment. Phase I treatments may produce anticancer effects and some patients have been helped by them.

♦ *Phase II* These studies determine the effect of a research treatment on various types of cancer. Usually, groups of 30 to 40 patients with one type of cancer— breast cancer that has become resistant to standard therapy, for example—receive a Phase II treatment. Side effects are assessed and, since more people receive the treatment than in Phase I, there is more chance to observe less common side effects. Patients are closely observed for anticancer effects and response rates are determined. If at least one-fifth of the patients respond, the treatment is judged to be active against the tumor type. A treatment that shows activity against cancer in this phase moves to Phase III.

♦ *Phase III* Trials in this phase require large numbers of patients—some trials enroll thousands—who are divided into groups. One group, called the "control" group, may receive the standard accepted treatment so the new treatment can be directly compared to it. The control group may receive the chemotherapy usually given for a certain type of cancer, for example, while another group receives the new treatment to see if it improves survival. All patients in Phase III trials are monitored closely for side effects, and treatment is discontinued if the side effects are too severe.

♦ *Adjuvant Trials* These are conducted to determine if an additional therapy—the adjuvant therapy—will improve the chance for cure in patients at risk for recurrence after the surgical removal of all visible disease. At one time, the standard therapy for breast cancer was surgery alone. Adjuvant trials of chemotherapy in women with breast cancer, in which one group received surgery and the other received surgery plus chemotherapy, showed that surgery plus chemotherapy is better than surgery alone. Surgery plus chemotherapy is now the standard treatment for many women with breast cancer.

Taking Part in a Clinical Trial Clinical trials offer patients the most up-to-date care available. Patients who take part in clinical trials have the first opportunity to benefit from new research and can make a very important contribution to medical science. The medical requirements for taking part depend on many factors. Patients who want to know more about clinical trials should talk with their doctors and ask them to print out PDQ's information on the design of clinical trials.

Patients should learn as much as they can about the trials before making up their minds about participating. A cancer specialist is often the best person to counsel a patient about the selection of a standard treatment option or a clinical trial.

Asking the Right Questions The important questions for anyone considering a clinical trial include:

♦ What is the purpose of the study?

♦ What does the study involve? What kinds of tests and treatments are done and how are they done?

♦ What is likely to happen in my case with or without this new research treatment?

♦ What are my other choices and their advantages and disadvantages? Are there standard treatments for my case, and how does the treatment in the study compare with them?

♦ How could participation in the study affect my daily life?

♦ What side effects can I expect?

♦ How long will the study last? Will it require an extra time commitment on my part?

♦ Will I have to be hospitalized? If so, how often and for how long?

♦ Will I have any costs? Will the treatment be free?

Medical Societies That List Their Physician Members in the PDQ Directory File

---

American Academy of Dermatology*
American College of Mohs Micrographic Surgery and Cutaneous Oncology
American College of Surgeons*
American Radium Society
American Society of Clinical Oncology
American Society of Colon and Rectal Surgeons
American Society for Head and Neck Surgery
American Society of Hematology
American Society of Pediatric Hematology and Oncology
American Society for Therapeutic Radiology and Oncology
American Urologic Association*
Association of Community Cancer Centers
Society of Gynecologic Oncology
Society of Head and Neck Surgeons
Society of Pelvic Surgeons
Society of Surgical Oncology
Society of Urologic Oncology

---

* Doctors who belong to these societies and spend a major portion of their time treating cancer are invited to submit their names for inclusion in the directory. The remaining societies list all of their physician members.

♦ If I am harmed as a result of the research, what treatment would I be entitled to?

♦ What type of long-term follow-up care is part of the study?

THE PDQ DIRECTORY

The directory contains the names, addresses, telephone numbers and medical specialties of more than 20,000 doctors who spend the majority of their time treating cancer patients.

The names of the doctors included in the PDQ directory have been compiled from the membership directories of 17 medical societies. Doctors conducting clinical trials that are included in the PDQ protocol file are also listed in the directory file. PDQ also lists more than 2,300 health care organizations that have organized programs of cancer care and more than 4,000 accredited breast cancer screening facilities.

The inclusion of individual doctors and organizations in the directory file does not imply endorsement by the National Cancer Institute.

ACCESS TO PDQ INFORMATION

Patients and others who want to know more about cancer and how it is treated can obtain PDQ information from their doctors or by contacting the NCI's Cancer Information Service (CIS). This service, staffed by trained information specialists, provides answers to cancer-related questions from the public, cancer patients and their families, as well as health professionals. Counselors who speak Spanish are available.

Individuals with questions can call toll-free 1-800-4-CANCER (1-800-422-6237) to be connected to the CIS office serving their area. The counselors at this number use PDQ to obtain information on state-of-the-art treatment and clinical trials for callers. The call and the information are free.

Publications The CIS supplies free publications to patients and families with specific questions on cancer and its treatment. The following is a partial list of helpful publications:

♦ Anticancer Drug Information Sheets
♦ *Advanced Cancer: Living Each Day*
♦ *Chemotherapy and You: A Guide to Self-Help During Treatment*
♦ *Eating Hints: Recipes and Tips for Better Nutrition During Cancer Treatment*
♦ *Facing Forward: A Guide for Cancer Survivors*
♦ *Radiation Therapy and You: A Guide to Self-Help During Treatment*
♦ *Taking Time: Support for People with Cancer and the People Who Care About Them*
♦ *What Are Clinical Trials All About?*

Organizations in the PDQ Directory File

American Association of Cancer Institutes
Association of Community Cancer Centers
Clinical and Comprehensive Cancer Centers funded by the National Cancer Institute
Clinical Cooperative Groups funded by the NCI and affiliates
Community Clinical Oncology Program (CCOP) grantees
Organizations with:

♦ Hospital cancer programs approved by the American College of Surgeons' Commission on Cancer

♦ Accredited mammography screening programs approved by the American College of Radiology

♦ *What You Need to Know About Cancer* (a series of disease-specific pamphlets)
♦ *When Cancer Recurs: Meeting the Challenge Again*

Publications on cancer prevention and early detection include:
♦ *Chew or Snuff Is Real Bad Stuff*
♦ *Clearing the Air: A Guide to Quitting Smoking*
♦ *Diet, Nutrition and Cancer Prevention: The Good News*
♦ *Why Do You Smoke?*
♦ *Breast Exams: What You Should Know*
♦ *Cancer Tests You Should Know About: A Guide for People 65 and Over*
♦ *Do the Right Thing: Get a Mammogram*
♦ *Questions and Answers About Breast Lumps*
♦ *Questions and Answers About Choosing a Mammography Facility*
♦ *Testicular Self-Examination*
♦ *The Pap Test: It Can Save Your Life*

There are also research reports that provide in-depth information on current knowledge about causes, prevention, symptoms, detection, diagnosis and treatment of various types of cancer, as well as an educational series for children with cancer. Some publications are available in Spanish. For a complete list of publications, write to the National Cancer Institute, Office of Cancer Communications, Building 31, Room 10A24, 9000 Rockville Pike, Bethesda, MD 20892.

How to Access the PDQ System A doctor can access the PDQ database directly. To do so, the doctor needs a computer equipped with a modem and telecommunications software, a CD-ROM reader or access to the Internet, a web of computer networks that reaches all over the world.

A modem and telecommunications software enable the user's computer to link up with the central computer that contains the PDQ system at the National Library of Medicine (NLM) or a commercial vendor over a standard telephone line. A CD-ROM reader lets the user's computer read PDQ information from an optical disk plugged into the computer. If a doctor's computer is linked to the Internet, he or she can also access the PDQ system through the NLM or other commercial database distributors. Although not essential, it is also highly desirable to have a printer so that a copy of the PDQ data appearing on the screen can be produced for the doctor and patient to review.

Online Access Through the National Library of Medicine (NLM) PDQ is available on the National Library of Medicine's computer network. This system, which is called MEDLARS—Medical Literature Analysis and Retrieval System—is available 24 hours a day, seven days a week to doctors with computers that communicate with the NLM system. Medical or hospital libraries that have access to databases on the MEDLARS system have access to PDQ. PDQ is particularly easy to use as implemented on the NLM MEDLARS system because it can be searched by making selections from a menu of choices.

To access PDQ through MEDLARS, the doctor must have a MEDLARS access code and a PDQ password. A doctor may request an access code by contacting the MEDLARS Management Service Desk at 1-800-638-8480.

Online access to PDQ on the NLM system costs $18/hr. These charges are prorated. In other words, if the user is connected to PDQ for only five minutes, he or she will be charged one-twelfth the cost of a connect hour. There is no initial fee or subscription charge, and a typical search requires only a few minutes of time. An online service operated by the European Organization for Research and Treatment of Cancer (EORTC) in cooperation with NCI makes PDQ treatment information available to European doctors. NCI also makes PDQ widely available to Latin American and Caribbean countries on the academic network BITNET.

Fax Access Through the NCI The NCI disseminates PDQ data in English and Spanish through its CancerFax service, which enables those without computers to obtain access to cancer treatment information with a fax machine. Users dial the CancerFax number (301-402-5874) from the telephone handset on their fax machine, request a contents list, enter a code number from the list for the desired information and follow the voice prompts to receive a faxed image of any of PDQ's state-of-the-art patient information or supportive care statements, bibliographic data or *News* articles.

The service is available 24 hours a day and there is no cost to the user other than that of the telephone call. CancerFax also provides information on NCI's scientific journals, patient education materials and commercial vendors that distribute PDQ.

Access Via the Internet PDQ's cancer information files are available on NCI's CancerNet, an electronic service that gives computer users the same information as CancerFax via the Internet 24 hours a day. CancerNet users send electronic mail messages containing the appropriate code to the NCI computer and receive the desired information in English or Spanish. As high-speed networks become more widely used, this technology is expected to play an ever more important role in disseminating NCI information services and products.

CancerNet has greatly improved foreign access to PDQ. One-third of the users accessing CancerNet on the Internet are from foreign countries. The complete PDQ system is also being made available on the Internet to members of the NCI's Information Associate's Program. For access to PDQ on the Internet, contact the National Cancer Institute's Information Associate's Program, Building 82, Room 123, 9000 Rockville Pike, Bethesda, MD 20892 or fax a request for information to (301) 480-8105.

Online Access Through Commercial Databases Commercial database distributors with online medical information systems also provide access to PDQ. More information on these vendors can be obtained from the NCI. Write to the PDQ Coordinator, National Cancer Institute, Building 82, Room 100, Bethesda, MD 20892, fax (301) 480-8105, or get a list of the distributors and their addresses from CancerFax.

Compact Disc Access PDQ is offered on CD-ROM by commercial database distributors. The advantage of a compact disc is that the user does not have to connect with another computer over a telephone line to search the PDQ system, but merely accesses the information on the CD from his or her computer. However, the user must have a compact disc player that can communicate with the user's computer.

Because the treatment information in PDQ changes each month, vendors must regularly send out a new disc to each user. Therefore, CD-ROM versions of PDQ are offered by annual subscription. Information on commercial distributors that provide PDQ on compact disc is also available from the NCI on CancerFax.

PART V:
TREATING THE COMMON CANCERS

ADRENAL GLAND

Malin Dollinger, MD, and Orlo H. Clark, MD

◇

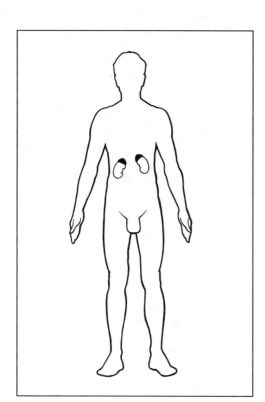

Functioning tumors of the adrenal gland are rare but incidentally discovered benign tumors involving the adrenal gland are discovered by CT scanning usually done for another purpose in 1.5 to 8 percent of patients.

The two glands, located just above each kidney (*see* page 446), produce a variety of hormones that are essential for life. The central part of the gland—the medulla—produces norepinephrine (noradrenalin), a substance necessary for the transmission of nerve impulses, and epinephrine. The outer part—the cortex—produces four hormones: aldosterone, which regulates salt and water balance; hydrocortisone, which is essential for body metabolism; and both androgens and estrogens, which are the sex hormones in males and females respectively.

When excessive amounts of these hormones are produced, a variety of clinical symptoms can result, including feminization in men, masculinization in women and the signs of excessive hydrocortisone production (Cushing's syndrome). Tumors of the cortex (aldosteronoma) or of the medulla (pheochromocytoma) produce excessive amounts of aldosterone or norepinephrine, respectively causing sustained or intermittent hypertension. Tumors that produce more than one hormone are frequently malignant.

The vast majority of adrenal tumors are benign, being discovered either because of the effects of hormone overproduction or by virtue of the ability of ultrasound, CT or MRI scanners to detect small adrenal tumors that are usually benign adenomas.

Malignant adrenal tumors are treatable and curable when still confined to the gland.

Types Primary tumors of the adrenal glands include a benign tumor (cortical adenoma), which may develop in up to 8 percent of people, often without any symptoms or clinical findings. Other types include adrenocortical carcinoma, pheochromocytoma, neuroblastoma, ganglioneuroma, as well as a variety of other benign tumors. The adrenal gland is also a common site for metastatic cancer, particularly lung and breast cancer and melanomas.

Benign adrenocortical adenomas are generally less than 2 in. (5 cm) in diameter

271

and, if functional, usually secrete a single hormone, such as hydrocortisone. The most common malignant tumors, adrenocortical carcinomas, tend to be large and to secrete several hormones. About 30 percent of these are non-functioning, meaning that they do not produce hormones. These tumors are usually recognized only after they have grown to a considerable size.

Pheochromocytomas, tumors of the adrenal medulla, can be either benign (85 percent) or malignant (15 percent). Either type can produce hormones or other substances that may cause significant health problems and sometimes fatal hypertension, but only the malignant tumor can spread to other places. Benign tumors, however, can be multifocal.

How It Spreads Adrenal tumors can directly invade nearby tissues and spread to regional lymph nodes. The most common sites for metastases are the lungs, liver, bone and the other adrenal gland.

What Causes It Unknown.

RISK FACTORS

People with neurofibromatosis and the Von Hippel-Lindau Syndrome as well as the multiple endocrine neoplasia (MEN II) syndrome are prone to develop pheochromocytoma. Patients with MEN I may develop adrenal cortical tumors. No specific preventive measures exist.

SCREENING

Because these tumors are so rare, no specific screening measures seem appropriate. A physician should suspect some type of adrenal tumor, however, if there are signs of Cushing's syndrome or high blood pressure in the presence of potassium deficiency, as well as unexplained hypertension, especially if it is severe or in patients with a family history of the above risk factors.

Patients with medullary thyroid cancer and hypertension always should be screened for pheochromocytoma prior to stressful procedures.

COMMON SIGNS AND SYMPTOMS

Non-functioning tumors—those that don't produce hormones—are frequently discovered by CT or MRI. Patients may also have abdominal masses, often with pain, weight loss or evidence of metastasis.

The hormonally active tumors produce a variety of symptoms. Women may have signs of masculinization (virilization) such as excess body and facial hair, a decrease in menstrual periods or enlargement of the clitoris. Breasts can become enlarged in men. Puberty may come early to children. The signs of Cushing's syndrome include swelling of the face and back of the neck, along with bruising and purple lines over the abdomen. Hypertension and signs of diabetes may appear.

People with a pheochromocytoma typically have attacks of anxiety and marked or sustained high blood pressure. Hypertensive crises may occur during minor operations or after trauma or exercise. The blood pressure often falls when the person rises from a sitting position. Other symptoms include headaches, sweating, palpitations and a rapid heartbeat.

Pheochromocytomas can produce other hormones besides norepinephrine, including ACTH, epinephrine and dopamine, so that some patients may also have Cushing's syndrome. If these tumors occur in both adrenal glands, this may represent a component of multiple endocrine neoplasia (MEN II), which includes medullary carcinoma of the thyroid gland (*see* "Thyroid") and multiple abnormal parathyroid glands.

DIAGNOSIS

With the use of ultrasound, CT and MRI scanning, adrenal tumors are being discovered at an earlier stage today. In fact, a diagnostic dilemma occurs when an adrenal mass is discovered on a routine scanning. Most of these masses are fortunately benign adenomas, but a diagnostic work-up should be done to discover whether the mass produces hormones or is cancer.

Pheochromocytomas can occur outside the adrenal gland and may be difficult to find. An extensive search is appropriate for anyone with typical signs and symptoms, even if scans of the adrenals are negative. Most of these tumors can be identified by MIBG scans.

Blood and Other Tests
♦ Endocrine studies (blood and urine tests).
♦ Serum chemistry profile.

Imaging
♦ CT, MRI, I-131-MIBG or ultrasound scans.
♦ Chest x-ray or bone scan to detect metastatic lesions.

Endoscopy and Biopsy
♦ A biopsy is necessary for a definitive diagnosis and is most useful for patients with suspected metastatic disease. The primary tumor may be biopsied surgically or with a CT- or ultrasound-directed needle biopsy or surgically after a metabolic workup reveals it is not a pheochromocytoma.
♦ Alternatively, an accessible metastasis in the lymph nodes or liver can be biopsied.

STAGING

Adrenocortical carcinoma is staged according to the TNM classification indicating the size of the tumor, the degree of invasion into adjacent tissues and whether it has spread to regional lymph nodes or distant sites.

There is no acceptable staging system for pheochromocytoma other than localized and benign versus malignant and metastatic.

TREATMENT OVERVIEW

Adrenocortical carcinomas are curable if the diagnosis can be made before the tumor is larger than 2 in. (5 cm) and has not spread outside the adrenal gland. At the time of diagnosis, however, most people with adrenal cortical carcinomas (70 percent) have Stage III or Stage IV disease. The initial treatment for all stages, even Stage IV, is to surgically remove the entire tumor and sometimes the adjacent kidney. Radiation and chemotherapy may be used as adjuvant treatment after surgery.

The 70 percent of these cancers that produce hormones have a better prognosis than those that don't, but this is probably because the symptoms of excess hormone production lead to an earlier diagnosis. Patients who respond to op-DDD (mitotane) also have a better prognosis.

Surgery Removal of the entire tumor is the only treatment that can lead to a cure. This may sometimes also require the removal of the adjacent kidney. As much of the primary tumor as possible is removed, even if all of it can't be, to decrease the amount of hormones produced.

Prolonged remissions have been reported after the removal of metastatic disease in the liver, lung and brain. As with the primary tumor, even if all the metastases cannot be removed, it may still be beneficial to remove most of them, for this will remove the source of the hormones and these cancers may grow slowly.

Surgery to remove pheochromocytomas requires specific preparation and management before, during and after the operation. The management of patients with these tumors is complex, and the surgical and medical teams have to be familiar with the specific medical and pharmacologic measures needed to minimize the risk to the patient and control the anticipated complications. The blood pressure may rise significantly during anesthesia or surgery, causing a life-threatening crisis.

 Radiation There may be an adjuvant role for radiation therapy after an early-stage tumor is removed, although this is still investigational. In more advanced disease, radiation therapy may shrink bone metastases.

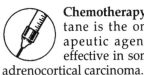 **Chemotherapy** The drug mitotane is the only chemotherapeutic agent known to be effective in some patients with adrenocortical carcinoma.

TREATMENT BY STAGE AND TYPE

ADRENOCORTICAL CARCINOMA

STAGE I
TNM T1, N0, M0
The tumor is less than 2 in. (5 cm) and does not invade other tissues.

Standard Treatment Complete surgical removal of the tumor.

Five-Year Survival 60 percent

Investigational
♦ Adjuvant radiation therapy.
♦ Adjuvant chemotherapy with mitotane.

STAGE II
TNM T2, N0, M0
The tumor is larger than 2 in. (5 cm) but is still not invasive.

Standard Treatment Complete surgical removal, similar to Stage I.

Five-Year Survival 30 percent

Investigational
♦ Clinical trials of new treatment combinations, especially with radiation therapy and mitotane, are appropriate for some patients.

STAGE III
TNM T1–2, N1, M0 or T3, N0, M0
The tumor has invaded outside the adrenal gland into fat but does not involve adjacent organs (T3), or the regional lymph nodes have become involved (N1).

Standard Treatment The tumor is completely removed, along with any enlarged lymph nodes.

Five-Year Survival 20 percent

Investigational
♦ Radiation therapy if the tumor cannot be removed but remains localized.
♦ Chemotherapy with mitotane reduces hormone production and tumor growth and/or recurrence in some patients.

STAGE IV
TNM Any T, any N, M1 or T3–4, N1, M0

Standard Treatment The goal of treatment for an adrenocortical carcinoma that has spread to adjacent organs (a T4 tumor) or has metastasized to distant sites is palliation rather than cure.

Chemotherapy with mitotane may lead to partial or complete remissions. Other treatment options are radiation therapy to bone metastases and/or the surgical removal of localized metastases, particularly those that produce hormones.

Five-Year Survival Less than 1 percent

Investigational
♦ Clinical trials are appropriate for patients with metastatic disease or with recurrent cancer.

♦ Cisplatin seems to benefit some patients with metastases and is being clinically evaluated.

PHEOCHROMOCYTOMA
LOCALIZED
Localized benign pheochromocytoma may be confined to one or both adrenal glands or situated in other (ectopic) locations.

Standard Treatment Before definitive treatment, pheoxybenzamine (Dibenzyline) is given to block the action of the hormones produced by the tumor. Because rather specific, specialized and vital medical management is essential before surgery or any other treatment is given, an endocrinologist is usually involved and the surgery is often done in a major medical center.

The standard treatment is removal of the tumor (adrenalectomy). Besides the essential preoperative management, blood pressure has to be controlled with specific drugs during surgery and patients vigorously hydrated to avoid hypotension (low blood pressure) once the tumor is removed.

Five-Year Survival Over 95 percent

METASTATIC
The pheochromocytoma has spread to nearby lymph nodes, adjacent tissues or to distant sites.

Standard Treatment If the pheochromocytoma has spread, it is still treated with aggressive surgery to remove all visible evidence of disease. This is to reduce the excess hormone production that causes many of the clinical problems these patients have. Long-term medical treatment decreases symptoms due to excess hormones. The same medical preparation used for patients with localized tumors is essential.

A variety of chemotherapy combinations have been used, including cyclophosphamide + vincristine + dacarbazine (DTIC), which may produce tumor regression and improve symptoms, biochemical markers and hypertension.

Radiation therapy may improve or palliate local complications caused by metastases.

Five-Year Survival About 40 to 45 percent

Investigational
♦ Clinical trials are under way to find more effective chemotherapy treatments.
♦ One therapeutic approach for patients whose tumors cannot be removed, have recurred or have metastasized is targeted radiation therapy with I-131-MIBG. This treatment has resulted in the shrinkage of tumors and a reduction in symptoms in some patients.

TREATMENT FOLLOW-UP
For adrenocortical carcinomas, treatment follow-up should include:
♦ Repeat CT, MRI or MIBG scanning to assess possible local recurrence or metastases.
♦ Measurement of specific hormones produced by the tumor.
♦ Studies—liver function tests, chest x-rays—to document the status of metastases.

Follow-up for pheochromocytomas should include:
♦ Measurements of hormones produced by the tumor by plasma and urine tests.
♦ Abdominal CT or MRI scans to assess the status of the primary tumor.
♦ Bone scans, chest x-rays and liver function tests to evaluate the status of metastases.
♦ Routine and regular blood pressure determinations to assess the effects of the hormone produced by the tumor.

RECURRENT CANCER

The selection of treatment for recurrent tumors depends on which therapy was initially used and the site of recurrence. Clinical trials evaluating new chemotherapy drugs should be considered for recurrent adrenocortical carcinoma. Recurrent pheochromocytoma is managed in the same way as metastatic disease.

THE MOST IMPORTANT QUESTIONS YOU CAN ASK

◆ What hormones is my tumor producing?

◆ Should an endocrinologist be involved in my care?

◆ If the tumor cannot be completely removed, would radiation therapy and chemotherapy be helpful?

◆ What is the role of mitotane in my treatment and what are its side effects?

◆ Can I live for a long time even if the tumor can't be removed?

◆ Should I be receiving antihypertensive therapy?

ANUS
Ernest H. Rosenbaum, MD

◇

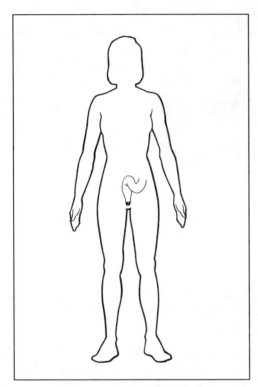

Cancer of the anus—the inch-long muscular tube where the rectum opens into the body surface—is less common than other bowel cancers, accounting for only about 1 to 2 percent of all cancers of the large bowel and its outlet. Fewer than 10,000 cases occur annually in the United States.

Anal cancer is highly treatable and often curable, especially in the early stages. The first sign of the cancer is often bleeding, which may be mistaken for hemorrhoids or benign anal disease. Anal cancers are often discovered by a pathologist in a specimen from a surgical operation done for apparently benign disease.

Types The vast majority—80 to 90 percent—of all primary cancers of the anus develop in the skin and are called squamous cell (epidermoid) carcinomas. These often first appear as an ulcer. An important subset is made up of tumors such as transitional cell, basaloid or cloacogenic cancer that can arise in the anal lining from embryonic tissue (cloacogenic) or the anal lining of transitional cells (basaloid tumors). There is also a squamous cell tumor within the anal lining (intraepithelial) called Bowen's disease that is a premalignant *in situ* squamous cell lesion of the skin around the anus. The third variety is mucoepidermoid anal cancer.

Anal cancers can also develop in a rare glandular tissue (adenocarcinoma). Less common lesions include small cell carcinomas, malignant lymphomas, sarcomas, melanomas or Paget's disease, an intraepithelial adenocarcinoma of the mucous or sweat glands. Melanomas have a poor prognosis, since they spread via the bloodstream.

Well-differentiated tumors have a more favorable prognosis than poorly differentiated tumors.

How It Spreads Anal tumors can extend directly into adjacent tissues, including the skin, sphincter muscle, or to local organs such as the prostate, bladder or vagina. Tumor cells can spread via the lymph system to lymph nodes in the groin (if the tumor is below the pectinate line) or to pelvic lymph nodes (if the tumor is above the pectinate line). Metastases can also travel through the bloodstream.

What Causes It Chronic irritation of the

anus is a primary cause. People who get anal cancer usually have a history of risk factors, one of which may be related to the human papilloma virus, especially type 16, or the trauma of anal intercourse. It is believed that invasive cancer is preceded by premalignant changes known as intraepithelial neoplasia, which include proliferation of anal basal-like epithelial cells that replace the squamous cells.

RISK FACTORS

At Significantly Higher Risk
♦ This cancer is more common in women over 40.
♦ Primary association with a history of chronic anal irritation—genital warts (condyloma), abscesses, fistulas, fissures, scars and infections such as chlamydia, trichomonas, genital herpes, gonorrhea and radiation dermatitis.
♦ Associated with venereal warts and the presence of the papilloma virus.
♦ Anal margin cancer (cancer encircling the anus) is more common in men.
♦ Increased incidence in cigarette smokers.
♦ Increased risk in homosexuals, probably related to anal intercourse and infections with a retrovirus such as HIV (human immunodeficiency virus) and HPV (human papilloma viruses).
♦ Persons with symptomatic HIV disease, lower CD4 (T4) blood counts.
♦ There is an increased incidence of anal cancer with cervical, vaginal and vulvar high-grade intraepithelial neoplasia (grade 3).
♦ Anal cancer may occur along with benign anal disease. It is more common in those with hemorrhoids, anal degenerative skin changes and white plaque (leukoplakia) on the mucous membranes.

SCREENING

A careful anal exam is an important part of a yearly physical. A digital rectal examination and anoscopy should be performed whenever there are rectal symptoms such as pain, bleeding, itching or hemorrhoidal complaints. All hemorrhoids, inflammation and local anal disease should be examined by a physician with a special interest in anal or rectal disease. And all lesions in the area should be biopsied no matter how benign-looking they are. In HIV+ patients an anal Pap smear; anoscopy if Pap smear is abnormal. Anal Pap smear: A large cotton swab is gently placed about 1 1/2 to 2 in. (4 to 5 cm) in the anus and rotated as it is withdrawn to obtain samples of tissue for analysis.

COMMON SIGNS AND SYMPTOMS

There are often no symptoms of anal cancer in its early stages. But there may be bleeding, discomfort or pressure, pain, itching or a palpable rectal mass. Small amounts of rectal bleeding not associated with anemia are often attributed to hemorrhoids.

Occasionally, a change in bowel habits, diarrhea or constipation may be noted and a bowel obstruction might develop. There may also be local pain or pressure that is not relieved by a bowel movement.

DIAGNOSIS

Physical Examination
♦ Digital rectal exam or an exam with local or general anesthesia if necessary.
♦ A small anal mass, often like hemorrhoids, may be found. Sometimes the mass protrudes and reaches a significant size.
♦ Physical examination for local invasion into muscle sphincter.
♦ Lymph nodes in the groin may be enlarged, indicating metastases.
♦ Perirectal and mesenteric lymph nodes are involved in 50 percent of patients.

Blood and Other Tests
♦ Complete blood count.
♦ Liver function chemistries (alkaline phosphatase, LDH, SGOT).
♦ CEA is normal in cloacogenic tumor, elevated in colorectal cancer.

- Tests of kidney function (creatinine).
- Papilloma virus culture or DNA test, if available.
- Test for hidden blood in the stools.
- Anal Pap smear.

Imaging
- CT and MRI scans of the pelvis to assess local invasion and whether the iliac and groin (inguinal) lymph nodes are involved (30 percent have inguinal metastases and 10 percent have liver metastases at the time of diagnosis).
- Rectal ultrasound may help assess local cancer and lymph node invasion.
- Pelvic and abdominal ultrasound.
- Abdominal CT scan if the liver is enlarged or if liver function tests are abnormal.
- Chest x-ray.

Endoscopy and Biopsy
- Anoscopy/proctosigmoidoscopy under local or general anesthesia if necessary.

STAGING
The stage of anal cancer describes whether the cancer has remained within the anus, has spread to lymph nodes near the anus or has spread to other sites, usually within the abdomen or other organs. The stage as defined by the TNM classification is important in determining the initial treatment options.

TREATMENT OVERVIEW
Surgery, radiotherapy and chemotherapy are all used to treat anal cancer.

The prognosis depends on the size and location of the tumor. The outlook is more favorable if the tumors are small (less than 2 in./5 cm), if there is no lymph node involvement or local extension and if the primary tumor is in the anal margin rather than the anal canal. Primary tumors less than 1 in. (2 cm) in size have a better prognosis, as do tumors that are well-differentiated (more mature) rather than undifferentiated or poorly differentiated.

Options by Size of Tumor The choice of conservative surgery or radiotherapy (with or without chemotherapy) for anal or perianal cancer depends on the size of the tumor, local invasion and/or lymph node involvement. Radical surgery (an abdominal-perineal resection) is often required for larger or more extensive cancers, and will result in a loss of anal function, a colostomy, and urinary and sexual malfunction. It is reserved for larger or residual cancers.
- Superficial in situ tumors—those that invade less than 1 in. (2 cm) can be treated with local excision or radiotherapy alone.
- Tumors 1 to 2 in. (2 to 5 cm) are *best* treated by chemotherapy (5-fluorouracil + mitomycin-C or 5-FU + cisplatin) plus radiotherapy, leaving surgery for "salvage" therapy. Some physicians still use just radiotherapy, but most oncologists today use combined chemotherapy and radiotherapy.
- Tumors larger than 2 in. (5 cm) are treated by chemotherapy, radiotherapy and surgery for residual disease.
- If the cancer is confirmed as local or is less than 1 in. (2 cm) in diameter and is well-differentiated, removal of the squamous anal verge or the anal canal will produce a high chance for cure, with 70 to 90 percent surviving five years. Removing the groin lymph nodes as a prophylactic measure does not improve these results and often contributes to lymphedema.
- A clinical trial is comparing radiation therapy with radiation plus 5-FU. High-dose radiation therapy alone (greater than 6,000 cGy) may be curative and has a five-year survival of greater than 70 percent and 80 percent control of small local tumors. Patients who relapse may require salvage surgery.

Options by Lymph Node Status The lymph nodes in the groin (inguinal), pelvis and perirectal area may become involved by anal cancer.

♦ When lesions are less than 1 in. (2 cm), nodes are not usually treated.

♦ When primary lesions are between 1 and 2 in. (2 to 5 cm), groin and pelvic nodes are treated prophylactically with radiation therapy.

♦ When lymph nodes can be felt, the treatment is chemotherapy and radiotherapy.

♦ Groin dissection has no prophylactic role, but is done for metastatic node involvement as palliation.

Combined Therapy Information from clinical trials supports the idea of using radiation therapy, or chemotherapy plus radiotherapy for the initial treatment of epidermoid cancer of the anus, reserving surgery for residual disease. Radiation therapy plus chemotherapy has been used as an alternative to surgery for patients with inguinal lymph node metastases.

External radiation therapy with chemotherapy is now the first line of therapy, resulting in a 90 percent local control. An alternative is interstitial implants of iridium with external radiation therapy, without chemotherapy.

The first choice of treatment should be radiotherapy with chemotherapy for small or even large, but not huge, lesions. Whether to give chemotherapy before radiotherapy or simultaneously is now being evaluated, although current reports recommend the simultaneous use of radiation and chemotherapy.

When all the tumor is eradicated by radiation and chemotherapy, careful follow-up is vital. The lymph nodes in the groin have to be watched carefully, since the most common site of local recurrence is in the pelvis and lymph nodes. If the tumor recurs, salvage surgery will be needed.

Treatment of the less common adenocarcinoma involving the upper portion of the anus (near the rectum) differs from treatment of squamous carcinoma. For smaller lesions, local excision or fulguration may suffice. For larger lesions, an abdominal-perineal resection may be required. Combined radiotherapy and chemotherapy is not as useful, although rectal adjuvant chemotherapy and radiotherapy programs can be employed. In selected cases, interstitial implants of iridium with external radiation therapy may be an alternative.

TREATMENT BY STAGE

STAGE 0
TNM Tis, N0, M0
Carcinoma in situ—a very early, microscopic, non-invasive cancer that has not spread below the membrane of the first layer of anal tissue.

Standard Treatment Surgical removal of the tumor.

Five-Year Survival 100 percent

STAGE I
TNM T1, N0, M0
A tumor less than 1 in. (2 cm) found only in the anal mucosa with no evidence of spread to lymph nodes or other organs. There is no sphincter muscle involvement.

Standard Treatment Small tumors of the skin around the anus and of the anal margin may be adequately treated by local excision with or without radiation therapy with preservation of the sphincter muscle.

When surgery that will preserve the sphincter is possible, both radiation and chemotherapy can be used before the operation to reduce the size of the tumor. Selected tumors may also be treated by implanting iridium in the tissue. Careful follow-up is mandatory.

When surgery would significantly impair anal sphincter functions, radiotherapy is an effective alternative, usually with chemotherapy.

External radiation therapy for small

lesions—with or without chemotherapy—may also be used to avoid surgery and/or avoid a colostomy. Surgery may be necessary for large lesions that do not shrink with radiotherapy and chemotherapy.

Combination chemotherapy with 5-fluorouracil (5-FU) + mitomycin-C with primary radiation therapy is more effective for larger lesions than radiation therapy alone in reducing the need for surgery and/or a colostomy. Cisplatin + 5-FU is an alternative treatment with radiotherapy. Both combinations seem to be equally effective.

The former standard approach—an abdominal-perineal resection (APR), which involves removal of the anus and rectum and requires a colostomy—is now rarely used except for recurrent disease. If there is still tumor in the anal canal after non-surgical treatment, the surgery that will be required ranges from a local sphincter preservation operation to a complete abdominal-perineal resection with colostomy.

Five-Year Survival Over 95 percent

STAGE II
TNM T2–3 N0, M0
The tumor is larger than 1 in. (2 cm) and has spread into the muscle wall of the anus (the sphincter muscle is involved), but does not involve lymph nodes or other adjacent organs.

Standard Treatment Current treatment is combination chemotherapy with 5-FU + mitomycin-C or cisplatin + 5-FU plus radiation therapy. When the response is not complete, the tumor can be removed surgically.

The result of treatment with 5-FU + mitomycin-C + radiotherapy is better than radiotherapy alone for all tumor stages. The omission of mitomycin-C reduced hematologic toxicity but gave lower primary tumor control.

The treatment options for anal cancer involving the sphincter are the same as for Stage I.

Five-Year Survival 75 percent

STAGE IIIA
TNM T4, N0, M0 or T1–3, N1, M0
The cancer has spread to nearby lymph nodes or has spread to nearby organs such as the vagina, urethra or bladder (it is often hard to determine Stage IIIA, since many patients clinically appear to be Stage II).

Standard Treatment Abdominal-perineal resection has been the treatment of choice in the past. Deciding whether to perform this operation may depend on whether the physical examination or the CT, ultrasound or MRI scans find that the perirectal lymph nodes are involved. The need for a biopsy of perirectal lymph nodes to differentiate between Stage II and Stage III disease may not be verifiable without surgery.

Chemotherapy and radiation given before surgery may not only improve the long-term results, but also permit sphincter preserving surgery by shrinking the tumor substantially before the operation.

Five-Year Survival 60 percent

Investigational
♦ Trials to evaluate postoperative external beam radiation to the involved area, which may improve local control and survival, are ongoing.
♦ Chemotherapy after surgery is also being evaluated.

STAGE IIIB
TNM T4, N1, M0 or any T, N2–3, M0
The cancer has spread to the internal iliac and/or groin lymph nodes on one or both sides or has spread to adjacent organs such as the vagina, urethra or bladder. Metastatic disease to the groin (inguinal) nodes is a poor prognostic sign and markedly reduces the chance for cure, although cure is still possible.

Standard Treatment Options include combination chemotherapy and radiation therapy as in Stage I, followed by surgical removal of the remaining disease at the primary site. This may involve either a local excision or an abdominal-perineal resection with colostomy. Removal of superficial and deep inguinal lymph nodes for residual tumor on one or both sides can be done in a separate operation.

Another option is an abdominal-perineal resection of the primary tumor as the initial treatment, with delayed removal of superficial and deep inguinal nodes.

Five-Year Survival 10 percent

STAGE IV
TNM Any T, any N, M1
The cancer has spread to the tail bone (sacrum), to distant lymph nodes within the abdomen far from the original cancer site or to other organs in the body such as the vagina, urethra, bladder, liver and/or lung.

Standard Treatment There is no standard treatment for patients with metastatic anal carcinoma. Relieving the symptoms produced by the primary cancer is the major consideration.

Palliation Treatment options include palliative surgery, palliative radiation and palliative combined chemotherapy and radiation.
♦ Abdominal-perineal resection is sometimes needed to control pain, bleeding or infection caused by tumor breakdown.
♦ Radiation has helped control pain and bleeding. The use of radiosensitizing drugs may improve local control.
♦ Endoscopic laser treatment has been used to reduce local tumor obstruction and also, sometimes, to control bleeding (*see* Chapter 9).
♦ Combination chemotherapy with 5-FU + mitomycin or 5-FU+ cisplatin as well as bleomycin or investigational combinations (see below) can be considered. For those who don't respond to these drugs, cisplatin + 5-FU therapy may be a good salvage program.

Five-Year Survival Unusual

Investigational Various chemotherapy drug combinations are being evaluated, including:
♦ mitomycin + Adriamycin + cisplatin
♦ 5-FU + bleomycin + lomustine (CCNU).

TREATMENT FOLLOW-UP
Careful follow-up is essential. This includes a history and physical examination every two to three months for three years after treatment, then every three to six months for the next three to five years.
♦ Careful observation for signs of enlarged inguinal lymph nodes.
♦ Chest x-rays and liver blood tests (alkaline phosphatase, SGOT) at follow-up visits.

RECURRENT CANCER
For a substantial number of patients, local recurrences of anal cancer after chemo-therapy and/or radiation therapy or surgery can occasionally be controlled by various treatments. Surgical removal of the recurrent tumor, the addition of various chemotherapy protocols with or without radiation and the use of radiosensitizers and endoscopic laser treatments can improve the local control.

Current investigational programs—including combinations of mitomycin + cisplatin + Adriamycin and bleomycin + lomustine (CCNU)—have been variably effective in controlling metastatic and/or recurrent disease.

THE MOST IMPORTANT QUESTIONS YOU CAN ASK
♦ How should anal cancer be evaluated?
♦ How do different pathologic types affect prognosis?
♦ How does staging affect prognosis?
♦ Can anal cancer be cured without surgery?
♦ What new advances in therapy are being used to reduce the need for a colostomy?
♦ What are the roles of local radiotherapy and of chemotherapy?

BILE DUCT

Alan P. Venook, MD

◇

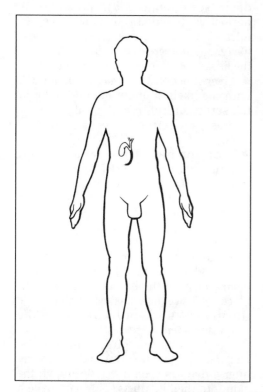

Bile is manufactured in the liver and helps the body digest fats. The bile ducts course throughout the liver collecting bile, then travel beyond the liver to connect with the gall bladder and small intestines (*see* page 406). Bile duct cancers may, therefore, arise in many locations in and around the liver.

Bile duct cancer—also called cholangio-carcinoma—is a rare cancer, and the prognosis depends largely on where the tumor begins and how large it has grown by the time of diagnosis. The only definitive treatment is the complete surgical removal of the tumor, which is not often possible. If the cancer cannot be entirely removed, the principal goals of therapy become the relief of symptoms caused by the accumulation of bile, and relief from pain.

Types The vast majority of these tumors develop in glandular tissue within the bile duct (adenocarcinoma). Other tissue types include squamous carcinomas and sarcomas. The therapy for all types of bile duct cancer is the same, depending on the extent of the tumor at the time of diagnosis.

How It Spreads Bile duct cancer tends to spread into the adjacent liver, along the bile duct surface and through the lymph system to lymph nodes in the region of the liver (porta hepatis). Tumors in the bile duct leading from the gall bladder to the common bile duct (cystic duct) can spread to involve the gall bladder. Ultimately, other lymph nodes may become involved, as well as other organs within the abdomen.

What Causes It The cause is unknown. People with chronic inflammatory pro-cesses, such as ulcerative colitis or parasitic infections of the bile ducts, are at higher risk for developing this cancer. But no one cause has been clearly demonstrated.

RISK FACTORS

At Significantly Higher Risk

♦ Chronic infection with the liver fluke Clonorchis sinensis, which is prevalent in parts of Southeast Asia. People may become infected with this parasite by eating raw or pickled freshwater fish from this region. Most people with this infection do not develop cancer, however.

♦ People with chronic ulcerative colitis

have a higher incidence of both benign inflammatory processes of the bile ducts (sclerosing cholangitis) and bile duct cancer.

♦ People with congenital abnormalities of the bile ducts (choledochal cysts) are more likely to develop bile duct cancer.

SCREENING

There are no screening methods to detect bile duct cancer at an early stage.

COMMON SIGNS AND SYMPTOMS

There are no signs or symptoms that indicate bile duct cancer. It usually develops slowly and the symptoms are often very subtle. Jaundice (the skin turning yellow) and itching are the most common signs. Jaundice is caused by the accumulation in the skin of a component of bile (bilirubin) that normally empties into the intestines after traveling through the bile ducts.

Bloating, weight loss, decreased appetite, fever, nausea or an enlarging abdominal mass are all signs that *may* be attributable to bile duct cancer. Pain usually signifies advanced disease.

DIAGNOSIS

Physical Examination

There are no specific findings on physical examination. Even if the findings associated with bile duct cancer are present, other explanations are far more likely. Findings may include:

♦ Jaundice.
♦ Fever.
♦ Tender mass below the ribs on the right side of the abdomen.
♦ Enlarged, hard lymph nodes.
♦ Swelling of the legs (edema) and fluid in the abdomen (ascites).

Blood and Other Tests

Diagnostic tests are usually done to determine the cause of jaundice. These tests may lead to the diagnosis of bile duct cancer, but a simple gallstone or other illnesses can cause the same problems and are much more likely to be the cause of the jaundice.

♦ A complete blood count may reveal a decrease in hemoglobin (anemia). A normal white blood cell count makes an infection in the bile duct (cholangitis) less likely, but an increased white count raises the likelihood of infection or cancer.

♦ Liver function tests may be abnormal, with the likeliest abnormalities being in the serum bilirubin and alkaline phosphatase, reflecting a blockage of flow within the bile duct.

♦ Prothrombin Time and Partial Thromboplastin Time (PT and PTT) are tests of clotting that may reveal a disorder in patients with poor liver function caused by an obstructed bile duct.

Imaging

♦ Abdominal ultrasound images of the gall bladder and bile ducts may reveal an enlargement of the bile ducts behind the blockage, since these channels will enlarge (dilate) when the pressure within the drainage system increases.

♦ PTC (percutaneous transhepatic cholangiography) involves taking an x-ray after a dye has been injected through the skin into the bile ducts. This can make a "road map" of the bile ducts within and outside the liver and may establish the site of the blockage.

♦ ERCP (endoscopic retrograde cholangiopancreatography) may be done to investigate the cause of an elevated bilirubin. This technically difficult procedure involves passing an endoscope through the mouth and into the small intestines. The physician operating this scope (endoscopist) identifies the site within the intestines where the bile and pancreatic ducts empty their contents. By injecting dye into this opening and doing an x-ray, a "road map" of the bile ducts may be made. PTC and ERCP may both be necessary to completely define the site and cause of an obstruction, and will correctly predict the presence of a cancer about 90 percent of the time.

♦ CT scanning assesses the extent of the tumor within the bile duct and its extension into the adjacent liver, lymph nodes or other structures within the abdomen. Often, bile duct cancer is not seen on a CT scan.

♦ Magnetic resonance imaging (MRI) may be helpful in determining if the bile duct cancer can be surgically removed.

♦ If the diagnosis of cancer is confirmed or suspected, a chest x-ray should be done to look for tumor nodules in the lungs that would confirm the distant spread of the cancer.

Endoscopy and Biopsy
♦ Biopsy, either with a fine needle (FNA) or regular needle, can be done through the skin without significant danger or through the scope when ERCP is done. The tumor cells may also be found in the bile; they are characteristic. Their presence may help decide whether surgery should be performed if the other studies also suggest the tumor has spread. It can be difficult to obtain an adequate biopsy sample because the tumors are often small and lie within normal liver tissue.

STAGING
A TNM staging system is used for bile duct cancer, but when deciding which treatment option to use there are really only two stages—localized and unresectable disease.

TREATMENT OVERVIEW
The optimal treatment for bile duct cancer is surgery. Unfortunately, by the time symptoms develop, the cancer has usually spread throughout the bile ducts and into the liver, meaning that the tumor cannot be entirely removed.

Chemotherapy and radiation therapy are occasionally useful to relieve symp-

toms. Although they have not been shown to be effective in curing the cancer, these measures can be taken to maintain the quality of life.

 Surgery The decision to take a surgical approach depends on the overall health of the patient and on the location of the tumor. If a patient is ill from complications of the cancer—jaundice or infection, for example—a drainage tube (stent) should be placed into the bile ducts to treat the complications. The patient then has to be allowed to recover before an operation is attempted.

If the tumor is in either the left or the right bile duct and hasn't spread to the lymph nodes, it may be possible to remove the tumor with its accompanying lobe of the liver because people with normal liver function do not need both lobes.

Tumors involving the junction of the right and left bile ducts (Klatskin tumor) create more problems. The tumor may not have spread, but its removal requires rebuilding the bile ducts. This can be done by removing all of the tumor and attaching a loop of intestine to the liver where the cut end of the bile ducts are draining (called a Roux-en-Y). This is a difficult operation and the overall health of the patient is an important factor in deciding whether to perform it.

Bile duct cancers can also occur at the far end of the duct, near where it empties into the intestine. Removing these tumors may also require a Roux-en-Y, as well as removal of parts of the intestines and pancreas (called a Whipple procedure). This extensive surgery is extremely complicated and has many side effects. It should be done only when a tumor has not spread beyond the local area.

 Chemotherapy Studies have not shown that chemotherapy can prolong survival, but the standard drugs used (mitomycin-C or 5-fluorouracil)

may cause tumors to shrink and help about 25 percent of patients. Even with tumor shrinkage, however, patients may not be better off after chemotherapy. The treatment has side effects and the tumor ultimately regrows.

There may be a role for chemotherapy after surgery, although this has not been studied systematically. In the hopes of finding a better chemotherapy treatment and improving survival, patients should be considered for clinical trials if chemotherapy is planned.

 Radiation Radiation is effective against bile duct cancers and may play a significant role. If the tumor is fairly small, it may be treated with radiation without causing much damage to the surrounding non-cancerous liver tissue.

Treatment may include placing a radiation-containing probe into the bile duct (brachytherapy). This therapy may also apply to patients with a small bit of tumor left after surgery or as a supplemental (adjuvant) therapy when the surgery is thought to have been complete. Studies evaluating the role of radiation therapy are ongoing.

Combined Therapy The combination of radiation and chemotherapy may play a role as adjuvant therapy. This treatment, which should be done as part of a clinical trial, may delay any recurrence of the cancer or even cure people who have already had surgery.

TREATMENT BY STAGE

LOCALIZED
At this stage, the cancer is confined to the bile duct. It is quite rare to find a bile duct cancer at this limited stage, for it would be unlikely to cause an obstruction of the bile flow when it is very small.

Standard Treatment Surgery can be done with hopes of a cure. The extent of surgery necessary depends on the tumor's location

and size. It may be possible to remove a tumor limited to a small portion of either the right or left bile duct with its surrounding liver in a routine operation. But cancers involving the bile ducts at their junction within the liver require removal of liver tissue and then the complicated reconstruction of the bile drainage system. Tumors close to the intestine and pancreas may demand even more difficult surgery.

Whatever the extent of the surgery, tubes may have to be left within the bile duct system for a time to insure against bile leakage or the formation of scar tissue within the bile ducts.

It is not known whether drainage tubes should be placed through the bile duct blockage before surgery. If patients are ill because of the obstruction—the bile has become infected, for example—then a stent should be inserted to enable the patient to be in better condition for the surgery. Radiation to the tumor site is an alternative if patients are too sick to have surgery.

Unfortunately, even with meticulous surgery and careful screening, the majority of tumors will regrow within the bile ducts, in the nearby liver tissue or elsewhere in the body. So it is generally agreed that treating the surgical area with radiation after the tumor has been removed is useful in that it may help to destroy any remaining tumor cells.

The chemotherapy drug 5-fluorouracil is often given at the same time as the radiation in an effort to improve the effectiveness of treatment. This combination therapy is felt to be better than other treatments.

Five-Year Survival Up to 25 percent

Investigational Various combinations of surgery, radiation and chemotherapy may be considered. But because this is such a rare disease, it is difficult to study the relative benefits of newer treatments.

UNRESECTABLE
The tumor cannot be removed because it

has spread to local lymph nodes, liver tissue or elsewhere in the body.

Standard Treatment There is no standard treatment, so chemotherapy and/or radiation therapy clinical trials should be considered.

Significant relief of symptoms may be achieved. Patients with symptoms such as itching or infection may benefit from a procedure to create a bypass system for the bile. Such a bypass tube (stent) can be placed through the skin during percutaneous transhepatic cholangiography or through a scope during ERCP.

With the ERCP stent placement, the tube may drain into the intestines and a collecting bag may not be needed. Occasionally, neither of these methods drains the bile successfully. In that case, surgery designed to create a bypass channel may be done.

Two-Year Survival Less than 1 percent

Investigational
♦ Clinical protocols designed to test the additive benefit of radiation and chemotherapy are ongoing.
♦ Newer forms of radiation, such as hyperthermia (the application of heat to the region) are also being studied.
♦ Patients who wish to try chemotherapy may be offered new drugs.

TREATMENT FOLLOW-UP

Careful follow-up is important after the surgical removal of a localized cancer because once a recurrent tumor is large enough to be seen on x-ray, it is probably too large to be cured.
♦ CT scans should be done every two to three months for the first year after curative surgery, since an early recurrence may still be removed if it is small enough at the time of diagnosis.

SUPPORTIVE THERAPY

♦ Problems associated with jaundice can

include severe itching and infections in the bile. If the drainage procedures described above are not effective, itching will often be relieved by Benadryl, Atarax or cholestyramine.
♦ Large doses of narcotics may be needed to relieve pain. Such drugs may have excessive side effects, since they are eliminated by the liver, which may not be functioning properly.
♦ Non-steroidal anti-inflammatory drugs may be surprisingly effective even against the pain associated with bile duct cancer.
♦ Frequent small meals may be necessary to get enough nutrition since an abdominal mass may reduce the size of the stomach.
♦ Water pills (diuretics) can reduce fluid in the abdomen or legs. They may cause significant imbalance in kidney function, however, and can create problems if not carefully monitored and adjusted.
♦ Nausea will often be relieved by standard medications, including suppositories.
♦ Loss of appetite may be helped by a drug called Megace.
♦ Sleep disturbances are common, but most sleeping pills are broken down by the liver, so they should be used carefully.

THE MOST IMPORTANT QUESTIONS YOU CAN ASK

♦ Should I see another physician to confirm that this tumor can or cannot be removed?
♦ Can the drainage of my bile ducts be done through my intestines so I won't have to have a tube coming out through my skin?
♦ Am I a candidate for an investigational therapy at another medical center?
♦ How sick will radiation and/or chemotherapy make me, and does the potential benefit make it worthwhile?
♦ Can anything be done to improve the quality of my life?
♦ Is the treatment worthwhile if the tumor is too advanced for surgery?

BLADDER

Alan Yagoda, MD

◇

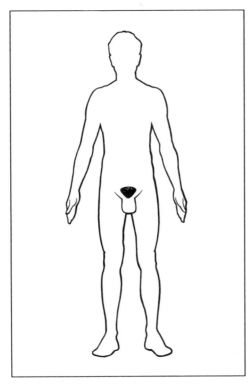

Bladder tumors account for about 4 percent of new cancers (51,200 cases) in the United States. Bladder cancer ranks as the fourth most common cause of cancer in men and ninth in women, and causes almost 3 percent of cancer deaths, about 9,900. It is the fourth leading cause of cancer deaths in patients over 75. While the average age of people who get bladder cancer is 68, this tumor is found in people as young as 45 to 55 years old.

Its origin is associated with certain chemical substances that induce or promote the growth of cancer (carcinogens). Men get it at a rate three times higher than women because of their greater exposure to such carcinogens in the workplace.

Five-year survival rates over the past 30 years have improved from 50 percent to over 70 percent, partly because the disease is being found in earlier stages when current therapies can be effective. Over 70 percent of cases are now being discovered with local tumors within the bladder. Only 20 percent have regional disease just outside the bladder, while 3 percent have distant metastases.

Types The urinary tract is lined with what are called transitional cells, and more than 90 percent of bladder cancers originate from these cells. The layer of three to four transitional cells lining the bladder can grow to six or more abnormal layers when they are irritated. Chemical carcinogens, chronic bladder infections, conditions called cystitis cysticia and cystitis glandularis, and chronic and repeated bladder trauma—repeated bladder catheterizations in paraplegics, for example—can cause cell changes that may turn into cancer.

This superficial layer of transitional cells is separated from the bladder muscle (which contracts to expel urine) by a thin, fibrous band called the lamina propria. The lamina propria separates tumors that are invasive (spreading into muscle) from those that are superficial (non-invasive). Treatment options depend on this distinction. Most bladder tumors are superficial and can be treated successfully.

Most of the remaining tumors—either alone or combined with transitional cell carcinoma—develop either in the glands of the bladder (adenocarcinoma) or in an embryonic remnant (urachal tumors, also adenocarcinoma). In men, adenocarcinoma occurs in the glands of the urethra near the prostate. The remaining bladder cancers are squamous cell carcinomas, which also are the most frequent type of urethral tumor in women. Tumors also develop in the pelvis of the kidney, where urine is formed, and in the ureters, the tubes that carry urine to the bladder. About 7 percent of all kidney cancers originate in the renal pelvis. The majority are transitional cell cancers, although the squamous cell type is noted more frequently in patients with a history of chronic stone problems.

There are also non-cancerous tumors called benign papillomas, labeled Ta, Grade I tumors. Fewer than 5 to 10 percent of patients with a benign papilloma will ever develop the more worrisome malignant superficial tumors (carcinoma in situ, or Tis) or muscle invasive tumors. Muscle invasive cancers may go through a Tis phase or may develop independently, so even though Tis does not invade muscle, the potential for invasion is implied. More important, Tis tends to recur again and again. Tis tumors, therefore, indicate an unstable, or sick, bladder lining.

How It Spreads Tumors can grow through the bladder muscle directly into the surrounding fat (perivesical) and into adjacent structures such as the prostate, vagina, rectum, uterus and pelvic bone. They also can directly enter the small blood and lymph vessels that supply the normal bladder wall. When they do, they can spread to local lymph nodes in the pelvis and farther up in the abdomen or be carried by the bloodstream to the lungs, bone and liver.

What Causes It Most of the time we are unaware of exposure to potent bladder carcinogens in our food and water supply, but some materials and the industries that use them have been strongly implicated with an increased risk for development of bladder cancer.

Bladder carcinogens include benzidine,

bracken fern (sometimes used in salads), naphthylamines and aromatic amines, nitrosamines, some cancer therapy drugs (cyclophosphamide, Alkeran), local radiation therapy, various dyes and solvents, chronic abuse of some pain medications such as phenacetin and acetaminophen, and particularly smoking cigarettes.

RISK FACTORS

The United States and Europe have the highest incidence of bladder cancer.

Cigarette smokers develop bladder cancers almost three times as often as non-smokers. Smoking may be responsible for 50 percent of bladder cancers in men and 40 percent in women. This relationship may be due to a substance called 4-ABP, a carcinogen found in tobacco smoke and the blood of smokers and which is known to induce bladder cancer. This substance disappears from blood within 90 to 120 days after a person stops smoking.

The relationship of tumors to the use of artificial sweeteners such as cyclamates and to coffee drinking is questionable. Recent studies have completely failed to find any risk above that of the general population.

Because chemical carcinogens and their breakdown products pass through the kidney down the urinary tract, the whole urothelial tract is exposed to these irritants and is at risk for forming new tumors. This is why people cured of one urothelial tract tumor have to be followed closely throughout their lifetime.

Those with a renal pelvis cancer, for example, are 21 times more at risk to develop another urinary tract tumor compared with the general population. Ten to 20 percent of those with a bladder cancer have been found to develop a superficial urethral tumor.

A good deal of work is now being done to evaluate agents that can prevent the development of such tumors. Much has been written about the testing of certain vitamin A derivatives for preventing

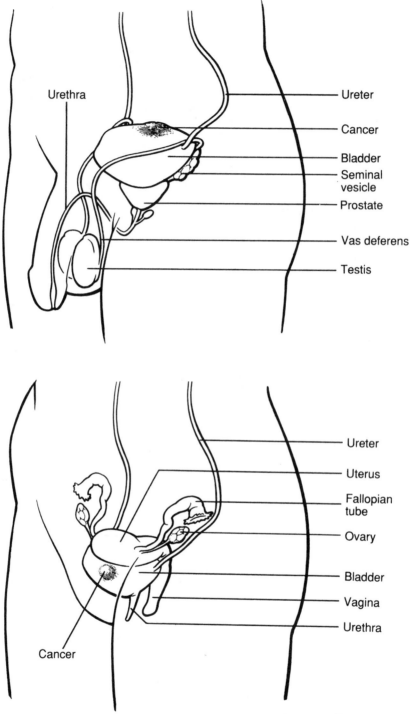

Urethra

Ureter

Cancer

Bladder

Seminal
vesicle

Prostate

Vas deferens

Testis

Ureter

Uterus

Fallopian
tube

Ovary

Bladder

Vagina

Urethra

Cancer

Overall view of pelvic organs showing bladder and surrounding structures

tumors and for making early tumors revert back to normal cells. But high doses of the derivatives now marketed (vitamin A itself or beta-carotene) should be avoided, since the doses needed to prevent new tumors produce severe liver toxicity.

At Significantly Higher Risk
♦ Smokers, especially of cigarettes.
♦ Beauticians, leather workers, machinists and metal workers, printers, rubber and textile workers, truckers and those exposed to industrial dyes.
♦ Abusers of certain pain medications.
♦ People taking alkylating agent chemotherapy drugs, such as Cytoxan, or who have had radiotherapy to the bladder.

SCREENING

A urinalysis to look for microscopic blood in the urine (hematuria) is the best screening test. Urine cytology (PAP) and ultrasound of the bladder are extremely useful in symptomatic cases, but are too insensitive and not cost-effective for general screening. Bladder monoclonal antibodies for testing urine and blood should be available in the mid-1990s.

COMMON SIGNS AND SYMPTOMS

Eighty percent of patients first go to their doctor because of blood and/or clots in the urine. Other urinary signs include increased frequency of urination, intermittent hesitancy, urgency, bladder spasms and pain or burning with urination (dysuria), difficulty passing urine and recurrent infections in the urinary tract. There are many more common reasons for such symptoms, however, such as an enlarged or inflamed prostate, stones, injury and various infections.

Late symptoms—loss of weight or appetite, fever, and pain in bones or the rectal, anal and pelvic area, for example—generally indicate more advanced disease.

DIAGNOSIS

Physical Examination
♦ There are few findings for early disease other than a bladder or pelvic mass discovered by digital rectal examination.
♦ With more advanced disease, there may be enlarged lymph nodes in the groin, abdomen or neck, a mass in the lower abdomen or an enlarged liver.
♦ Feeling the bladder with both hands while the patient is under anesthesia to determine the depth and extent of tumor penetration.

Blood and Other Tests
♦ Urinalysis for blood in the urine (hematuria).
♦ Complete blood count (CBC) to evaluate anemia.
♦ Chemistry profile to evaluate kidney, liver and bone abnormalities.
♦ Vigorous washing of the bladder for examination of the cells (cytology, or PAP) and flow cytometry.
♦ Flow cytometry—which can measure the number of chromosomes in tumor cells—can help evaluate the effectiveness of therapy and tumor aggressiveness more accurately.

Cells having more chromosomes than the usual number of two are called nondiploid or aneuploid cells and have a worse prognosis. The disappearance of tumor cells after anticancer drugs are placed inside the bladder is associated with a prolonged complete response.
♦ In the near future, bladder monoclonal antibodies, alone and combined with flow cytometry, should help in screening, diagnosis, predicting the potential for metastases, and response to therapy.

Imaging
♦ Intravenous pyelogram (IVP).
♦ Abdominal and pelvic CT scans and chest x-rays can help find metastases to lymph nodes, liver, lungs and surrounding bladder structures.

♦ MRI and ultrasound images of the abdomen and rectal and urethral areas are not very useful.

♦ Bone scans and bone x-rays are used before surgery only when there is bone pain.

Endoscopy and Biopsy

♦ Cystoscopy is the direct visualization of the bladder by passing a small rigid or flexible tube through the urethra into the bladder. Biopsy of tumor masses can be done at the time of cystoscopy.

♦ A new investigative staging procedure uses laparoscopic surgery in patients suspected of local tumor extension because CT and MRI scans are inaccurate in almost one-half of cases of high-grade (Grade 3–4) cancers that deeply invade bladder muscle or fat surrounding the bladder, or when cancer cells are found in the small blood and lymphatic vessels within the bladder muscle. With laparoscopic surgery, it is possible to remove selected lymph nodes and tissues to rule out the possibility that tumor extends outside the bladder. If tumor is found in lymph nodes, surgery would not be performed, and patients would be offered radiation therapy alone or chemotherapy followed by either radiation therapy or surgery.

STAGING

The TNM staging system is generally used for bladder cancer, although an alternative—the Jewett-Strong-Marshall system—is also used. There are slight differences in the two methods.

A major problem in clinical staging is the inaccuracy rate of 30 to 50 percent in determining precisely the extent of muscle and lymph node involvement when compared with the surgical or pathological staging of a tissue specimen.

In 20 to 40 percent of cases, high-grade (Grade 3) and high-stage (T3 and T4) lesions have lymph node metastases found at the time of surgery.

TREATMENT OVERVIEW

Treatment depends on the stage of disease. For superficial tumors that do not invade muscle, resection (cutting out), fulguration (burning out with heat or laser) or intravesical therapy (placing drugs directly into the bladder by a catheter inserted through the urethra) are the treatment options.

Therapy for muscle invasive lesions (Stages B and C) depends on the extent of invasion, the grade of the tumor and how involved the local lymph nodes and the blood vessels of the bladder are.

Surgery Removal of the tumor can often lead to cure. In selected cases where a single, relatively low grade tumor is found without carcinoma in situ, removing the tumor along with the adjacent portion of the bladder wall that guarantees an adequate margin (partial cystectomy) is appropriate.

But if the bladder shows evidence of "instability"—a tendency to continuously form new tumors as shown by the repeated presence of carcinoma in situ—a radical cystectomy is the treatment of choice. Radical cystectomy involves removing the entire bladder, the fat and tissue surrounding the bladder (perivesical) and the pelvic lymph nodes. In men, the prostate and seminal vesicles are removed. In women, the uterus, tubes, ovaries, anterior vaginal wall and urethra are removed.

Cystectomy raises many quality-of-life issues, especially concerning its effect on sexual function because of the nerves controlling penile erection being cut and the need for an ileal conduit (a piece of the gut or small bowel) leading to a large plastic bag outside of the body to collect urine.

Both problems have now been attacked and the various alternatives have to be discussed with a urologist. For instance, newer pouches (Kock, Indiana, Camay,

Mainz, etc.) have a large internal reservoir and a small external opening (nipple) that requires self-catheterization to remove urine only two or three times a day. This is much more appealing cosmetically because the external nipple can be left uncovered or be covered with an adhesive bandage. In some cases in males, a "neopouch" can be used—an attachment of a piece of bowel directly to the urethra—requiring no external pouch or catheterization at all. The neopouch cannot be used in females because of their short urethra.

Sexual function in males can also be improved by penile implants or by medication injected into the penis or inserted into the urethra before sex.

 Radiation External radiation can be used for more advanced stages of bladder cancer. Overall, the five-year survival rate for muscle invasive disease with surgery is 30 to 40 percent; for radical external radiation therapy, 20 to 30 percent.

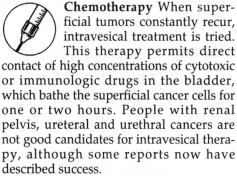 **Chemotherapy** When superficial tumors constantly recur, intravesical treatment is tried. This therapy permits direct contact of high concentrations of cytotoxic or immunologic drugs in the bladder, which bathe the superficial cancer cells for one or two hours. People with renal pelvis, ureteral and urethral cancers are not good candidates for intravesical therapy, although some reports now have described success.

There have been more studies of chemotherapy with single and combination drug regimens, before and/or after surgery or radiation therapy. If used before surgery (neoadjuvant), the aim is to decrease tumor size, increase the chance for a surgical cystectomy, destroy any tiny metastases that later seed the body but cannot be seen on x-rays or other imaging

studies, predict good-risk versus poor-risk cases, lead eventually to bladder preservation (no need for removal of the bladder and creation of a pouch) and, more important, increase survival.

Some studies in limited numbers of patients suggest benefit with neoadjuvant chemotherapy combined with either surgery or radiation therapy, but others have found only increased toxicity. The value of preoperative chemotherapy is being tested in the United States and Europe. Until the results are known, preoperative chemotherapy must still be considered investigational.

Patients with large bladder lesions (T4), nodal involvement (N+) or disseminated disease (M+) should be offered chemotherapy.

 Laser Therapy Superficial cancers can be treated by laser vaporization-coagulation with Nd:YAG or carbon dioxide (CO_2) lasers.

Combination Therapy Therapy with preoperative and/or postoperative radiation has not been found to be as effective in improving survival as previously thought and has been abandoned in many cancer centers. The real problem after a cystectomy is the appearance of distant metastases in over two-thirds of patients despite excellent local pelvic control of the cancer. High-grade, high-stage bladder cancers must be thought of as a disseminated disease. More systemic, instead of local, therapy will be required to improve survival.

 Biological Therapy The best immunological drug is BCG vaccine (used for tuberculosis vaccination) given by catheter inside the bladder (intravesical) weekly for six consecutive weeks. Cystoscopy and urine cytology with flow cytometry at six weeks after the last dose are used to evaluate effectiveness. If a partial response is seen, that is, fewer lesions are found than previously, another course may be given. BCG is completely effective in more than 60 percent of cases and has been proven to be better than no therapy and cytotoxic drugs.

People who respond completely to BCG not only have fewer superficial tumor recurrences but also develop fewer muscle invasive cancers requiring surgery. They also live significantly longer than non-responders.

BCG toxicity includes temporary local bladder irritation, fever and, in very rare cases, a type of tuberculosis infection that can be treated successfully with antitubercular drugs.

TREATMENT BY STAGE

STAGE 0
TNM Tis, N0, M0
Ta, N0, M0
In the Jewett-Strong-Marshall staging system, Stage 0 means the tumor is very superficial and does not even invade the lamina propria. It has not spread to lymph nodes and there are no metastases.

Tumors can be either a papillary exophytic mass (Ta or like a bunch of grapes on a thin stalk) or a flat Tis (Tumor in situ).

There is some controversy about the designation of Grade I (very well-differentiated) Ta lesions, since the malignant potential for spreading into lymph nodes or metastasizing is almost non-existent. Many urologists believe Ta Grade I tumors should be designated as non-cancerous benign papillomas, in contrast to Grades II and III Ta masses that are true cancers having the potential to invade their stalk and travel down into the lamina propria and then into muscle. People who develop one papilloma have about a 30 percent chance of developing another, while those with two or more have a 70 percent chance. Flat Tis lesions are considered aggressive.

Standard Treatment Surgery is the first treatment of choice and is generally curative. There is almost no requirement for a total cystectomy for benign papillomas. In selected cases, however, a segmental or partial cystectomy may be appropriate.

Intravesical therapy with BCG is used for recurrent papillomas, mostly as a preventive agent. Other effective anticancer drugs include thiophosphoramide (Thiotepa), doxorubicin (Adriamycin), mitomycin-C and, in Europe, epodyl (Ethoglucid) and epirubicin. Complete tumor prevention succeeds in 20 to 45 percent of cases given cytotoxic drugs and 65 percent given BCG. More important, none of these drugs seem to be cross-resistant with each other or with immunological drugs.

Patients with diffuse recurrent Tis or who fail one or more trials of intravesical therapy should be considered for cystectomy.

In the United States, external radiotherapy, radiation seeds or needles and intraoperative radiation therapy have not yet been proven effective in controlling or in preventing Stage 0 disease.

Five-Year Survival Over 90 percent

Investigational
♦ New immunological drugs—interferon, interleukin-2, tumor necrosis factor, keyhole-limpet extract—are being evaluated.
♦ New cytotoxic drugs such as epirubicin and mitoxantrone are being tested.
♦ Photodynamic laser therapy uses a photosensitizing material called hematoporphyrin that is similar to that found in red blood cells. Hematoporphyrin is unique in that it goes into all cells but remains for a prolonged time only in cancer cells and a laser will change the hematoporphyrin into a toxic drug. This technique is still experimental. A new study now suggests that vitamins A, C, E and beta carotene may be beneficial with BCG in preventing new tumors.

STAGE I or A
TNM T1, N0, M0

The tumor is superficial. It does not invade through the lamina propria and cannot be felt. There is no spread to lymph nodes and no metastases.

Standard Treatment Same as for Stage 0.

Five-Year Survival Over 75 percent

Investigational Same as for Stage 0.

STAGE II or B1
TNM T2, N0, M0

The tumor invades through the lamina propria into the inner half of muscle. Using two hands, the physician can feel the tumor before surgery.

Standard Treatment Surgery via the cytoscope can cure low-grade T2 lesions in highly selected patients. A partial or segmental cystectomy when the bladder is otherwise normal can be curative too. However, staging errors approach 50 percent, and if the T2 tumor is high grade (Grade III) or invades blood vessels it probably should be considered as a higher stage T3 or B2 lesion. In that case, a radical cystectomy is the preferred treatment, as it is for most T2 cancers.

Radiation therapy after complete removal of a T2 tumor with removal of the bladder at first sign of local relapse (salvage cystectomy) is another option that has produced almost similar results.

Five-Year Survival 55 to 70 percent, depending on tumor grade and the accuracy of staging

Investigational

♦ Combinations of cystectomy or of radiation therapy plus chemotherapy with cisplatin, and more recently with three and four drug chemotherapy regimens—called CMV, MCV (followed by radiation plus cisplatin) and M-VAC—look very promising. Some early results have described 60 to 70 percent complete remission rates with bladders being preserved in limited numbers of cases. These rates were discovered clinically (by cystoscopy), however. Only 15 to 30 percent have been found to be truly tumor-free with pathological staging after surgery.

Results of the ongoing randomized clinical trials will have to be reviewed before these combinations are accepted as superior to the "gold-standard" of cystectomy.

STAGE III or B2 and C
TNM T3, N0, M0

A tumor that invades deeply into muscle (more than halfway through) is designated as T3a, or B2 by the Jewett-Strong-Marshall system. If it invades into perivesical fat, it is a T3b, or C by the Jewett-Strong-Marshall system.

About 35 percent of clinical Stage III cases show tumor invasion outside the bladder at the time of surgery, so survival statistics vary. For those having tumors outside the bladder, survival is low—about 20 percent—with most relapsing from distant metastases. Survival rates are much better—30 to 50 percent—for true Stage III cases that have a lower grade and in those cases where the tumor can be downstaged (reduced) after preoperative radiation therapy or chemotherapy alone or after radiation therapy plus cisplatin.

Standard Treatment Cystectomy.

Five-Year Survival 20 to 40 percent

Investigational Treatment for this stage is becoming controversial. Since most patients do not do well with cystectomy alone, many investigators are entering patients into clinical trials that will answer the important question of how effective neoadjuvant therapy is in increasing survival.

♦ Two national protocols under investigation are: chemotherapy with M-VAC versus no chemotherapy before cystectomy; and MCV chemotherapy followed by combined radical (doses of 7,000 cGy) radiation therapy plus cisplatin.

Preliminary results suggest that patients downstaged from a T3 to a much lower stage tumor fare better. Patients are urged to participate in these studies so that correct answers to the true value of neoadjuvant therapy can be discovered.

STAGE IV or D
TNM T4, N0, M0
Any T, N1–3, M0
Any T, any N, M1
The tumor invades adjacent organs such as the prostate, uterus and vagina alone (T4a, N0, M0 / D1), or it spreads to the pelvic bone and abdominal wall (T4b, N0, M0 / D1), to pelvic lymph nodes (any T, N1–3, M0 / D1), to abdominal lymph nodes (any T, N4, M0 / D2) or to other organs (any T, any N, M1 / D2).

Almost half of Stage IV cases will be found, during surgery, to have lymph node involvement. The cystectomy fails because metastases occurred before the operation. Over 50 percent of patients with D2 disease die within one year, over 80 percent within two years, and less than 5 percent survive five years.

Standard Treatment Patients with extensive nodal disease should first be treated with chemotherapy. Only if the tumor completely disappears should cystectomy be considered as an adjuvant form of therapy.

Cystectomy, with or without radiation therapy, can be beneficial in a very limited number of T4a, N0–1, M0 cases, but if more than microscopic nodal involvement is found, adjuvant chemotherapy could be used. There is still no clear-cut proof that adjuvant chemotherapy is beneficial, but the prognosis for Stage IV is so poor that some form of additional treatment could be tried, preferably within the context of a clinical study.

Five-Year Survival 5 percent

Investigational
♦ Chemotherapy and chemoradiation therapy programs.

RECURRENT OR METASTATIC CANCER

Cisplatin, methotrexate, doxorubicin (Adriamycin) and vinblastine are active single chemotherapy agents and have been combined into a number of programs. Popular regimens include:
♦ Methotrexate + vinblastine + Adriamycin + cisplatin (M-VAC). Studies have proven that M-VAC is better than both CISCA and cisplatin alone and is the treatment of choice. Thirty-five to 70 percent of patients will respond, with 15 to 35 percent having a complete tumor regression that sometimes lasts more than five years in 10 to 15 percent.

The use of M-VAC is limited, however, by the need to maintain good kidney function (cisplatin and methotrexate are both excreted by the kidney) and the requirement that the patients cannot have significant cardiac abnormalities because of Adriamycin toxicity. CMV can be given to those who cannot take Adriamycin. Even when kidney and heart function are normal, full doses of Adriamycin or M-VAC can result in major complications in almost a quarter of cases.
♦ Investigational studies suggest that toxicity can be decreased and even higher M-VAC doses can be given when combined with granulocyte macrophage-colony stimulating factor (GM-CSF) or granulocyte-colony stimulating factor (G-CSF).
♦ carboplatin + methotrexate + vinblastine ± Adriamycin
♦ cisplatin + methotrexate + vinblastine (CMV or MCV)
♦ 5-fluorouracil + interferon
♦ Other single drugs that show some antitumor activity against bladder cancer include 5-fluorouracil, ifosfamide, carboplatin and gallium nitrate. Therapy remains limited for adenocarcinomas, although some respond to 5-fluorouracil

combinations.

♦ Radiation therapy can be palliative for bone and brain metastases.

♦ Immunological agents have not yet been adequately tested for this tumor.

THE MOST IMPORTANT QUESTIONS YOU CAN ASK

♦ What stage is my cancer?

♦ Do I need surgery, and how extensive would it be?

♦ What type of pouch is planned?

♦ What is the role of radiotherapy or chemotherapy?

♦ When do you place drugs into the bladder instead of doing surgery?

♦ How can I control my urine after my bladder is removed?

♦ How can I function sexually?

♦ If my bladder doesn't have to be removed, how often do I need to have cystoscopy performed?

♦ What is the role of antioxidant vitamins A, C, E and beta carotene?

BRAIN TUMORS: ADULT

Malin Dollinger, MD, James Fick, MD, Michael W. McDermott, MD, and Charles B. Wilson, MD

◇

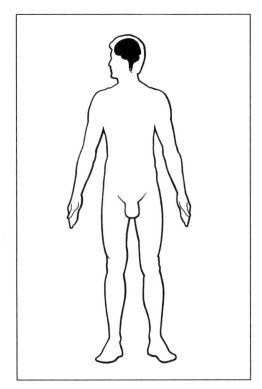

Primary brain tumors—those that arise in the brain itself—account for 1 percent of all cancers or 12,000 cases of brain tumors in the United States each year. As most of these tumors are malignant, they will cause 2.5 percent of all cancer-related deaths. They most commonly occur in the fifth and sixth decades of life but are the second most common form of cancer in childhood next to leukemia.

Tumors arising in some other part of the body may also spread to the brain (metastases). These most commonly come from cancers of the lung, breast, kidney and skin (malignant melanoma). Metastatic tumors to the brain are usually multiple, although a solitary metastasis can mimic a primary brain tumor.

Types Brain tumors can arise from many different types of cells within the brain, with tumors of the supporting cells more common than nerve cell tumors. A tumor is named for the cell from which it arises. Tumors derived from astrocytes are called astrocytomas and those from the ependymal cells are called ependymomas, for example. Tumors of the neurons include neuroblastomas, neurocytomas and ganglioneuromas. Meningiomas are tumors that originate from cells in the linings of the brain called the meninges. Other tumors include those derived from specialized brain structures such as the pineal gland, pituitary gland or choroid plexus.

What Causes It Most brain tumors have no known cause. The field of molecular genetics is devoted to understanding the changes that occur in cells that allow them to acquire malignant characteristics and form tumors. Although many of these cell alterations have been identified, the process of how these changes lead to the development of tumors is not yet well understood.

A variety of statistical and environmental associations have been made, but no chemical or environmental agent has been definitely shown to cause brain tumors.

Some inherited conditions predispose a person to the development of brain tumors. Patients with neurofibromatosis, tuberous sclerosis and familial polyposis have a tendency to develop astrocytomas.

Viruses are known to produce genetic changes in cells that in laboratory animals can induce the formation of a tumor.

There is an association in people infected with the Epstein-Barr virus and primary central nervous system lymphoma, although a definite causal relationship remains to be established. Central nervous system lymphoma frequently develops in immunosuppressed patients, such as those who have received an organ transplant or those who have AIDS.

Radiation can produce genetic damage in cells and induce tumors. It was once standard medical practice to use low doses of radiation to treat ringworm of the scalp in children. Years later it was found that children treated this way had an increased chance of developing tumors of the scalp, skull and brain. These radiation-induced tumors have a much greater likelihood of being malignant than do the forms that occur spontaneously.

SCREENING

There are no useful screening measures in healthy people. If a physician suspects a tumor on the basis of characteristic clinical signs, careful neurologic evaluation as well as CT or MRI scanning will lead to an earlier diagnosis and the best chance for long-term control or cure.

COMMON SIGNS AND SYMPTOMS

A brain tumor can produce neurologic symptoms and signs in two ways. The first is by increased pressure within the skull. As a tumor grows it occupies space and causes swelling in the surrounding brain. Since the brain is housed within a rigid and unyielding skull, only a limited amount of tumor mass and swelling is tolerated before symptoms are produced. The symptoms produced by increased intracranial pressure include:

♦ Headaches, which are frequently described as pressure at the top of the head and behind the eyes. These are usually made worse with exertion and are most severe at night or early in the morning.

♦ Nausea, which may be associated with vomiting.

♦ Lethargy, which may progress to the point where a patient spends most of the day sleeping.

♦ Confusion and disorientation.

The second category of symptoms are those that occur because of localized brain dysfunction. A tumor may invade or compress the surrounding brain. Depending on the extent or location of the tumor, the normal function of the brain at that location may be impaired. This loss of function may be noticed as numbness or weakness of an arm or a leg, loss of vision, difficulties with speech, and impaired memory and judgment. Such symptoms of neurological deficit can help to determine the location of a tumor.

♦ Symptoms also depend on age. Children may have vomiting, double vision, difficulty walking, and poor coordination of the arms and legs. Adults may have headaches, seizures, weakness or personality changes.

Seizures People with brain tumors often have seizures. They result when the brain is irritated, producing abnormal electrical activity locally and in the surrounding brain tissue.

♦ If this activity remains confined to a small area of brain, the result is a focal seizure. During this type of seizure, a patient remains conscious and may experience a strange sensation, such as a smell or taste, or have a brief episode of uncharacteristic behavior. Another common type of focal seizure includes the uncontrolled movement of an arm or leg. These seizures usually last from seconds to minutes and a complete recovery occurs within the same time period.

♦ A generalized seizure occurs when the electrical activity spreads throughout the brain. When this occurs, the patient loses consciousness, falls to the ground and may have uncontrolled movements of the body, arms and legs. Control over the

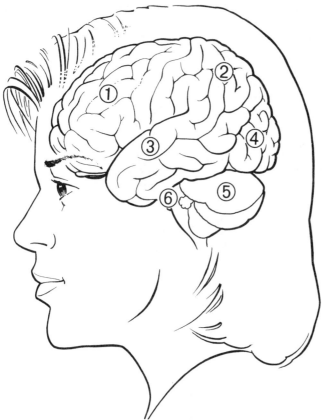

①	Frontal lobe
②	Parietal lobe
③	Temporal lobe
④	Occipital lobe
⑤	Cerebellum
⑥	Brainstem (Pons, Medulla)

Areas in the brain that develop brain tumors

bowel and bladder may be lost. The seizure can go on for several minutes, then it may take several hours for the person to awaken.

When a seizure occurs for the first time in an adult, a thorough evaluation, which includes a neurological examination and a diagnostic brain scan, should be done. Daily medication will be administered to prevent the seizures. Blood tests are performed to monitor the anticonvulsant drug level in the blood to make sure that it remains within the therapeutic range.

DIAGNOSIS

A neurologist or neurosurgeon often needs to evaluate the patient. Although an excellent tentative location can be suggested on the basis of a careful history (from the family as well as the patient) and neurologic evaluation, CT and MRI scans will usually confirm the suggested location. These scans are also used by the neurosurgeon and radiation oncologist to plan treatment.

Physical Examination
♦ As well as a complete neurologic examination, specific tests such as visual field determinations and hearing tests are sometimes useful.

Blood and Other Tests
♦ Routine blood tests will be performed as a baseline.

♦ Some tumors secrete substances that can be measured in the blood and cerebrospinal fluid (CSF). This fluid is removed by lumbar puncture (spinal tap), a procedure similar to spinal anesthesia. CSF may also be examined for malignant cells from tumors that have a tendency to spread from the brain into the spinal cord or its covering. A lumbar puncture may be risky when there is increased intracranial pressure. This risk has been largely removed now that CT or MRI scans can determine if there is enlargement of the fluid cavities within the brain (ventricles) or major pressure shifts within the brain.

Imaging
♦ Radiological evaluation plays an important role in both the diagnosis and management of brain tumors. The images are used by the neurosurgeon to decide whether a biopsy or a surgical resection of the tumor should be performed. The scans are repeated during the course of treatment to assess how the tumor is responding. The exact study chosen will depend upon the preferences of the treating physicians and may be influenced by the results of an initial scan.
♦ MRI and CT scans are the most often used. MRI images provide better definition between normal brain and tumors and can better depict the swelling associated with these tumors. MRI scans produce a three-dimensional image of the brain but can take over an hour to complete. The patient must hold very still in a tight space, which some find uncomfortable and confining.

A CT scan takes only minutes to complete but does not provide images with as much detail as MRI. CT scans provide superior images of calcified tumors and the skull. Contrast substances injected into a vein just before an MRI or CT scan is performed will cause some tumors to be enhanced so that they can be better defined. When a tumor is suspected, scans are usually performed both before and after contrast has been given.
♦ A tumor may be found near important blood vessels or have characteristics that suggest that it could be derived from a blood vessel. In these circumstances, a blood vessel study (angiogram) is performed. Dye is injected into the major feeding arteries of the brain and x-rays are taken.

Biopsy
♦ The diagnosis can be suggested by the above tests, but tumor tissue must be obtained by biopsy or surgery to confirm the tumor type and grade.
♦ Sometimes the tumor is small or in an area of the brain where it cannot be easily approached or safely removed. In such cases a special procedure called a stereotactic biopsy can be performed. A computer is used to plot a pathway to the tumor based upon a CT or MRI image. A small-caliber needle is then passed through the brain to the site of the tumor and a biopsy is obtained. This approach has proved to be very safe and effective in establishing a tissue diagnosis. In many cases it can be performed under local anesthesia. Patients can usually be discharged from the hospital the following day.
♦ When the tumor is accessible, a neurosurgeon may recommend an open operation (craniotomy) to attempt to remove some or nearly all of the tissue. Tumor samples will be sent for diagnosis at the time of the craniotomy.

STAGING

It is rare for primary brain tumors to spread outside the nervous system, so staging procedures of organs in the rest of the body are not routinely performed.

Certain brain tumors have a tendency to spread not only in the brain but also into the spinal cord. These tumors include lymphomas, medulloblastomas, pinealblastomas, germinomas, ependymomas and tumors of the choroid plexus. When they are diagnosed, staging of the spinal cord is also required. This staging process includes scans of both the brain and spine and a lumbar puncture to obtain cerebrospinal fluid for microscopic evaluation.

When a metastatic tumor of the brain is discovered, a thorough staging of the rest of the body should be performed. Treatment for a patient with a metastatic brain tumor will depend on the extent of spread of the primary tumor.

TREATMENT OVERVIEW

Several characteristics of brain tumors distinguish them from other types of tumors.

♦ Even the most malignant brain tumors rarely metastasize outside the nervous system.

♦ The location of a tumor often determines whether a neurological deficit occurs.

♦ The most common brain tumor, the astrocytoma, ranges from a low- to high-grade type (the grade of each tumor is based on its microscopic features and determines type of treatment and prognosis).

♦ Even tumors regarded as slow growing or more benign can produce symptoms as severe and life-threatening as malignant tumors. This is because they may occur in a vital area of the brain or because when they reach a critical size there is no room for them to expand within the surrounding skull. This puts significant pressure on key structures.

♦ The brain has no lymphatic blood vessels to remove the products of tumor dissolution, so the tumor may not appear to shrink on CT or MRI scans even if treatment is successful.

♦ Treatment of a tumor can result in a new neurological deficit. A temporary or permanent loss of function can occur after surgery and problems of brain swelling can occur during radiation treatments, for example.

♦ Unless a dramatic, early and sustained improvement occurs after therapy, it may be difficult for a long time to determine the response to treatment. Treatments may themselves produce temporary neurological deterioration that might take weeks or months to clear.

 Surgery Surgery is the front line treatment for primary brain tumors. The goal of surgery is to confirm the diagnosis and remove as much of the tumor as possible without causing a loss of neurologic function. Some tumors can be completely removed and the patient cured, but surgery alone is not sufficient to cure a patient with a malignant tumor and other forms of treatment will be required. Surgically reducing the size of the cancer may improve the efficiency of other therapies.

The surgical removal of tumors can improve a patient's neurological condition. Increased intracranial pressure is usually reduced and a focal neurological deficit may improve or resolve. The frequency of seizures may also be reduced. Tumors can block the fluid pathways in the brain, leading to buildup of fluid, called hydrocephalus, which can be associated with symptoms of increased intracranial pressure. To relieve these symptoms, it is sometimes necessary to place a permanent shunting device into the fluid cavities to divert the fluid to another part of the body where it can be absorbed.

Specialized equipment used during surgery includes a microscope to magnify the operative field, an ultrasonic aspirator that helps break up the tumor, lasers that vaporize tumor tissue, ultrasound localizing equipment and computer-based navigational equipment to help the surgeon define the tumor boundaries.

Specialized techniques are used to remove a tumor located near speech or motor brain regions. The surface of the brain can be stimulated with an electrical current to obtain clues about the function of a particular part of the brain. This is referred to as speech or motor "mapping." The process is painless and produces only mild speech disturbance or twitching of the part of the body served by that area of the brain. A decision can then be made about whether it is safe to remove that part of the tumor. Speech mapping is done under sedation and local anesthesia and requires a cooperative patient. Motor mapping can be performed under general anesthesia.

 Radiation Radiation is effective in the treatment of both primary and metastatic brain tumors. The treatments are designed to maximize the lethal effects on the tumor and minimize the harmful effects to the surrounding brain. Computer-generated models are used to plan the dose and field of irradiation.

Treatments are generally given five days a week. Some patients may become fatigued or develop neurological problems related to radiation-induced brain swelling. This problem is usually brief and is treated with steroid medication to alleviate the swelling. A full course of conventional radiation can be administered only once. Exposing the brain to further extensive radiation could produce brain injury and create a disabling or a life-threatening problem.

New methods of delivering additional radiation to brain tumors are being used in investigational treatment protocols across the country. One of these approaches is to administer the radiation several times each day. Using these "hyperfractionated" schedules, a higher dose can be safely administered. Radiation-sensitizing drugs can be given in an attempt to increase the effect on a tumor.

Two techniques have been developed that provide a focal boost of radiation to a tumor after a conventional course of radiation has been given.

♦ With interstitial brachytherapy, radioactive seeds are placed, with computer guidance, directly into a tumor mass.

♦ Stereotactic radiosurgery ("gamma knife") directs many precisely focused external radiation beams at a tumor.

Using these techniques, a high dose of radiation may be given to a tumor while the surrounding brain is spared the adverse effects. These approaches require that the tumor be small to medium-sized and in an area of the brain that could tolerate a radiation injury without causing the loss of an important function. This approach has shown promise in the treatment of both primary and metastatic tumors and will likely play an increasing role in the future.

 Chemotherapy Chemotherapy can be effective when used before or after surgery and radiation. It can be used at the time of diagnosis and for a recurrence. Some tumors in the brain can be exquisitely sensitive to chemotherapy, including germinomas, lymphomas and oligodendrogliomas.

A roadblock to treating brain tumors with chemotherapy is that the drugs do not easily pass through the blood vessels in the brain into the brain substance where the tumor is located. Some experimental approaches have investigated ways to open this blood-brain barrier with drugs, while others have attempted to directly inject drugs into the major arteries feeding a tumor. Research is focused on developing drugs that have increased specificity for brain tumors and that can easily cross the blood brain-barrier.

Biological Therapy Gene therapy is a new approach to treating brain tumors and relies on the transfer of a new gene into tumor cells. The tumor then receives a new set of instructions.

One approach uses a virus to infect the tumor and insert a gene into the cancer cells. The infected cells become susceptible to an anti-viral medication and they die when treated with it. This technique has shown great promise and efforts are under way to begin treating humans.

Advances in the field of immunology have led to ground-breaking work in using the immune system to fight tumors. Methods have been developed to insert new genes into immune cells that will improve their tumor-fighting abilities. New research is focusing on using interferon, a compound that stimulates the immune system, to attack brain tumors.

TREATMENT BY TUMOR TYPE

ASTROCYTOMA

Astrocytomas are categorized by their grade of malignancy. Most classification schemes include low-grade astrocytoma (Grade I/II), anaplastic astrocytoma (Grade III) and glioblastoma multiforme (Grade IV).

Standard Treatment In children, low-grade astrocytomas can sometimes be cured with complete surgical removal. Radiation is reserved for recurrent tumors. In adults, these tumors infiltrate the brain and cannot be completely removed, so radiation therapy is recommended.

Treatment for the anaplastic astrocytoma often includes surgery, radiation and chemotherapy.

The glioblastoma multiforme is a very aggressive tumor that grows quickly and invades into the surrounding brain. Complete surgical removal is uncommon. Surgery and radiation are rarely curative.

Five-Year Survival 50 percent for low-grade astrocytomas. For the anaplastic astrocytoma, the two-year life expectancy is 50 percent. For the glioblastoma multi-

forme, the average life expectancy is one year.

OLIGODENDROGLIOMA

People with this tumor often have a history of seizures.

Standard Treatment Oligodendrogliomas are treated in a similar manner to astrocytomas, with surgery and radiation the favored methods. They can also be successfully treated with a chemotherapy regimen consisting of procarbazine, lomustine and vincristine. Many of these tumors also have a component of an astrocytoma. It is standard practice to grade these mixed tumors by the component that predominates. Like the astrocytomas, the higher-grade oligodendrogliomas have a poor prognosis.

BRAIN STEM GLIOMA

This tumor is an astrocytoma that occurs in the brain stem. Brain stem gliomas can cause incapacitating neurological deficits. They have a very characteristic appearance on an MRI scan, and treatment is often performed without first obtaining a tissue diagnosis.

Standard Treatment These tumors are treated with radiation and sometimes chemotherapy. Surgery is rarely useful. The radiation is often given twice a day and in a higher dose than is used for other brain tumors.

Five-Year Survival 20 to 30 percent

MEDULLOBLASTOMA

This tumor occurs more often in children than in adults. Most cases occur in those under 16 years of age.

Standard Treatment Surgery followed by irradiation to the brain and spine. Chemotherapy is used after surgery in children too young to undergo irradiation or in cases where tumor remains after surgery and irradiation.

Medulloblastomas tend to spread throughout the nervous system. Scans of the brain and spine, along with cerebrospinal fluid cytology, are used to follow the condition of the tumor. Survival depends on whether it has already spread when diagnosed.

Five-Year Survival 60 percent when the tumor can be completely removed, but this drops dramatically if there is residual tumor after surgery or if the tumor has spread throughout the nervous system.

MENINGIOMA

Most meningiomas are benign tumors in the covering of the brain. Some have malignant features and behave aggressively. They produce symptoms by compression of the surrounding brain and by the swelling that they incite.

Standard Treatment Many meningiomas can be cured by surgical removal alone. Radiation can be an effective treatment for incompletely removed tumors and malignant or recurrent forms, but repeated surgical resections are sometimes required. Meningiomas that grow along the skull base are very difficult to remove and often require a combination of surgery and radiation to control the tumor.

PITUITARY ADENOMA

The great majority of pituitary tumors are benign. They can cause visual loss (which occurs when the tumor compresses the nearby optic nerves), fluid and electrolyte imbalances and endocrine problems caused by an excessive amount of pituitary hormones in the bloodstream. The most common hormonal problems include:

♦ an excess of prolactin hormone, leading to impotence in men and excessive lactation in women;

♦ an excess of growth hormone that can lead to an enlarged heart, growth of the hands and feet and a change in facial features;

♦ an excess of cortisol, which can lead to weight gain, diabetes and high blood pressure.

Standard Treatment The drug bromocriptine can successfully treat a prolactin hormone-producing pituitary tumor. Treatment of other tumors is with surgery known as a transphenoidal hypophysectomy. In this procedure, the tumor is removed through the sphenoid sinus at the back of the nasal cavity so the skull does not have to be opened (craniotomy).

Some tumors can be cured with surgery alone. Others require postoperative treatment with medication and irradiation.

If visual loss has been present only for a short time, some recovery of vision can occur after surgery relieves the pressure on the optic nerves.

PRIMARY CENTRAL NERVOUS SYSTEM LYMPHOMA

These tumors are especially seen in patients whose immune systems have been suppressed. This suppression may be because of inherited immunosuppressive diseases, after therapy for organ transplantation or other acquired conditions that suppress immunity such as tuberculosis, blood vessel inflammation (vasculitis), lupus erythematosus and Epstein-Barr (EB) virus infection. Primary lymphoma of the central nervous system has become a common manifestation of AIDS.

Standard Treatment The role of surgery is usually to establish a tissue diagnosis, since there are usually multiple lesions that are inaccessible and surgery is not curative.

Radiation produces improvement, but relapse may occur in one to two years.

Studies are evaluating various chemotherapy combinations. It is clear that remissions can be produced, but it is not yet known which therapy is the most effective.

Five-Year Survival Unusual

METASTATIC CANCER TO THE CENTRAL NERVOUS SYSTEM

The number of patients with metastatic intracranial tumors exceeds the number of those with primary brain tumors by a factor of 10. Brain metastasis can occur in 25 percent of all people with cancer. Since cancer patients are now living longer, it is expected that the number of people with metastatic tumors will continue to increase. The finding of brain metastases will radically change the intent and direction of therapy. This generally takes precedence over almost any other complication.

When someone with cancer develops headaches, drowsiness, personality changes or problems with speech, strength or balance, a brain metastasis should be suspected. Although a single metastasis can occur, it is more common for there to be multiple tumors. MRI scans are best able to detect multiple metastases.

A primary tumor in the body can cause no signs or symptoms. When a tumor in the brain is discovered, a physician will always consider the possibility that it could represent a metastasis.

If there are multiple brain tumors, there is a greater chance that they are metastatic rather than primary. A screening evaluation may then be performed to look for other tumors in the body. This evaluation includes blood tests, a chest x-ray and CT scans of the chest and abdomen. Initial therapy usually includes corticosteroid hormones such as Decadron to immediately reduce the pressure in the brain and thereby relieve symptoms.

Standard Treatment Many metastatic tumors are located over the surface of the brain and can be safely removed. Radiation is given after surgery. If there are multiple tumors, surgery is deferred and the treatment is irradiation.

Even when small, these tumors can cause considerable swelling. In most cases, radiation is given to the entire brain with the hope of eliminating any small tumor deposits not yet seen on a scan. This can lead to memory loss and a decline in intelligence, so in most patients the highest radiation dose is limited to the tumor site. Avoiding these side effects is important for those with tumors with a fairly good prognosis, such as breast cancer.

The treatment of intracranial metastasis with stereotactic radiosurgery has shown great promise. This focused radiation can successfully control tumor growth. It offers the advantage of being able to treat multiple tumors at one time and can be repeated if new lesions develop.

Metastatic tumor cells can line the fluid cavities and surface of the brain. This is called carcinomatous meningitis. It can be disabling, and is treated by instilling chemotherapy into the spinal fluid. This can be done by lumbar puncture, or a specialized catheter can be placed into the ventricle of the brain and then connected to a small plastic reservoir placed under the skin. Drugs can then be injected into the reservoir to circulate throughout the spinal fluid.

TUMORS OF THE SPINAL CORD

Tumors can develop in the spinal cord just like in the brain. The most common are astrocytomas, ependymomas and meningiomas. They are more often low grade than high grade. They also lead to neurological deficits when they invade or compress the spinal cord. MRI imaging is becoming more valuable for accurately evaluating spinal cord tumors.

These tumors are usually slow growing, and the problems they cause develop over months or years. These problems include sensory loss and pain, paralysis, incontinence of the bowel and bladder and impotence in males.

Cancers arising elsewhere can metastasize to the spine or spinal cord and produce pressure symptoms such as pain, weakness or loss of sensation (numbness). Diagnostic methods are similar to those for primary spinal cord tumors.

Standard Treatment Surgery is the preferred method of treatment. Ependymomas can often be completely removed. Radiation is used if there is residual tumor.

Astrocytomas have infiltrating margins and usually cannot be completely removed. They are biopsied or the solid component removed, then they are irradiated. Meningiomas can often be completely removed. If there is residual tumor and it is benign, a series of clinical and radiographic evaluations will be performed. A repeat operation or radiation is used if the tumor grows and causes new problems.

A fluid-filled cavity can develop within the spinal cord near a tumor. This is called a syrinx, and it can grow to a large size and cause pain and loss of spinal cord function. It can also lead to wasting of the affected muscles. An operation to shunt the fluid from this cavity can improve the neurological condition and alleviate symptoms.

TREATMENT FOLLOW-UP

The response of a brain tumor to treatment may not be immediately apparent. A series of scans may be required to determine whether the tumor is growing. The changes that are seen on a brain scan after surgery can resemble residual tumor, and the swelling that occurs in response to the surgery can be identical in appearance to that caused by a tumor. Serial scans are performed with the goal of detecting a recurrent tumor early.

SUPPORTIVE THERAPY

♦ Swelling of the brain can persist after treatments have been completed. Swelling also often accompanies recurrent tumors. It can cause neurological deficits and create symptoms of increased intracranial pressure. The corticosteroid medication dexamethasone (Decadron) is used to decrease this swelling.

♦ A few patients need a very low maintenance dose of corticosteroid hormones even if the tumor is not active or has been controlled. In such cases, some of the original symptoms, such as headache, nausea or neurological abnormalities, may recur if the steroid hormones are discontinued.

♦ Medications are sometimes needed to eliminate nausea and relieve pain.

♦ The risk of seizures can persist over the patient's lifetime. Medications are given to prevent this from happening. The drugs used most often include phenytoin (Dilantin), carbamazepine (Tegretol) and phenobarbital. Blood tests are performed to measure the amount of the drug in the blood. The dose required to control seizures varies from patient to patient. Sometimes two different drugs have to be used.

♦ Neurologic status may change or deteriorate because of the cascade of secondary effects on the brain rather than because of tumor growth. Factors causing apparent neurologic deterioration may include lowering the steroid dosage too rapidly, mineral or electrolyte imbalance, complications such as infections or metabolic problems, other medications, particularly for pain, and the effects of radiation therapy.

Tumor destruction from radiation may briefly produce waste products that may irritate the brain. Because the brain lacks lymphatic blood vessels, there is no efficient method of removing the waste materials, which is why tumors responding to treatment may not appear to change in size for a long time.

♦ Tumors cause neurological problems that can persist well after all treatments have been completed. The speed and extent of any recovery will depend on how severe the deficits are. Rehabilitative therapies can speed the recovery along, improve overall endurance and maintain muscle tone and strength. Children, young adults and the elderly can all benefit from rehabilitative therapies.

RECURRENT CANCER

The earlier a recurrent tumor is found, the more options there are for treatment and the greater the chance that treatment will be successful. Health permitting, surgery is the most effective treatment for a recurrent tumor. A focal boost of radiation to the tumor using radioactive implants or stereotactic radiosurgery can be effective. Chemotherapy is often used to treat recurrent tumors.

THE MOST IMPORTANT QUESTIONS YOU CAN ASK

♦ What type of brain cancer do I have?
♦ How does it usually behave?
♦ What type of surgery is most useful and what are the risks?
♦ Will I need radiation afterwards?
♦ Is there a role for chemotherapy?
♦ Will my symptoms go away?
♦ What medications do I need?
♦ How functional can I expect to be?

BREAST

Malin Dollinger, MD, Ernest H. Rosenbaum, MD, Christopher Benz, MD, William H. Goodson, III, MD, Gary Friedman, MD, Edward A. Sickles, MD, Lawrence W. Margolis, MD, T. Stanley Meyler, MD, and I. Craig Henderson, MD

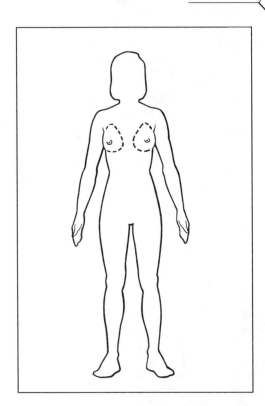

Breast cancer is the most common malignancy in women, affecting about one woman in 9. About 180,000 women will develop breast cancer in the United States in 1994, and about 45,000 will die of it. Breast cancer is most treatable when detected in its earliest stages, and there is great interest in screening healthy women—beginning when they are between 30 and 40 years old— with mammography and periodic physical examinations. These measures will detect breast cancers at a much earlier stage, resulting in earlier treatment and a better chance for cure.

For decades, breast cancer was treated by the Halsted radical mastectomy or a modified radical mastectomy. Women whose cancer was inoperable or who had residual or recurrent local disease were given radiotherapy. Those with metastatic disease were given chemotherapy and radiotherapy. Over the past 20 years, the approach to evaluating and treating breast cancer has changed considerably.

Types Breast cancers are divided generally into two types: invasive cancers and non-invasive or in situ cancers. Invasive cancers are generally divided into lobular and ductal cancers. Lobular cancers start in the many small sacs in the breast that produce milk. The much more common ductal cancers start in the tubes that carry milk from the lobules to the nipple. Within these broad categories, there are over 30 histologic types as seen under the microscope. About half are infiltrating ductal cancers, meaning that they spread through the duct wall. Another 28 percent are combinations of infiltrating ductal cancers and other types, including mucinous, papillary and lobular.

Infiltrating lobular carcinoma (5 to 10 percent of breast cancers), which is often detected as a thickening of the breast tissue rather than as a lump, may be found in many places, not only in the same breast but also in the opposite one.

Other infiltrating cancers include Paget's disease, a cancer that begins in the area of the nipple and is associated with bleeding, redness, itching and burning (this is not the same as Paget's disease of bone, which is a chronic benign process), and inflammatory breast cancer, which shows up as a hot, red, swollen area having the appearance of an infection or inflammation. This sub-type has a worse prognosis, because the red color and warmth of the skin indicate that tumor cells have already spread into many lymphatic vessels.

In situ cancers are confined within the lining of the ducts or lobules. These are early cancers or precancerous lesions that have not developed the ability to become invasive. They are generally of two types. Ductal in situ carcinomas (also called intraductal or ductal carcinoma in situ [DCIS]) do have the ability over a long period to become invasive cancer if untreated. So these tumors have to be completely removed. In situ lobular cancers (also called lobular carcinoma in situ [LCIS) are best understood as markers for the risk of developing cancer. It is not usually possible to remove all lobular carcino-

mas in situ without removing all of both breasts. This is excessive treatment in most situations, so very careful follow-up is often recommended after removal of the in situ lesion. Treatment at the time of diagnosis may also include radiotherapy (for DCIS only).

Nearly all breast cancers arise from glandular tissue (adenocarcinomas), although other types also occur, including squamous cell carcinomas, sarcomas, carcinosarcomas, cystosarcoma phylloides and sweat gland carcinomas. There are several less common types which have a generally better prognosis than infiltrating ductal cancer such as medullary carcinoma (6 percent of cases), mucinous (2.5 percent) and tubular (1 percent). Each type has prognostic and therapeutic implications.

How It Spreads After cancer starts, it may be several years before a lump appears.

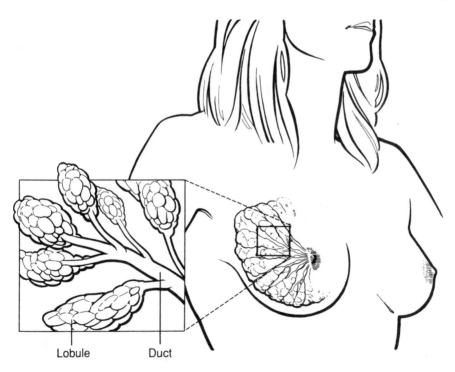

Lobule   Duct

Normal breast structures in which cancers may develop

There are wide differences in the way a breast cancer behaves. It may remain confined to the breast for a long time, or, in other cases, spread to nearby lymph nodes and distant organs early in the disease.

What Causes It No definite cause has been established, although genetic factors, personal history and diet all play a role.

RISK FACTORS

At Significantly Higher Risk
♦ History of previous cancer in one breast, especially if it occurred before menopause.

At Slightly Higher Risk
♦ Increasing age.
♦ Family history of breast cancer, primarily in parents, daughters and sisters, but also in second-degree relatives such as aunts, cousins and grandmothers. This is true for relatives on the father's side as well as the mother's. (Genetic markers are becoming available to screen for some forms of familial breast cancer.) The risk is about 6 times greater if a mother or sister had breast cancer before menopause, and up to 10 times greater if the cancer was in both breasts. A specific gene for familial breast cancer has been discovered (17q21).
♦ Carriers of the familial breast cancer gene BRCA-1, which is associated with a high risk of developing breast cancer and transmitting this risk to offspring.
♦ Some premalignant breast lesions may be associated with development of breast cancer, including multiple papillomatosis, atypical hyperplasia and, occasionally, very large cysts in the breast (not the more common and smaller fibrocystic breast condition). Most women with fibrocystic changes are not at increased risk because of them. There is no relation between these palpable breast changes and the risk of cancer.
♦ There is a slightly higher risk for women who have never carried a term pregnancy or who were first pregnant after age 30.

♦ Early onset of menstruation and late onset of menopause.
♦ Excessive radiation, with an increased risk for women who were given radiation for postpartum mastitis, received prolonged fluoroscopic x-ray evaluations for tuberculosis or were exposed to a large amount of radiation before the age of 40.
♦ Women with a family history of cancer of the cervix, uterus or colon have a slightly increased risk of developing breast cancer.
♦ Female descendents of European Jews have a higher than normal risk.
♦ Obesity with excess caloric and fat intake (three times the usual risk).

At Lower Risk
♦ Term pregnancy under age 18.
♦ Early menopause.
♦ Surgical removal of the ovaries before age 37.
♦ Japanese ancestry (but not if born in America and adopting American dietary habits).

Factors That May Affect Risk, but Whose Role Is Unclear
♦ Taking female hormones such as postmenopausal estrogens or premenopausal contraceptives. Some studies have suggested an increased risk with early oral contraceptive use or many years of estrogen replacement at menopause. Other studies have *not* shown an increased risk with either oral contraceptive use or estrogen replacement therapy. These findings need further study.
♦ A low-calorie, low-fat (especially animal fat), high-fiber or Oriental-style diet may decrease risk.
♦ Controversy continues regarding breast feeding. Some studies suggest that breast feeding may reduce the risk of breast cancer, particularly in cultures where prolonged breast feeding (several years for each child) is the norm.

Factors Not Related to Breast Cancer
♦ Fibrocystic breasts.

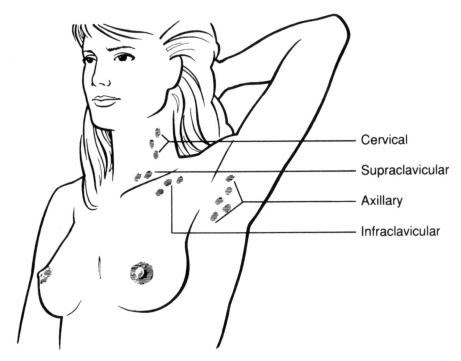

Cervical

Supraclavicular

Axillary

Infraclavicular

Regional lymph nodes important in breast cancer

♦ Multiple pregnancies.
♦ Coffee or caffeine intake.

SCREENING

A thorough breast examination should be part of every routine physical and be included with a yearly gynecologic checkup. There are three well-proven methods for detecting early breast cancer.

Mammography for Apparently Healthy Women There is now widespread agreement that mammography (low-dose x-ray imaging of the breasts) can discover cancers at least a year before—and sometimes as much as four years before—they can be felt. The scientific evidence is most convincing for screening women over age 50, but there is evidence that it may be beneficial for younger women.
♦ The American Cancer Society recommends that women have mammography every year or two between age 40 and 49

and yearly thereafter. Yearly mammograms are recommended beginning at age 30 when the risk of breast cancer is very high (because of prior breast cancer, history of premenopausal breast cancer in a mother or sister or a breast biopsy showing atypical hyperplasia).
♦ The smallest lump usually felt is about 1/3 in. (1 cm) and contains 1 billion cancer cells. Routine mammography can detect smaller cancers, some even less than 1/5 in. (0.5 cm). It is estimated that five-year survival is 20 to 25 percent better for cancers detected by mammography than for those diagnosed after a lump has appeared. Women screened regularly with modern mammography (after 1985) have only a 10 to 30 percent rate of axillary node metastasis, compared to 50 percent for women who do not undergo screening.
♦ Some concern has been expressed

about the risk of frequent x-ray imaging, but the potential benefits far outweigh the risks. The x-ray dose of a mammogram today is about one-tenth that of 25 years ago and is about the same as the cosmic radiation received during a transcontinental airplane flight. The risk of mammography causing a tumor has been compared to the risk of getting lung cancer from smoking one cigarette.

Breast Self-Examination Monthly breast self-examination (BSE) is widely advocated and taught although scientific evidence supporting its use is still being developed. BSE can detect cancers earlier than no screening at all. To be useful, BSE should be done regularly, preferably every month. BSE can be taught by trained physicians and nurses, and most communities have centers to teach women how to perform this examination. BSE identifies a large number of breast lumps that are not cancer, more so than either mammography or physical examination.

Breast Examination Examination of the breasts is a component of routine physical checkups. Benign lumps and masses as well as areas of thickening occur from time to time in most women, and repeated examinations by a physician may call attention to areas that deserve further testing. Physicians often draw in their records diagrams of areas of change or concern, which makes it easier to detect small changes at the next examination.

Although mammography is the most effective screening method, about 10 to 15 percent of cancers will be missed by mammography yet found by physical examination, including BSE. Complete breast cancer screening involves all three methods.

COMMON SIGNS AND SYMPTOMS

Breast lumps are found in most patients, although sometimes the lump is seen only on mammography and no mass can be felt. The cancer is often hard and irregular and may feel different from the rest of the breast. There may also be a persistent lump in the armpit (axilla), a symptom of enlarged lymph glands. Pain in the breast is more often due to a benign condition, but medical evaluation is advised.

Spontaneous discharge from the nipple of one breast may indicate breast cancer but most discharges are from benign conditions and most cancers do not have a discharge. There may be irregularity or retraction of the breast skin or nipple. Scaling of the nipple may indicate Paget's disease, a form of local nipple cancer.

In advanced cases, there may be significant swelling or distortion of the skin or breast. Skin pores may be accentuated because of lymphatic involvement, creating an appearance resembling the skin of an orange, known medically as peau d'orange. This may indicate the advanced stage called inflammatory breast carcinoma, which may also be signaled by redness, swelling or increased heat in the skin.

Breast cancer may occasionally first appear as metastatic disease, with signs or symptoms related to whatever other organ is involved—pain in an area of bony metastasis, swelling in the neck, lung nodules seen on chest x-rays or liver enlargement.

DIAGNOSIS

It may be difficult to clinically distinguish malignant from benign breast masses such as fibrous tumors (fibroadenomas), fatty collections, inflammatory masses, infections or cysts. In premenopausal patients, it is common for benign lesions to enlarge just before menstrual periods and then shrink.

It is often helpful for the physician to draw an exact diagram with a description of a newly detected mass. Mammography and/or biopsy may be useful, but if these are not done the mass should be re-examined one or two months later if there is any suspicion that it might be cancer. If the mass persists, mammography and biopsy should be considered.

Physical Examination
♦ Physical examination of the breast is conducted with the patient in various positions and with careful recording of any suspicious masses or abnormal findings.
♦ This should be accompanied by a complete physical, including a pelvic examination and evaluation for signs of cancer in other locations such as the skin, lymph nodes and liver.

Blood and Other Tests
♦ Blood counts and chemistry panel to determine organ function and detect metastases, including liver function tests (alkaline phosphatase, LDH and SGOT).
♦ Tumor marker blood tests—including serum carcinoembryonic antigen (CEA) and CA 15-3—may be performed to help determine prognosis and response to therapy.
♦ Tumor tissue tests, including hormone receptors, DNA and other protein markers with potential diagnostic and prognostic value (*see* below).

Imaging
♦ Mammography is helpful in evaluating a suspicious mass, especially if it is new or persistent. It is also useful in women whose breasts are large and difficult to examine or who have had implants. Mammography is also used to locate precisely the position and extent of a known tumor. A standard two-view mammogram and specialized views, including magnified images, can provide vital information, but mammography is not a definitive diagnostic test since 10 to 15 percent of cancers are not detectable by this technique. A suspicious palpable mass should be biopsied even if mammography does not show cancer.
♦ Mammograms may detect an abnormality elsewhere in the same or opposite breast. These images may show microcalcifications suspicious for cancer (even if no mass is palpable) or a smaller, non-palpable but still suspicious mass. In this situation, a biopsy must be done, usually guided by mammography, to determine whether the lesion is cancer.
♦ Mammography may also be used to evaluate women with precancerous breast conditions, to evaluate yearly the opposite breast of women with known breast cancer (as there is a higher risk of developing cancer there) and to evaluate women with metastatic adenocarcinoma from an unknown primary source. Sometimes the primary source is a hidden breast cancer. This last point is especially important because breast cancer may respond to chemotherapy or hormonal therapy not used to treat other forms of metastatic cancer.
♦ Ultrasound evaluation (breast ultrasonography) may be used to diagnose cysts. The accuracy of ultrasonography in determining whether a mass is cystic (containing fluid) or solid approaches 100 percent. This may eliminate the need for more complex procedures. Some physicians prefer to withdraw fluid from all cysts with a simple needle and syringe (aspiration). If clear fluid is removed and the mass completely disappears, no further treatment or evaluation is needed.
♦ Tissue should be removed by biopsy for microscopic examination if a mass is still present after fluid is removed, if blood is removed, if abnormal cells are found in the fluid, if no fluid can be aspirated or if the mass returns two weeks later (*see* biopsy diagram, page 22.)
♦ Chest x-rays will assess lungs, ribs and the spine for metastases. Specialized x-rays of other areas may be done if there are specific bodily complaints.
♦ Bone scan will rule out bone metastases. This is often not necessary with small cancers.

♦ An abdominal CT scan may be done to evaluate the liver, especially if the serum alkaline phosphatase (a bone and liver enzyme) is elevated.

Biopsy

♦ Almost all biopsies of suspicious breast masses used to be open surgical biopsies, but fine needle aspiration (FNA) biopsy is being used more often. This simple office procedure can usually give a definitive answer about the possibility of cancer, but interpretation by a specially trained cytologist or pathologist is necessary to evaluate the tissue correctly. About 1 in 20 aspirations does not confirm a malignancy when one is known to be present (false negative), so either a repeat FNA, a needle-guided biopsy or an open surgical biopsy should be done if mammography or physical findings are suspicious and the initial FNA is negative.

♦ Mammography may help guide the surgeon to do an open biopsy of the correct area. This is especially important for non-palpable lesions. A needle is placed within or adjacent to the lesion under x-ray guidance (needle localization). A mammogram is then done to make sure the suspicious area has been removed.

♦ Stereotactic fine-needle biopsy and core biopsy are specialized mammography procedures, similar to needle localization, that rely on computer assistance to allow a biopsy needle to be positioned even more precisely. These techniques are used mainly for small non-palpable lesions detected by mammography alone.

STAGING

Stage is directly related to prognosis and determines the type of treatment to be offered, especially when several therapies are available. The TNM classification system is used to stage breast cancer according to the size of the primary tumor (T), the involvement of the lymph nodes in the armpit (axillary nodes) next to the affected breast (N) and the presence or absence of metastasis (M). The clinical stages range from Stage I to IV. Stage 0 is in situ cancer, which is still localized to the point of origin and has not yet begun to invade outward or spread. TNM staging for breast cancer is shown on page 326, 328, 330 and 331.

FACTORS AFFECTING PROGNOSIS AND TREATMENT DECISIONS

The prognosis and selection of therapy are influenced by the size, type and stage of the cancer, the microscopic appearance and tumor grade, the involvement of axillary lymph nodes and the number of nodes involved, and the woman's age and her menopausal status (natural or surgically induced) at the time of diagnosis. The larger the cancer, the more likely it has spread to axillary lymph nodes and metastasized.

They are also influenced by several other increasingly important prognostic factors. These tests offer predictive information about the risk of recurrence or metastasis. This may make it possible to identify women with a worse prognosis who should be offered earlier and/or more aggressive therapy. Prognostic markers also help oncologists tailor the most appropriate forms of adjuvant chemotherapy to each individual. These tumor tissue tests include:

♦ The measurement of protein receptors for two types of female hormones that affect breast cancer tissue—estrogen and progesterone. The tumor content of these receptors—positive or negative—correlates with prognosis and response to hormonal therapy.

♦ Flow cytometry for analysis of the tumor's DNA content. The average amount of cellular DNA in the chromosomes of the tumor—DNA ploidy—strongly correlates with the cancer's aggressive activity. Poorly differentiated tumors tend to have abnormal DNA content (aneuploid), and patients with these tumors will not generally do as well as those whose tumors have the correct amount of chromosomal DNA (diploid).

♦ Cell cycle analysis. Both normal and malignant cells go through a complete cell cycle known as mitosis. During one phase of the cycle (the S-phase), new DNA is

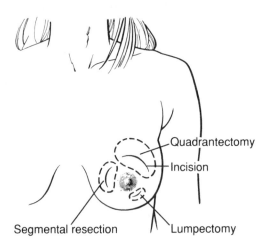

Types of limited surgery, showing typical incisions and amount of tissue removed

synthesized in preparation for the division of one cell into two. Flow cytometry as well as other techniques are used to measure the S-phase fraction, or growth rate.

The percentage of tumor cells in this S-phase is an indication of how rapidly a tumor is trying to grow. As might be expected, tumors with a high S-phase fraction (over 7 percent when measured by flow cytometry)—in other words, growing rapidly—have a less favorable prognosis. The S-phase fraction for breast cancer can range from less than 1 percent to more than 20 percent of the cells.

♦ Immunohistochemical detection of abnormal tumor proteins, including secreted enzymes and stress proteins, are under investigation. Lower levels of the enzyme cathepsin-D or specific "heat-shock" proteins, for example, are associated with better survival in some studies.

There are also abnormal oncogene and growth factor-related products. The product of the HER-2/*neu* oncogene is overproduced in about one-third of breast cancers. The overproduction appears to be associated with earlier tumor relapses and lower survival rates. Another promising marker is the epidermal growth factor (EGF) receptor.

♦ Several studies have shown that the number and density of tiny blood vessels in the tumor could be correlated with the risk of metastasis.

Years of clinical testing will be needed to confirm how many of these tests add to our ability to identify individuals with a higher risk of relapse and reduced chances for survival. It is expected, however, that during the next few years many additional tests will be discovered and routinely performed on all breast tumors.

TREATMENT OVERVIEW

It is now standard practice for primary physicians, surgeons, radiation oncologists and medical oncologists to work together to plan and carry out each patient's treatment. Any one of these physicians can assume the role of "quarterback," serving as the leader for decision-making and conveying information to the patient and family and other members of the medical team.

 Surgery The basic principle of breast cancer treatment is to remove the identifiable cancer and a rim of surrounding normal tissue to make sure that there is a "margin" of safety around the tumor. The degree of excision depends on

POST-MASTECTOMY BREAST RECONSTRUCTION

Women who have had a mastectomy have a number of options to restore their normal physical appearance, including wearing a breast prosthesis. A number of scientific medical papers, however, have concluded that breast reconstruction greatly improves an overall feeling of wholeness, elevating a sense of well-being and female image. This also eliminates the need for an external prosthesis and decreases the number of clothing restrictions.

Post-mastectomy breast reconstruction is one of the most significant advances in plastic surgery over the past two decades. There are now several ways to reconstruct the breast, each with its advantages and disadvantages. Improved techniques are now also available for reconstructing the nipple. The opposite breast may have to be reshaped or have its size altered to provide the best symmetry. A team approach—where the plastic surgeon works with the primary care physician, general surgeon and radiation and/or medical oncologist—generally leads to the most satisfactory result.

The first question to be decided is whether to reconstruct the breast immediately after a mastectomy or to delay the procedure.

The immediate approach of creating a breast mound at the same time as the mastectomy has the advantage of being less psychologically disruptive ("mourning" for the lost breast). Immediate reconstruction is appropriate for women with small cancers and without spread to axillary lymph nodes who wish to avoid an extra operation but realize that under certain circumstances or if spread is likely there may be a slightly higher risk of healing problems. But if the tumor is large, immediate reconstruction is usually not performed. The primary goal is always curing the cancer. Breast reconstruction is always a secondary goal.

The delayed approach has certain advantages. It allows the surgical wound to heal completely, so the reconstruction does not compound possible post-mastectomy healing problems. The surgical specimen and axillary lymph nodes are evaluated by a pathologist, allowing both patient and physician to make the most appropriate decisions about the various options for reconstruction.

Reconstruction is also generally delayed if radiation therapy and chemotherapy are undertaken immediately after surgery. Both can cause low blood counts and impaired immunity, increasing the risk of infection, compromised wound healing and other complications. Reconstruction is usually delayed for four to six weeks after radiation therapy is completed and two to three months after chemotherapy ends.

Other than timing, the various techniques of reconstruction must be considered. Some use silicone implants, others use a woman's own tissues in addition to or instead of a silicone implant.

Over the past few years, isolated cases of possible reactions to silicone gel leading to autoimmune diseases have been reported. While these reports are being investigated, silicone gel implants are no longer available for routine breast reconstruction and augmentation. Except for a limited number of gel-filled implants used by specific clinical investigators, inflatable silicone implants filled with saline (sterile salt water) are now being used.

The most common complication following silicone breast implantation has historically been capsular contracture. In certain individuals (up to 50 percent), the normally thin layer of scar tissue surrounding the smooth surface of the implant thickens and contracts. This creates an abnormal firmness and sometimes pain and/or distortion of the breast. This problem has been particularly prevalent when the implant is placed on top of rather than underneath the chest wall muscle. Capsular contraction often can be corrected with additional plastic surgery.

One-Stage Silicone Breast Reconstruction On rare occasions, a permanent small breast implant can be placed under the chest wall muscles at the end of the mastectomy operation. This can be done in some small-breasted women who have had a minimal amount of breast skin removed with their mastectomy.

Advantages
♦ Re-establishes the completed breast mound with minimal additional surgery.

Disadvantages
♦ Can be used only to produce a relatively small breast contour that may not have as natural a shape as that produced by other techniques.
♦ As with any silicone implant, there is a low but definite risk of complications, which could lead to further surgery.

Tissue Expansion Technique An inflatable silicone prosthesis is placed under the muscles of the chest wall and is gradually inflated with saline (sterile salt water). This is usually done bi-weekly in the doctor's office. Two to three months are generally needed before the breast reaches the size needed to match the opposite breast. The expander implant may be used as a permanent prosthesis or may be exchanged in a simple operation for a permanent implant. (*See* diagram page 322.)

Advantages
♦ The technique is simple and can be done on an outpatient basis under local or general anesthesia.
♦ This approach is particularly applicable to immediate reconstruction since minimal additional time or dissection is required for the placement of the expander.
♦ Patients may also be less psychologically stressed since they have an immediate visible result of the reconstruction procedure rather than the absence of the breast.

Disadvantages
♦ This multi-staged procedure requires many office visits and two to three months to complete.
♦ There are the usual risks associated with silicone implants.

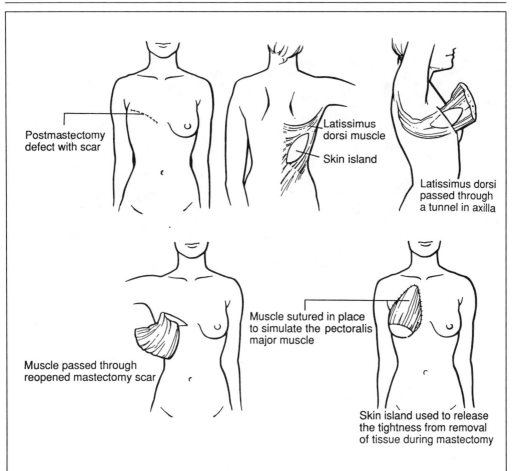

Postmastectomy defect with scar

Latissimus dorsi muscle

Skin island

Latissimus dorsi passed through a tunnel in axilla

Muscle passed through reopened mastectomy scar

Muscle sutured in place to simulate the pectoralis major muscle

Skin island used to release the tightness from removal of tissue during mastectomy

LATS breast reconstruction, using skin flap from back muscle

Latissimus (LATS) Flap Technique This technique became very popular in the late 1970s and early 1980s. It is most useful when the lower chest wall tissues are tight or thin or when there has been some localized radiation damage after the mastectomy.

A breast implant is generally used along with the broad, fan-shaped back muscle (latissimus dorsi) and a segment of overlying skin, which is rotated around to the chest wall to replace tissue removed during the mastectomy.

Advantages
♦ Adds fullness to the lower portion of the breast where it is most needed to produce a natural-looking breast.
♦ Generally produces a better-defined lower breast crease than the expansion technique.

Disadvantages
♦ Skin from the back may be a different shade or texture.
♦ Creates an additional chest scar and a visible scar on the back.
♦ Transferring this back muscle may impair muscle power for some athletic activities.

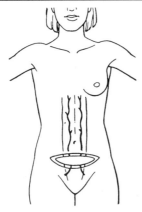

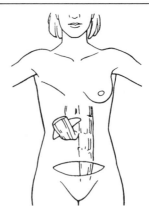

1. After mastectomy, designated abdominal skin and underlying fat are isolated along with a segment of muscle that maintains the blood supply to the elliptical skin island.

2. The tissue (including skin, fat, blood vessels and one or both of the abdominal muscles) is tunneled up beneath the upper abdominal skin and placed in the breast area.

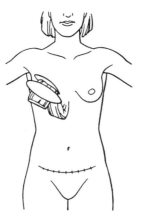

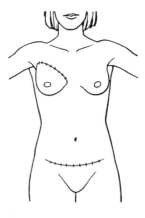

3. The flap of muscle, skin and fat is shaped into a breast.

4. The nipple is often formed with tissue from the new breast mound or from the opposite nipple. The skin around the nipple is later tattooed to make the areola. The resulting abdominal incision is similar to that from a "tummy tuck."

TRAM flap technique

TRAM (Transverse Rectus Abdominus Myocutaneous) Flap Technique This is the most complex of the commonly used techniques and is not appropriate for all patients. But with experience over the past decade, complication rates have dropped to a satisfactory level and most breast reconstruction surgeons now routinely perform the technique. It has also become more popular as concerns about silicone implants have increased.

A portion of the vertical muscle in the center of the abdomen (the rectus abdominus) and a large ellipse of skin and fat from the lower abdomen are transferred onto the chest wall and shaped in the form of a breast.

Microsurgical Free Flap Technique Just as with the standard TRAM flap, this technique uses a similar skin and fat ellipse from the lower abdomen transferred to the chest wall and shaped into a breast mound. The free flap technique, however, requires only a small portion of the rectus muscle, which contains the major blood vessels responsible for nourishing the flap.

When the free flap is transferred to the chest wall, the divided blood vessel ends are joined directly to an appropriate chest wall artery and vein by microsurgical technique. This eliminates the need for the full length of rectus muscle (which surrounds the nourishing vessels) to be twisted and turned upward as the flap is repositioned onto the chest wall.

Patients who have had their abdominal muscles cut during previous surgery (a gall bladder operation, for example) would not be acceptable candidates for a standard TRAM flap, but a free TRAM flap could be safely used in such cases.

With either technique, it is imperative that any smoking stop completely for one month before and after surgery.

Advantages
♦ Cosmetic results are generally pleasing. Skin transferred from the abdomen to the chest wall is usually a good match in color and texture.
♦ A silicone prosthesis is usually not required.
♦ A "tummy tuck" follows the transfer of skin and fat from the lower abdomen.

Disadvantages
♦ Possible weakness or hernia of the abdominal wall.
♦ Additional scars across the upper chest and lower abdomen.
♦ Involves a major, lengthy surgical procedure under general anesthesia.
♦ A plastic surgeon with microsurgery skills is required for the free flap technique.
♦ There may be a higher risk of complications.

the individual. The surgeon and the pathologist evaluate the extent of the cancer and its location within the tissue that has been removed.

Very small tumors can be treated with lumpectomy. Most early breast cancers can be treated with segmental resection. Only larger tumors require a quadrantectomy.

If a tumor is advanced or has spread throughout the breast, complete removal of the cancer will remove a large portion of the breast itself and it may be advisable to proceed with a mastectomy. The judgment as to the amount of tissue that can be removed before it is wiser to do a mastectomy must be discussed between a patient and her surgeon. Radical operations such as the Halsted radical mastectomy (which removes muscles on the chest wall) should be used only in very

advanced situations where a cancer is attached to the muscle.

Lymph nodes are generally removed as part of the surgical procedure to determine the extent of the cancer. Cancer present in the lymph nodes indicates a significant risk of microscopic (and, therefore, undetectable) metastases outside the breast and the axillary (armpit) area, possibly in the lung, liver or bones. The finding of positive lymph nodes usually means that additional adjuvant therapy—hormonal or chemotherapy—is required. If the lymph nodes do not contain cancer, the likelihood of distant metastases is lower. Removal of the lymph nodes *per se* does not make a difference to survival.

It is now also recognized that axillary lymph nodes are not an effective barrier to tumor spread. The nodes are removed not as a curative measure but mainly to provide information about the risk of recurrence and metastasis and to better define the need for adjuvant therapy. Removing all or some of the lymph nodes in the armpit—called axillary lymph node dissection and sampling, respectively—may be performed with either a separate incision during the primary operation or as a completely separate surgical procedure. Sampling is done in most patients, being omitted only if treatment decisions would not be influenced by the results.

◆ *Breast Reconstruction* Another role for surgery is reconstructing a breast after one has been removed. This is being done more often than it used to be. It is also being done earlier and with techniques that produce a more cosmetically acceptable result. An experienced plastic or reconstructive surgeon may see the

patient before primary surgery to give advice and assistance, but is more often consulted near the end of therapy if the patient wants her breast reconstructed.

 Radiation Radiotherapy is often part of standard treatment for breast cancer to treat the remaining breast tissue after the primary tumor has been removed. This is based on the frequent risk of microscopic (and undetectable) cancer cells remaining in the breast. For smaller breast cancers, the combined treatment with surgery (lumpectomy or segmental resection) and subsequent radiotherapy has been shown to be equivalent to the modified radical mastectomy.

Another use of radiation therapy as primary treatment is in postmastectomy radiation to the chest wall. This may be

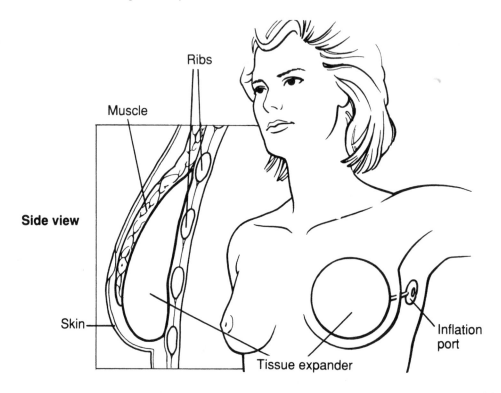

Breast reconstruction using inflatable tissue expander

done if the tumor was found at surgery or after tissue examination to invade the skin or chest wall muscles, if it was very large or if many lymph nodes were involved. The assumption is that there may be hidden tumor cells in the chest wall or armpit (axilla) after surgery that can be eradicated effectively by radiation. In addition to the chest wall, the area treated (the radiation field or port) sometimes includes the lymph nodes in the armpit or over the collarbone (supraclavicular nodes).

In patients who later develop chest wall recurrence, radiation therapy is often used (if the area was not previously treated with radiation), usually with a wide margin to kill the presumed microscopic tumor implants that could also be nearby. This therapy to localized recurrences may achieve permanent control over the cancer in up to half of patients.

Radiation is given daily, usually five days a week, over about six weeks. The usual technique involves external beam radiation to the entire involved breast, sometimes with an additional booster dose to the tumor area. This boost may be given by an external beam or with radiation seeds surgically implanted directly into the tumor area (brachytherapy). There is no increased risk of a secondary malignancy or a breast cancer on the opposite side as a result of radiotherapy.

♦ *In Metastatic Disease* Radiation is often used in treating metastatic disease, both to shrink tumors and to relieve local symptoms such as pressure or pain. If metastatic bone lesions occur in a weight-bearing bone such as the leg, for example, the bone may fracture with very little injury. This is called a pathologic fracture. Such areas are usually given radiation to help heal the bone, decrease pain and control local spread of the tumor.

If a bone lesion is extensive, there may be a significant risk of pathologic fracture during the next several months it might take to complete radiation therapy and healing. An orthopedic surgeon is often called in to determine if a fixation device—such as a rod or plate surgically placed over the cancerous bone to stabilize it—should be used to minimize the risk of fracture during this time.

Similarly, pain in the spine or spinal lesions seen on a bone scan or x-ray should be promptly investigated. If a metastatic tumor is present, there may be a risk of compression fractures of the vertebrae (even on simple walking) or of pressure on the spinal cord by the tumor, which can result in paralysis. Tumors that spread to the neck are especially worrisome because compression and fractures there can lead to paralysis of both arms and legs (quadriplegia) as well as loss of bladder and bowel control (incontinence).

Pain is often produced by tumors pressing on nerves, and radiation may help relieve the pain by shrinking these tumors. As is true in other types of cancer, the radiation dosage has to be kept low in some locations because of the limited tolerance of normal tissues.

Side effects of radiotherapy may include tiredness and skin changes, but with modern techniques major complications are infrequent (*see* Chapters 6 and 17).

 Chemotherapy Chemotherapy may be used either as an adjuvant therapy for high-risk patients following surgery or to treat metastases.

♦ *Adjuvant Therapy* Adjuvant or prophylactic chemotherapy and/or hormonal therapy is now given to many patients after surgery to try to prevent or minimize the growth of microscopic deposits of tumor cells that might grow into a recurrent tumor. Some patients with no obvious metastases at the time of surgery but who are at high risk for such micrometastases may be rendered disease-free. Premenopausal patients at high risk for residual microscopic metastases are usually given chemotherapy. Common drug combinations include Cytoxan + methotrexate + 5-fluorouracil

(CMF), Adriamycin + Cytoxan (AC) and Cytoxan + Adriamycin + 5-fluorouracil (CAF). Tamoxifen is often given to most high-risk postmenopausal women, whether chemotherapy is added or not.

Some uses of adjuvant therapy are now clearly defined and accepted. In other areas there are differences of opinion. There may be several acceptable alternatives depending on the preferences of physician and patient. Adjuvant therapy is a constantly evolving field, so an experienced and up-to-date medical oncologist should be involved in treatment planning from the time of diagnosis to explain and implement the latest developments.

♦ *In Metastatic Disease* A variety of treatment combinations have a significant chance of causing metastatic tumors to shrink or stop growing. Cure is not usually possible in this situation, although improvement in symptoms and tumor shrinkage may last for months and often many years. More aggressive and effective combinations are being developed in clinical trials.

♦ *Intensity of Treatment* In the past, chemotherapy was often omitted if the white blood cell or platelet counts dropped moderately (even if there were no symptoms or significant risk) or when minor gastrointestinal or other side effects occurred. Sometimes a dose of chemotherapy would be modified or postponed because of holidays or inconvenience. It is now recognized that these practices are generally unwise.

For metastatic disease and especially for adjuvant treatment, *it is important to give full doses and to avoid postponing regularly scheduled doses for minor reasons or for less than significant toxicity.*

Attempting to be "kind" to a patient by making toxicity as tolerable and minimal as possible can decrease the chances of a good result from the treatment. The kindest thing a physician can do is make sure the dose is as close to the theoretical maximum safe dose as possible and is also given on time. One study of the standard

CAF program (Cytoxan + Adriamycin + 5-fluorouracil), used as adjuvant therapy, showed that with high-dose-intensity therapy, 75 percent were free of recurrence of the cancer three years later, compared with only 64 percent of those given low-dose-intensity therapy.

Hormonal Therapy The lining of the ducts and lobules in the breast change under the influence of hormones, and hormonal manipulation and therapy play an important role in managing breast cancer. A variety of methods were once used to manipulate the hormone balance— removing the ovaries or adrenal glands and sometimes the pituitary gland, for example. Many women responded to these manipulations, others did not. Those who responded not only seemed to have disease that was less aggressive but if they relapsed they could be treated by another hormonal maneuver with an increased chance of response.

More recently, it was discovered that the amount of estrogen and progesterone receptors in a tumor signifies that tumor's dependence on these hormones. This measurement has become important in determining tumor behavior and treatment. Tumors are classified as positive or negative based on the amount of receptor protein present. Tumors with positive receptors are associated with a better patient prognosis and longer survival.

Estrogen receptors may be found in up to two-thirds of patients, while only 40 to 50 percent have progesterone receptors. Postmenopausal women are more likely than premenopausal women to have receptor-positive tumors.

About half of patients with receptor-positive tumors, especially older, postmenopausal women, will respond to hormonal treatment using a drug such as tamoxifen, which blocks the action of estrogen in the tumor cells. It is taken orally and has few major side effects except for occasional hot flashes.

Tamoxifen should be taken for at least two years, and indirect evidence suggests that it will be more effective when taken longer (five years). (Clinical trials are in progress.) Sometimes the progestational hormone Megace is used, and occasionally the androgenic agent Halotestin. Both are usually given after tamoxifen no longer effectively arrests tumor growth. Another agent, Cytadren, is sometimes used to decrease hormone production, especially if metastatic disease is present. Recently, gonadotropin releasing hormone analogs (lupron or zoladex, for example) have been used in premenopausal women to decrease female hormone production.

Patients whose tumors lack both estrogen and progesterone receptors have a low response rate to hormonal therapy. Therefore, they generally do not receive agents such as tamoxifen on an adjuvant basis or as treatment of metastatic disease.

Since hidden breast cancer cells may remain in the body after initial treatment, *it is extremely important that before any female hormones of any kind are taken by a woman who has had breast cancer, she should discuss the potential risk with her oncologist.*

♦ *Hormonal Therapy in Special Situations* Tamoxifen may be the primary tumor treatment in some very special situations—for elderly patients who cannot have or refuse to have surgery, for example, or for patients with estrogen receptor positive tumors who can't have surgery or chemotherapy because of medical problems. In older patients, especially those over 80, tamoxifen will often shrink tumors. Except in such special circumstances, tamoxifen should not be considered an alternative to established primary therapy.

Investigational Women who have many positive axillary lymph glands at primary surgery are at very high risk for recurrent disease. Women with Stage IV cancer have a low cure rate with conventional therapy, including aggressive chemotherapy. Both conventional dose chemotherapy and

tamoxifen benefit these patients. The prognosis in both situations might be improved if extremely high doses of chemotherapy could be given. But there is as yet no evidence that higher doses of chemotherapy will prolong the survival of patients at high-risk for recurrence (for example with 10 or more positive axillary lymph nodes). Recent investigational programs using high-dose chemotherapy and stem cell or bone marrow protection have tried to overcome this problem, but there is no evidence yet that cure is more likely with very high-dose chemotherapy and bone marrow or stem cell protection than with high-dose chemotherapy alone.

♦ The use of autologous bone marrow transplantation (ABMT) for metastatic and even high-risk early-stage breast cancer is currently under study. This is riskier than the usual treatment with chemotherapy. Because the patient's own stem cells or marrow is used, the risk is not related to the grafting problems seen in allogeneic bone marrow transplants where marrow comes from another donor (*see* Chapter 12). Rather, it relates to the fact that blood counts become very low for many weeks, during which time there is a high risk of bleeding and/or infection. A small percentage of patients (less than 10 percent) will not survive treatment with ABMT. Clinical studies are trying to determine if ABMT offers an increased chance of long-term disease control, especially important when considering the expense and risk for breast cancer patients.

Current studies are trying to determine the curative advantage of ABMT as an adjuvant therapy for patients with 10 or more involved lymph nodes. In one study, 80 percent of such patients were free of evidence of disease three years after treatment, but their overall survival was identical to that of matched patients in an identical study. Until randomized comparative trials are carried out, the role of ABMT will not be clarified.

♦ Another technique to combat the life-threatening problem of low blood counts (with possible serious infections) associated with chemotherapy is to give colony-stimulating factors such as G-CSF. These stimulate the rapid production of blood cells and minimize the period of white blood cell depression (*see* Chapter 8). It is too soon to know if the use of these agents will be translated into improved survival.

♦ To attempt to *prevent* breast cancer in women at high risk, an investigational trial of tamoxifen is being conducted by the National Cancer Institute.

TREATMENT BY STAGE

STAGE 0 (in situ)
TNM Tis, N0, M0
Non-invasive or in situ cancers consist of lobular carcinoma in situ and ductal carcinoma in situ (intraductal carcinoma). These cancers are often small and may be discovered incidentally by mammography before a mass can be felt. They may also be in several locations in one or both breasts. In situ cancer can also be found in the presence of invasive cancer, in which case the cancer is staged and treated according to the invasive cancer.

Standard Treatment Both types are generally curable.
♦ For intraductal carcinoma, conventional therapy is a wide excision of the tumor. It is critical to remove an additional area around the initial biopsy if the edges of the biopsy showed tumor cells. Axillary lymph nodes were usually removed in the past, but several studies have shown that positive nodes are rare for this type of cancer. Accordingly, axillary sampling is usually omitted.

Following surgical excision of the tumor, radiation therapy is usually given to the remaining breast tissue, since this significantly reduces the chances of additional cancer developing in the same breast. Another option is to remove the entire breast tissue (total mastectomy), with or without axillary dissection especially in cases where there may be several primary cancers.
♦ In situ lobular cancer—a form that more commonly occurs in both breasts—is thought by some to be less malignant, but patients with this lesion have a 25 percent risk of developing some form of invasive cancer in either breast over many years.

There are some differences of opinion about management of these patients. Standard treatment can include periodic examinations (including mammography) and follow-up without any additional therapy. This may be adequate if the patient is aware of the long-term risk of developing invasive cancer and will participate in the frequent evaluations. Axillary lymph node dissection is not necessary.

An alternative is total mastectomy on both sides. This choice is often appealing to women who don't want to have examinations several times a year, mammograms once or twice a year and the constant worry that invasive cancer may be found during their next visit to the doctor.

Five-Year Survival Over 95 percent

STAGE I
TNM T1, N0, M0
The tumor is 3/4 in. (2 cm) or less in size, without any evidence of spread to nearby lymph nodes or distant sites.

Standard Treatment This stage is most often curable with surgery. The treatment plan may use radiotherapy and chemotherapy or hormone therapy as well as surgery, and has to be tailored to the individual, taking the risks and benefits of each plan into account.

The surgical procedure used depends on the tumor's size and location, the size of the breast and whether the patient prefers a more extensive operation (probably without radiotherapy) or feels strongly about preserving her breast with a more limited procedure. Options include:

♦ Excisional biopsy and/or lumpectomy with a separate axillary node dissection. With a lumpectomy, there is a significant risk of residual microscopic cancer, and radiotherapy is given to the breast to minimize the possibility of residual tumor cells growing. This often requires an external radiation boost or internal implant as well as the usual external beam therapy to the entire breast.

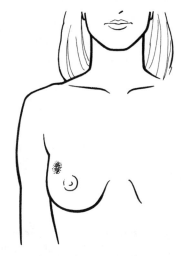

♦ Removal of a larger wedge or portion of the breast, again with an axillary node dissection and radiation to the breast. This has a lower failure rate than lumpectomy with radiation. For both lumpectomy and wedge resections, the margins *must* be free of cancer. If they are not, there is a much higher local failure rate. Sometimes (less than 10 percent of the time for Stages I and II) a tumor seems small, but with microscopic study is found in multiple sites or is found to be so extensive that a mastectomy may be needed to remove all cancer and improve the chance for cure.

♦ Modified radical or a total mastectomy, with removal of axillary lymph nodes. Radiotherapy is sometimes used after a modified radical mastectomy in patients at high risk for microscopic residual tumor that could lead to a recurrence in the area of surgery. If possible, however, the surgeon

will ensure that the tissues at the edge of the surgical incision are free of cancer cells. If radiotherapy is used, it is 90 to 95 percent effective in eliminating these cells and preventing tumor recurrences in the skin of the chest, which is a very troublesome, hard to manage problem that is far easier to prevent.

Removing the tumor and a portion of surrounding tissue while conserving a major part of the breast, usually if followed by radiation therapy, provides a cure rate about the same as the modified radical mastectomy.

The conventional recommendation has been to remove the axillary lymph nodes, since about one-third of patients who do not have obviously enlarged nodes still have microscopic involvement (positive nodes reclassifies the disease as Stage II, a treatment category requiring adjuvant chemotherapy or hormone therapy).

Adjuvant Therapy For many years it was not customary to treat Stage I breast cancer with chemotherapy or hormone therapy. These patients generally have a good prognosis, with only about one chance in four of further tumor spread. For cancers smaller than 1/2 in. (1 cm) in diameter, the chance of recurrence is less than 10 percent within 10 years of diagnosis. The National Institutes of Health Consensus Conference on Treatment of Early Stage Breast Cancer in June 1990 suggested that it is reasonable not to give adjuvant treatment to patients with these very small tumors unless they are part of a clinical trial or high-risk factors are involved.

Recent trials suggest, however, that many other Stage I patients will benefit from adjuvant therapy. Two large trials by the National Surgical Adjuvant Breast Project (NSABP) showed significant reduction in recurrences in the opposite breast at four-year follow-up for estrogen receptor negative patients given chemotherapy and for estrogen receptor positive patients treated with tamoxifen.

Although there is an early benefit for adjuvant treatment in patients with negative axillary lymph nodes, studies are continuing to see if there will be an improvement in survival. It will be several years before it is known what the benefits of such therapy are and which patients should be considered for it. A careful discussion with each patient is appropriate.

Adjuvant therapy with chemotherapy for estrogen receptor negative patients and tamoxifen for estrogen receptor positive patients usually begins within four to six weeks of surgery. There are several effective programs, with other drug combinations and hormonal therapies under clinical evaluation.

Five-Year Survival 85 percent

STAGE II

TNM T0, N1, M0 or T1, N1, M0 or T2, N0, M0 (IIA)

T2, N1, M0 or T3, N0, M0 (IIB)

Stage IIA implies either a small primary lesion (less than 3/4 in./2 cm) and positive axillary lymph nodes or a larger primary lesion (between 2 and 5 cm) without positive nodes.

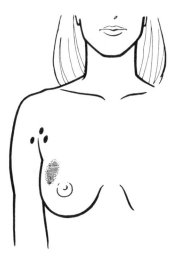

Stage IIB consists of a primary lesion between 3/4 and 2 in. (2 - 5 cm) and posi-

tive axillary nodes or a very large tumor [greater than 2 in. (5 cm)] with no axillary metastases.

Standard Treatment Stage IIA and IIB cancers can often be cured with various surgical procedures. Conservative surgery that removes only a portion of the breast, followed by radiation therapy, has been shown to be equivalent to more radical surgery for tumor control [for tumors smaller than 1 1/2 in. (4 cm)].

The same considerations for selection of the surgical procedure apply as in Stage I, including the size of the cancer, the size of the breast and concerns about breast preservation. The indications for axillary dissection are similar to those in Stage I. Surgical options are also similar, namely:

♦ Excisional biopsy or lumpectomy, with an axillary node dissection, followed by radiation therapy to the breast. For tumors larger than 2 in. (5 cm), chemotherapy may be given before surgery ("neoadjuvant" chemotherapy).

♦ A wedge or partial breast resection, again with axillary node dissection and postoperative radiation. The limitations on tumor size and tumor-free margins again apply. Radiation therapy consists of external radiation and sometimes an implant or, alternatively, an optional booster dose of external radiation. Local recurrence rates are lower than with lumpectomy alone.

♦ Modified radical or total mastectomy. In a few patients with large tumors [larger than 1 1/2 in. (4 cm)] or extensive tumors (invasion of the chest wall muscles, for example), a modified radical or even a Halsted radical mastectomy may be required to remove all of the tumor. Postmastectomy chest wall radiation is given in selected patients with muscle invasion, residual tumor in the chest wall, or a high risk for tumor cells close to the surgical margins. Some physicians irradiate patients with more than four positive axillary nodes with very large tumors, or if lymphatic vessels within the breast are involved.

Patient survival with Stage II cancer depends on controlling tumor cells that have likely already spread throughout the body. Starting adjuvant chemotherapy promptly after surgery is critical since the major risk to life is the possibility of hidden metastases. Radiotherapy, which may limit drug dosages, can begin later, as early as three months after chemotherapy has begun or even after six months when chemotherapy has been completed. While radiotherapy to the chest wall decreases the chance of local recurrence it does not affect tumor cells that may be elsewhere in the body. The exact timing of radiotherapy is a question still being addressed by clinical studies.

The Conservative Surgical Option The June 1990 NIH Consensus Conference (*see* "Stage II") held that breast conservation treatment—with close follow-up to detect local recurrences early—is appropriate primary therapy for most women with Stages I and II breast cancers and is preferable because it provides the surgical equivalent to total mastectomy while preserving the breast.

Conservative surgery followed by primary radiation therapy depends upon careful patient selection, however. Not all women with early-stage cancer are good candidates for this approach.

♦ It is sometimes not used in patients with a large tumor in small breasts where excision would produce a significant loss of breast tissue and compromise symmetry.

♦ Conservative surgery plus radiotherapy is not suggested if there are multiple malignant or in situ tumors in one breast, widespread microcalcifications on mammography or a history of collagen vascular disease. The latter patients often develop scar tissue (reactive fibrosis) with radiation therapy, undesirable breast changes that might require additional surgery.

♦ Patients with lesions in the extreme edge of the breast may be better candidates for this option, since if a mastectomy were done, it might require removing additional portions of the chest wall.

♦ A small percentage of patients will develop a recurrence in the breast area following limited surgery to conserve the breast. Mastectomy may still be able to control the disease in most cases.

♦ Radiotherapy should not be given during pregnancy because of the hazard to the fetus.

Adjuvant Chemotherapy and Hormone Therapy After surgical treatment to control local disease in the breast, adjuvant chemotherapy is recommended to reduce the risk of recurrence.

♦ Drug combinations shown to produce a survival advantage include CMF (Cytoxan + methotrexate + 5-fluorouracil [5-FU]) with or without VP (vincristine + prednisone), and CAF (Cytoxan + Adriamycin + 5-FU).

♦ Earlier combinations that have been tried include L-PAM (Alkeran) + 5-FU for premenopausal women and L-PAM + 5-FU + tamoxifen for postmenopausal women with receptor positive tumors. Recent studies suggest that shorter courses of Cytoxan + Adriamycin (AC) may be at least as good as CMF given for six months.

♦ Adriamycin (doxorubicin) can produce cardiac toxicity, a form of heart muscle weakness. This can be disabling and life-threatening, but the risk can be reduced by giving the drug slowly via continuous intravenous infusion over one or more days and by limiting the total dosage.

♦ Adjuvant chemotherapy has been shown to prolong the disease-free interval and survival of Stage II premenopausal patients with positive axillary lymph nodes. The treatment lasts four to six months in most programs.

♦ There may be some benefit in giving adjuvant chemotherapy to postmenopausal women with positive axillary nodes, but the results are less impressive than in premenopausal patients.

♦ Postmenopausal women whose lymph nodes and hormone receptors are both positive are usually given adjuvant tamoxifen therapy, which can be as effective at prolonging disease-free and overall survival as chemotherapy is in premenopausal patients. Tamoxifen is given for at least two years. More than two years and as long as five years may be more beneficial. Beyond five years, treatment is investigational. Patients receiving tamoxifen who have not had a hysterectomy require some observation for potential slight increased risk of uterine cancer.

♦ It may be appropriate to give chemotherapy in postmenopausal patients with positive nodes and negative hormone receptors. However, other studies suggest that tamoxifen may be beneficial.

♦ Patients with negative lymph nodes and larger (T2 or T3) tumors have the same considerations as those with Stage I cancers. Both premenopausal and post-menopausal patients benefit, but as is true for Stage I cancers, the benefit of hormonal treatment is most significant in women over 50.

Five-Year Survival 66 percent

STAGE IIIA
TNM T0–2, N2, M0 or T3, N1–2, M0
The hallmark of Stage III is a big tumor [over 2 in. (5 cm)] with involvement of the axillary lymph nodes on the same side as the cancer or with fixation of the lymph nodes to one another or to other structures. If the lymph nodes inside the chest are involved or the tumor extends into the chest wall or involves and ulcerates the skin, the lesion is Stage IIIB.

Standard Treatment This stage is generally regarded as operable and is treated aggressively. Control for long periods is possible, but more often than not the

tumor ultimately recurs. Treatment plans often use surgery, radiation and chemotherapy in varying sequences.

Initial surgical treatment is a modified radical or radical mastectomy. Several months of chemotherapy may be given before surgery to try to shrink or eliminate the tumor and make it easier to remove surgically, and this may improve survival. Combinations that have been extensively used in this manner include CMF (Cytoxan + methotrexate + 5-FU) and CAF or FAC (Cytoxan + Adriamycin + 5-FU).

Chemotherapy and radiotherapy are generally given after surgery.

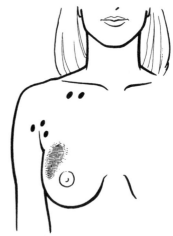

STAGE IIIB
Any T, N3, M0 or T4, any N, M0

Standard Treatment This stage, which includes inflammatory carcinoma, is generally regarded as inoperable. Surgery is usually limited to the initial diagnostic biopsy, with treatment of the local tumor by chemotherapy or radiation. Chemotherapy is often used because over 50 percent of patients have hidden metastases. If a good response is obtained with chemotherapy and/or radiation, surgery may be helpful to remove residual tumor.

Because all three therapies are used but their best sequence has not yet been determined, newly diagnosed patients with Stage IIIB cancer should be considered for clinical trials. Complex treatment programs involving integrated chemotherapy (with or without autologous bone marrow transplantation) and radiotherapy followed by surgery are under study. If a clinical trial is not available, consideration should be given to one of the current aggressive combined treatment protocols.

Five-Year Survival 41 percent

STAGE IV
TNM Any T, any N, M1
There are distant metastases (to bone, liver or lung, for example) or skin and chest wall involvement beyond the breast area.

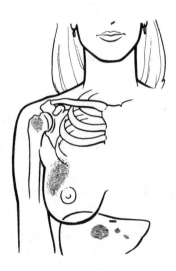

Standard Treatment Surgery is generally limited to a biopsy to prove the diagnosis and tumor cell type, as well as provide hormone receptor levels. The primary tumor may have to be treated with surgery or radiation, but this problem is generally overshadowed by the need to control metastases.

Chemotherapy and/or hormonal therapy are the principal treatments. Tumor shrinkage is common in about 60 percent of patients, although only in 10 to 20 percent does the tumor completely disappear for a long time.

◆ If the metastasic disease is not immediately life-threatening or doesn't involve such critical internal organs as the liver, hormonal management is usually tried before starting chemotherapy. This may involve tamoxifen or removal of the ovaries for premenopausal patients, and progestins, androgens, Cytadren, estrogens or tamoxifen for postmenopausal patients. Hormonal manipulation may be especially useful for those with predominantly bone metasteses.

◆ If metastases involve vital organs or are life-threatening, chemotherapy combinations similar to those used in earlier stages are given. Again, the risk of Adriamycin-induced cardiac toxicity may limit the amount of drug that can be given.

Five-Year Survival 10 percent

Investigational
◆ All patients are candidates for clinical trials, which may involve new drugs in Phase I, II or III trials, new biologic agents, autologous bone marrow transplantation (ABMT), treatment with monoclonal antibodies, or high-dose chemotherapy with growth factor (such as G-CSF) support. The use of ABMT for advanced disease shows some early promise (20-25 percent after two years) but the final role of ABMT is uncertain.

BREAST CANCER IN MEN

Male breast cancer is rare, but one out of every 150 cases of breast cancer involves a man, usually one over 60 years old. There is a higher frequency of Stage III disease, principally because of skin involvement by the tumor.

Although a painless breast lump is the most common sign, most breast lumps in men are benign and are related to some other cause, such as medications or liver disease.

Standard Treatment Both simple and radical mastectomies have been done, but no statement can be made about a standard method. Skin grafting may be required.

Radiation therapy is often used postoperatively to decrease the risk of local recurrence. Some centers are now treating male breast cancer patients with chemotherapy or hormonal therapy because nearby lymph nodes are commonly involved and because adjuvant chemotherapy has had such good results in women. Preliminary data are encouraging.

It is customary to obtain hormone receptors in these patients, although most male tumors are hormone receptor positive and respond to hormone manipulation, such as tamoxifen.

Sometimes there is delay in seeking therapy, which is perhaps due to low awareness by the public and doctors of the possibility of this diagnosis.

TREATMENT FOLLOW-UP

Careful follow-up after treatment is essential for two purposes—to detect recurrences and to monitor the response to treatment. The standard procedure involves:
♦ Regular physical examinations and mammograms.
♦ Blood chemistry panel (liver, kidneys) and tumor markers (e.g., CEA, bone, CA15-3) if they were positive initially. (Some insurance plans may not cover these markers.)
♦ Bone scan, especially if the initial bone scan was positive, pain develops or the serum alkaline phosphatase level is elevated.
♦ Chest x-ray and x-rays of positive areas on bone scan.
♦ Special studies such as endoscopy or fine needle aspiration of recurrent masses.

Detecting Recurrence Hidden metastases can lie dormant for a long time after surgery. In unusual cases, recurrences have been noted 15, 20 or even more years after the primary cancer developed. Lifelong close and comprehensive follow-up is therefore required to be sure that recurrences are detected and treated early.

During the first two years after initial treatment, the intervals tend to be short—every two to four months. If no evidence of recurrence is found, the intervals are lengthened during the next few years, usually to about every three to six months.
♦ Any abnormal studies, such as bone scans, x-rays (including CT) or blood tests, are repeated at appropriate intervals. Tumor markers such as carcinoembryonic antigen (CEA) and CA 15-3 are often included if they were positive at the time of diagnosis, since they are then useful in detecting a recurrence of metastatic cancer and for monitoring therapy.

Monitoring Response to Treatment For either recurrent or metastatic disease, appropriate studies are done to determine response to treatment. Before any significant change in therapy—a new chemotherapy program, for example—it is essential to establish baseline information, documenting current status by blood tests, examinations, measurements and x-rays.

Objective clinical response is ordinarily defined as at least a 50 percent shrinkage in the greatest diameter of a metastatic lesion.

A metastatic tumor in the lung 1 1/2 in. (4 cm) in diameter would have to shrink to 3/4 in. (2 cm) for this to be called a significant response, with such shrinkage being classified as a partial response. A complete response or remission occurs when all visible and detectable disease disappears.

"Stable disease" suggests disease that does not grow in any area or shrinks by less than 50 percent in diameter (also called minimal response).

Disease progression means that at least one lesion increases in size during treatment.

♦ It is easy to assess lung metastases. Measurements can be made with a ruler held against a chest x-ray.

♦ Lesions in the liver can be monitored by liver function tests, especially the alkaline phosphatase, but also by direct measurement of metastatic tumors seen on abdominal CT or ultrasound images.

♦ Skin lesions and the size of lymph nodes can be measured directly.

♦ Measuring response in bone lesions takes longer and is more difficult because most metastatic breast cancers produce a softening or dissolving of the bone with the appearance of a "lytic" spot that looks like a hole. If treatment is successful, the lytic lesion will fill in with new bone, but this takes many months.

For determining the response to chemotherapy or hormonal therapy, a bone lesion that has not received radiation therapy has to be chosen as a marker. Obviously, if a lesion given radiation heals and hormone therapy or chemotherapy is also being given, it would be impossible to know which treatment brought about the healing.

Bone lesions require that an x-ray be done before treatment and another as soon as the treatment has been given an adequate trial.

Following bone scans for evidence of response to treatment may not be as useful as conventional x-rays of lytic bone lesions. Scans may show "hot spots" in any abnormal area, and these spots may also indicate healing. They may also be produced by inflammation, metabolic diseases or severe arthritis. The area could remain positive for months or a few years with successful therapy.

In a few patients with positive bone scans but without any lesions on x-rays, response may be signified by no new lesions developing. If the bone scan is unchanged after six months, especially if pain lessens, the positive areas can be presumed to indicate healing.

♦ In some breast cancer patients, the bone lesions themselves produce extra bone (blastic lesions) instead of "holes" in the bone (lytic lesions). Here it is not possible to determine healing by looking at x-rays because healing is *also* associated with the laying down of extra bone. Again, healing may be signified by the failure to develop any new lesions elsewhere.

The "Flare" Response Hormone treatment and also chemotherapy can sometimes produce worse bone pain during the first few weeks of therapy, and the serum calcium level may also rise. This endocrine "flare" may be early evidence that the cancer is responding to the hormone treatments.

If possible, pain medication is given to allow therapy to continue while the elevated calcium level is evaluated and treated. Usually the calcium returns to normal and the pain decreases, confirming a response.

Similarly, the bone scan sometimes becomes temporarily worse in a patient who is clinically improving. The increased uptake on the scan may represent healing of the diseased bone. The x-ray appearance may not change for several months even in patients with a good response to treatment and whose pain has decreased.

In a similar way the tumor markers CEA or CA 15-3 may rise temporarily in patients who respond.

RECURRENT CANCER

Recurrent breast cancer may be in the area of the breast surgery or in the chest wall. Alternatively, it may be metastatic disease anywhere in the body.

A recurrence in the skin or chest wall near the surgical site most often indicates that more widespread metastatic disease will occur in the future, although it may be the only site of recurrence in a small group of patients. For these patients, local additional surgery and/or radiation therapy may be used.

Most patients with even small local recurrences, however, will eventually develop other areas of metastasis despite aggressive local treatment. After treatment of an isolated local recurrence, only 30 percent of patients have developed *no* other evidence of spread by 5 years, 7 percent by 10 years. These figures apply to patients who develop chest wall recurrence after aggressive surgery such as a modified radical mastectomy. The prognosis is much better if a recurrence occurs in the breast after conservative surgery followed by radiation therapy.

Standard Treatment

♦ If there is no internal disease and recurrence is confined to the area of the original tumor, surgery and/or radiation therapy is used, plus tamoxifen in selected cases.

♦ If there is no life-threatening disease involving major internal organs, if it has been at least two years since mastectomy and if hormone receptors are positive or unknown, the standard treatment is tamoxifen or removal of the ovaries for premenopausal patients, and tamoxifen, estrogens, androgens, Cytadren or progestin therapy for postmenopausal patients.

♦ If patients respond to hormonal treatment and then relapse, other forms of hormonal therapy are used, including Cytadren, hypophysectomy, androgen therapy and corticosteroids.

♦ If major internal organs such as the liver are involved, hormone receptors are negative or it has been less than two years between the primary treatment and the recurrence, chemotherapy is usually given. Standard combinations include CMF, CAF and CMFP (*see* "Stage IIIA" and "Stage IV"). Cyclophosphamide + Adriamycin appears to produce similar results but has been studied less extensively. Other combinations include mitomycin-C + Velban as well as Velban + Adriamycin + thiotepa + Halotestin (VATH). Taxol may be of value in patients who fail to respond to Adriamycin (doxorubicin).

♦ Combination chemotherapy with or without hormone management for patients who recur after initial response to hormonal manipulation.

Investigational

♦ If there is major organ involvement and negative hormone receptors or if less than two years has elapsed since primary treatment, clinical trials of combination chemotherapy, newly developed chemotherapy agents and biologic treatment should be considered (*see* Chapter 36).

♦ Leuprolide is also undergoing clinical trial as a method of hormonal manipulation.

♦ Examples of drugs in clinical trial are anthrapyrazoles, taxotere, topotecan and monoclonal antibodies.

THE MOST IMPORTANT QUESTIONS YOU CAN ASK

♦ Can I save my breast? Is this wise?

♦ Will I need radiation therapy?

♦ Will the radiation therapy produce any damage to the skin or any deformity? What are the other side effects?

♦ If I need chemotherapy, what are the choices? How long will it last and what are the side effects?

♦ When can I have breast reconstruction done and what are my choices? What will I look like afterwards?

♦ Why do I have to stop taking female hormones?

♦ What can you give me to help me with my hot flashes?

♦ Will I lose my hair? When will I start losing it and how long will it take to come back?

♦ How often do I need to be examined afterwards? What tests will I have?

♦ How often should I have a mammogram?

♦ When will I be sure that my cancer will not come back?

CANCER OF AN UNKNOWN PRIMARY SITE (CUPS)

Raphael Catane, MD, and John D. Hainsworth, MD

◇

Cancer of an unknown primary site (CUPS) is a metastatic tumor with no obvious source. It is detected by a biopsy that shows cancer from a part of the body that does not produce that type of malignancy, and no site of origin is identified despite a thorough physical examination, blood tests, x-rays and other imaging studies.

No primary site of origin can be identified in 2 to 9 percent of patients diagnosed with metastatic cancer. This is often because the primary tumor is so small that it is undetectable or the primary site is difficult to see directly or by using imaging techniques.

Since by definition the disease is diagnosed at a metastatic stage, the prognosis is generally poor. A significant percentage of patients, however, can have symptoms relieved and can occasionally be cured. For example, germ cell tumors, choriocarcinoma, lymphoma and certain sarcomas are potentially curable even in their metastatic stages. Other tumors such as prostate cancer, breast cancer and endometrial carcinoma are amenable to hormonal therapy.

Unfortunately, the most common origins of CUPS are lung and pancreatic cancers. These two tumors are generally incurable at the metastatic stage, with an average survival of about three or four months and with only 25 percent and 10 percent alive after one and five years respectively.

FINDING THE PRIMARY SITE

In trying to discover the primary site, there are two important considerations.

1. Some primary cancers are much more treatable than others. These include cancers of the breast, prostate, thyroid and ovary, lymphomas (including Hodgkin's disease), as well as germ cell tumors similar to those that develop in the testes. Great efforts are made to determine if one of these is the primary site. Not only is the prognosis much better with these types of cancer, but the treatment has to be specific for that cancer. The usual non-specific combination chemotherapy programs for CUPS have a low rate of response.

2. There are important clues your doctor can use to discover the primary site.

♦ One clue is the location of the metastases. A woman with a tumor that develops in glands (adenocarcinoma) and is found in the lymph nodes of the armpit, for example, is more likely to have carcinoma of the breast. A woman who develops fluid in the abdomen (ascites) or has a tumor involving the lining of the abdominal cavity (peritoneum) should be suspected of having ovarian cancer.

♦ The most common sites of CUPS are metastases to the lung, lymph nodes, bones and liver. When CUPS is found in the upper part of the body (above the diaphragm), the most common source is the lung. When it appears in the liver, the usual primary site is the gastrointestinal tract, including the pancreas.

♦ Another clue is the type of pathology. If a person has epidermoid carcinoma in lymph glands high in the neck, for example, the primary site is most often in the nasopharynx, the throat or the tonsils. Special endoscopic procedures and biopsies can be used to look for the primary site and even if it is not found, such people are often treated for head and neck cancer. Epidermoid cancer involving low

cervical nodes is usually of lung origin. Cervical lymph nodes with metastases of other pathological appearance may repre-

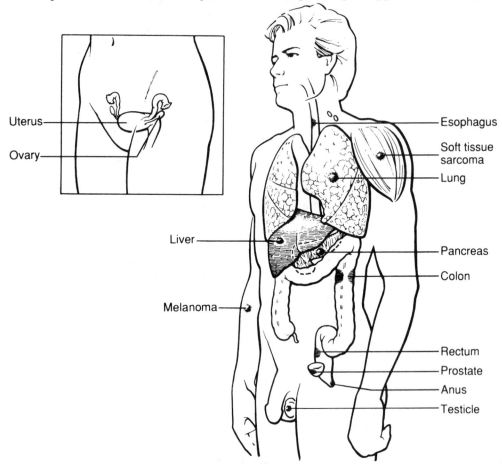

Possible primary sources of cancer first diagnosed in a metastatic site

TABLE 1: TREATABLE CANCERS THAT MAY PRESENT AS CUPS

Potentially curable	Chance of significant remission
Germ cell tumors	Breast cancer
Hodgkin's disease	Some lymphomas
Lymphoma	Ovarian cancer
Trophoblastic tumors	Head and neck cancer
Thyroid cancer	Small cell lung cancer
Ovarian cancer	Prostate cancer
	Sarcoma
	Bladder cancer

sent breast cancer, lymphoma, melanoma or other tumors (*see also* "Special Pathologic Methods" on this page).

DIAGNOSIS

People with CUPS undergo certain standard methods of medical evaluation to discover the primary site (if possible) and other potential areas of spread. Evaluation will include a history as well as a specific work-up for the major potential sites of the cancer's origin that can be treated—breast cancer, germ cell tumors, lymphomas and cancers of the head and neck, lung (especially small cell), prostate, thyroid and ovary. A consensus about the minimal investigation that has to be performed includes the following.

Physical Examination

♦ When CUPS is found in high cervical lymph nodes, a thorough examination of the nasopharynx, throat and upper respiratory tract should be done, usually by an ear, nose and throat specialist.

♦ A gynecological examination, including a rectal examination, Pap smear and a pelvic ultrasound or CT, should be done for any woman with CUPS, especially if the inguinal (groin) lymph nodes are enlarged or there is fluid in the abdomen (ascites).

Blood and Other Tests

♦ Complete blood counts.

♦ Urinalysis to check for blood.

♦ Test for hidden (occult) blood in the stool.

♦ Blood chemistry tests to assess liver and kidney function.

♦ Tests for serum tumor markers that may be elevated with specific cancers, such as CEA (colon), CA-125 (ovary), CA 15-3 (breast), CA 19-9 (pancreas), prostatic specific antigen (prostate), alpha-fetoprotein (hepatoma, germ cell tumors), βHCG (choriocarcinoma, germ cell tumors) and thyroglobulin and calcitonin (thyroid gland).

Imaging

♦ Chest x-ray may reveal the most common tumor origin, carcinoma of the lung. It is often impossible, however, to distinguish between a primary lung cancer and a metastatic lesion within the chest. Sometimes chest CT is also helpful.

♦ Mammograms for all women diagnosed with CUPS. Fifty percent of females with isolated metastases in the lymph nodes in the armpit will have a breast cancer primary. This will not always be seen on a mammogram, however (a false negative result).

♦ It is not helpful to do extensive x-rays—bowel x-rays, for example—to look for a primary site unless there is a specific complaint in that area, such as constipation or gastrointestinal bleeding.

The following imaging study is frequently done:

♦ Abdominal CT scan, especially if there are metastases in the liver. The scan may reveal the presence of the second most common malignancy causing CUPS, pancreatic cancer.

The following imaging studies are occasionally done:

♦ CT, MRI and ultrasound studies of the area of known tumor and likely primary sites.

♦ Nuclear scans of bone, liver and thyroid.

Endoscopy and Biopsy

♦ Endoscopic evaluation of the colon, urinary tract and lung is performed when indicated by results of the previous studies.

♦ Biopsy of suspicious lesions identified by x-rays may establish a primary site; breast, prostate, pancreas may need special studies on biopsy; hormone receptors, DNA, other studies.

SPECIAL PATHOLOGIC METHODS

The pathologist has a crucial role in the diagnosis, evaluating the biopsy specimen and determining not only if it is malignant but, on the basis of his or her experience and the tissue's appearance under the microscope, the most likely source.

The pathologist is often consulted before the biopsy is done because some special immunohistochemistry studies require frozen tissue or tissue may have to be specially prepared for examination by an electron microscope. These methods were not generally available even five years ago. They offer a significant advantage in obtaining an accurate diagnosis of the primary site of origin. The limited material obtained with a needle biopsy may not be adequate for specialized pathologic studies. In such cases, an excisional biopsy is recommended.

Immunohistochemistry Along with the usual tissue stains used to examine the tumor tissue under the microscope, special stains using monoclonal antibodies are directed against specific tumor antigens. These can often determine the likely primary site, thereby allowing therapy to be more specific and improving the chance of remission or even cure.

Electron Microscopy (EM) Regular microscopes magnify tissues up to 1,000 times. The electron microscope can magnify tissues 50,000 to 100,000 times. Very small structures inside and on the surfaces of cells, often characteristic of certain types of cancer cells, can be seen. There are structures characteristic of squamous cell cancers, cancers of neuroendocrine origin, muscle tumors and most melanomas. Besides suggesting likely sites, EM studies are useful in eliminating certain tumor types.

Polymerase Chain Reaction (PCR) This new method detects minute amounts of genetic material (DNA or RNA). PCR may detect abnormal DNA or RNA structures in the biopsy specimen. A few of these abnormalities are specific for certain can-

TABLE 2: SPECIAL STAINS USED FOR SPECIFIC TISSUES

♦ The presence of keratin, a protein found in epithelium (surface tissue), indicates the tumor is a carcinoma rather than a sarcoma or lymphoma.

♦ S-100, a protein found in neuroectodermal tissues, is useful in the diagnosis of melanomas or nerve tumors.

♦ Neuron-specific enolase is positive in small cell (oat cell) lung cancer.

♦ Leukocyte-common antigen found on the surface of leukocytes is positive in leukemia and lymphoma.

♦ Prostate-specific antigen (PSA) is positive in prostate cancer.

♦ Human chorionic gonadotropin is often positive in germ cell tumors such as testis cancer and in choriocarcinoma.

♦ Alpha-fetoprotein is present in primary liver cancer and certain germ cell tumors.

♦ Estrogen receptors are present in breast cancer and cancer of the lining of the uterus (endometrial cancer). Finding estrogen receptors not only helps in the diagnosis but suggests that hormonal therapy may be useful.

Many new tissue stains are being developed and are rapidly enlarging the diagnostic capability of the modern pathologist.

cers and, thus, will suggest the origin of the tumor.

STAGING

The actual tumor origin is the most important thing in planning treatment and assessing the prognosis. By definition, all CUPS are in an advanced stage because the cancer has already metastasized. It has been suggested that doctors caring for patients with CUPS should refrain from extensive investigations, since the cost of the evaluation financially and with respect to time and discomfort is not worth the results and may not affect survival anyway.

The results of exhaustive tests are also sometimes misleading. The tests may sometimes seem to show a positive finding when none is really there (false positive) or may instead fail to show an abnormality that is present but not detectable (false negative).

TREATMENT OVERVIEW

There is no generally recommended treatment for *all* patients with CUPS. Whenever there is a likely primary origin, based on the opinion of the pathologist as well as the clinical, laboratory and imaging studies, the treatment will be given according to that probable diagnosis.

The prognosis for people with CUPS is highly variable because so many different tumors may be involved.

Standard Treatment While no specific standard therapy is generally agreed upon for people with CUPS with no definable primary sources, these patients are sometimes treated with combination chemotherapy programs. If the disease appears to be localized, complete surgical removal or radical radiotherapy may occasionally result in a cure. But when the tumor has spread, investigational protocols might be considered.

Investigational
♦ Combination chemotherapy (frequently including cisplatin).
♦ Hormonal therapy.
♦ New chemotherapeutic agents such as carboplatin (paraplatin) alone or in combination with other drugs.

TREATMENT FOR SPECIFIC PRESENTATIONS

Certain rules have been recommended for a number of specific presentations of CUPS.

"MIDLINE" TUMORS
These tumors originate in the middle part of the body such as the mediastinum (chest) or midabdominal lymph nodes. Some people with these tumors who are under 50 years of age, have lung and lymph node metastases and have a poorly differentiated histology respond well to combination chemotherapy that contains cisplatin and etoposide.

Sixty percent of the patients in one such group had a significant response to therapy and 15 percent were apparently cured. Some of these patients had blood or tissue markers (HCG or AFP) suggesting that they had a germ cell tumor.

CUPS IN THE NECK LYMPH NODES
When epidermoid (squamous) carcinoma is found in the neck (upper cervical) lymph nodes, patients should be treated as if they had a tumor of the upper respiratory area even though a thorough ear, nose and throat evaluation—including blind biopsies of the base of the tongue and the nasopharynx—may have been negative.

Treatment is potentially curative and may include:
♦ Radical radiotherapy to the cervical lymph nodes.
♦ Surgery to remove the lymph node group involved.
♦ A combination of surgery and radiotherapy.

♦ Chemotherapy, usually with a cisplatin combination.

CUPS IN THE ARMPIT LYMPH NODES

In males, the most likely diagnosis is incurable lung cancer.

In females, 50 percent may have a treatable breast cancer. Treatment will emphasize:
♦ Surgery, including removal of all axillary nodes in the involved site.
♦ Partial or total mastectomy.
♦ Radiation to the axilla and the breast, if not removed.
♦ Hormonal therapy, especially if hormone receptors are present.
♦ Chemotherapy should be considered as suggested for breast cancer.

CUPS INVOLVING THE PERITONEUM

In women, CUPS involving the lining of the abdominal cavity should be treated following the recommendations for ovarian cancer, even if the ovaries are normal or have been removed. Treatment will include:
♦ Initial exploratory surgery with removal of all tumor possible.
♦ Chemotherapy, usually with carboplatin and cytoxan.

CUPS IN A SINGLE LYMPH NODE

Any single lymph node site may represent melanoma. A cure may be achieved in 15 percent of cases by completely removing the lymph nodes in the involved area, even when the primary site is never found.

MULTIPLE SKELETAL LESIONS

In males, a prostatic cancer should be suspected. If there are no other clues, hormonal therapy might be given, because it will be beneficial for a cancer with a prostatic origin and is quite harmless.

In females, breast cancer is a possibility. In both sexes, a thyroid cancer should be kept in mind, since both tumors may be treated effectively even in the metastatic stage (by hormonal therapy and chemotherapy for breast cancer and with radioiodine for thyroid cancer). Metastatic thyroid cancer that does not resemble normal thyroid tissue (poorly differentiated or undifferentiated), however, can seldom be treated with radioactive iodine.

THE MOST IMPORTANT QUESTIONS YOU CAN ASK

♦ How much investigation is really needed to increase my chance of survival or to improve my quality of life?
♦ Has the pathologist used any of the special studies described here?
♦ What is the most probable diagnosis?
♦ Can I benefit from surgery, radiotherapy, chemotherapy or hormonal therapy?

CARCINOIDS OF THE GASTROINTESTINAL TRACT

Ernest H. Rosenbaum, MD, Malin Dollinger, MD, and Larry K. Kvols, MD

◇

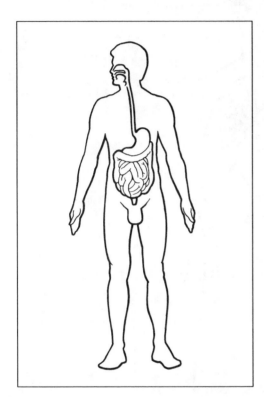

Carcinoid tumors are unusual cancers. Although they can develop in other organs, especially the lung, they generally arise in the intestinal tract, including the stomach, small bowel, appendix and rectum. They are the most common tumors of the appendix, occurring in one out of every 300 appendectomies. They make up 30 percent of small bowel tumors but less than 2 percent of all gastrointestinal malignancies.

In their early stages, carcinoid tumors are highly treatable and often curable. They are usually slow growing and behave like benign tumors. The risk of metastasis is related to the size of the primary tumor.

Carcinoids may occur in multiple sites (about 20 percent have multiple tumors) and, except for those of rectal origin, may produce an endocrine substance called serotonin. In most cases there are no symptoms, so many carcinoid tumors are discovered incidentally during abdominal operations performed for other reasons. The survival of most people with carcinoid tumors is quite good, although symptoms may develop when the tumor cannot be removed, when it recurs after treatment or when there is metastatic disease.

Types There are no meaningful cell type (histologic) variations that help predict the clinical course of these tumors. Carcinoids are broadly classified as neuroendocrine or APUD (amine precursor uptake and decarboxylation) tumors. The APUD type is associated with the MEN (multiple endocrine neoplasia) type I syndrome (pancreas islet cell carcinoma). Malignant carcinoids may produce at least two hormones, serotonin and substance P, but many carcinoid tumors are nonfunctional and do not release any substances.

How It Spreads Carcinoid tumors spread by direct invasion of underlying layers of tissue (submucosally). They can also spread via lymphatics to regional lymph nodes and through the bloodstream to the liver, lungs, bone or other organs.

The site of origin and size of the primary tumor are important in determining whether the carcinoid tumor is likely to spread. A tumor less than 1/2 in. (1 cm) rarely metastasizes. But 88 percent of

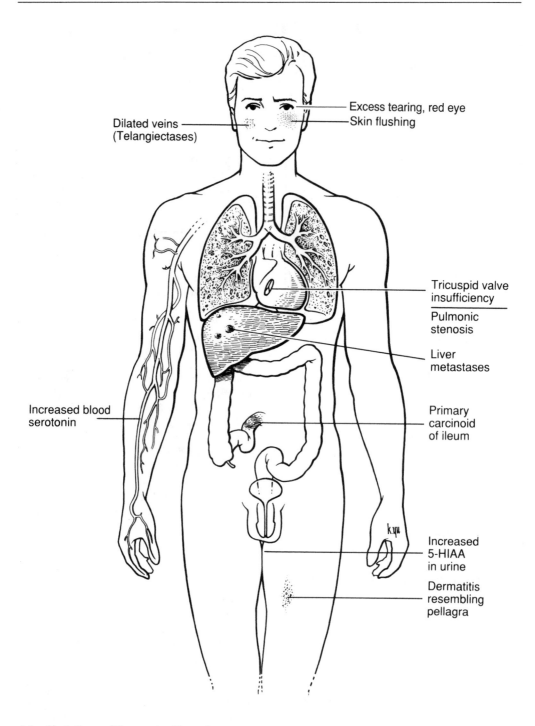

Manifestations of the carcinoid syndrome

patients with tumors larger than 3/4 in. (2 cm) have metastases, and 18 percent of these develop the carcinoid syndrome (*see* "Common Signs and Symptoms").

What Causes It Unknown

RISK FACTORS

None known. It is exceedingly rare for carcinoids to be hereditary.

SCREENING

There are no effective screening methods.

COMMON SIGNS AND SYMPTOMS

Symptoms are unusual in the early stages. When symptoms do occur, the tumor has already spread in 90 percent of patients. The most common symptoms are periodic abdominal pain, intermittent intestinal obstruction and kinking of the bowel. Gastrointestinal bleeding is uncommon and ulcerations of the tumor are rare.

In addition to the symptoms caused by the tumor, there may be symptoms of the carcinoid syndrome. This is characterized by facial flushing, wheezing, diarrhea and cardiac valvular disease. It is caused by abnormal amounts of the two hormones produced by malignant carcinoids, serotonin and substance P, and other biologically active substances. The syndrome occurs in about 10 percent of patients with carcinoid tumor, almost always because of carcinoid metastases in the liver.

DIAGNOSIS

Physical Examination
♦ Abdominal mass and enlarged liver.
♦ Prominent skin veins (telangiectasis).
♦ Signs of the carcinoid syndrome—heart murmur, wheezing on expiration and flushing of the skin.

Blood and Other Tests
♦ Metastatic carcinoid tumors may be diagnosed by elevated levels of 24-hour urinary 5-hydroxyindolacetic acid (5-HIAA), a metabolic product of the serotonin produced by the tumor. False positive 5-HIAA tests can be caused by foods such as bananas, avocados and pineapple and by certain drugs. The laboratory should provide a complete list of foods to be avoided during urine collection.

Imaging
♦ X-rays of the chest and gastrointestinal tract (small bowel and barium enema).
♦ CT or MRI scan of the abdomen to detect liver metastases.

Endoscopy and Biopsy
♦ Liver biopsy, if indicated.

STAGING

There is no accepted staging system for carcinoids.

TREATMENT OVERVIEW

Surgery is the standard therapy, but the extent of spread is important in deciding the initial treatment options.

 Surgery Surgical removal of the tumor is the standard treatment for cure. If the primary tumor is localized and can be removed, the five-year survival rate is in the range of 70 to 90 percent. Since carcinoid tumors are usually slow growing, even patients with tumors that can't be removed have an average survival of several years. Surgery often offers excellent relief from symptoms, for example, by removing the liver metastases causing the carcinoid syndrome, resecting or bypassing intestinal obstructions. Such surgery may add years to a patient's life, an uncommon result of surgery for other types of liver metastases.

Radiation Radiation therapy may be used for palliative treatment of metastases.

Chemotherapy There has been modest success with chemotherapy. Drug combinations of 5-fluorouracil and streptozocin have had responses of about 30 percent.

Palliation Drugs such as Periactin, alpha and beta adrenergic blocking agents, chlorpromazine and corticosteroids may be used to alleviate the symptoms related to the carcinoid syndrome.

A relatively new drug, octreotide (Sandostatin), is very effective in preventing the secretion of serotonin and can help relieve symptoms of the carcinoid syndrome. Interferon-alpha can also alleviate symptoms and occasionally cause tumor shrinkage.

TREATMENT OF LOCALIZED TUMORS BY SITE

APPENDICEAL CARCINOID

Appendiceal tumors account for 22 percent of all carcinoids. They are treated by appendectomy and, in fact, are usually diagnosed for the first time at surgery. Lesions less than 5/8 in. (1.5 cm) in diameter are essentially 100 percent curable.

Appendiceal tumors larger than 3/4 in. (2 cm) are rare and treated like a carcinoma of the colon. For these larger tumors, removal of the right side of the colon and the lymphatics is recommended.

Five-Year Survival 99 to 100 percent

RECTAL CARCINOID

These account for a quarter of all carcinoids. Rectal carcinoids less than 1/2 in. (1 cm) can be treated adequately by local excision (fulguration), with cure rates approaching 100 percent.

Carcinoid lesions larger than 3/4 in. (2 cm) are treated surgically. As with carcinoma, an abdominal-perineal resection may be necessary, but sphincter-preserving surgery may be performed in some cases.

Lesions between 1/2 and 3/4 in. (1 to 2 cm) receive individualized treatment depending on extent of invasion. The cure rate is excellent.

Five-Year Survival 76 to 83 percent

SMALL BOWEL CARCINOIDS

Small bowel tumors make up 28 percent of all carcinoids. Conservative local excision is sufficient for tumors less than 1/2 in. (1 cm) in diameter. For larger tumors, a wedge of the tissues supporting the bowel (mesentery) containing the regional lymph nodes should also be removed.

Anyone with a tumor larger than 3/4 in. (2 cm) should be followed closely for a minimum of 10 years. The follow-up program should include an annual CT scan of the abdomen and annual or semiannual measurements of urinary 5-HIAA levels.

Five-Year Survival 54 percent

TREATMENT OF INVASIVE AND METASTATIC CARCINOIDS

REGIONAL GASTROINTESTINAL CARCINOIDS

Carcinoid tumors with regional metastasis or local extension should be treated by aggressive surgery. If all visible malignant disease can be removed, long-term survival rates will be excellent.

No surgical adjuvant treatment is known to be helpful.

If the regional disease can't be removed, palliative surgery—to remove all the accessible disease, for example—should be carried out.

Chemotherapy is not required until significant symptoms occur, for these patients frequently have many months or even years of comfortable life without further treatment.

METASTATIC CARCINOID TUMORS

A number of standard treatment options are available for metastatic carcinoid tumors.

 Surgery This may sometimes be of considerable value when there are large liver metastases involving surgically accessible areas of the liver. Liver metastases that recur after surgery should be considered for another resection if they are in an area where the operation can be done with minimal complications.

♦ For very carefully selected patients with slowly progressive disease and symptomatic carcinoid heart disease, heart valve replacement may be indicated.

♦ For patients with bulky or symptomatic liver metastases, one treatment option is tying off the hepatic artery, placing a tube (catheter) into the artery and injecting a material that blocks the blood flow to the tumor nodules in the liver. For optimal effectiveness, this is followed by chemotherapy. This can lead to substantial tumor regression. It can also cause severe toxic effects—abdominal pain, fever, nausea and a short-term worsening of the syndrome—but many patients do experience substantial relief from symptoms.

 Radiation The role of radiation therapy in managing carcinoid tumors with distant metastasis is restricted to relief from symptoms, most commonly of bone involvement. However, localized metastasis will occasionally respond to radiation therapy.

Supportive Therapy There are a number of ways to manage symptoms from metastatic disease with medication.

♦ Diarrhea will frequently respond to standard antidiarrheal medications such as Lomotil or tincture of opium and to dietary changes such as restricting consumption of foods high in fat.

♦ The somostatin analogue octreotide (Sandostatin) has recently been shown to be useful in improving symptoms of the carcinoid syndrome and may be life-saving in carcinoid crisis (sudden exacerbation of symptoms).

♦ Interferon-alpha preparations may have a role in controlling symptoms of the carcinoid syndrome and/or in arresting tumor growth.

♦ Monoamine oxidase inhibitors such as procarbazine (Matulane) and tranylcypromine sulfate (Parnate) are drugs to be avoided. They will exacerbate the carcinoid syndrome by inhibiting the breakdown of serotonin.

♦ Acute symptoms—carcinoid crisis—may be prevented and controlled by pretreatment with octreotide. Some specific drugs are to be avoided in these patients because of the risk of causing the release of vasoactive substances. This is especially true during surgery and in the treatment of low blood pressure.

Chemotherapy Although activity with a variety of single agents and drug combinations has been reported—5-fluorouracil (5-FU), doxorubicin (Adriamycin) and dacarbazine (DTIC) or 5-FU + streptozocin—response rates seldom exceed 30 percent. Complete responses are uncommon, and the duration of the response may be short, if chemotherapy is used alone.

Chemotherapy should be used for palliation in patients with symptoms and in the case of liver metastases, after blocking the hepatic (liver) artery and then giving chemotherapy (chemoembolization).

Investigational

♦ Protocols using new drugs may be considered (*see* "Recurrent Cancer"). One study showed a three-fold increase in survival of patients treated with octreotide compared to chemotherapy, but further studies are needed to confirm results and prove that the improved survival is significant.

TREATMENT FOLLOW-UP

Patients should be evaluated every 3 to 12 months. The evaluation should include:
◆ Physical examination.
◆ 24-hour urine 5-HIAA levels.
◆ Chest x-ray.
◆ Abdominal CT scan, if required.

RECURRENT CANCER

The selection of further treatment depends on many factors, including the therapy initially used, the site of the recurrence and individual considerations.

Since some tumors grow rather slowly, attempts to remove them again or multiple operations to remove liver metastases or slowly growing tumors are worthy of consideration. Reducing tumor volume may provide long-term relief of symptoms.

Investigational treatments are appropriate and should be considered when standard treatment fails.

THE MOST IMPORTANT QUESTIONS YOU CAN ASK

◆ How are carcinoids different from the usual cancers of the bowel?
◆ What tests are needed to follow my progress after surgery?
◆ What does a rising urine 5-HIAA mean?
◆ What are the toxic side effects of chemotherapy?
◆ What is the role of repeated surgeries for recurrent carcinoid cancers?
◆ Am I eligible for any research or investigational protocols?

CERVIX
Jeffrey L. Stern, MD

◇

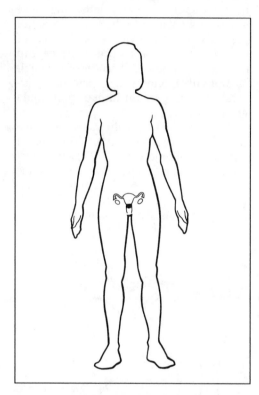

Invasive cervical cancer accounts for 2.3 percent of all cancers that afflict women in the United States. About 13,500 cases of invasive carcinoma of the cervix are diagnosed in the United States each year, while there are at least 50,000 new cases of a pre-invasive cancer—known as carcinoma in situ—where the cancer cells are confined to the surface skin of the cervix.

But since 1940, there has been a steady decrease in the incidence of carcinoma of the cervix because most women with no symptoms are screened with cervical and vaginal Pap smears. The probability at birth that a white woman will eventually develop cervical cancer dropped from 1.1 percent in 1975 to 0.7 percent in 1985. Similarly, for African-American women the probability dropped from 2.3 percent in 1975 to 1.6 percent in 1985.

Types Over 90 percent of cervical carcinomas start in the surface cells lining the cervix and are called squamous cell carcinoma. About 5 to 9 percent start in glandular tissue (adenocarcinoma). Adenocarcinomas are more difficult to diagnose, but they are treated the same way as squamous cell carcinomas and the survival rate, stage for stage, is similar.

There are several types of adenocarcinoma. About 60 percent are the endocervical cell type, 10 percent are each of endometrioid and clear cell carcinomas and 20 percent are adenosquamous carcinoma.

There are two rare types of cervical cancer known as small cell carcinoma and cervical sarcoma. Both have a poor prognosis.

How It Spreads Most scientists believe that cervical warts or pre-invasive cervical cancer may develop over a period of months or years after the cervix is infected with the human papilloma virus (HPV). This early tumor—known as low-grade SIL (squamous intraepithelial lesion) or as mild dysplasia or cervical intraepithelial neoplasia (CIN) Grade 1—can progress to moderate dysplasia (CIN-2) or high-grade SIL, then to high-grade SIL or severe dysplasia and carcinoma in situ (CIN-3) and eventually to invasive carcinoma. Most physicians believe that about two thirds of all cases of severe dysplasia progress to invasive cancer if left untreated. This transformation takes anywhere from 3 to 30 years, about 10 years on the average.

Once the cervical cancer becomes invasive, it can spread locally to the upper vagina and into the tissues surrounding the upper vagina and the cervix (the parametrium). Eventually it grows toward the pelvic sidewall, obstructing the tubes (ureters) that drain urine from the kidney to the bladder. It can also spread directly to the bladder and rectum.

Cervical tumor cells can invade the lymphatic system and spread to the lymph nodes in the pelvic wall. Eventually they may spread to the iliac lymph nodes higher in the pelvis, the aortic lymph nodes, the nodes above the collarbone and occasionally to the groin nodes.

Metastases can also spread through the bloodstream to the outer vagina, vulva, lungs, liver and brain. Invasion of the pelvic nerves is common in advanced cases. There may also be spread within the abdomen when the tumor penetrates the full thickness of the cervix.

What Causes It There is much evidence that cervical carcinoma is venereal in origin. Most researchers believe that the human papilloma virus is either the cause or a strong cofactor in the development of pre-invasive and invasive carcinomas of the cervix, as well as pre-invasive and invasive squamous cell cancer of the vagina and vulva. Ninety to 95 percent of cervical cancers contain human papilloma virus DNA.

The virus is a sexually transmitted disease. There are more than 50 types of human papilloma virus (HPV) that infect humans. Types 6 and 11 usually cause warts, while types 16, 18, 31 and 33 usually result in high-grade SIL (CIN-2 and 3) and carcinomas. The virus infects the tis-

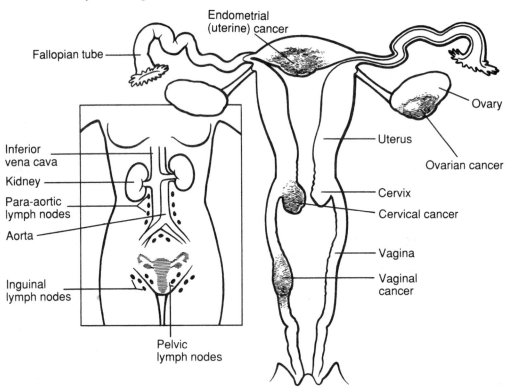

Cancers of female pelvic organs

sues of the lower genital tract and may produce obvious genital warts or mild, moderate or severe dysplasia and carcinoma in situ. Genital warts are associated with cervical, vaginal and vulvar dysplasia and invasive carcinoma in about 25 percent of cases.

RISK FACTORS

The average age of women with invasive cervical cancer in the United States is between 45 and 50, but the average age of women with carcinoma in situ is between 25 and 35. The difference is attributed to the long latent period of progression of an in situ to an invasive cervical cancer.

The risk factors for pre-invasive cervical cancer (cervical dysplasia) and cervical cancer are the same. Circumcision is no longer believed to lower the risk of cervical carcinoma.

At Significantly Higher Risk
♦ Suppression of the immune system from corticosteroids, kidney transplants, therapy for other cancers, or AIDS.
♦ A history of genital warts.
♦ A history of herpes simplex virus infection.
♦ Low socioeconomic status.
♦ Early age at first intercourse.
♦ Multiple sexual partners.
♦ Women whose male partner(s) either have or have had penile warts, have had multiple sexual partners or whose previous partners had cervical cancer.

At Slightly Higher Risk
♦ Multiple pregnancies.
♦ Cigarette smoking.

SCREENING

The American College of Obstetricians and Gynecologists recommends that a Pap smear be done for all women by age 18 or who are sexually active, regardless of age. Women who have multiple sexual partners should be screened annually, but those in long-term, stable relationships who have had negative Pap smears three years in a row may be screened less often.

A major problem with the Pap smear is that it is often thought to be normal when it is actually abnormal. The pathologist examining the cells can make an error, the health care provider may not sample the cervix adequately or an infection might obscure the results. The estimated false negative rate is about 20 percent, half of which can be attributed to faulty sampling techniques.

Adenocarcinomas and adenosquamous carcinomas are also more difficult to detect on Pap smears since they start high up in the cervical canal and may not be sampled by the Pap smear. Because of the high false negative rate, routine annual screening is strongly recommended to decrease the likelihood that cervical warts, dysplasia or cancer will be missed.

COMMON SIGNS AND SYMPTOMS

In many cases—and in almost all cases of carcinoma in situ—there are no symptoms. The most common symptoms that do appear include abnormal vaginal bleeding or discharge, bleeding after intercourse and pain.

DIAGNOSIS

Physical Examination
Most women with cervical cancer will have a normal general physical examination.
♦ Careful evaluation of the vulva, urethra and vagina.
♦ Lymph nodes in the groin and above the collarbone should be examined to detect any enlargement.
♦ Examination of the abdomen to look for an enlarged liver, a mass or excessive abdominal fluid (ascites).
♦ A gynecologic pelvic and rectal examination is important to detect disease in the tissue surrounding the cervix and vagina and the pelvic lymph nodes.

Blood and Other Tests
♦ Complete blood count.
♦ Liver function chemistries.
♦ Kidney function chemistries.
♦ The levels of the serum squamous cell carcinoma antigen (SCCA) and the serum carcinoembryonic antigen (CEA) in the blood should be measured. SCCA is elevated in 50 percent of all women with cervical cancer. CEA is elevated in about 20 percent of all cervical carcinomas. Although CEA and SCCA are not accurate enough to use for screening, they are useful to monitor the response to treatment and for follow-up to detect recurrent disease.

Imaging
♦ Chest x-ray.
♦ CT and MRI scans of the abdomen and pelvis.

Endoscopy and Biopsy
♦ Cystoscopy.
♦ Sigmoidoscopy.
♦ All women with an abnormal Pap smear or cervical lesions should undergo an office colposcopic examination. A colposcope is an instrument that can magnify the cervix from 7.5 to 15 times.
♦ The definitive diagnosis is made on a biopsy. Early cancers are occasionally diagnosed by a large biopsy of the cervix, known as a cone biopsy. A cervical conization should be done when colposcopy cannot determine if there is not an invasive cancer, when there are no obvious lesions on the cervix and the Pap smear is consistently abnormal, when a colposcopically directed biopsy does not adequately account for abnormal cells found on a Pap smear, when a diagnosis of microinvasion (early invasion) is found on the biopsy or when a cervical intraepithelial neoplasia is identified by a scraping from the cervical canal (endocervical curettage).

STAGING

Most gynecologic oncologists use the FIGO (International Federation of Gynecology and Obstetricians) classification. This divides the disease into five stages, with further divisions in each stage. A carcinoma in situ is Stage 0. The cancer is confined to the cervix in Stage I and, in Stage II, either extends beyond the cervix but not to the pelvic sidewall or involves the vagina but not the lower third. A Stage III carcinoma extends to the pelvic sidewall, involves the lower third of the vagina or obstructs one or both of the ureters. In Stage IV, the cancer has spread to distant organs beyond the true pelvis or involves the lining of the bladder or rectum.

TREATMENT OVERVIEW

Squamous cell carcinoma and adenocarcinoma are generally treated in similar ways. Radical surgery and radiation therapy are equally effective treatments for early stage disease (Stage Ia, Ib and small IIa).

For carcinomas more advanced than Stage IIa, treatment is with radiation therapy alone or radiotherapy and chemotherapy. Higher stages are generally treated with higher doses of radiation therapy as well.

 Surgery For younger women surgery is usually recommended because it preserves ovarian function and it avoids the atrophy of the upper vagina and the vaginal scarring that can result from radiation. There is also a small chance that women who survive many years after radiation therapy will develop a second malignancy in the radiated area.

Radical exenterative surgery—removal of the rectum and/or bladder and the cervix, uterus and vagina—is reserved for recurrent carcinoma confined to the central pelvis.

Surgery may also be used to stage the disease, since other methods, even using CT and MRI scans, are notoriously inaccurate in detecting lymph node metastasis and intra-abdominal spread in the more advanced stages. Unfortunately, there is no reliable way to diagnose microscopic metastases to the pelvic and para-aortic nodes without removing them. Therefore, many gynecologic oncologists will occasionally recommend a surgical staging procedure before any radiation therapy is given to evaluate the intra-abdominal surfaces and the status of the pelvic and aortic lymph nodes.

Surgical staging is done through an approach outside the lining of the abdominal cavity or occasionally via a laparoscope. This does not involve the manipulation of the intra-abdominal organs as much as an intra-abdominal operation and results in fewer complications following radiation therapy.

The incidence of cancerous pelvic and para-aortic nodes increases with more advanced disease and there may be a survival advantage to removing the involved nodes. About a third of the time, women with microscopic metastases to the pelvic and aortic nodes can be cured if the nodes are removed and radiation therapy is then given.

Women with positive para-aortic nodes may have distant metastases to the lymph nodes above the collarbone (10 to 20 percent of cases). If the neck nodes are positive, then only palliative therapy is warranted.

 Radiation Several radiation techniques may be used depending on the stage of the disease—external beam therapy or the insertion of radioactive substances into the cervix (intracavitary radiation) or into the tumor (interstitial radiation).

Women with metastatic cancer of the para-aortic lymph nodes are usually treated with external beam radiation.

 Chemotherapy This treatment is currently being investigated for women at high risk for recurrent disease (regardless of the stage) or for those with multiple pelvic lymph node or aortic lymph node metas-

tases. It is also being used simultaneously with radiation therapy in women with large cancers. These studies are too recent to determine the effectiveness of chemotherapy.

TREATMENT BY STAGE

STAGE 0 (Squamous cell carcinoma)
Carcinoma in situ (intraepithelial carcinoma).

Standard Treatment There are five treatment options for this early-stage tumor.

Freezing the cervix (cryotherapy) can be performed in the doctor's office and has a negligible complication rate.

Loop electrical excision (LEEP) is becoming more popular because of its diagnostic accuracy, technical ease and low cost.

Laser therapy is usually done for larger lesions.

A cervical conization not only is for cure but is often performed in women in whom colposcopy cannot distinguish between dysplasia and an underlying invasive carcinoma. A LEEP cone biopsy can be done in the doctor's office with a local anesthetic.

For women who have completed their childbearing or have several recurrences, the removal of the uterus and cervix (hysterectomy) is often recommended.

STAGE 0 (Adenocarcinoma)

Standard Treatment Adenocarcinoma in situ (confined to the surface of the cervix) is often difficult to diagnose. The diagnosis is usually made with a cervical biopsy or an endocervical curettage. In all cases a conization is required to rule out a truly invasive lesion.

For women who want to remain able to have children, a cone biopsy may cure the disease if the surgical margins, or edges, do not show any evidence of disease. Even so, adenocarcinoma in situ or an invasive adenocarcinoma is occasionally found in the residual cervix even if the cone biopsy has negative margins.

For those who have completed child-bearing, the treatment of choice is a simple hysterectomy.

Five-Year Survival 100 percent

STAGE Ia1
Stage I is a cancer confined to the cervix. Stage Ia involves a carcinoma of the cervix diagnosed only microscopically. This is further divided into two stages based on the depth of invasion of the cervix. In Stage Ia1, there is only minimal, microscopic invasion.

Standard Treatment Women with this stage of disease are usually treated with a cone biopsy or a hysterectomy.

Five-Year Survival 100 percent

STAGE Ia2
The depth of invasion is less than 5 mm from the surface and less than 7 mm wide.

Standard Treatment When the depth of invasion is less than 3 mm from the surface and there is no vascular space involvement, an abdominal hysterectomy is usually performed. It is not necessary to remove the ovaries in younger women. Five-year survival is 100 percent.

Women with cancer invading greater than 3 mm into the cervix or with cancer less than that, but with blood vessel involvement are treated like women with Stage Ib disease.

Five-Year Survival 80 to 90 percent

Investigational Cervical conization may cure women with lesions that invade less than 3 mm of the cervix and have no blood vessel involvement, if the edges, or margins, of the cone biopsy do not have evidence of disease. This is appropriate therapy for women who want to preserve their fertility or avoid a hysterectomy.

STAGE Ib
Lesions are larger than in Stage Ia2 but are still confined to the cervix.

Standard Treatment There are two options for treatment. A radical hysterectomy may be done, with removal of the pelvic lymph nodes on both sides. An alternative is external beam radiation (total dose of 4,000 cGy given in divided doses five days a week for five weeks) followed two weeks later by an intracavitary cesium insertion for two days and usually by a second one two weeks later. Both options result in an equal rate of cure. The choice depends on available local expertise, the age of the patient and her medical condition.

Small lesions are usually operated on while large ones are treated with radiation. Women who have metastatic disease in the removed pelvic lymph nodes are frequently treated with five weeks of external beam radiation therapy to the pelvis following surgery.

Large lesions confined to the cervix may be treated with external beam radiation five days a week for five weeks, followed by a cesium insertion two weeks later, followed six weeks after that by an abdominal hysterectomy and surgical staging.

Five-Year Survival 80 to 90 percent

STAGE IIa
A Stage II cancer is one that either extends beyond the cervix (but not to the pelvic sidewall) or involves the vagina (but not the lower third). In Stage IIa there is no obvious involvement of the tissue surrounding the cervix (parametrial), but there is involvement of the upper two thirds of the vagina.

Standard Treatment Treatment with either a radical hysterectomy and removal of the pelvic lymph nodes or external beam radiation therapy followed by either one or two insertions of intracavitary cesium is standard.

Women with large lesions of the cervix

are sometimes managed with preoperative radiation therapy (4,000 cGy external beam radiation therapy, given in divided doses over five weeks, followed two weeks later by a 72-hour cesium insertion), followed by an abdominal hysterectomy and selective node sampling.

Women who have metastatic disease in the pelvic lymph nodes are often given five weeks of external beam radiation therapy to the pelvis after surgery.

Five-Year Survival Approaching 75 to 80 percent

STAGE IIb
There is obvious parametrial involvement, but no extension to the pelvic sidewall.

Standard Treatment External beam radiation therapy may be given in divided doses over five weeks, followed by two 36- to 48-hour cesium insertions two weeks apart.

Five-Year Survival 65 to 70 percent

Investigational
♦ Radiation therapy given at the same time as chemotherapy (cisplatin + 5-fluorouracil + mitomycin-C or bleomycin + mitomycin-C).
♦ Interstitial radiation therapy—with radioactive iridium temporarily implanted directly into the tumor—is being investigated.
♦ Hyperthermia, a technique using radiation therapy and heat, is also being studied.

STAGE IIIa or IIIb
Stage III is defined as a carcinoma that extends to the pelvic sidewall, involves the lower third of the vagina or obstructs one or both ureters. Stage IIIa means there is no extension to the pelvic sidewall, but the tumor involves the lower third of the vagina. In Stage IIIb, there is extension to the pelvic sidewall, obstruction of one or both ureters, or there is a non-functioning kidney.

Standard Treatment External beam radiation therapy followed by two insertions of intracavity cesium or interstitial iridium.

Five-Year Survival 40 to 60 percent

Investigational Same as for Stage IIb.

STAGE IVa
Stage IV is defined as cancer that has spread to distant organs beyond the true pelvis or involves the lining of the bladder or rectum. Stage IVa means that a biopsy has shown that either the lining of the bladder or the rectum have become involved.

Standard Treatment This stage is usually treated with radiation therapy or by the surgical removal of the uterus, the vagina and the bladder and/or rectum (pelvic exenteration).

Five-Year Survival 20 to 30 percent

Investigational Radiation therapy given in conjunction with chemotherapy.

STAGE IVb
In Stage IVb there is spread to distant organs.

Standard Treatment Radiation may be used to relieve the symptoms of pelvic disease or isolated distant metastases.

Several chemotherapy drugs are useful for treating cervical cancer, but they are rarely curative. They include cisplatin or carboplatin, which has a response rate of 15 to 25 percent, and ifosfamide, which has a response rate of 30 percent.

Combination chemotherapy, including cisplatin + etoposide + bleomycin, has a response rate of 50 percent. Other drug combinations that have been used in women with metastatic disease include mitomycin-C + 5-fluorouracil + cisplatin, Velban + bleomycin + cisplatin and cisplatin or carboplatin + ifosfamide + bleomycin.

Investigational Many of the drugs used in the standard treatment are being tested in different combinations and doses.

TREATMENT FOLLOW-UP

A Pap smear and a careful examination of the pelvis, abdomen and lymph nodes is performed every three months for the first two years after treatment, and then every six months for three more years.

◆ Routine chest x-rays and pelvic and abdominal CT scans are not warranted in the absence of symptoms.

◆ The blood levels of carcinoembryonic antigen and/or squamous cell carcinoma antigen (SCCA) will often be measured at each visit if they were elevated before treatment.

RECURRENT CANCER

Symptoms of recurrent cervical carcinoma may include vaginal bleeding or discharge, pain in the pelvis, back or legs, leg swelling (edema), chronic cough and weight loss.

◆ If radiation was not given previously, recurrences that are confined to the pelvis may be treated with external beam radiation and intracavitary or interstitial radiation therapy.

◆ If radiation therapy was already given, the only option is the removal of the vagina, uterus and the bladder and/or rectum with the creation of an artificial bladder—a pelvic exenteration. The five-year survival rate after a pelvic exenteration is about 50 percent.

◆ Women with recurrent tumors that can't be surgically removed or with metastatic disease are usually treated with chemotherapy. Commonly used drugs include single agent cisplatin or carboplatin. Other regimens include cisplatin or carboplatin + ifosfamide, vincristine + mitomycin-C + bleomycin + cisplatin and bleomycin + mitomycin-C + 5-fluorouracil.

◆ Those with unresectable pelvic disease may be re-irradiated with or without heat or given pelvic arterial chemotherapy.

THE MOST IMPORTANT QUESTIONS YOU CAN ASK

◆ What qualifications do you have for treating cancer? Will a specialist in gynecologic oncology be involved in my care?

◆ What is the advantage of surgery versus radiation therapy?

◆ Why or why won't a staging surgery be performed?

◆ Is adjuvant chemotherapy with radiation therapy beneficial?

CHILDHOOD CANCERS

Jerry Z. Finklestein, MD

◇

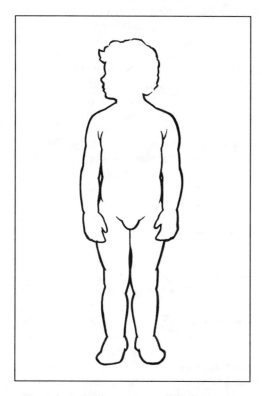

Cancer in children is a rare disease. For every 120 adults who develop cancer there is one child. Yet next to accidents, cancer is the second most common cause of death in children between the ages of one and 14. In the United States, about 10,000 new cases of cancer are diagnosed in children under 18 each year. Recent evidence suggests that the incidence of cancer in children has increased during the past two decades by about 4 percent. However, the overall mortality rate in children younger than 15 has decreased by 38 percent.

Childhood cancers are different from those in adults. The growth pattern is different and the tumors react differently to treatment. Most important, the problems seen in a child differ from those of an adult.

Fortunately, with the development of new drugs, new treatment methods, better diagnostic tools and the involvement of multidisciplinary medical teams, the outlook for childhood cancers has improved dramatically over the past few decades. More and more children with cancer are now being cured.

Types The most common childhood cancer is leukemia, accounting for about one-third of all cancers seen. The most common types in children are acute lymphoblastic leukemia and, less frequently, acute non-lymphoblastic leukemia. A smaller number of children may develop chronic granulocytic leukemia.

Brain tumors—gliomas, medulloblastomas and ependymomas—are the second most common type of cancer in children. A new term has recently been designated for certain types of brain tumors—PNET, which stands for primitive neuroectodermal tumors.

Some cancers of children are rare in adults. A cancer of the sympathetic nervous system known as neuroblastoma may occur in the adrenal glands located on top of the kidneys or may originate anywhere there is a particular kind of nerve ending known as a sympathetic nerve ending—the chest, the abdomen, the pelvis and, rarely, other sites. A cancer of the kidney known as Wilms' tumor is also particular to children, occurring most commonly in children two to four years of age and rarely in those over 16. It may occur in one or both kidneys.

Other childhood tumors that are

uncommon in adults are a tumor of the membrane at the back of the eye, the retina, called retinoblastoma; a muscle tumor called rhabdomyosarcoma; teratomas, which are tumors of young cells known as germ cells; and a tumor of the liver known as hepatoblastoma.

Bone tumors such as osteogenic sarcoma, Ewing's sarcoma or chondrosarcoma occur in children, particularly teenagers. Histiocytosis X or Langerhans cell histiocytosis is not a malignancy but is often cared for by physicians who specialize in pediatric cancer therapy.

Children, like adults, develop lymphomas known as Hodgkin's disease and non-Hodgkin's lymphoma. They may also have tumors of the liver (hepatomas), skin cancer (melanoma, which is rare) and cancers of the thyroid, adrenal glands and blood vessels.

Over 80 percent of cancers in adults develop in the glands or lining tissues of the breast, lung, intestinal or urinary tract and are called carcinomas. But over 90 percent of cancers of children are malignancies of muscle, bone, supporting tissues or blood vessels and are called sarcomas. The types of cancer seen in children, therefore, differ from those in adults not only in name but in their microscopic appearance.

What Causes It We do not know why children develop cancer. Occasionally there are clues from the environment or from a genetic inheritance pattern that a child may be at risk. But specific causes have not been identified. However, children with certain diseases do have an increased incidence of cancer (*see* "Risk Factors").

For more than 30 years there have been reports of "clusters" or concentrations of childhood cancer developing in certain geographic areas. There were clusters of children with leukemia in Niles, Illinois, in 1963, in Woburn, Massachusetts, in 1979, and in central California in the early 1990s. But physicians have not been able to figure out the significance of these clusters.

It is believed that children are more likely than adults to develop leukemia as a result of exposure to radiation. Children exposed to the radiation of the atomic bomb blasts in Japan had an increased risk of acute leukemia in childhood, with the peak occurring about five years after exposure. A higher incidence of leukemia in children exposed to radiation after the accident in Chernobyl, USSR, is expected. Radiation treatment is useful in the treatment of many cancers in children, but there is risk that children cured of their first cancer may develop a second one partly related to the use of radiation therapy.

A number of cancer-causing chemicals or industrial processes are all around us. Their role in causing childhood cancers is the subject of ongoing research.

There has also been recent publicity about electromagnetic waves produced by high-tension power lines as a possible cause of cancer in children. Various reports have either supported or refuted the claim, and further research is being done in the United States to determine whether these electromagnetic waves do in fact play a role in causing cancer. In recent years, new information has been released about causation with discoveries in the field of molecular genetics. Oncogenes (tumor-promoting genes) have been found in certain childhood cancers. Anti-oncogenes (tumor-suppressing genes) have been found in association with other childhood tumors.

For parents it is frustrating to acknowledge that there is very little we can do to protect our children from an environmental or genetic factor. Research is continuing, however, and one day we shall probably have better means of protection.

RISK FACTORS

The cancer rate for Afro-American children in the United States is about 80 percent of that seen in white children; children who are black do not have the same incidence of common cancers such as acute lymphocytic leukemia and lymphomas as children who are white. Black children rarely have Ewing's sarcoma, but there is a suggestion that they have a higher incidence of Wilms' tumor, retinoblastoma and the bone tumor known as osteogenic sarcoma.

Several cancers in children—leukemias and Wilms' tumors, for example—peak in incidence between the ages of two and four years. Others, such as lymphomas and bone cancer, have a peak incidence in older children.

At Significantly Higher Risk

♦ Previous exposure to radiation.
♦ Children who do not have an iris—the colored circle in their eye—have a higher incidence of developing the kidney cancer called Wilms' tumor.
♦ Children whose body is bigger on one side than the other (hemihypertrophy) have a higher incidence of Wilms' tumor.
♦ Males with an undescended testicle (cryptorchidism) are at higher risk for testicular cancer.
♦ Children with the skin disease xeroderma pigmentosum have a higher risk of developing skin cancer.
♦ Children with the immune disorder ataxia telangiectasia, Down's syndrome, Fanconi's anemia and Bloom's syndrome are at higher risk for developing leukemia.

SCREENING

A number of tests screen for cancer in adults but very few such tests exist for children. In Japan, Quebec and some other parts of North America, there is an attempt to screen the urine of very young children to detect the presence of abnormal amounts of the chemical group known as catecholamines in the hope that earlier detection of neuroblastoma will result in an improved cure rate.

The child with a risk factor for developing cancer should be evaluated carefully by his or her physician. The screening may be as simple as a blood test in an identical twin of a child with leukemia or a series of ultrasound examinations of the abdomen for many years in a child with hemihypertrophy.

COMMON SIGNS AND SYMPTOMS

Many of the symptoms and signs of childhood cancers are very common and only health professionals with sufficient training will be able to tell whether a complaint is due to a normal childhood disease or a rare disease such as cancer.

Tiredness and paleness are usually the result of nothing more than the flu but could also signal the onset of leukemia. Fever is often noted in a child with an infection, but recurrent fever, especially with bone pain, may be a symptom of leukemia or a bone tumor.

Children who have headaches with vomiting may have nothing more than an upset stomach, but recurrent headaches with vomiting that do not to go away with time require a physician to make sure there isn't a brain tumor.

Children who have a mass in their abdomen are probably just constipated, but the mass could be Wilms' tumor, neuroblastoma, lymphoma or a liver tumor. Lumps in the neck are usually due to an infection, but if they don't respond to antibiotics, a lymphoma is a possibility. Drainage from the ear is usually due to an ear infection and only rarely due to some tumor.

Weight loss is rare in a young child, although it is something teenagers often desire. If the weight loss is not controlled, however, there may be psychological reasons involved or a lymphoma such as Hodgkin's disease.

Obviously, children's complaints are usually the result of normal childhood diseases. But when parents are concerned that their child has a persistent problem, then they should take him or her to the doctor. The findings of a physical examination may suggest that special tests are necessary to discover whether the child does in fact have a cancer.

Some signs and symptoms are not common. Any newborn child with a cat's eye—a white dot in the center of the eye—should be seen by a physician, since the dot may indicate a retinoblastoma. It is also very rare for children to have blood in their urine, so any child with this complaint should be seen by a physician. Blood in the urine may be the result of an infection, but may also be caused by Wilms' tumor.

DIAGNOSIS

Physical Examination
♦ A complete physical examination should include the groin area, the testicles, the skin and the nervous system. A rectal examination may also be performed to rule out a tumor in that area.
♦ Enlarged liver and/or spleen or a mass in the abdomen may indicate a tumor.
♦ Lumps in the neck that are firm, non-movable and have not responded to antibiotics may be due to lymphomas, leukemias and other cancers.
♦ The eyes may be examined, a procedure that requires the child's cooperation. A special instrument for looking into the eyes (ophthalmoscope) lets the physician see if there is increased pressure in the brain, which is often due to a brain tumor.

Blood and Other Tests
♦ A simple blood test examining the red cells, white cells and platelets will usually let the doctor decide whether acute leukemia is a serious possibility.
♦ Other tests such as a special type of urine test will be helpful in cases of suspected neuroblastoma.

Imaging
♦ X-rays and CT and MRI scans help the physician decide whether there are tumors in the brain, chest, abdomen or extremities.

Endoscopy and Biopsy
♦ Some suspected tumors may have to be biopsied for a definitive diagnosis.

STAGING

Many so-called solid tumors of childhood—those that do not develop in the blood—are often staged by a system that classifies the disease by whether it can be completely removed surgically. The involvement of lymph nodes and spread to distant sites are also considered. Greatly simplified, Stage I usually refers to local disease that can be entirely removed by a surgeon. Stage II could still be a local disease that may also be removed but has extended beyond the immediate area of the tumor. Stage III disease tends to be more extensive but localized in one particular region of the body, and Stage IV disease is widespread, having spread though the blood or lymphatic system to produce new tumors (metastases) in other organs.

Leukemia is often defined according to its potential for relapse as low risk, average risk and high risk. The child with low-risk leukemia has an excellent chance of responding to therapy in the long term and the best chance of being cured. On the other hand, a child with high-risk leukemia may still respond to therapy and may still be cured, although he or she may need more intensive treatment.

TREATMENT OVERVIEW

The treatment of a child's cancer may involve surgery, chemotherapy, radiation therapy, immunotherapy and various supportive measures.

The special problems seen with childhood cancers mean that a child should not be treated only by a single physician. A team approach is required, with physicians assisted by many specialists including psychologists and experts in nursing, social services, nutrition, physical therapy, occupational therapy, pharmacy, child life, and other fields. They should all be involved in designing the appropriate treatment and support program for the child and his or her family.

This kind of multidisciplinary approach can be accomplished only in a "center of excellence," an approved pediatric cancer specialty unit. In the United States and Canada there are two cooperative groups known as The Children's Cancer Group and The Pediatric Oncology Group. Over 90 percent of children younger than 15 with cancer are treated at an institution that is a member of one of these two groups. Families of adolescents and young adults between 16 and 21 are encouraged to seek a referral to one of these centers.

When a child is diagnosed with cancer in most of these centers, his or her case is presented to a Tumor Board, a meeting of physician specialists, subspecialists and other members of the treatment team who evaluate the child, discuss the options and agree to a proposed treatment plan.

Clinical Trials Cancer in children is rare. Each year in the United States, slightly over 3,000 children develop leukemia, 2,000 develop various kinds of brain and nervous system tumors. Approximately 500 children develop neuroblastoma and fewer than 500 develop Wilms' tumor. Rhabdomyosarcoma, retinoblastoma, osteosarcoma and Ewing's sarcoma are less common. Obviously, if progress is to be made on more effective treatment methods, physicians throughout the nation have to work closely together in designing therapies.

Accordingly, all children with cancer who are treated in a center of excellence are asked to participate in a clinical research program. It is because of these programs that we have made such gratifying progress in the treatment of childhood cancer over the past few decades. Parents and their children are encouraged to participate in them.

Phase III Trials A child may be a candidate for a research program known as a clinical protocol, which will compare one form of treatment to another. The research protocol will be explained and parents will be asked to agree to participate with their child in the program.

The program may involve "randomization," meaning that which one of the several potentially effective treatments the child receives will be decided by chance. Parents are often upset when they learn that if they participate in a research program the decision about which treatment their child will receive will not be chosen by their child's physician. But parents should understand that their child's physician would not participate in the program unless he or she were comfortable that *all* the various treatment choices are reasonable, appropriate and offer the child an excellent chance of attaining a response.

The initial treatment programs designed to answer which treatment program is best are often known as Phase III studies. Sometimes a research protocol is not available, and then the physician chooses the best-known effective treatment available for the disease and presents it as the proposed treatment plan.

Most children respond very well to the initial treatment of their cancer. The opportunity to cure a child with cancer may be as high as 80 to 90 percent for some children with acute lymphoblastic leukemia and Wilms' tumor, but unfortunately less in most other tumors. The patient's physician will be able to describe in detail the treatment being proposed and the chances of the child being cured.

Phase II Trials Unfortunately, not all children respond to therapy. Even those who do may relapse. These children may still have their disease controlled and cured.

Children with recurrent disease are often asked to participate in Phase II protocols, treatment programs in which the dose and many of the side effects of a particular drug or treatment are known. The goal of treatment is to determine how effective the treatment is for certain kinds of childhood cancer.

If this kind of study is available and the child and parents are asked to participate, the physician will describe in detail the proposed treatment, the risks involved and the possible advantages of the child working with the physician in this research approach.

Phase I Trials Occasionally there are drugs to be tested in children for the first time. Research protocols involving new drugs are called Phase I studies. The goal is to find the appropriate dose to be used, with the hope that the children will respond to the treatment.

Investigational Treatments There is a long list of investigational protocols for most childhood cancers. These protocols are devised after close cooperation and collaboration among investigators working in The Children's Cancer Group or Pediatric Oncology Group or at specific centers of excellence.

The protocols may involve new drugs that have rarely been used in children, such as interferon or IL-2 (interleukin-2). Or they may involve new types of radiation therapy such as high-dose radiation given in a series of small doses (fractionated radiotherapy).

Most pediatric cancer experts do not consider such programs experimental but rather investigational. They consider these protocols an opportunity for the child and his or her family to participate on the frontier of medicine. A child with cancer should be treated with the methods being devised today that will possibly improve the chances for a cure tomorrow.

Bone Marrow Transplantation Several treatment programs for childhood cancer use the concept of bone marrow transplantation, although with many concerns, it is still considered an investigational treatment under evaluation (*see* Chapter 12).

Allogeneic bone marrow transplantation—which involves giving the child who has cancer bone marrow taken from a donor, ideally a close relative such as a brother or a sister—is being used very often in children with acute non-lymphoblastic (granulocytic) leukemia. It is also used quite frequently in children with acute lymphoblastic leukemia who have had a relapse.

In autologous bone marrow transplantation, the patient's own bone marrow is used. A portion of the bone marrow is stored in the laboratory while the patient receives treatment, and then returned in the form of an intravenous infusion of bone marrow cells. These cells circulate throughout the body and settle into the bone marrow compartment from which they came. They subsequently grow and regenerate the bone marrow.

Newer approaches have also recently been devised. It is now known that bone marrow cells may circulate throughout the blood, and machines that can remove some of the circulating cells are being developed, raising the possibility of removing bone marrow cells from a vein rather than by drawing them out of bones through a needle.

In high-dose rescue therapy—also known as autologous rescue—the patient's bone marrow cells are stored while high-dose chemotherapy is given. The cells are then reinfused. The higher doses of chemotherapy may kill cancer cells more effectively but might also seriously damage the bone marrow if rescue therapy were not performed.

SUPPORTIVE THERAPY

Throughout the course of the child's treatment, there will be a need for many kinds of support therapies.

♦ Transfusions of blood products, platelets and white cells may be needed.

♦ Infections are common in children and may require specific antibiotics. Exposure to contagious disease is likely to occur, so the child may require specific gamma globulin.

♦ Supportive measures can include nutritional support such as artificial feedings through a vein (hyperalimentation). Access to a vein may be a problem so central venous catheters are often used, such as the Broviac or Hickman catheters or the Port-a-Cath.

♦ Drugs, other agents and psychological support techniques may be necessary to help children with anticipatory nausea, or nausea and vomiting after radiation or chemotherapy treatments.

TREATMENT FOLLOW-UP

Whatever the treatment a child with cancer is receiving, he or she will be followed closely by the pediatric oncologist, other physician specialists and the multidisciplinary team assembled to work with both the child and the family.

Since the child will be on a research protocol in most cases, the physician will be able to outline for the parents an organized plan for follow-up evaluations. These may include specific liver function tests, urine tests for children with neuroblastoma, specific x-rays, psychologic testing or other tests that can help follow the progress and effects of the disease and the response to treatment.

Even when a child finishes a course of treatment, he or she will require long-term follow-up by a pediatric cancer expert. This is not only because some treatments have long-term side effects, but also because children who are cured of a first cancer do have a small risk of developing a second one. So even the child who fin-

ishes therapy and is apparently cured should be followed by a specialist for the rest of his or her life.

SOME OF THE MOST IMPORTANT QUESTIONS (AND ANSWERS) FOR YOU AND YOUR CHILD

FOR THE CHILD

♦ *What do I have?*
It is now known that children do better when they are told the truth about their illness. We no longer hide from them the fact that they have cancer. We explain the nature of their disease, tell them about the therapy and ask them to work with physicians and other experts to help them attain a cure. Honesty is the best way to help a child with cancer face the serious problems of the disease.

♦ *Why did this happen?*
We do not know why children develop cancer. Although there are some environmental or genetic clues that a child may be at risk, specific causes have not been found in the same way that streptococcus bacteria causes a sore throat.

It is important for the child—and the parents—to realize that having cancer is not a punishment. Cancer occurs in children throughout the world. Parents should not feel guilty. Their strength and optimism is needed by their child, who is facing a serious disease and requires their support to conquer the cancer and win the battle for his or her life.

♦ *Will my hair grow back?*
Most children lose their hair temporarily after chemotherapy. In rare cases, such as when very intensive radiation treatments are used, hair may not grow back. But in most cases the child develops a beautiful head of hair after the temporary period of baldness. Many children use wigs to help them with their self-image during these periods.

♦ *What will happen with the acne and chubby face I have when I'm getting prednisone treatment?*

Prednisone and other steroids such as dexamethasone do cause a temporary gain in weight and may cause facial acne. Once these drugs are stopped the weight gain and the puffiness of the face disappear and the skin improves dramatically. There are very few if any permanent side effects of these treatments. Occasionally stretch marks may be seen in the abdomen, but otherwise the child's complexion and facial configuration do return to normal.

FOR THE PARENT

♦ *When will I get my child back?*

When a child is diagnosed as having cancer, he or she may experience a change in personality. The child's spirit, temperament and behavior pattern may change substantially. The initial treatment may require a long period of hospitalization and even if the child is seen as an outpatient there are frequent visits that may include uncomfortable injections. It may take a while before the family pattern gets back to normal. Parents have to be patient. It may take several months before their child's behavior returns to what it was before the illness.

♦ *How about school?*

For a child, school is the normal working environment. Just as an adult wishes to return to work and continue his or her normal activities, so too the child wishes to get back to the normal routine. Multidisciplinary programs will offer the family support to work with the school system so that the child with cancer can re-enter his or her normal environment. School administrators, teachers and others are becoming more familiar with the fact that children in their classrooms may be undergoing cancer therapy. For the most part, school personnel are understanding. They can develop flexible schedules that permit the child to take advantage of the maximum number of educational opportunities while continuing with treatment programs.

♦ *How can we help relieve the nausea, vomiting and other side effects of chemotherapy?*

Unfortunately, many cancer chemotherapy drugs cause nausea, vomiting, mouth sores, constipation, skin rashes, sore eyes and generally a lower resistance to infection. Physicians can offer other medications that will help the child tolerate some of these side effects. The medications themselves will often cause tiredness. Prompt attention should be given to the constipation caused by vincristine.

♦ *What are the long-term effects of therapy?*

A number of long-term effects of childhood cancer therapy are currently being studied. Radiation therapy to the brain may leave some children with certain deficits in intellectual or motor development, which is why psychometric testing is so important as part of the general treatment follow-up.

Some children may have growth problems. Some may have an organ abnormality because of the effects of radiation therapy or surgery. Rehabilitation may be necessary, such as a new bladder to urinate or an artificial limb. Some drugs also affect the way organs such as the lungs and heart work. Children with cancer may have to be followed for many years to discover whether some of the treatments used to cure the disease will result in organ problems later on in life.

♦ *What are the chances for my child being cured?*

A physician will be able to explain to the child and the parents the chances of attaining not only remission—control of the disease—but actual cure. These "chances" are statistical averages, however, and children are not statistics. A family can concentrate on the negative or on the positive. As long as there is an opportunity for a cure, it makes more sense to concentrate on the positive and focus the family's energy on the possibility that their child will be cured and will grow up and live a normal life span. Most children with cancer *are* cured and become healthy adults, parents and productive members of society.

♦ *What happens if my child does not respond?*
There are children who do not respond to treatment and unfortunately the disease may take their life. If it appears that this is going to happen, the child's physician will be the first to explain to the parents the nature of the problem and the reason why it looks as though the child is not going to have his or her life saved. The health care team will make sure that the child is comfortable and treated in a humane, caring manner. The physician and other members of the multidisciplinary team will work with the family to provide emotional, psychological and spiritual support.

"CLIMBING THE MOUNTAIN"
For the child with cancer and his or her parents there are two basic choices. They can choose the pessimistic road, which goes downhill and expects that the cancer will cause the child to die. They can choose the optimistic road, an admittedly uphill road leading to the top of a mountain.

The curves in the mountain road are many. They are the many problems that have to be handled during treatment, which may include:
♦ Recurrent admission to the hospital for fevers and infections requiring intravenous antibiotics.
♦ Side effects of chemotherapy such as hair loss, nausea, vomiting, mouth ulcers, stomach ulcers, blood in the urine and rectal ulcers.
♦ Side effects of radiation therapy such as hair loss, skin irritation, nausea, vomiting and fatigue.
♦ Side effects of surgery including discomfort and organs that do not work in a normal way.
♦ Allergic reactions to blood, blood products or antibiotics.
♦ Changes in plans to attend school or social functions or to go on family trips.
♦ Therapies that are only partially successful.
♦ Special kinds of treatment such as investigational protocols or bone marrow transplantation.

Each and every one of these problems or curves can be difficult to manage. But each and every one has been managed successfully by other children and other families of children who have cancer. Sometimes, a curve can't be maneuvered and it is necessary to move onto the pessimistic road. But for most children with cancer, the curves can be managed and the climb up the mountain is successful. Treatment may be for six months or a year or even two, three or more years, but the top of the mountain can be reached.

The goal for all children with cancer is that they will be cured. More and more children with cancer are attaining this goal and are growing up to be healthy adults. So children and their parents should be optimistic. Knowing that cure is a possibility, each child and his or her family should plan on climbing the mountain and reaching the top. On the top, the sky is blue and the sun is shining.

CHILDHOOD CANCERS: BRAIN TUMORS

Malin Dollinger, MD, and Mark Greenberg, MB, ChB

Primary brain tumors—those that start in the brain rather than spreading there from other parts of the body—are the most common "solid" tumors children get. They pose a major treatment challenge that has to be met by the coordinated efforts of a variety of health care professionals, including specialists in pediatric neurosurgery, radiation therapy and oncology, as well as neuroradiologists and neuropathologists. Significant emotional stresses and problems may occur, requiring intervention by specialized health care professionals.

Many tumors are controllable or curable with treatment, and over half of the children diagnosed with brain tumors will live more than five years. Every child's therapy should be aggressively planned with the intent to cure if possible. This is true even in situations where the same tumor occurring in an adult would not likely be cured.

As is true of all pediatric cancers, but especially with brain tumors, most advances in treatment have been produced by clinical trials of new methods. Various major cancer centers and cooperative groups such as the Pediatric Oncology Group and the Children's Cancer Study Group have clinical treatment protocols available for many tumors, and consideration should be given to enrolling children in such trials. They generally represent the most advanced and promising methods of treatment.

Types Brain tumors are classified by the appearance of their cells under the microscope (histopathology) and their location in the brain. The types that occur in children are generally similar to those seen in adults, although there are a few types that

are much more common in children.

There is a structure in the back part of the brain, a roof-like membrane called the tentorium. This is just above the cerebellum (the portion of the brain having to do with balance and coordination) and the brain stem. There are significant differences in the types of tumors occurring above and below this membrane, as well as in the methods used to make a diagnosis and follow the results of therapy.

About half the brain tumors in children occur below the tentorium, most being in the cerebellum or the nearby cavity called the fourth ventricle. This area of the skull cavity is the posterior fossa. Tumors in the region include astrocytomas, medulloblastomas, ependymomas and brain stem gliomas.

The area above the tentorium, which makes up most of the brain, is called the supratentorial region. Tumors in this area include astrocytomas, cerebral neuroblastomas, ependymoma, craniopharyngioma, meningioma, germ cell tumors, optic nerve glioma, pineal tumors and choroid plexus tumors.

There may be many different names for these tumors, especially as newer classification systems are more descriptive or accurate.

How It Spreads Brain tumors rarely spread outside the central nervous system, but can spread within the brain and the spinal cord.

What Causes It Unknown, although some genetic disorders have been associated with an increased risk.

SCREENING

There are no effective screening measures.

COMMON SIGNS AND SYMPTOMS

Symptoms related to the increased pressure in the brain as the tumor expands include headache, nausea, vomiting (which may or may not not accompany nausea) and seizures. Symptoms related to the tumor's location and the pressure it puts on nearby structures include weakness or changes in sensation in various parts of the body, difficulties in coordination or balance, vision and speech problems and seizures.

DIAGNOSIS

Physical Examination
♦ Complete neurologic examination.
♦ Evaluation for optic tract glioma includes neuro-ophthalmological testing, including visual fields. Subtle changes in the tumor that may not be apparent with CT or MRI scanning can be measured in this way. Young children may have a test called visual-evoked response for diagnosis and follow-up.

Blood and Other Tests
♦ Bone marrow may be analyzed for tumors that spread outside the central nervous system (medulloblastoma).
♦ For tumors that may spread to the spinal cord or through the cerebrospinal fluid (medulloblastoma, ependymoma, intracranial germ cell tumors, pineal tumors, cerebral neuroblastoma—PNET), spinal fluid should be examined for malignant cells.
♦ For intracranial germ cell tumors, tumor markers including alpha-fetoprotein (AFP) and human chorionic gonadotropin (HCG) are measured in the blood and cerebrospinal fluid. The same markers are also measured in pineal tumors to exclude the possibility of a malignant germ cell tumor.

Imaging
♦ Imaging has been conventionally done by CT for the brain and myelography for the spinal cord. Recently, MRI imaging with gadolinium enhancement has been shown to be extremely sensitive, useful and simpler for both the brain and spinal cord.
♦ Images of the entire brain and spinal cord should be done for tumors that may spread to the spinal cord (medulloblastoma, ependymoma, intracranial germ cell tumors, pineal tumors, cerebral neuroblastoma—PNET).
♦ Bone scans and bone marrow examinations are sometimes done in medulloblastoma because this tumor may spread outside the central nervous system, especially to bone and bone marrow.

Endoscopy and Biopsy
♦ Tumors of the brain stem, the medulla and the pons (brain stem glioma) may be biopsied. The procedure is risky. They cannot be removed surgically (radiation therapy is the standard treatment). Stereotactic needle biopsy techniques may enable biopsy to be done when it could have an effect on treatment—for example, if it is not certain that a mass in this area is malignant, if the tumor grows outwards and protrudes into the ventricles or if there is a need to remove part of the tumor because of pressure symptoms.
♦ Biopsy of optic tract glioma is not always possible because it is difficult to expose the area surgically.

STAGING

There are no generally useful staging systems for most brain tumors, although some are classified according to grade. With brain stem glioma, for example, tumors in the higher region—the midbrain—are more likely to be lower grade and have a higher chance of long-term survival than tumors lower down in the pons and the medulla (40 percent versus less than 20 percent).

A variety of staging systems have been used for medulloblastoma. The Pediatric Oncology Group and the Children's Cancer

Study Group have divided this tumor into low and high stages. Essentially, low-stage implies smaller tumors without metastasis, in which the tumor remaining after surgery is smaller than 1.5 cubic cm. High-stage refers to larger tumors with evidence of metastatic spread or brain stem involvement and tumor over 1.5 cubic cm remaining after surgery.

TREATMENT OVERVIEW

Treatment includes surgery, with or without radiation therapy, and for some tumors, chemotherapy. Radiation therapy of pediatric brain tumors is very complex and should be carried out in facilities with extensive experience.

Chemotherapy has recently shown some activity in children with recurrent brain tumors and in children with high-stage medulloblastoma treated with chemotherapy prior to relapse. There is great interest in using chemotherapy after surgery as the only therapy in children under age three, since radiation therapy to the brain in this age group may seriously impair brain development.

Clinical Trials All children with brain tumors should be considered for entry into clinical trials. This form of cancer is rare in children and trials offer the advantage of the pooled experience of pediatric cancer centers around the country.

Pediatric clinical trials are designed in two ways. One method divides the children into two groups, with one receiving the best currently accepted standard treatment and the other receiving the new therapy that appears promising. The other method is to evaluate a single new treatment in all patients and then compare the results with those obtained with existing therapy, often in the same institution.

TREATMENT BY TUMOR TYPE

MEDULLOBLASTOMA
This is also called primitive neuroectodermal tumor (PNET). It arises in the cerebellum and may spread to adjacent tissues. It also can spread via the cerebrospinal fluid to the rest of the brain or the spinal cord and very rarely to sites outside the nervous system.

Standard Treatment An attempt is made to surgically remove as much tumor as possible. Studies are done during and after the operation to define the risk of relapse, and treatment is given according to the best estimate of low-stage or high-stage disease.

For low-stage disease, standard therapy after surgery is a high dose of radiation to the tumor area and a lower dose to the entire brain and spine. Lowering the dosage of radiation to reduce problems with nervous system development reduces the chance for cure. Children under three should be entered in studies that use chemotherapy and probably delayed or modified radiation therapy.

Treatment of high-stage disease involves chemotherapy in addition to surgery and radiation therapy similar to that given in low-stage disease.

These patients should be considered for entry into clinical trials to establish the best combination and sequence of chemotherapy.

Five-Year Survival About 60 percent

Recurrent Cancer Medulloblastoma that recurs after radiotherapy should be considered for treatment with investigational protocols using new agents. Fewer than one-third of those patients respond and long-term control of disease is unusual.

CEREBELLAR ASTROCYTOMA
These are generally low-grade tumors in the cerebellum. Spread is unusual.

Standard Treatment The primary treatment is surgical removal of the tumor, which is successful in removing all the tumor in most cases. In contrast to most other brain tumors, some patients with microscopic and even larger residual tumor after surgery may survive a long time without any symptoms or tumor growth even without postoperative therapy. This may be significant because a second operation may produce neurologic problems.

The use of radiation therapy for patients with residual tumor after surgery is under discussion. Some radiation oncologists treat all patients with residual disease, others withhold treatment until the tumor starts to grow.

Ten-Year Survival About 80 percent

Recurrent Cancer Cerebellar astrocytoma that recurs is treated, if possible, with another surgery. If this is not possible, local radiation is used. If it recurs in an area where it can't be removed and has already received maximum radiation, chemotherapy should be considered. Since there is little information available about the role of chemotherapy, Phase I and Phase II clinical studies should be considered.

INFRATENTORIAL EPENDYMOMA
These tumors arise from the cells lining the fourth ventricle (a cavity within the brain), as well as those lining a cavity in the center of the spinal cord. They can occur anywhere in the brain or spinal cord, but 60 percent of them start in the part of the brain in the back of the skull, the posterior fossa. The prognosis depends on the grade and size of the tumor and the degree of spread. These tumors may spread via the spinal fluid pathways.

Standard Treatment Surgical excision followed by high-dose radiation to the back part of the brain is the usual treatment.

Radiotherapy to the entire brain and spinal cord is controversial, being used most commonly in high-grade tumors.

There is no clear benefit for adjuvant chemotherapy, although consideration should be given to using chemotherapy to delay or modify radiation therapy in very young children.

Five-Year Survival 25 to 60 percent

Recurrent Cancer This tumor is seldom controlled permanently if it recurs after surgery and radiotherapy. About one-third of patients respond to cisplatin, so Phase I and II clinical trials should be considered.

BRAIN STEM GLIOMA
Tumors arising in the brain stem are often astrocytomas, a tumor of neuron-support cells. These are also referred to as brain stem gliomas. They may be low-, intermediate- or high-grade.

Standard Treatment The usual treatment is high-dose radiation therapy (over 5,500 cGy). Higher doses may be possible using twice-daily (hyperfractionated) treatment.

The role of chemotherapy is not well defined. Some patients may be candidates for surgical removal. Children younger than three may be given chemotherapy to delay or modify radiation therapy to reduce the risk of neurologic impairment.

Two-Year Survival Varies with site and grade of tumor

Investigational
♦ The use of chemotherapy before the standard radiotherapy treatment.

Recurrent Cancer There is no standard therapy for recurrent brain stem glioma. These children cannot have surgery, have already received maximum radiation therapy, and there are no standard chemotherapy drugs that have significant results. They should be entered in a Phase I or Phase II clinical drug trial.

CEREBRAL ASTROCYTOMA
LOW GRADE
These tumors may sometimes be completely removed surgically, in which case they have a favorable prognosis. These tumors spread by extension to the adjacent brain and sometimes occur in multiple sites.

Standard Treatment The treatment for low-grade supratentorial astrocytoma is surgery. If the tumor cannot be completely removed, radiotherapy is given after the operation. In some centers, radiotherapy is withheld until progression of disease is shown. The role of chemotherapy is not defined but initial results are promising.

Five-Year Survival 50 to 80 percent

Recurrent Cancer Patients may benefit from chemotherapy if tumors recur after maximum surgery and radiation therapy. No standard agents have a high degree of response, although cyclophosphamide, cisplatin and the nitrosoureas may be useful. Carboplatin has shown promise. Consideration should be given to clinical trials.

CEREBRAL ASTROCYTOMA
HIGH GRADE
Sometimes called anaplastic astrocytoma or glioblastoma multiforme, these tumors often grow rapidly and involve portions of the brain that cause major neurological problems.

Standard Treatment Treatment includes surgery, radiation therapy and chemotherapy. Radiation is given after as complete a surgical resection as possible to an area that encompasses the entire tumor and sometimes the whole brain.
A Children's Cooperative Group study with radiation therapy and three chemotherapy agents (vincristine + lomustine + prednisone) produced a 40 percent survival of three years compared

with 13 percent for children treated with radiation therapy alone. Again, children under the age of three may receive chemotherapy to delay or modify radiotherapy. A number of clinical trials are evaluating the role of chemotherapy.

Two-Year Survival Less than 25 percent. The prognosis may be better if the tumor can be totally removed. Younger patients and those with lower grade tumors may do better.

Recurrent Cancer Chemotherapy is given if relapse occurs after radiation therapy. Since no standard agents have a high degree of activity, entry on a clinical trial should be considered.

SUPRATENTORIAL EPENDYMOMA
These ependymomas arise outside the posterior fossa (back of the skull), usually within and adjacent to the ventricles.

Standard Treatment Surgery followed by radiation therapy. In low-grade tumors, the primary tumor area is given radiation. With high-grade tumors, the entire brain and spinal cord are treated.
Adjuvant chemotherapy is under evaluation. Consideration should be given to its use in very young children to delay or modify radiation therapy.

Two-Year Survival About 40 percent

Investigational
♦ Various radiotherapy trials, with and without chemotherapy.

Recurrent Cancer This tumor is seldom controlled if it recurs after surgery and radiation therapy, although one-third of patients respond to cisplatin. Phase I and II clinical studies should be considered.

CRANIOPHARYNGIOMA
These benign tumors arise in the central portion of the brain and produce prob-

lems primarily because of their location. Since they are benign, metastasis is unknown.

Standard Treatment Surgery is the treatment of choice and produces a high rate of control in most patients. For recurrent unresectable tumors, radiotherapy is recommended. There is no reported role for chemotherapy.

Ten-Year Survival About 80 percent

INTRACRANIAL GERM CELL TUMOR

Germ cell brain tumors—there are a number of sub-types—usually arise in the central portion of the brain. Under the microscope, they resemble more common germ cell tumors of the testis and ovary. The prognosis relates to the cell type and is especially favorable in patients with germinoma.

Standard Treatment The role of surgery is usually a biopsy to establish the diagnosis, since the location of these tumors usually prevents complete removal. Germinoma may be treated with radiation therapy to the brain and spinal cord, with high doses to the tumor and somewhat lower doses to the rest of the nerve tissue. There is emerging evidence that local radiation therapy plus chemotherapy produces equivalent cure rates.

Advanced or disseminated germinomas, as well as the various germ cell tumors other than germinoma, are usually treated with radiation to the brain and spinal cord. There are several views about the dosage and areas that should be treated.

Non-germinoma germ cell tumors may respond to a variety of chemotherapeutic agents, including bleomycin, cisplatin, etoposide, cyclophosphamide and vincristine. The role of adjuvant chemotherapy, in addition to radiation, is not yet determined for these tumors that arise within the brain, although chemotherapy is extremely effective in these tumors elsewhere in the body.

Survival Variable

Recurrent Cancer Intracerebral germ cell tumors may be responsive to the same type of chemotherapy combinations used against germ cell tumors in other locations—PVB (cisplatin + vinblastine + bleomycin) and VAC (vincristine + dactinomycin + cyclophosphamide).

If the tumor recurs after treatment with these programs, Phase I and II clinical studies should be used to try to find agents that may be useful in treating this tumor, which is often responsive to chemotherapy.

PINEAL TUMORS

This undifferentiated tumor resembles medulloblastoma, but it develops in the region of the pineal gland in the center of the brain. The prognosis depends upon the size of tumor and its degree of spread.

Standard Treatment The usual treatment is radiation therapy. There is some controversy about the possibility of surgical removal, although biopsy is recommended whenever possible to establish a diagnosis. A high dose of radiation is given to the tumor, with a lower dose to the brain and spinal cord.

Studies are exploring the role of chemotherapy for poorly differentiated pineal tumors, although well-differentiated tumors may be treated with simple local radiation therapy. Young children may be given chemotherapy to delay or modify the radiation treatments.

Two-Year Survival Less than 50 percent

OPTIC TRACT GLIOMA

These tumors grow along the optic tracts of the brain that carry visual impulses. They are low-grade and slow-growing astrocytomas that produce visual symptoms.

Standard Treatment Radiation therapy is the usual treatment for optic tract gliomas that are growing. Some tumors that do not appear to be growing and have no symptoms may be observed without treatment.

Chemotherapy has not been used as an adjuvant to radiation therapy as part of standard treatment, but the previous considerations about the risks of radiation in children under the age of three apply. The use of vincristine and other drugs of relatively low toxicity has enabled radiation therapy to be delayed in more than 80 percent of children and is being further evaluated.

Five-Year Survival Over 75 percent

CEREBRAL NEUROBLASTOMA— *Supratentorial Primitive Neuro-ectodermal Tumor (PNET)*

There are a variety of names for these tumors. They are poorly differentiated tumors, which microscopically may have features of various primitive tumors of other cell types. Prognosis depends upon the extent of disease.

Standard Treatment The usual treatment is high-dose radiation therapy. Many radiation oncologists also radiate the entire brain and spinal cord because of this tumor's tendency to spread to the rest of the central nervous system through the cerebrospinal fluid. Chemotherapy has been used in several clinical trials, especially in younger children. It appears to produce good control and has particular

value in younger children to delay or avoid the use of radiation therapy. Carboplatin may be a particularly useful drug.

Two-Year Survival 30 to 50 percent

TREATMENT FOLLOW-UP

♦ Repeated clinical evaluation, emphasizing initial neurologic signs and symptoms.
♦ Repeated CT or MRI scanning.
♦ Repeated studies of any other abnormal tests, such as cerebrospinal fluid or visual fields.
♦ Since radiotherapy can affect growth hormone production and brain development, careful endocrine and neurologic follow-up is very important.

THE MOST IMPORTANT QUESTIONS YOU CAN ASK

♦ What type of brain tumor does my child have?
♦ How does it usually behave?
♦ What is the chance of cure?
♦ What is the standard treatment and how successful is it?
♦ Should radiotherapy be used? When?
♦ Should chemotherapy be used? When?
♦ If the treatment is not completely effective or my child relapses later, what else can be done?

CHILDHOOD CANCERS: RETINOBLASTOMA

Jerry Z. Finklestein, MD

Retinoblastoma is a malignant tumor of the retina, the membrane at the back of the eyeball. About 200 children in the United States develop this cancer each year, most diagnosed before they reach the age of five. The tumor may be in one eye (70 percent) or both eyes (30 percent).

How It Spreads The tumor may be confined to the retina or extend directly to other parts of the eye. In its later stages, it may spread to the central nervous system or other parts of the body.

What Causes It There are hereditary and non-hereditary forms of retinoblastoma. When there is disease in both eyes, it is almost always the hereditary form. The retinoblastoma gene has been identified and, therefore, families of children with retinoblastoma should have genetic counseling.

DIAGNOSIS

Most children in the U.S. are diagnosed while the tumor remains within the eye. The tumor is detected by shining a light into a child's eye and looking for what is called a cat's eye—a white spot in place of the dark pupil. There may also be symptoms such as poor vision or malfunctioning of the eye.

It is important for children with retinoblastoma to be seen in a specialized center where physicians have experience in evaluating the size of the tumor and the extent of the disease.

STAGING

Several staging systems are used, but for purposes of treatment retinoblastoma is divided into intraocular (within the eye) and extraocular (spread beyond the eye) disease.

TREATMENT OVERVIEW

Standard Treatment In some cases, it may be possible to destroy the tumor within the eye by using light treatments (photocoagulation), freezing (cryotherapy) or laser therapy. Treatment may include an enucleation, meaning that the eye is removed and eventually replaced with an artificial eye. High-dose radiation also has a role.

Which of these procedures is used depends on the size of the tumor and whether the child has potentially useful vision.

The use of chemotherapy requires additional investigation, although tumors generally respond in a satisfactory manner to a number of chemotherapy drugs.

Five-Year Survival Over 90 percent if disease is confined to the eye; less than 10 percent if it has spread beyond the eye.

TREATMENT FOLLOW-UP

Children with retinoblastoma, especially the hereditary form, have an increased risk for developing other malignancies later in life and so should be followed closely. Up to 8 percent, for example, may develop bone tumors after 18 years, and the percentage may be higher with longer follow-up. Second cancers may develop spontaneously or be the result of treatment.

CHILDHOOD CANCERS:
SOFT TISSUE AND BONE SARCOMAS
Arthur Ablin, MD, and Malin Dollinger, MD

Cancers involving muscle, bone, blood vessels and other supporting tissues in the body are termed sarcomas. They are different than carcinomas, which are malignancies of the tissues lining or covering the body's internal organs and passageways. Of all the cancers of solid tissues, children most frequently have sarcomas. Carcinomas are much more frequent in adults.

Types Rhabdomyosarcoma of muscle is the most common soft tissue sarcoma in children, accounting for slightly more than half of all soft tissue sarcomas. Many different tissue types account for the rest. They may be located in nerves or their covering sheaths, blood vessel walls, joint linings, fatty tissues or muscles.

Other sarcomas in children occur in or around bone. The most common is osteogenic sarcoma, which is a cancer of the bone tissue itself. The second most common is Ewing's sarcoma and the closely related primitive neuroectodermal tumors. Although they occur in or around bone, these tumors probably originate from the nerve tissue in these locations.

In the United States, an estimated 500 to 700 children under 18 are diagnosed with rhabdomyosarcoma each year. Osteosarcoma strikes 450 to 600 young people, Ewing's sarcoma affects 350 to 400, and fewer develop primitive neuroectodermal tumors.

The rarity of these tumors emphasizes the need for treatment by a small number of physicians in a limited number of children's cancer centers so that the most experienced physicians and expert care can be available. This also allows the most rapid accumulation of knowledge about treatment, since it facilitates cooperative studies between institutions. The great progress made in treating these tumors over the past two decades has been in large part due to cooperative clinical studies designed to find the most effective treatments.

What Causes It Unknown.

RHABDOMYOSARCOMA

This tumor is almost always found in muscle areas that can be controlled voluntarily, such as the eye, bladder, arms and legs. (Involuntary muscles are those that work automatically, such as the heart or the wall of the intestinal tract.) The head and neck is the most common site, followed by the genito-urinary area—the vagina in girls, near the testes or prostate in boys, and the bladder. The trunk, chest or back of the abdomen are less frequently involved.

How It Spreads The tumor can spread directly into surrounding tissues, through the lymphatic vessels to regional lymph nodes or through the bloodstream to the lung, bone, bone marrow and the central nervous system.

Symptoms Symptoms vary according to the location. The tumor is often painless but produces symptoms when it impinges on nearby tissues. The first sign may be a painless lump in or around the eye, on a limb or in the abdomen. A small mass may extrude from the vagina. When the tumor is in the bladder, there may be difficulty urinating or blood in the urine. Back or abdominal pain or jaundice can develop when the tumor is large enough to cause pressure or obstruction.

Diagnosis and Staging Other entities can produce the same symptoms as rhabdomyosarcoma, so a biopsy is always necessary to establish the diagnosis with certainty. X-rays, MRI scanning and bone marrow examinations are used to determine the extent of the disease.

Treatment Overview Surgery, radiation and chemotherapy are combined in the treatment of this diverse tumor. The order in which they are given, which combination of drugs is used and how and how much radiation is delivered vary according to the location, tissue type and extent of the disease. Putting together the many variables about each tumor—staging—allows a specific treatment plan and the most accurate estimate about outcome to be formulated.

TREATMENT BY GROUP

GROUP I
No evidence of tumor remaining after surgery.

Standard Treatment Surgery, followed by chemotherapy and, possibly, radiation. The tumors with the best outlook are those around the eye or testes that can be completely removed and have no evidence of spread. Patients are given vincristine and actinomycin, sometimes without radiation therapy.

The next best outlook is for tumors in the head, neck and pelvic areas, other than the bladder and prostate, that can be completely removed. Vincristine or actinomycin or both may be given with cyclophosphamide, etoposide or ifosfamide and radiation.

Five-Year Survival 75 to 95 percent

GROUP II
Microscopic tumor remaining after surgery.

Standard Treatment These tumors are treated in the same manner as Group I lesions.

Five-Year Survival 65 percent

GROUP III
Tumors cannot be removed at initial surgery because they have infiltrated into surrounding tissues or lymph nodes, but have not shown evidence of spread to distant sites.

Standard Treatment These patients are treated with similar combination chemotherapy and radiation after surgery, but may have a second opportunity at surgery to remove the tumor completely after it has decreased in size.

Five-Year Survival 45 percent

GROUP IV
The tumor has spread to distant sites at the time of diagnosis.

Standard Treatment New combinations of drugs are used in the hope of finding effective agents that are then combined with standard combinations of vincristine, actinomycin and cyclophosphamide and radiation.

Five-Year Survival 20 percent

RECURRENT CANCER

Several options are available if there is a relapse or inadequate response to initial therapy. Extremely intensive treatment with radiation and chemotherapy, which would not normally be possible because of severe damage to the bone marrow, can be followed by bone marrow transplantation. Alternatively, investigational drugs or biologic agents are often available for trial at children's cancer centers. Supportive treatments are always available, especially for dying patients, who should never be allowed to feel that treatment is stopping.

OTHER SOFT TISSUE SARCOMAS

There are many types of sarcoma, and any single one occurs very rarely. Treatment varies from one patient to the next and can vary from simple surgical excision alone to extensive surgery and aggressive chemotherapy, with and without radiation. In general, staging and treatment are similar to rhabdomyosarcoma. Treatment can be somewhat less aggressive for small, completely excised tumors.

Type	Most Common Location
Fibrosarcoma	
Congenital	Extremity and trunk
Adult form	Thigh and knee
Neurofibrosarcoma	Extremity, back of abdomen, trunk
Synovial sarcoma	Around but not in joints
Hemangiopericytoma	Head, neck, back of abdomen
Malignant fibrous histiocytoma	Extremity
Liposarcoma	Extremity, back of abdomen

OSTEOGENIC SARCOMAS

These highly malignant tumors are composed of abnormal cancerous bone cells. They can spread throughout the body, producing new masses.

Osteogenic sarcoma occurs most commonly during or just after the years of rapid growth, in the teens and early twenties.

Symptoms There is usually swelling and persistent pain in the involved bone, which is most commonly just above or below the knee, in the hip or in the arm at the shoulder. Any bone may be involved, however. Because of the weakening of the bone by the tumor, there may be a fracture at the cancer site.

Diagnosis and Staging An x-ray may lead to suspicion of an osteogenic sarcoma, but a biopsy is needed for a diagnosis. Determining the extent of disease—staging—is done by looking at the most likely areas of spread with CT, MRI and bone scans. These areas include the lung, other bones and the central nervous system.

TREATMENT BY STAGE

LOCALIZED

This stage of the disease is highly treatable and often curable. The surgeon, radiation oncologist and pediatric oncologist, along with the pathologist and radiologist, meet to plan the overall approach to therapy.

Standard Treatment Some years ago it was customary to recommend amputation for bone sarcomas involving the arms or legs. Nowadays it may be possible to save the extremity (limb salvage) by the use of a combination of several treatment methods, often including a prosthesis, which is surgically inserted to replace the bone that must be removed. Often the first intervention is chemotherapy using drugs such as platinum, doxorubicin, methotrexate and cyclophosphamide or ifosfamide in an attempt to shrink the tumor. Whether a limb-saving surgery or amputation is performed depends on many factors, including the location of the tumor, response to chemotherapy, age and the wishes of the patient and family. Further chemotherapy is given after surgery, sometimes with the same drugs used preoperatively.

Five-Year Survival 60 to 70 percent

METASTATIC
When the tumor has spread through the blood, the disease is still treatable and occasionally curable.

Standard Treatment The most aggressive chemotherapy approaches are used. Radiation may be given to sites of metastases, most commonly the lungs. Surgery may also be necessary to remove lung metastases as well as the original tumor.

More intense chemotherapy, made possible by the use of bone marrow stimulating factors and optimum supportive care measures for complications such as infections and bleeding, may improve survival.

Five-Year Survival 10 to 20 percent

RECURRENT CANCER

When a metastasis occurs in the lung many months after treatment has been completed and no other disease exists, surgery with or without chemotherapy or radiation therapy can be curative. When new metastases develop soon after initial treatment begins, however, the outlook for cure is markedly reduced.

EWING'S SARCOMA AND PRIMITIVE NEUROECTODERMAL TUMORS

This is the second most common bone cancer in adolescents and young adults, occurring usually in those between 5 and 20 years of age. It may also occur in soft tissue (extraosseous Ewing's sarcoma). A more differentiated or mature form of this tumor can develop in either bone or soft tissue, especially in the chest wall, and is called a peripheral primitive neuroectodermal tumor.

Symptoms The most typical sign of the disease is persistent bone pain in one place, most commonly in an extremity, the pelvis or rib.

Diagnosis and Staging Bone x-rays and CT or MRI scans can strongly suggest a diagnosis of Ewing's sarcoma, but definitive diagnosis depends on a biopsy. Chromosome analysis of tumor tissue is sometimes helpful in establishing the diagnosis.

A bone scan, bone marrow analysis, a CT scan of the chest and, perhaps, an MRI scan of the brain are necessary to determine the extent of disease.

TREATMENT BY STAGE

LOCALIZED
The tumor has not spread beyond the site of origin.

Standard Treatment When the tumor is in a bone that can be removed without causing a significant physical handicap, the bone is surgically removed. Unlike treatment for osteogenic sarcoma, major bones are not removed and amputations are not generally recommended because the tumor is sensitive to radiation therapy.

Since most patients have microscopic tumor spread even if this does not show up on imaging studies, chemotherapy is given after initial treatment. Combinations of vincristine, actinomycin, cyclophosphamide or ifosfamide and etoposide are used.

Five-Year Survival 60 to 80 percent

METASTATIC
The tumor has spread, usually to the lungs, other bones and the bone marrow.

Standard Treatment The initial treatment is similar to that for localized disease, but more aggressive chemotherapy is used and radiation therapy is given to metastases.

Supportive care measures, such as

administering bone marrow growth factors, preventing infections and intensively treating fever, are important parts of the treatment plan.

Two-Year Survival 30 to 50 percent

RECURRENT CANCER

This serious complication is even worse if it occurs while the initial treatment is being given. If combination chemotherapy causes the tumor to shrink, consideration should be given to very high dose chemotherapy combined with radiation therapy. This would require a subsequent bone marrow transplant to replace the bone marrow destroyed by these treatments. No reliable figures are yet available to predict the outcome of this approach.

THE MOST IMPORTANT QUESTIONS YOU CAN ASK

♦ What are the details of treatment that will allow my child to receive optimum care?

♦ What can I do to minimize side effects of chemotherapy or radiation?

♦ How can I help my child, especially teenagers, to cooperate with the treatment program?

♦ Is a limb salvage operation or amputation the best procedure and how will each affect survival?

♦ Are further surgical procedures likely if a limb salvage procedure is done?

♦ Does my child understand that the disease is not his or her fault and that no one else can catch it?

COLON AND RECTUM

Ernest H. Rosenbaum, MD, Malin Dollinger, MD, and Michael A. Friedman, MD

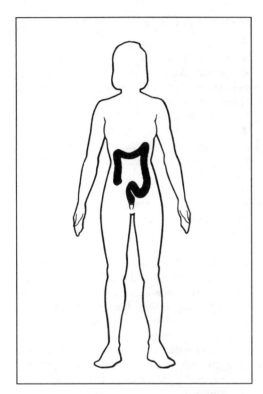

Cancer of the large bowel, or colon and rectum—the last 7 ft. (2 m) of the intestine—is a highly treatable and often curable disease when it is localized and diagnosed in its early stages. But when it spreads through the bowel wall to lymph nodes or nearby organs, the chances for cure are reduced.

Thirteen percent of all cancers in the United States involve either the colon or the rectum. An estimated 149,000 colorectal cancers will be diagnosed in 1994, 107,000 in the colon and 42,000 in the rectum. Taken together, they are second only to lung cancer as a cause of cancer deaths in the United States (56,000 deaths).

These tumors may be common because about half the population over 40 are thought to have clumps of tissues protruding from the inner layer (mucosa) of the colon or rectum. These mushroom-like growths are called polyps, and while most are benign, at least one type—adenomatous polyps—may be a precursor to cancer. About 90 percent of colorectal cancers are thought to arise from these polyps, and a person with a colorectal adenoma runs three times the risk of developing colorectal cancer. Overall, the lifetime risk of developing colorectal cancer is 6 percent (one out of every 20 Americans).

The colon and the rectum look similar and are connected to each other—the rectum is the final 5 in. (12 cm) of the colon above the anus—but there are *major differences* in the way colon and rectal tumors are treated.

Almost half of all patients with colorectal cancer can be cured with surgery, the primary treatment method. Adjuvant chemotherapy can improve the survival for colorectal cancer. Adjuvant radiotherapy and chemotherapy can be used to improve survival for rectal cancer.

The chance for cure is clearly related to how far the tumor has invaded through the bowel wall and whether it has spread to the nearby lymph nodes. For those people whose lymph nodes are invaded by cancer, a major problem is that the tumor can come back after surgery. Recurrent cancer is the ultimate cause of death in one-third of cases.

Types Most colorectal cancers develop in the glands of the inner lining or mucosa and are called adenocarcinomas. Other kinds of tumors—lymphomas, melanomas and carcinoids—occur much less frequently.

How It Spreads Colorectal cancer spreads directly from the mucosa or inner lining through the muscle wall of the bowel and into adjacent tissues. The tumor may metastasize through the lymphatic system to nearby lymph nodes, to the liver through the portal vein and, less frequently, by the bloodstream to the bones or lungs.

What Causes It Environmental factors thought to contribute to the development of colorectal cancers include diet (high in saturated fat, low in fiber and possibly low in calcium) and lack of exercise. It is most common in industrialized countries with high standards of living. It is becoming more common in Japan as consumption of fats increases.

One percent of colon cancers are related to an inherited condition called familial polyposis in which multiple polyps begin to appear in childhood and adolescence. Given enough time, most affected individuals will develop cancer.

Several genetic factors linked to colorectal cancer have been found. *Ras* gene mutations, largely in the *Ki-ras* gene resulting from environmental causes rather than being passed on genetically, are found in half of all people with colorectal adenomas and cancers. The tumor-suppressor gene p53 on chromosome 17 seems to be inactivated in most cases. A second tumor-suppressor gene—called "DCC", for Deleted in Colon Cancer—has been found on chromosome 18, and other genetic abnormalities have been found on chromosome 5. These may be important for tumor suppression. A defective gene dubbed MSH2 has been located on chromosome 2. It has been postulated that this gene defect is responsible for up to two-thirds of the inherited forms of colon cancer. It is possible that when these genetic

defects are fully evaluated, family members could be screened and tested for detection of early colon cancer. Once a polyp has one of these chromosome changes, other "hits" to the cell may cause cancers to develop.

RISK FACTORS

At Significantly Higher Risk
♦ Advancing age, usually over age 40.
♦ Family history of colorectal cancer, especially among first-degree relatives (Lynch syndrome Type I). The risk is two to three times the risk of an average person.
♦ "Cancer Family Syndrome" (Lynch syndrome Type II), with a higher risk for colon cancer and other adenocarcinomas such as cancers of the ovary, endometrium, breast and pancreas.
♦ A personal or family history of multiple adenomatous polyps after age 10 (familial polyposis).
♦ Previous polyps of the colon and rectum.
♦ Inflammatory bowel disease such as ulcerative colitis and ileitis (Crohn's disease). With ulcerative colitis, the risk of cancer is about 20 times the average. Cancer may also develop in the flat surface of the mucosa rather than in polyps. Increased risk for ulcerative colitis occurs in gynecologic cancer, prostate or pelvic cancer, and pelvic cancer following radiation therapy.
♦ Diets high in fat and low in fiber and calcium. Animal rather than vegetable fat is believed responsible. One study indicated that women eating red meat (beef, lamb and pork) daily had 2 1/2 times the risk of those who eat red meat less than once a month. Those eating fish and chicken without the skin were at lesser risk.
♦ High consumption of charcoal-broiled foods.
♦ Inactivity and constipation.
♦ Asbestos exposure.
♦ European (Ashkenazy) Jews.

At Lower than Average Risk
♦ Seventh Day Adventists, lacto-vegetari-

ans who do not drink alcohol or smoke, and Mormons, who abstain from alcohol, tobacco, coffee and tea and eat meat in moderation.

♦ Mediterranean and lower European (Sephardic) Jews.

♦ Hispanics.

SCREENING

Since this cancer is highly curable in the early stages, several techniques for early detection are recommended. These apply to the general population but are especially recommended for people with first-degree relatives with colorectal cancer.

Screening for adenomas that may become carcinomas after 10 or 15 years should begin at age 40, with screening for cancer beginning at age 50. A digital rectal examination should be an annual routine for those over 40, along with testing stools for hidden blood. About 3 percent will have a positive hidden blood test, and anywhere from 20 to 50 percent of these will be positive for polyps or cancer (10 percent will have cancer, 20 to 30 percent will have adenomas). These tests have rates of 2 percent false positives and 30 percent false negatives. False negatives are high because colorectal cancers bleed intermittently and the test may be done between bleedings. The chance of a false positive test can be reduced by not consuming red meat, vitamin C and iron—avoiding cantaloupe, broccoli, parsnips, cauliflower, mushrooms, potatoes, cucumbers, red radishes and horseradish—for 24 hours before the test. A test called HemoQuant has fewer false positive results.

The sigmoid colon and rectum should be examined with a flexible or rigid tube (sigmoidoscopy) every three to five years after age 50 (after two negative sigmoidoscopies one year apart). Colonoscopy will examine the entire colon. It takes about five years for an adenomatous polyp to grow to the size where a cancerous change may occur.

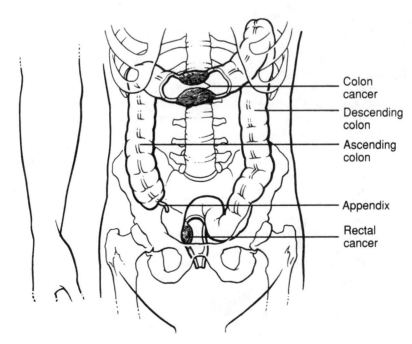

Colon and rectal cancers

Measuring the level of the carcinoembryonic antigen (CEA) in the blood can detect a few early cancer cases, but it is not a good test for screening.

Soon genetic studies will improve screening for people at high risk for developing rectal cancer. Recent research has identified a gene responsible for an inherited form of colon cancer. It is hoped that a blood test will soon be available to identify individuals at high risk.

Screening is costly but may be effective. Finding colorectal cancer before it invades tissues or spreads to lymph nodes will improve the cure rate. The American death rate from this cancer fell 5.5 percent from 1973 to 1985, but there are still 57,000 deaths per year.

COMMON SIGNS AND SYMPTOMS

Colon cancer symptoms depend on the location of the tumor—right colon or left colon.

Cancers of the larger and more pliable right colon frequently bleed, causing anemia, but do not usually block the colon because the stool is still liquid in the right side of the colon.

Cancers in the left colon may obstruct the bowel, causing a change in bowel habits and stool size. There may be dark red rectal bleeding or blood in the stools, which may be long and narrow.

Cancers in the rectum may cause an obstruction, causing a change in bowel habits (including constipation) and in the size of stools, which may become long and narrow. There may also be rectal bleeding. Other symptoms include abdominal or pelvic pain, gas, vomiting, persistent constipation or diarrhea, weight loss and weakness. Pain is a worrisome problem with rectal cancer, since it often means the tumor is growing into nerves.

DIAGNOSIS

Physical Examination
♦ Digital rectal examination to feel for lumps.
♦ Abdominal exam for a mass or an enlarged liver (hepatomegaly).
♦ Enlarged lymph nodes over the left collarbone and in the groin (inguinal) area.

Blood and Other Tests
♦ Test for hidden blood in the stools (stool tests for bleeding may be negative in half of colorectal cancer cases).
♦ Complete blood count (CBC).
♦ Urinalysis.
♦ Serum chemistry profile, including liver enzymes, cholesterol, calcium and serum iron or ferritin (for anemia).
♦ Test for carcinoembryonic antigen (CEA), a serum tumor marker that may be elevated with primary or recurrent colorectal cancer. Very high levels of CEA may indicate more advanced disease. The CEA level should be measured before surgery and, if elevated, periodically (every 3 to 6 months) after surgery.
♦ Beta-2 microglobulin or CA 19-9 may be a sensitive indicator for tumor bulk and may indicate metastases when the CEA level is normal.

Imaging
♦ Barium enema x-ray.
♦ Ultrasound of the abdomen and, if indicated, within the rectum. Endorectal ultrasonagraphy can accurately show tumor invasion and enlarged lymph nodes outside the rectum, but cannot indicate if enlarged lymph nodes actually contain metastatic tumor.
♦ Abdominal CT and MRI scans to identify distant metastases before surgery.
♦ Chest x-ray may reveal lung metastases.
♦ PET (positron emission tomography) scanning, if available (experimental) can help assess the early response of liver metastases to chemotherapy by showing changes in sugar metabolism.
♦ Radioimaging body scan before surgery with CYT-103 monoclonal radiolabeled indium antibodies may help detect hidden metastatic disease in about 12 percent of cases. This experimental method can complement CT scans, increasing their diag-

nostic sensitivity for finding hidden metastatic sites in the pelvis and other areas outside the liver. Other monoclonal antibody and imaging tests are being developed. Current monoclonal antibody scans are not completely reliable in the detection of liver metastases.

Studies with anti-CEA monoclonal antibodies have shown a high accuracy in detecting tumors smaller than 1/2 in. (1 cm). This may be helpful to the surgeon. The usefulness of these radioisotope scans is not yet certain.

Endoscopy and Biopsy

♦ Examination of the entire colon with a colonoscope (colonoscopy), or the lower part of the colon and rectum with a flexible tube (proctosigmoidoscopy) and biopsy of any mass found.
♦ If there is a rectal mass, a bladder evaluation, for example cystoscopy and IVP (intravenous pyelogram), may be required.

STAGING

The stage of colorectal cancer describes whether the cancer has remained within the bowel or has spread to other sites. As with all cancers, the appropriate therapy can be decided only when the stage of the cancer has been defined.

There have been a number of staging systems for colorectal cancer. The original system developed by Dr. Dukes in 1932 has been modified several times. Since 1985, a staging system based on the Tumor/Nodes/Metastases (TNM) classification that corresponds directly with the Dukes system has been used. This allows an improved definition for the number of lymph nodes involved, a factor that can affect the prognosis. The 1990 National Cancer Institute Consensus Panel recommended using the TNM system to help identify people at highest risk because it better describes the tumor size and degree of invasion and the number of lymph nodes involved. The staging system is described in detail in the treatment section.

TREATMENT OVERVIEW

Surgery is the primary treatment, resulting in the cure of about 50 percent of patients. Adjuvant chemotherapy (for colorectal cancers) and radiation therapy (for rectal cancers) probably increases survival. Most researchers now believe that adjuvant radiotherapy decreases local rectal recurrence without any improvement in survival. Combined radiotherapy and chemotherapy increases disease-free survival for rectal cancer more than radiotherapy alone and probably long-term survival as well It should be recommended for people with high-risk tumors who are not candidates for participation in clinical trials.

The prognosis depends on how far the tumor has penetrated through the bowel wall or to adjacent structures and on whether the cancer has spread to local lymph nodes. In node-negative patients, local recurrence is about 5 to 10 percent for Stage I and 25 to 30 percent for Stage II.

Recent studies indicate that the number of local lymph nodes involved is important. When one to four nodes are involved, survival is significantly better than when more than four nodes are involved.

Poor prognostic factors for both colon *and* rectal cancer include:
♦ The tumor has penetrated the bowel wall.
♦ The tumor has perforated the bowel wall.

There are several features of rectal cancer that suggest an unfavorable outcome:
♦ The tumor is fixed, has invaded, or adheres to other parts of the pelvis or adjacent tissues.
♦ The tumor has perforated the bowel wall.
♦ The tumor is deeply ulcerated.
♦ The tumor penetrates through the bowel wall or encircles the rectal wall.
♦ The tumor is larger than 2 1/2 in. (6 cm).

There are several conditions found at the time of diagnosis of colon cancer that suggest an unfavorable outcome:
♦ Pelvic nodes (rectal) or abdominal nodes (colon) are involved.
♦ There is a large bowel or rectal obstruction.

♦ The veins or lymphatic vessels of the bowel have been invaded.
♦ The tumor cells are poorly differentiated under the microscope.
♦ The chromosome pattern is abnormal.
♦ The level of carcinoembryonic antigen (CEA) in the blood is high before surgery.

♦ The cancer cell DNA is abnormal (investigational).

Caution is needed when planning treatment for rectal cancers because the rectum lacks the covering layer of the bowel (the serosa). Thus, treatment of these tumors differs.

COLON

 Surgery Tumors of the colon should be removed whenever practical, even if there are metastases, because complications—blockage of the bowel or bleeding—frequently will develop.

The standard operation is designed to remove the portion of the bowel with the tumor along with the entire lymph node drainage. This requires removing the vessels that supply blood to a considerable portion of the bowel, so most of the time about one-third to one-half of the colon is removed even if the tumor itself is relatively small. This procedure is easier, safer and more likely to provide surgical margins—areas around the tumor—that are free of cancer. The bowel is then reconnected (anastomosis).

Sometimes, in patients who have tumors in the left side of the colon and who have a partial or complete obstruction, reconnecting the bowel is not possible because there is too much stool or contamination in the area. These patients receive a temporary colostomy, which is removed 6 to 10 weeks later (*see* Chapter 21).

Local excision may be used for small lesions or the removal of polyps, with a wedge resection for larger tumors.

Radiation Therapy In selected cases of invasive cecal tumors (where the small bowel joins the colon), radiotherapy may help reduce local recurrences. Palliative radiation is primarily used for localized metastatic tumors and painful liver metastases.

 Chemotherapy For metastatic colon cancer, 5-fluorouracil (5-FU) can be used as a single agent (given by rapid injection or continuous infusion) or as part of combination chemotherapy.

For over 25 years, adjuvant chemotherapy trials have tried to improve the surgical cure rate of colon cancer. 5-FU has been combined with other agents such as leucovorin and/or levamisole. Combination therapy is better than 5-FU alone, and recent reports show an increase in survival and a decrease in recurrence.

Trials for Stage II patients (Dukes' B2 and B3) are comparing 5-FU + leucovorin and 5-FU + leucovorin + levamisole, a drug that may work as a "biochemical immune modulator" to make 5-FU more effective at killing cancer cells.

For people with Stage III (Dukes' C) colon cancer with positive lymph nodes who are unable to enter a clinical adjuvant trial, the combination of levamisole or leucovorin and 5-FU has shown a clear benefit, with reduced rates of both recurrence and death.

Reports on using 5-FU and interferon-alpha (chemoimmunotherapy) for metastatic colon cancer (Stage IV) have shown an increased response rate, and new studies are trying to confirm these preliminary reports. This combination program has increased toxicity, however, with such side effects as fatigue, fever, diarrhea and sore mouth.

 Laser Therapy In certain cases, treatment with lasers may be appropriate for people with colon cancer, primarily for palliation. These cutting beams of light can reduce the bulk of a tumor causing an obstruction in the bowel and can also be used to stop bleeding. Lasers have not been as successful at relieving pain (*see* Chapter 9).

COLON CANCER TREATMENT BY STAGE

STAGE 0 (Dukes' Stage 0)
TNM Tis (Tumor or carcinoma in situ)
This is a very early cancer that has not spread below the limiting membrane of the first layer of colon tissue (mucosa).

Standard Treatment Treatment may be local excision of the tumor or polyp or a "wedge resection" involving the removal of a portion of the colon. Standard surgery, however, involves removing the tumor along with at least a 2 in.(5 cm) margin of normal colon on either side of the tumor site, and the nearby lymph nodes and veins. Because of the way blood is supplied to the colon, it is necessary to remove either the entire right side or the entire left side of the colon. This decreases the chance for local recurrence and increases the safety of the operation.

Five-Year Survival 95 percent. This should be 100 percent curable with earlier detection.

STAGE I (Dukes' A, B1)
TNM T1-2 N0, M0
The cancer is confined to the lining or muscular wall of the colon and has not yet spread anywhere else.

Standard Treatment This stage is highly curable. Radical surgery is the primary treatment and results in a high cure rate. According to the 1990 Consensus

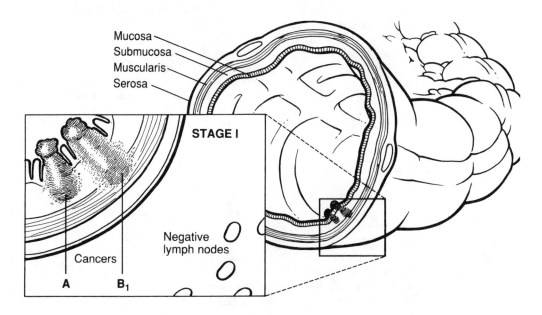

Mucosa
Submucosa
Muscularis
Serosa

STAGE I

Negative lymph nodes

Cancers

A   B₁

Conference on Colon Cancer, no adjuvant therapy is warranted for this stage because of the low risk for recurrence.

Five-Year Survival 85 to 95 percent, depending on whether the muscular wall has been invaded.

STAGE II (Dukes' B2 or B3)
TNM T3-4, N0, M0

The cancer has spread through the muscular wall of the intestine or has extended to adjacent organs through the structures, but has not spread to lymph nodes. Dukes' B2 extends through the bowel wall; B3 involves adjacent structures.

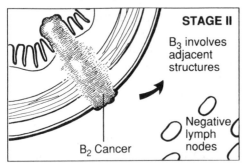

STAGE II

B_3 involves adjacent structures

B_2 Cancer

Negative lymph nodes

Standard Treatment Surgical removal of the primary tumor, with or without adjuvant chemotherapy. Specific adjuvant therapy cannot be recommended for intermediate risk tumors outside a clinical trial. But since a significant percentage of Stage II patients will develop recurrences, they should be considered candidates for clinical trials of adjuvant therapy. Higher-risk tumors are those where there is bowel wall perforation, involvement of adjacent structures and abnormal chromosomes (an aneuploid tumor).

Current adjuvant chemotherapy programs include 5-FU + leucovorin or 5-FU + levamisole. The side effects of treatment with 5-FU + levamisole are few and are primarily associated with 5-FU. Levamisole alone has mild toxicity, mainly gastrointestinal, causing nausea, vomiting, diarrhea or upset stomach, as well as neurotoxicity.

Alcohol is to be avoided, as levamisole has an Antabuse-like effect. 5-FU + leucovorin may cause severe diarrhea without low white blood cell counts, and fluids may have to be replaced intravenously in the hospital because of dehydration.

Five-Year Survival 30 to 70 percent, depending on whether adjacent tissues are involved.

Investigational
♦ Adjuvant chemotherapy clinical trials of various combinations including 5-FU and leucovorin or chemoimmunotherapy with 5-FU and levamisole.
♦ Evaluation of the combination of 5-FU + levamisole for Stage II (Dukes' B2) patients will need another one or two years of study to determine its effectiveness. The number of patients treated so far with the combination has been too low to provide a final answer.
♦ 5-FU + PALA (an immune adjuvant drug) or 5-FU and leucovorin may be given for one year after surgery.
♦ Postoperative local radiation therapy may help control tumors that have spread to tissues adjacent to the colon or lesions in the pelvis.

STAGE III (Dukes' C1, 2, 3)
TNM Any T, N1-3, M0

The cancer has spread outside the intestine to one or more lymph nodes near the bowel. Dukes' C1 is within the bowel wall, C2 is through the bowel wall, and C3 involves adjacent structures.

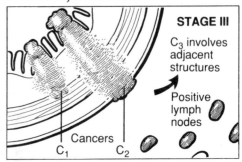

STAGE III

C_3 involves adjacent structures

Positive lymph nodes

Cancers
C_1 C_2

Standard Treatment This stage is highly treatable and often curable with standard therapy, but patients should be considered candidates for adjuvant clinical trials.

The standard treatment is to remove a wide section of the colon and rejoin the remaining ends (anastomosis), followed by adjuvant chemotherapy with 5-FU + levamisole. Clinical trials of new treatments are also appropriate.

More than half the patients with colon cancer have tumors that penetrate the serosa (B2) or have positive lymph nodes (C). It is estimated that about 20 to 25 percent of those with Dukes' B2 and 40 to 90 percent of those with Dukes' C who are treated with surgery will have recurrences and so need adjuvant chemotherapy.

Dukes' C patients now commonly receive a combination of levamisole + 5-FU (which was recommended by the U.S. National Institutes of Health's Consensus Conference on Colon Cancer in May 1990). One study of treatment with levamisole + 5-FU for Dukes' C starting within five weeks of surgery did show decreased recurrences and prolonged survival. Another trial showed a 41 percent decrease in the rate of recurrence and a 33 percent decrease in the death rate.

Five-Year Survival 10 to 60 percent with positive regional lymph nodes, 40 to 60 percent when the tumor is within the bowel wall (C1), 20 to 40 percent when the tumor extends through the bowel wall (C2), 10 to 30 percent when adjacent structures are involved (C3). These data do not reflect adjuvant therapy programs.

The Consensus Conference used positive lymph nodes for determining prognosis with previous therapy. If one to four nodes are positive, 55 to 60 percent may be cured. When five or more nodes are positive, only 33 percent will be cured. Adjuvant therapy will improve all the old prognostic figures.

Investigational
♦ Adjuvant therapy trial comparing 5-FU + PALA with 5-FU + levamisole with 5-FU + levamisole or interferon.
♦ Trials to see if 5-FU + leucovorin + levamisole is superior to conventional therapy are ongoing.
♦ 5-FU + leucovorin. (*See also* Stage II.)

STAGE IV (Dukes' D)
TNM Any T, any N, M1
The cancer has spread beyond the colon to distant sites or organs, possibly including the liver or lungs.

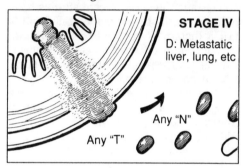

STAGE IV
D: Metastatic liver, lung, etc
Any "N"
Any "T"

Standard Treatment Cancer at this stage is not usually curable, but removal of a large section of the colon and reconnection of the bowel is still the standard treatment so that major problems such as obstruction, bleeding or bowel perforation can be avoided. In some cases, tumors that are blocking the colon may be bypassed.

It should be noted that 80 percent of colon cancer patients die of liver failure. And, if there are metastases in only a portion of the liver, removal of the metastases by removing part of the liver can cure 20 to 40 percent of such patients. The prognosis is better if there are fewer lesions—one lesion is better than three—and there is *no* survival benefit unless all lesions are removed. Non-curative surgery has the same prognosis as no surgery at all. In selected cases, both the colon cancer and the liver metastases (if there are three or fewer) can be removed at the same surgery.

Liver metastases may be reduced if chemotherapy, with 5-FUDR (floxuridine) delivered by infusion pump through the main hepatic artery, is given after surgery (*see* Chapter 5).

There are new and innovative treatment methods. Treating liver metastases with intra-arterial chemotherapy— 5-FUDR—by infusion pump can improve the response rate to about 50 percent. But several studies have shown side effects—increased liver toxicity, scarring of the bile duct (biliary sclerosis) and liver function abnormalities, gastritis, diarrhea and pain—that required dose reductions in about 40 to 50 percent of patients (*see* "Metastatic Cancer"). Recent studies have reduced toxicity by alternating 5-FU and 5-FUDR therapy. Response to 5-FUDR intra-arterial therapy often occurs even in patients who failed to respond to intravenous 5-FU or who are no longer responding.

The infusion can be delivered on an outpatient basis by a surgically implanted pump (Infusaid) connected to the hepatic artery. Although the response rate is high, increased survival has not yet been proven.

Hepatic artery 5-FUDR given through a catheter inserted through the skin into an artery in the arm or groin also has a high response rate. This method isolates the blood supply to the cancer and then releases chemotherapy into the isolated area. There may be local toxicity, including liver function abnormalities and biliary tract scarring (sclerosis).

 Palliation Radiation therapy may be given to help control the size of the tumor and/or pain, and both radiation and chemotherapy with 5-FU alone or 5-FU + leucovorin may be used for palliation of advanced cancer.

The 5-FU + leucovorin combination usually provides little benefit, however, to someone who has relapsed after treatment with 5-FU alone. The current treatment recommendation is to begin therapy with 5-FU + leucovorin or an investigational protocol. Other drugs with some anti-cancer activity that might be considered include mitomycin-C, BCNU and CCNU.

Another method of delivering 5-FU is by continuous intravenous infusion using a portable or bedside pump. A study comparing intermittent 5-FU injections with continuous long-term (two to four weeks) low-dose infusions showed a high response rate for the infusion, although the survival outcomes were identical. A later report showed a 45 percent response rate to 5-FU infusion in patients who were resistant to other therapy.

Five-Year Survival 5 percent, rising to 20 to 30 percent if liver metastases can be removed surgically.

Investigational

♦ Chemoembolization is a method of treating liver metastases. This process involves injecting and filling the artery leading to the tumor with a plastic-sponge mixture containing chemotherapy (*see* "Metastatic Cancer").

♦ Biological therapies using specific antibodies are being evaluated, with several protocols under investigation especially using interferon just before 5-FU + leucovorin. Injections of 5 to 10 million units of interferon three times a week in conjunction with 5-FU by infusion and direct injection has shown a high response rate (greater than 50 percent). This therapy may not be effective if it is used after the disease has progressed on 5-FU.

♦ Trials are comparing 5-FU + PALA versus 5-FU + interferon-alpha versus 5-FU + leucovorin. PALA + 5-FU has been reported to have responses better than 5-FU alone.

♦ Trials with monoclonal antibodies (MAbs) are now being started, with MAbs against colon cancer tagged to a radioisotope being used to locate hidden cancer sites before and during surgery. Preliminary results seem promising, although the eventual role of MAbs is yet to be determined (*see* summary of Consensus Conference on Colon and Rectal Cancer, on page 393).

♦ Investigational drugs, such as CPT-11 (*see* Chapter 36).

TREATMENT FOLLOW-UP

Recommendations for following patients after treatment to detect recurrences may include:

♦ History and physical examination every two to three months.

♦ Chest x-ray every 6 to 12 months for three to five years.

♦ CT scans of the abdomen and pelvis once or twice a year for one to two years if CEA or liver function tests are abnormal or liver becomes enlarged, then yearly as required.

♦ Barium enema as required.

♦ Complete blood count and serum chemistry profile every 3 months.

♦ Measurement of the CEA level in the blood every 6 to 12 weeks for 3 to 5 years, since a rise in the level may occur before other clinical, x-ray or laboratory tests show recurrence. If the CEA rises above normal, about one third of patients may have a recurrent tumor that can be totally removed with surgery and so may be cured.

♦ Periodic proctosigmoidoscopy or colonoscopy at least every year, or more often, depending on staging. If there are polyps, colonoscopy should be done one to three times a year. There is three to four times the risk of developing new tumors.

Recommendations for follow-up after the successful surgical removal of Dukes' A, B and C tumors include:

♦ History and physical examination every three months for detection of tumor recurrence.

♦ Complete blood count, serum chemistry profile and CEA tests every three to six months.

♦ Colonoscopy (rather than a barium enema) every year to detect recurrent or new polyps or cancer.

♦ Since family members share the same genes and/or diet, first-degree relatives should be tested for hidden blood in the stool and have colonoscopy after age 30.

RECURRENT COLON CANCER

Cancer may recur in the colon or any part of the body, including the liver or lungs. Unfortunately, those who have a recurrence will usually die of cancer.

Treatment for recurrent colon cancer is essentially the same as for Stage IV, although therapy also depends on the site of the recurrence.

♦ When there is only one area of recurrence such as the liver or lung and surgery is possible, the lesion should be removed to increase the chance of cure or prolong survival.

♦ Occasionally, the cancer will come back only where sections of the bowel have been sewn together. These local suture line recurrences can be removed with a reasonable chance for cure.

♦ Chemotherapy with single drugs (10 to 20 percent response), combinations (30 to 40 percent response) or investigational drugs have been used for palliation.

♦ Trials involving the administration of the drugs into an artery with implantable infusion pumps and access devices have been conducted for recurrence in the liver.

Investigational

♦ Recent chemotherapy programs show an improved response rate and may improve survival. Promising developments include: 5-FU + leucovorin, 5-FU + interferon-alpha, 5-FU + PALA, 5-FU + levamisole and 5-FU + levamisole and leucovorin or interferon or PALA.

♦ Dosages of chemotherapy drugs may be significantly increased with the use of hematopoietic growth factors (GM-CSF).

♦ Studies are evaluating adjuvant radiation therapy with chemotherapy and monoclonal antibodies directed against colon associated antigens.

THE MOST IMPORTANT QUESTIONS YOU CAN ASK

♦ What are the symptoms of colon cancer?

♦ Does rectal bleeding always suggest colon cancer?

♦ What are the guidelines for screening for colon cancer?

♦ Can I live a normal life after colon surgery?

♦ Should radiotherapy be used for colon cancer?

♦ What is a good nutritional support dietary program?

♦ When is surgery effective for colon can-

cer that has spread to the liver or lungs?

♦ When will I know if I am cured? What kind of follow-up will you be doing after my therapy?

♦ What is the role of adjuvant chemotherapy and of chemotherapy for metastatic disease after a colostomy?

♦ How does the immunochemotherapy combination approach work? Can it cure colon cancer?

♦ Can laser treatment cure colon cancer?

RECTUM

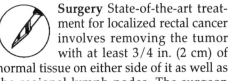 **Surgery** State-of-the-art treatment for localized rectal cancer involves removing the tumor with at least 3/4 in. (2 cm) of normal tissue on either side of it as well as the regional lymph nodes. The surgeon and the surgical pathologist should examine the rectal margins in the surgical specimen for the presence or absence of tumor. If the tumor is small, it may be removed with a local wedge resection.

In some patients with a tumor that is low in the rectum, high-dose radiation given before the operation may reduce the size of the tumor, allowing it to be removed while still leaving enough bowel below the tumor site for the surgeon to sew the bowel back together. This will spare the rectum and the sphincter muscle, thereby avoiding the need for a colostomy in up to 85 percent of patients with rectal cancer.

Mortality for this operation is less than 7 percent, but there is a 25 to 40 percent incidence of impotence or urologic problems. About 10 to 15 percent of patients have a late local recurrence of cancer in the pelvis, particularly when sphincter-preserving operations have been used for low-lying tumors.

But the main concern should be removing all the tumor and a reasonable margin on either side—which leads to cure—

rather than preserving the sphincter.

In rare cases of non-invasive tumors—those confined to the top layers of the rectal lining (mucosa and submucosa)—it is sometimes possible to remove the tumor from below, entering through the anus and using a cold probe (cryotherapy), electrofulguration or simple excision of the tumor without removing part of the bowel. Radiotherapy before or after the operation may decrease the incidence of local pelvic recurrence.

In tumors that are very low in the rectum—within 2 to 2 1/2 in. (5 to 6 cm) of the anus—once the tumor and its lower edge have been removed there is no rectum left to sew back together. In these cases the surgeon performs an abdominal perineal resection, the standard treatment for invasive cancer. The rectum and the anus with all its muscular attachments are removed, leaving the patient with a permanent colostomy (*see* Chapter 21).

Ongoing clinical trials are attempting to identify patients who may be spared this extensive surgery. This investigative approach treats selected patients with a local excision of the tumor (as long as the margins show no evidence of cancer), along with radiation to the pelvis and often chemotherapy as well.

A novel stapling device to join the ends of the bowel may sometimes allow the surgeon to perform what is called a low anterior resection in some patients with low rectal cancers. This will also help avoid a colostomy.

Where there is no evidence of gross pelvic disease after local excision with negative margins, adjuvant pelvic radiation may be an alternative to abdominal perineal resection. This may help reduce local recurrence, which is associated with significant symptoms. Follow-up studies are in progress.

 Radiation Therapy Radiation given before or after surgery has been used to treat rectal cancer. High-dose preoperative therapy in selected high-risk cases—selection depends on the size and location of the tumor—will improve survival, reduce local recurrence and allow the sphincter to be preserved even in low rectal cancers.

Placing the radiation source inside the rectum (intraluminal radiation therapy) may result in a high cure rate in some cases, as with a well-differentiated tumor less than 3 to 4 cm above the sphincter, for example. This may preserve the sphincter.

Adjuvant Radiation Therapy Radiation therapy given after surgery may be more effective in rectal cancer than in colon cancer because of the increased tendency for tumors to grow back locally. Several trials of adjuvant radiation and chemotherapy after an abdominal perineal resection have suggested a decrease in the rate of local recurrence with a small increase in disease-free and overall survival.

Adjuvant Chemotherapy Stage I (Dukes' A and B1) tumors have a high cure rate with surgery alone and there is no need for adjuvant chemotherapy for these stages. But for more advanced tumors (Dukes' B2 and C), the use of chemotherapy alone has shown some improvement in survival. Combination therapy, using chemotherapy plus radiation, is better

than either therapy alone and should be started within 6 weeks of surgery.

Combined Therapy Disease-free survival has recently been extended in patients with Dukes' B2 and C rectal cancer treated with both chemotherapy and radiation, compared with those treated with radiation therapy alone.

Clinical trials are now evaluating 5-fluorouracil (5-FU) with radiation therapy or 5-FU + leucovorin or levamisole or both for Stages II and III (Dukes' B2 and C) rectal cancer. Combined chemotherapy and radiation therapy have been reported to improve disease-free and overall survival, with clear benefit having been shown for combination therapy with 5-FU given before and during radiotherapy.

 Palliation With advanced cancer that cannot be cured, radiation therapy may be used for palliation in most cases when it was not used before or after surgery to remove the tumor. 5-FU is often used with radiotherapy.

Short-term palliation may also be achieved with chemotherapy in about 20 percent of patients, although there is little evidence that chemotherapy significantly improves survival for those with advanced (Dukes' D) disease.

Laser therapy may be a very effective way to relieve an obstruction or control localized bleeding (*see* Chapter 9).

RECTAL CANCER: TREATMENT BY STAGE

STAGE 0
TNM Tis (Tumor in situ)
This superficial, non-invasive carcinoma in situ is a very early cancer that has not spread below the membrane (mucosa) of the first layer of rectal tissue.

Standard Treatment Because of its superficial nature, limited rather than radical surgery, as well as other procedures, may be used. Surgery may involve only cutting out the tumor itself (enucleation) of the tumor and a small wedge of tissue.

Other options include electrocoagulation and external or internal (inside the rectum) radiation therapy for rectal sphincter preservation.

Five-Year Survival Over 95 percent.

STAGE I (*see* Stage I colon cancer diagram)
(Dukes' A, BI)
TNM T12, N0, M0
The cancer is confined to the lining or muscular wall of the rectum and has not yet spread anywhere else. In Dukes' A, the tumor is limited to the mucosa. In Dukes' B1, it is within the bowel wall.

Standard Treatment Surgery will generally result in a cure.

When the tumor is in the upper rectum, a wide margin of tissue may be removed and the bowel reconnected (anastomosis).

When the tumor is near the anus, an abdominal perineal resection and colostomy is the standard treatment. Local transanal resection can be done in selected patients.

Radiation inside the bowel (intraluminal) may be used in selected patients. This technique requires special equipment and experience, but the results are equivalent to surgery and can preserve the sphincter muscle.

There is a 5 to 10 percent chance of a local recurrence with this stage of cancer.

Five-Year Survival 85 to 95 percent (95 percent for Dukes' A, 85 to 90 percent for Dukes' B1). ·

Investigational Results from clinical trials of radiation therapy and electrocoagulation are promising.

STAGE II (*see* Stage II colon diagram)
(Dukes' B2, B3)
TNM T34 N0, M0
The cancer has penetrated all layers of the

bowel wall with or without extension to adjacent tissues (uterus, ovaries or prostate), but has not spread to lymph nodes. Dukes' B2 extends through the bowel wall: B3 involves adjacent structures such as the uterus, ovaries, bladder or prostate.

Standard Treatment Stage II rectal cancer is highly treatable and often curable. There are several options for treatment, including:
♦ Removal of a wide margin of tissue and reconnection of the bowel to the rectum (anastomosis) when the tumor is in the upper rectum.
♦ The same surgical procedure followed by chemotherapy and radiation therapy, which has shown an increased disease-free survival compared with surgery alone or surgery and radiation. 5-FU and radiation can improve remission and prolong survival.
♦ Continuous-infusion 5-FU chemotherapy together with radiation therapy, especially for high-risk Stage II and Stage III cancers.
♦ An abdominal perineal resection and colostomy, with or without adjuvant radiation and chemotherapy, for tumors near the anus.
♦ Those with B2 tumors will benefit from adjuvant chemotherapy if they have features that point to a recurrence (abnormal chromosomes by DNA analysis, invasion of the outside wall, perforation, adhesion to organs or invasion of adjacent organs).
♦ For B3 lesions, the pelvic organs (bladder, uterus or prostate) may be removed (pelvic exenteration) when that is necessary to remove all the cancer, with or without adjuvant chemotherapy.
♦ Adding postoperative radiation and chemotherapy will reduce pelvic recurrences and improve chances of survival (there is 25 to 30 percent chance of local recurrence with this stage).
♦ For tumors near the anus, radiation

therapy followed by surgery may allow sphincter function to be preserved.

Preoperative or postoperative radiation therapy has resulted in fewer local recurrences but has never been definitely shown to affect survival.

Five-Year Survival 30 to 70 percent (50 to 70 percent for Dukes' B2, 30 percent for Dukes' B3).

Investigational New adjuvant programs may increase survival by 10 to 15 percent.
♦ Adjuvant 5-FU + leucovorin and radiotherapy.
♦ 5-FU + levamisole and 5-FU + PALA.
♦ Giving radiation during surgery (intraoperative radiation therapy) is being evaluated for locally advanced disease.

STAGE III (*see* Stage III colon diagram) **(Dukes' C1, 2, 3)**
TNM Any T, N1-3, M0
The cancer has spread within or outside the rectum and one or more lymph nodes are involved. A Dukes' C1 tumor is within the bowel wall, C2 is through the bowel wall and C3 involves adjacent structures.

Standard Treatment The number of lymph nodes that are positive for cancer needs to be known because patients with one to four positive nodes have a better prognosis than those with five or more involved nodes.

The standard therapy for a tumor near the anus is an abdominal perineal resection with or without adjuvant chemotherapy and/or radiotherapy.

For tumors in the upper rectum far from the anus, a wide margin of tissue may be removed and the bowel reconnected to the anus, with or without adjuvant chemotherapy and radiation therapy.

Removal of the pelvic organs (pelvic exenteration) may be necessary to remove all the cancer and may be followed by adjuvant chemotherapy and/or radiation therapy when the level of penetration has reached the C3 stage.

For tumors near the anus, radiation therapy followed by surgery may allow the sphincter function to be preserved.

There is a 50 percent chance of recurrence with this stage of disease.

The 1990 consensus conference on colon and rectal cancers noted that if one to four lymph nodes are positive, 55 to 60 percent will be cured. If five or more are positive, only 33 percent will be cured. Current adjuvant therapy will improve all of the old prognostic figures.

Five-Year Survival Up to 60 percent (40 to 50 percent for Dukes' C1, 15 to 25 percent for C2, 10 to 20 percent for C3). These data do *not* reflect current adjuvant therapy programs.

Investigational
♦ Survival rates may be increased by 10 to 15 percent with new adjuvant chemotherapy programs such as 5-FU + leucovorin and/or radiation therapy.
♦ Intraoperative radiation therapy (IORT) is also being evaluated in patients with locally advanced disease.
♦ 5-FU + levamisole and 5-FU + PALA are being evaluated.

STAGE IV **(Dukes' D)**
TNM Any T, any N, M1
The cancer has spread outside the rectum to distant areas, including organs such as the liver or lungs.

Standard Treatment This stage of cancer is largely incurable. Treatment is directed basically toward palliation, although there can be long-term disease-free survival if isolated metastases in the liver or lung can be removed.

Treatment options include:
♦ Palliative removal of the primary tumor in some cases, with radiation thera-

py for local disease that can't be removed.

♦ Removal of isolated liver, ovary or lung metastases for possible cure. Liver metastases (if there are three or fewer) can be removed at the same surgery to remove the rectal cancer in selected cases.

♦ Patients can be treated either with chemotherapy programs such as 5-FU alone or 5-FU combined with leucovorin or interferon or be considered candidates for clinical trials for new chemotherapy or biological agents. Mitomycin-C, BCNU and CCNU have been used, with a mild response.

♦ Palliative chemotherapy, possibly with the continuous infusion of a low daily dose of 5-FU.

♦ There are a number of other standard and investigational methods of treating Stage IV (Dukes' D) rectal cancer. These closely resemble those described earlier for colon cancer on pages 383 - 386 which should be consulted.

Five-Year Survival Less than 5 percent (*see* summary of Consensus Conference on Colon and Rectal Cancer, on page 393)

TREATMENT FOLLOW-UP

Rectal cancer has a much higher rate of local recurrence than colon cancer. Close follow-up may lead to the earlier diagnosis of recurrent disease and improved treatment. After treatment for rectal cancer, follow-up should include:

♦ Physical examination every two to three months for at least five years.

♦ Chest x-ray every 6 to 12 months for three to five years as indicated.

♦ Abdominal and pelvic CT scans twice a year for one to two years, then yearly.

♦ Serum chemistry profiles and CEA levels every 6 to 12 weeks (when operated on for a rising CEA level, 30 to 40 percent may have a recurrent rectal cancer which may be successfully removed for cure).

♦ Barium enema as indicated.

♦ Sigmoidoscopic examinations every 3 to 6 months and yearly colonoscopy.

RECURRENT RECTAL CANCER

Rectal cancer can recur locally or often in the liver or lungs, and it is important to determine if the recurrence is only local or metastatic. Treatment depends on the site of recurrence as defined by physical and x-ray examinations and scans.

♦ If local disease can be removed, there is a potential chance for cure.

♦ Often the recurrence can be in one area such as the rectal area, liver or lung, where surgical removal may possibly lead to a cure or significantly prolonged survival.

♦ Alternatively, intra-arterial chemotherapy with an implantable portable pump can sometimes give significant palliation (*see* "STAGE IV").

♦ Hepatic intra-arterial chemotherapy with 5-FUDR for liver metastases has been studied. This approach has been shown to produce a higher overall response rate without significant improvement in survival. In several studies, there is increased local toxicity including liver function abnormalities and biliary sclerosis (*see* "STAGE IV").

♦ As in Stage IV, chemotherapy with single-agent 5-FU or 5-FU in combination with leucovorin, or with interferon with or without leucovorin (investigational), may improve survival and achieve significant palliation. Various doses are used. Lower-dose leucovorin + 5-FU has the same response and survival as high-dose leucovorin + 5-FU. 5-FU + levamisole has no role in recurrent colorectal cancer.

Standard Treatment Removal of liver metastases may be done in selected cases. The five-year survival rate for patients with solitary metastases exceeds 20 percent. The chances for cure are improved when there are only two or three metastases to be removed. Non-curative removal provides no benefits to patients who have no symptoms, since survival is not affected.

Both palliative radiation therapy and palliative chemotherapy may be given for recurrent disease.

Investigational
♦ Biologic therapy with 5-FU + interferon, monoclonal antibodies or interleukin-2.
♦ 5-FU + PALA, Phase I and II agents.

THE MOST IMPORTANT QUESTIONS YOU CAN ASK
♦ How does the Dukes' staging affect my prognosis?
♦ How extensive does my surgery need to be? Will I need a colostomy?
♦ How do you know who needs adjuvant chemotherapy?
♦ When should radiotherapy be used?
♦ What is the role of combination chemotherapy and radiotherapy?
♦ How can one screen for rectal cancer? What should family members do if there is a history of colorectal cancer in a close relative?

CONSENSUS CONFERENCE ON COLON AND RECTAL CANCER:

SUMMARY
A Consensus Conference on Colon and Rectal Cancer was held at the National Institutes of Health in April 1990. The treatment recommendations of the panel were:

1. Stage I Colon and Rectal
No adjuvant therapy is warranted, since there is a low risk of recurrence.

2. Stage II Colon
Specific adjuvant therapy cannot be recommended routinely for intermediate-risk tumors outside a clinical trial. Those with larger tumors (T3 or T4), an elevated preoperative CEA level, poorly differentiated tumors and abnormal DNA, are candidates for adjuvant chemotherapy.

3. Stage III Colon
There is a high risk for recurrence, and treatment with levamisole and 5-FU is recommended.

4. Stages II and III Rectal
Adjuvant combined radiotherapy and chemotherapy is recommended postoperatively. This will improve local control and survival.

5. Future Research
Further clinical trials focussing on adjuvant chemotherapy and immunotherapy are needed both to improve the effectiveness of current treatments and try to understand drug and immune mechanisms. Studies are also needed to determine the optimum role of radiotherapy in rectal cancer.

FOR DIETARY PREVENTION OF COLORECTAL CANCER
RECOMMENDATIONS
♦ The diet should stress high fiber and low fat.
♦ Increased growth rate of colon membrane cells may precede colon cancer. Chemoprevention is being tested with micronutrients—vitamins and minerals.
♦ Calcium may help by regulating cell overgrowth.
♦ Other factors are stool acidity (pH) and the effect of bile and fatty acids on the colon's lining (mucosa). Depending on acidity, calcium may help regulate the cancer-promoting role of bile acids and fatty acids.
♦ A women's trial has shown a 2 1/2

times normal risk of colon cancer when red meat (pork, beef, lamb) is eaten daily (animal fats) rather than a few times a month. (Vegetable fat was not a risk factor.)

♦ 1,200 - 2,000 mg daily calcium intake (in skim milk or substitute, food or pills) to help reduce colorectal cell growth, especially if a polyp has already been found.

♦ Eat the most colorful fresh fruit and vegetables, which may contain chemopreventive agents (vitamins, minerals and fiber). Cruciferous vegetables such as broccoli and brussel sprouts are especially important.

♦ Bran (oat or wheat) has a role in high fiber diets but the results are uncertain. Recent studies show that fiber probably plays a role in colon cancer prevention.

♦ Wheat bran supplements may help inhibit polyp formation, but this has to be confirmed. It is possible that fiber in natural foods (fruits and vegetables) is better for cancer prevention.

ESOPHAGUS

Ernest H. Rosenbaum, MD, Carlos Pellegrini, MD, T. Stanley Meyler, MD,
Lawrence Margolis, MD, Malin Dollinger, MD, and David R. Byrd, MD

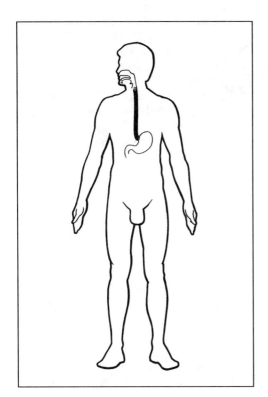

The first recorded case of esophageal cancer was described in China 2,000 years ago. It was called *ye ge*, which seems to have been a polite way of referring to difficult swallowing (dysphagia) and belching. It is a treatable and sometimes curable cancer, although most patients have a poor prognosis because the cancer is usually advanced by the time symptoms appear.

Special attention to good nutrition is an important part of treatment, especially since people in good physical condition with minimal weight loss have a better prognosis. Overall five-year survival for cases amenable to surgery is about 5 to 20 percent; only 25 to 40 percent of cases are amenable to surgery. Earlier diagnosis and treatment can improve survival. Recent improvements in radiation therapy and chemotherapy results are somewhat encouraging.

Esophageal cancer is relatively uncommon in the United States, affecting about 11,000 Americans each year, with an estimated 10,400 deaths in 1994. It is responsible for 1.5 percent of all cancers in the U.S. and 7 percent of gastrointestinal cancers.

Types Sixty percent of esophageal cancers appear in the cells lining the esophageal tube (squamous cells), usually in the upper two-thirds of the esophagus. About 40 percent develop in the glands (adenocarcinoma) in the lower third. One to 2 percent are relatively rare tumors, such as melanoma, primary lymphomas or tumors in the smooth muscles, among others. Barrett's esophagus is a premalignant condition thought to be caused by chronic inflammation where the normal squamous epithelium (lining of the esophagus) is replaced by glandular (columnar) epithelium resembling the stomach lining.

How It Spreads Carcinoma of the esophagus usually starts on the surface layer, invades the surrounding tissue and grows to cause an obstruction that makes swallowing difficult. It spreads through the lymph system to lymph nodes. The most common sites for metastases are the lymph nodes, lungs, liver, brain, adrenal glands and bones.

What Causes It Alcohol and tobacco abuse are the most common causes in

North America. Contributing factors in other parts of the world include exposure to environmental carcinogens such as nitrosamines and diets deficient in riboflavin, magnesium, nicotinic acid and zinc. Betel nut chewing and bidi smoking are major factors in India.

Who Gets It Esophageal cancer is much more prevalent in China, Singapore, Iran, Puerto Rico, Switzerland and France than in North America. On this continent, it is most prevalent among men over sixty, smokers, drinkers and blacks. In the United States, men with esophageal cancer outnumber women by 3-to-1 and blacks outnumber whites 3.5- to-1.

RISK FACTORS
At Significantly Higher Risk
♦ Men over 60.
♦ Long-term drinkers, especially in whites.
♦ Long-term smokers (more common in blacks than in whites).
♦ Smokers who drink alcohol (more common in blacks than in whites).
♦ Pickled vegetable consumption.
♦ Individuals with muscle spasm (achalasia) or chronic stricture.
♦ Barrett's esophagus with esophagitis—inflammation of the esophagus related to a chronic backup of stomach acid with bile (gastric reflux) causing "heartburn." This may also develop from a malfunction of the

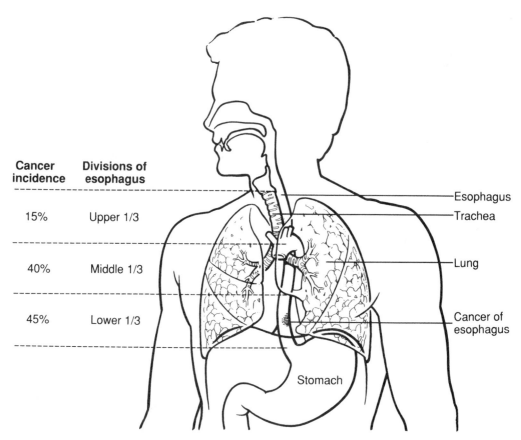

Cancer incidence	Divisions of esophagus
15%	Upper 1/3
40%	Middle 1/3
45%	Lower 1/3

Esophagus
Trachea
Lung
Cancer of esophagus
Stomach

The esophagus and nearby organs

gastroesophageal valve that results in back-up (reflux) of stomach acid. The male-to-female ratio is 5-to-1 for adenocarcinoma.

♦ Other causes of esophageal injury, such as lye ingestion or long-term consumption of very hot beverages.

At Lower Risk

♦ Mormons and Seventh Day Adventists who monitor their diets and neither drink nor smoke.

SCREENING

Screening programs aren't common in North America because of the low incidence of esophageal cancer. But high-risk individuals (such as those with Barrett's esophagus) can be screened every 3 to 12 months by passing a brush through a nasogastric tube or by endoscopy. Cell analysis (cytology) has a 75 percent detection rate and may be considered for patients with Barrett's esophagus.

COMMON SIGNS AND SYMPTOMS

The most common symptom of esophageal cancer—occurring in 90 percent of patients—is difficulty or pain in swallowing foods and liquids (dysphagia). Other symptoms include weight loss, which can be severe (cachexia), heartburn, hoarseness, pain in the throat or back, vocal cord paralysis, pneumonia and coughing up blood.

DIAGNOSIS

Physical Examination

♦ Enlarged lymph nodes, particularly over the left collarbone.

♦ The vocal cords may be less mobile or paralyzed.

♦ Tapping the spinal area may cause pain in the vertebrae.

♦ Rarely, thickening and scaling of the palms and soles.

Blood and Other Tests

♦ Cells for analysis similar to a Pap smear cytology may be scraped off a swallowed balloon or obtained with a brush inserted through an endoscope or a nasogastric tube.

♦ Blood counts and serum chemistry profile.

♦ Serum liver function tests to measure alkaline phosphatase and LDH. Elevated levels may suggest metastases to liver or bone.

♦ An elevated CEA (carcinoembryonic antigen) may indicate liver metastases.

♦ Analysis of cell DNA and DNA histograms are under evaluation as investigational diagnostic tools and may help identify patients with Barrett's esophagus who are about to develop cancer. Preliminary data suggest that a tumor with abnormal chromosomes has a poorer prognosis.

Imaging

♦ A barium swallow and x-ray of the esophagus may reveal a tumor.

♦ A chest x-ray can detect masses in the midchest area and the lungs.

♦ CT scans of the whole lung (mediastinum) and abdomen (liver) will define the size and lateral extent of the tumor so that the stage can be identified accurately. (CT scans will also highlight lymph nodes, although these may not be cancerous.)

♦ Esophageal endoscopic ultrasound of the surrounding tissue will assess the size and depth of the tumor's invasion of the esophagus and evaluate the status of nearby lymph nodes.

Endoscopy and Biopsy

♦ Esophagoscopy is the key test because it allows both visualization and biopsy. A flexible fiberoptic tube is passed through the mouth and down the esophagus. A piece of tissue may be removed with forceps (punch biopsy and cytology). About 25 to 40 percent of patients have a narrowing of the esophagus, which does not permit an endoscope to be passed, so an esophageal dilation may be needed.

♦ For tumors near the place where the trachea (central air passage) divides into the right and left bronchi, it is advisable to include bronchoscopy.

♦ A mediastinoscopy (inspection of center of the chest through a thin telescope) may be needed occasionally to assist in staging, for biopsy and to help decide on surgery.

STAGING

The esophagus is not an accessible organ. Although CT and MRI are very helpful, clinical evaluation and staging are difficult. Clinical staging is correct only about half the time, so biopsy and other invasive procedures are usually necessary. The TNM classification system is used to describe the stage.

TREATMENT OVERVIEW

All forms of treatment—radiation therapy, surgery, laser therapy, combination chemotherapy—have been of modest help.

Cancers in the lower two-thirds of the esophagus are generally treated with surgery. Tumors in the upper third (which may have invaded the trachea or larynx) seem to respond better to radiation, but patients with cancers in that area have a poorer prognosis. Unfortunately, 80 to 90 percent of patients have local tissue or lymph node invasion. Nutritional support is necessary. Those with more than a 10 percent weight loss have a poorer prognosis, with an average survival of six months.

 Surgery Since most patients in North America have advanced (Stage III) esophageal cancer before diagnosis, only 25 to 40 percent have tumors that can be removed

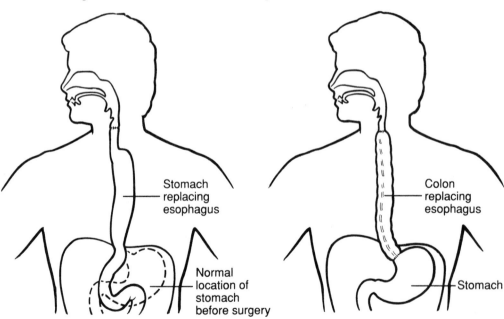

STOMACH "PULL-UP" | Stomach replacing esophagus | Normal location of stomach before surgery

COLONIC RECONSTRUCTION | Colon replacing esophagus | Stomach

Two types of surgery to replace a cancerous portion of the esophagus

in an attempt at cure. Before surgery, an evaluation for metastases is performed.

Radical surgery for cure involves removing the entire esophagus (or a good part of it) and the surrounding tissues and lymph nodes. If the lesion is in the lower esophagus near the stomach, the top of the stomach has to be removed as well. Once the esophagus is removed, the stomach can be brought all the way up to bridge the gap (esophagogastrostomy). A portion of the colon may be used instead. This operation is rather demanding of both patient and surgeon. It should be performed only in major medical centers because complex care will be needed during and after surgery.

Mortality ranges from 5 to 10 percent, but the removal of the esophagus relieves swallowing problems in over 90 percent of patients and is the only method with a chance of cure.

Tumors in the upper half of the esophagus have usually invaded the trachea or larynx, so reconstruction (with a high risk of complications) will be required.

♦ *Palliative surgery* Bypassing the tumor and creating a new swallowing tube may help some patients whose tumors have invaded the trachea, but otherwise this operation is not recommended for relief of symptoms. A prosthetic indwelling (Celestin) tube inserted through the esophagus may ease swallowing for four to six months. In general, surgery may improve swallowing better than radiotherapy, although the results of chemotherapy and radiation are equal to surgery.

Laser therapy, administered through a flexible tube inserted through the mouth, may open (evaporate) the blockage and relieve dysphagia temporarily. The procedure usually has to be repeated every four to six weeks.

For Barrett's esophagitis with a symptomatic reflux that persists despite potent antacids, H-2 blockers or omeprazole (Prilosec), some medical centers are now investigating antireflux surgery, which may help control symptoms and prevent chronic reflux. Whether this will prevent cancer has not been proven. In patients with progressive Barrett's esophagus who have abnormal changes in the cells that indicate cancer might develop (mucosal dysplasia), the esophagus may be removed as a prophylactic measure.

Combined Therapy Surgery is now often used in combination with chemotherapy and radiation therapy. Combined therapy helps prevent the cancer from recurring and slows the spread of metastases. Chemotherapy may be given before surgery to try to decrease the size of the tumor and reduce metastases. Radiotherapy decreases the incidence of local recurrence, and chemotherapy may decrease the incidence of metastatic disease. Using radiochemotherapy before surgery has prolonged the median survival.

 Radiation Therapy The earlier the cancer is diagnosed, the better the results of radiation therapy. Radiation may cure a small number of selected patients, but lesions must be no larger than five centimeters. Generally, radiotherapy is used preoperatively or for relief of symptoms. It is used for palliation if the tumor is larger than 2 in. (5 cm) or if there are distant metastases.

Preoperative radiation can eliminate almost one-third of esophageal cancers but will make only 40 to 67 per cent of tumors operable. Very precise treatment planning with use of an x-ray simulator is important for the best results, with CT scans used to plan treatments accurately.

Chemotherapy with 5-fluorouracil (5-FU) infusions and cisplatin will improve the effect of radiation, although adenocarcinoma (Barrett's esophagus) may not be as sensitive to radiotherapy and chemotherapy. Several investigative programs are currently being tried using multidrug chemotherapy, including 5-FU, VP-16 and/or mitomycin-C with radiation therapy.

Intraluminal radiation using a radiation source placed inside the esophagus (brachytherapy) may complement external radiation. The average five-year survival is 5 to 10 percent for radiation treatment alone.

Adjuvant Chemotherapy Chemotherapy alone is of little benefit. But 5-FU + cisplatin chemotherapy before surgery, will reduce the size of the tumor, allowing a more complete resection (Stages I and II) and may eliminate small metastases. Other chemotherapy programs (5-FU + cisplatin, cisplatin + vinblastine or Bleomycin, 5-FU + mitomycin-C, or cisplatin + 5-FU/leucovorin + VP-16 for neoadjuvant therapy) have shown response to treatment. Studies thus far suggest that carboplatin is less effective than cisplatin and should not be substituted, although it is less toxic.

The role of chemotherapy and radiation therapy is being evaluated. To date, there is significant increased survival from chemotherapy and radiation therapy versus radiation therapy alone. Recent studies of 5-FU + mitomycin-C with radiotherapy have shown an improved survival for Stages I and II disease with almost twice the survival as radiotherapy alone. Tumors of the gastroesophageal junction are treated with combination chemotherapy after surgery, as in stomach cancer (*see* "Stomach").

 Laser Therapy Endoscopic laser therapy (ELT) has been used over the past few years to relieve swallowing problems. Lasers can vaporize the tumor and cut a hole through a blockage in the esophagus, although the hole will last only a few weeks to three months. The procedure can be repeated to keep the obstruction open, but repeated laser treatments may be more difficult.

Esophageal dilation with ELT can be used to reopen the food channel when surgery or radiation therapy are not practical or when treatment with mechanical methods (by balloon dilators or mercury-filled rubber dilators) fails. Esophageal rupture is a possible complication of dilation.

With laser therapy there are dangers of perforation, bleeding and fistula formation. Lasers can also treat tumors only inside the esophagus, not tumors outside the esophageal wall (*see* Chapter 9).

TREATMENT BY STAGE

STAGE 0
TNM Tis (Tumor in situ)
This very early cancer has not spread below the lining of the first layer of esophageal tissue. It is unusual for cancer to be found at this stage in Western countries, though it's not unusual in China, where esophageal cancer is seen frequently and screening programs are common.

Standard Treatment Early-stage esophageal cancer can be cured with surgery. Radiotherapy could be an option in poor-risk patients.

Five-Year Survival The prognosis is excellent if the tumor is treated surgically or with radiotherapy.

STAGE I
TNM TI, N0, M0
The tumor involves less than 2 in. (5 cm) of the esophagus, does not penetrate the muscular wall, and there is no spread to lymph nodes, adjacent structures or other organs. While patients may have some difficulty swallowing, there is no obstruction of the esophagus.

Standard Treatment Stage I cancer is treatable and occasionally curable. Surgical removal of the tumor is the treatment of choice, with the highest success rate for cancer in the lower third of the esophagus. About 4 in. (10 cm) of the esophagus and the adjacent lymph nodes are removed. With surgery, there is a 5 to 10 percent mortality rate and a 15 to 30 percent complication rate.

Radiation therapy may effectively control and sometimes cure small tumors. Side effects of radiation therapy can include a short-term inflammation of the esophagus and the development of a benign stricture (30 percent), which can be dilated.

There is no standard chemotherapy, but recent studies suggest that combined radiation and chemotherapy (with 5-FU + cisplatin or 5-FU + mitomycin-C) may possibly achieve a clinical remission and cure for Stages I or II cancers. This may be in conjunction with or instead of surgery.

Palliation Surgery and radiation therapy can relieve swallowing problems in about 80 percent of cases.

Five-Year Survival Over 50 percent

Investigational
♦ Protocols using combinations of chemotherapy and radiosensitizers, along with radiation therapy before or after surgery, are being evaluated.

STAGE II
TNM T2, N+, M0
The tumor involves more than 2 in. (5 cm) of the esophagus and may involve the entire circumference in one area, causing blockage problems. The cancer has not spread to adjacent organs but may have spread to regional lymph nodes. Most cancers larger than 2 in. (5 cm) have positive lymph nodes.

Standard Treatment Combination therapy with radiation (3,000–5000 cGy) and a chemotherapy infusion of 5-FU and mitomycin-C or cisplatin has produced local response rates of up to 80 percent. Treatments are toxic and side effects require intense medical management. About 20 percent of patients had complete remission locally, meaning that no tumor was found at surgery. There is an average survival of one and a half years and up to 3 years for patients who experienced complete remission before surgery.

Surgery holds out some potential for cure, but there is high operative mortality. Stomach reflux and inflammation are common side effects. It should also be noted that because the esophagus has unusual lymphatic drainage, metastatic tumors may be found quite distant from the primary tumor.

Palliation Successful surgery will alleviate swallowing problems for two to three months in 90 percent of patients; radiation therapy will provide relief for 70 percent. Overall survival is about 11 months.

External beam radiation therapy may be palliative for larger tumors or with celiac lymph node involvement (for the lower esophagus) and supraclavicular lymph node involvement (for the upper esophagus).

A radiation source (iridium) may be inserted into the esophagus and left at the tumor site for several hours (intraluminal brachytherapy). Side effects can include inflammation of the esophagus (but rarely the heart or spinal cord), bleeding or a hole from the esophagus into the lungs (esophagobronchial fistula). This may also happen as part of the disease process, especially for the middle third of the esophagus.

Five-Year Survival 10 to 15 percent

Investigational
♦ Radiation therapy given for two weeks before surgical removal of the esophagus may eliminate some of the tumor cells that have spread and make some inoperable tumors operable.

♦ There are several trials being conducted using combinations of chemotherapy (5-FU and cisplatin) and radiosensitizers along with radiation before or after surgery.

♦ Various chemotherapy programs to increase resectability are being evaluated. Chemotherapy may not increase the number of tumors that are operable, but those who respond to chemotherapy live longer than those who don't (12 months versus 6.2 months).

♦ A new laser approach—photodynamic therapy—involves the injection of a substance that makes tissue more sensitive to light. This is followed by the burning of a hole with a laser through the esophageal obstruction. This is safe and may temporarily help to control tumors and allow eating. (*See* Chapter 9.)

♦ An interferon + 5-FU/leucovorin + cisplatin program is under study.

STAGE III
TNM T3–T4, any N, and M0
The tumor has spread outside the esophagus and there is extensive lymph node involvement, but there are no metastases.

Standard Treatment Multiple approaches are used with Stage III cancer. Radiation therapy and chemotherapy are used for palliation (5-FU + cisplatin, 5-FU, 5-FU + cisplatin + Adriamycin or 5-FU + mitomycin-C).

Nutrition is a major concern, because patients cannot swallow. A nutritional support program should be instituted with an enteral feeding tube or hyperalimentation. Lasers may be used to open up a blocked esophagus or an eating tube may be inserted.

Five-Year Survival Less than 10 percent when the cancer has spread to adjacent structures but not to other organs

Investigational
♦ Various combinations of chemothera-

py, radiation and surgery may be attempted. Radiation and chemotherapy without surgery is being evaluated for patients who are inoperable, have refused surgery or are over 80 years old.

♦ 5-FU + interferon-alpha has shown significant activity.

♦ One study showed improved survival for patients with non-resectable tumors if radiation, chemotherapy and heat treatments (hyperthermia) were given after part of the esophagus was removed.

♦ Laser therapy may be used to reduce obstruction (photodynamic protoporphyrin therapy and dilation). Patients with severe weight loss or anorexia are generally poor risks for therapy.

STAGE IV
TNM Any T, any N, M1
The tumor has spread to other organs (distant metastases).

Standard Treatment There is no standard treatment for Stage IV esophageal cancer. Standard palliative approaches—including external radiation with chemotherapy, with or without the insertion of an eating tube and dilation—are used. All patients may be considered candidates for investigational protocols evaluating new approaches to treatment, including promising chemotherapy combinations.

Five-Year Survival Unusual

Investigational
♦ Chemotherapy and radiotherapy treatments as outlined in Stages II and III.

SUPPORTIVE THERAPY

People with esophageal tumors often have a poor nutritional status. Attempts to correct weight loss may help reduce the complications of surgery, radiotherapy, chemotherapy and combined treatments.
♦ A nasogastric feeding tube (if there is

no obstruction) or a gastrojejunostomy may be used for enteral nutrition.

♦ Parenteral hyperalimentation may be necessary for support during therapy.

♦ Esophageal dilation with or without laser therapy to maintain an open esophagus may help maintain nutrition.

TREATMENT FOLLOW-UP

Patients who have had treatment for cure should visit their physician every few months for close follow-up. The adequacy of treatment can be assessed and any needed palliative treatment—radiation or laser therapy—can begin.

RECURRENT CANCER

All such patients may be treated with standard or palliative chemotherapy described for Stages II and III or should be considered candidates for clinical trials.

Palliation is difficult and nutritional support and pain control are helpful.

PREVENTION

♦ Avoid drinking alcohol and smoking.

♦ For Barrett's esophagus, it is important to try to heal the esophagitis and prevent the reflux of stomach acids.

Reflux may be managed by using H-2 blockers to relieve symptoms, by changing the pressure in the lower esophagus with metoclopramide (Reglan) and by not eating for several hours before sleep. Losec (omeprazole), a new drug that has antisecretory properties that suppress gastric acid, may not only help heal esophagitis but also may heal or normalize a Barrett's esophagus. Dietary restrictions—avoiding fats, chocolate and peppermint—opiates, calcium-channel blockers and anticholinergic drugs may also help control reflux.

THE MOST IMPORTANT QUESTIONS YOU CAN ASK

♦ What are the criteria for surgery? for radiation therapy?

♦ How does the stage of disease relate to the chance for cure?

♦ How does squamous cell cancer differ from adenocarcinoma of the esophagus?

♦ What is the role, treatment and prognosis of radiation therapy, the role of surgery, and chemotherapy in treatment of cancer of the esophagus?

♦ How can I obtain nutritional support?

GALL BLADDER

Alan P. Venook, MD

◇

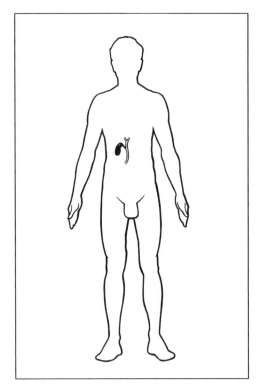

The gall bladder stores bile, which aids in the digestion of fat-containing foods. It is a non-essential organ and can be removed without significant consequences. Gall bladder cancer—also called carcinoma of the gall bladder—is extremely rare. And unless it is very small and found when the gall bladder is removed for other reasons, the treatment now available is not particularly effective.

Because it is so uncommon and because its symptoms mirror those of far more common ailments, cancer of the gall bladder is usually not found until it is at an advanced stage and cannot be surgically removed. In the advanced stages, pain relief and the restoration of normal bile flow from the liver into the intestines are the principal goals of therapy.

Types The majority of gall bladder tumors are found in glandular tissue within the gall bladder (adenocarcinoma). Others originate in the connective tissue (sarcoma) or other tissues (squamous carcinoma). The management for all gall bladder cancer types is the same, always depending upon the extent of the tumor at the time of diagnosis.

How It Spreads Gall bladder cancer tends to spread to nearby organs and tissues such as the liver or intestines. It also spreads through the lymph system to lymph nodes in the region of the liver (porta hepatis). Ultimately, other lymph nodes and organs can become involved.

What Causes It No one factor has been clearly shown to cause gall bladder cancer. Although it occurs most often in people with gallstone disease, it is extremely rare even in such patients. It is not known if bouts of gallstones predispose people to developing this cancer.

RISK FACTORS

At Significantly Higher Risk

♦ About 85 percent of people with gall bladder cancer have a history of gallstones (cholelithiasis). Sometimes, although not often, the gall bladder becomes hardened (calcified) from repeated inflammation as gallstones are passed. People with this "porcelain gall bladder" have a higher risk of developing this cancer than do others. The typical patient with gall bladder cancer is an elderly woman with a history of gall bladder problems.

At Slightly Higher Risk
♦ Gallstone disease without a "porcelain gall bladder."

SCREENING

No screening tests are available to detect this cancer at an early stage. But, since the gall bladder isn't essential, people with a calcified gall bladder may consider having it removed as a preventive measure.

COMMON SIGNS AND SYMPTOMS

There are no clinical signs or symptoms characteristic of gall bladder cancer. Jaundice (the skin turning yellow), bloating, abdominal pain, weight loss, decreasing appetite, fever, nausea or an enlarging abdominal mass are all signs that *may* be attributable to gall bladder cancer. Frequently, jaundice is a late development and the other symptoms have been present for a long time. Itching may result from the buildup in the skin of a derivative of bile, bilirubin, which turns the skin yellow. This symptom usually reflects advanced disease.

DIAGNOSIS

Physical Examination
There are no specific findings for gall bladder cancer on physical examination. Even if the following are found, gall bladder cancer would still not be the prime suspect because it is so uncommon:
♦ Fever.
♦ Tender mass below the ribs on the right side of the abdomen.
♦ Enlarged, hard lymph nodes.
♦ Jaundice (the skin turning yellow).
♦ Swelling of the legs (edema).

Blood and Other Tests
Diagnostic tests are notoriously inaccurate in their ability to pinpoint gall bladder can-

cer before surgery. A standard evaluation, however, would include:
♦ A complete blood test, which may be normal or may reveal a decrease in hemoglobin (anemia). The white blood cell count may be normal or increased.
♦ Liver function tests may be abnormal. The most likely abnormalities are in the serum bilirubin and alkaline phosphatase, indicating a blockage in the bile duct leaving either the liver or the gall bladder.
♦ Prothrombin Time and Partial Thromboplastin Time (PT and PTT) are tests of clotting that may reveal a disorder in patients with poor liver function related to a blocked bile duct.

Imaging
♦ An abdominal ultrasound study to view the gall bladder area without exposure to x-rays can confirm that the gall bladder wall has thickened and provide information about the size and characteristics of any mass in the region.
♦ Swallowing pills with dye that travels to the gall bladder, enabling it to be seen on x-ray (oral cholecystography), or the injection of dye into the bile ducts through the skin followed by an x-ray of the area (percutaneous cholangiography) may be done because of symptoms or an elevated serum bilirubin level. While both studies may document an abnormality within the bile ducts or gall bladder, neither can reliably distinguish between inflammation of the gall bladder (cholecystitis) and gall bladder cancer.
♦ A CT scan may help determine the extent of the tumor within the gall bladder bed and the possible involvement of other organs.
♦ Magnetic resonance imaging (MRI) may be helpful in determining if the cancer can be surgically removed, but it is usually not necessary because the CT scan shows similar information.
♦ If the diagnosis of cancer is confirmed or suspected, a chest x-ray should be obtained. A finding of tumor nodules in

the lungs would mean that the disease is already metastatic.

Endoscopy and Biopsy

♦ If cancer is suspected in a situation not involving gall bladder surgery for other reasons, a biopsy, either with a fine needle (FNA) or regular needle, is always required. This can be done through the skin without significant danger.

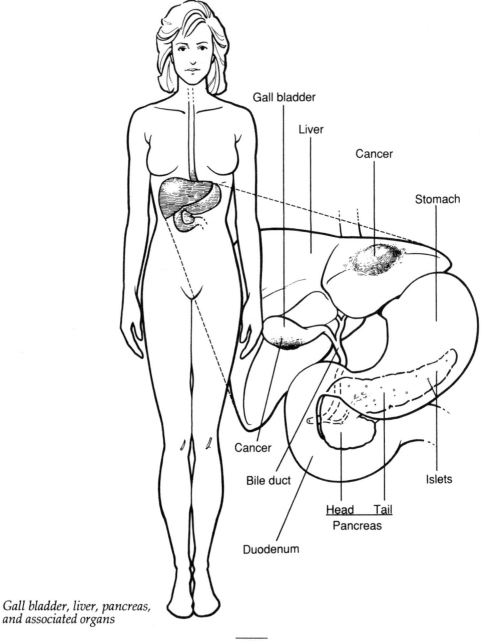

Gall bladder, liver, pancreas, and associated organs

STAGING

A TNM staging system exists for gall bladder cancer, but for the purposes of deciding on which therapeutic option to use there are only three stages—localized resectable, localized unresectable and advanced disease.

TREATMENT OVERVIEW

Gall bladder cancer can be cured only when it is localized enough to be removed surgically. Unfortunately, virtually the only people with such localized disease are those whose cancer is found unexpectedly when the gall bladder is removed for other reasons.

The goal of the diagnostic work-up is to determine if the cancer can be entirely removed. This is rarely possible because the tumor usually spreads to local regions early in its course. More effective chemotherapy and radiation therapy than are available today are under investigation. These treatments are occasionally useful to relieve symptoms related to the cancer. Although patients with advanced gall bladder cancer have a poor prognosis, measures can be taken to maintain the quality of life.

 Surgery Surgery is the only possible cure. If there is no distant tumor spread, the gall bladder as well as the draining lymph nodes and a wedge of normal underlying liver tissue may be removed. This may cure a patient, can help relieve symptoms and may improve the quality of life.

If a gall bladder cancer is found unexpectedly in the pathology specimen after surgery performed for problems not thought to involve cancer, a second operation may be required. If the tumor is limited to only the superficial layers of the gall bladder, observation may be adequate. If the cancer has spread into the surrounding tissues, lymph nodes or blood vessels, however, a second operation may be performed to remove other tissues that may be involved.

When the tumor cannot fully be removed, it may still be necessary to create a drainage system for the bile from the obstructed gall bladder or bile ducts. This may require surgery, although draining of the gall bladder by a tube placed through the skin by a radiologist or through a tube in the stomach and small intestines usually suffices.

The presence of tumor anywhere else in the body—in the lung, bone or lymph nodes, for example—is a clear indication that surgery will not be curative. If the disease has already spread, there is rarely a need to remove a gall bladder cancer, for such surgery involves a difficult recovery period and so may be more damaging to the patient.

 Chemotherapy Studies have not yet shown that chemotherapy can prolong the survival of patients with gallbladder cancer. The standard drugs used—5-fluorouracil or mitomycin-C—may cause tumor shrinkage in about 25 percent of patients. Even with tumor shrinkage, however, patients may be in a worse condition afterward because the tumor usually regrows quickly and the treatments have some side effects.

There is no proven role for adjuvant chemotherapy after a cancerous gall bladder has been removed, but it is logical to consider chemotherapy. In the hopes of finding drugs that may work better than the chemotherapy now used, patients should be entered into a clinical trial if chemotherapy is planned.

Radiation The usefulness of radiation in gall bladder cancer is limited by the damage it causes to the surrounding noncancerous liver tissue. Radiation may help patients who have small bits of tumor remaining after surgery or in those who have had large tumors removed.

Patients who are not candidates for surgery may also benefit from radiation to the gall bladder area, although they are still likely to have recurrent tumors. The toxicity of such radiation may also worsen existing symptoms such as nausea and loss of appetite.

Combined Therapy The combination of external beam radiation and chemotherapy may play a role after surgery, perhaps prolonging the period before the cancer returns or even curing people who have undergone surgery without complete tumor removal. This treatment, however, is still being studied.

TREATMENT BY STAGE
LOCALIZED RESECTABLE
In this stage, the cancer is confined to the superficial layers (mucosa and submucosa) of the gall bladder. Cancers at this limited stage are generally found when the gall bladder is removed because of other problems.

Standard Treatment Experts disagree over the extent of surgery needed for a localized gall bladder cancer. Studies are ongoing, but most experts would recommend:
♦ removal of the gall bladder
♦ a lymph node dissection of all the draining lymphatic vessels in the region
♦ the removal of a wedge of about 1 1/2 in. (4 cm) of apparently normal liver.

Such surgery is the most likely treatment to render a patient cancer-free. If the cancer is not recognized until after surgery, the need for a second operation is considered. A patient with a truly limited cancer (superficial) may just be observed closely, but because of the poor prognosis should the cancer recur, it is difficult to argue against the aggressive approach outlined above.

Five-Year Survival About 80 percent. Those with cancers that are still very small but cause symptoms have a somewhat lower five-year survival rate.

Investigational
♦ There is no certain role for adjuvant chemotherapy. Although chemotherapy such as 5-fluorouracil (5-FU) or mitomycin-C is often recommended, no studies have shown that the chance of cure can be increased.
♦ Radiation is often given to the liver area after surgery but has never been proven to be beneficial.
♦ The use of a combination of 5-FU and radiation therapy following complete removal of the cancer is now being studied.

LOCALIZED UNRESECTABLE
Despite being a localized mass, the tumor cannot be removed because of the particular way it has spread to local lymph nodes or adjacent liver tissue.

Standard Treatment There is no standard treatment. Patients should be considered for clinical trials aimed at prolonging survival and relieving the symptoms associated with the tumor.

Two-Year Survival Less than 5 percent

Investigational
♦ Protocols designed to test the additive benefit of combining radiation with chemotherapy are ongoing and should be offered to patients with this condition.

ADVANCED
The cancer has metastasized to distant sites.

Standard Treatment No standard therapy is known to prolong survival in patients with advanced gall bladder cancer. The usual approach is a trial of chemotherapy with a single agent such as 5-FU or mitomycin-C. Even if the tumor shrinks, patients may not benefit because of the side effects of the chemotherapy and because the tumor usually regrows very quickly.

Two-Year Survival Less than 1 percent

Investigational
♦ Combination chemotherapy or new drugs may prove to be better in the treatment of advanced gall bladder cancer than therapies now available. Because the side effects are likely to be greater than those caused by single-agent chemotherapy, such treatment should be done in a clinical protocol.

TREATMENT FOLLOW-UP
Careful follow-up is important after the removal of a localized gall bladder cancer, although once a recurrent tumor is large enough to be seen on an x-ray it is probably too large to be cured. Follow-up should include:
♦ CT scans every two to three months for the first year after surgery, since another small tumor may still be resectable at the time of diagnosis.

SUPPORTIVE THERAPY
♦ Symptoms associated with jaundice can include severe itching and a general sense of poor health. These symptoms can generally be managed with a drainage procedure to bypass the blockage in the biliary tract. This procedure may include placing of a tube through the skin or through the stomach. Surgery is rarely necessary to bypass an obstruction.

If such drainage is ineffective, itching may be relieved by the use of Benadryl, Atarax or cholestyramine.
♦ Pain relief may require large doses of medication. Narcotics must be used carefully, however, since they may have excessive side effects and are metabolized by the liver, which may not be working properly.
♦ Non-steroidal anti-inflammatory drugs may be surprisingly effective even against the severe pain associated with gall bladder cancer.
♦ The use of water pills to reduce fluid in the abdomen or legs may be helpful, but may cause significant imbalance in kidney function and can create major problems if not monitored carefully.
♦ Nausea can be treated with standard medications, including suppositories.
♦ Sleep disturbances are common, but sleeping pills should be used carefully since most are metabolized by the liver.
♦ Frequent small meals may be necessary since an abdominal mass may encroach on the size of the stomach.
♦ Patients with the severe loss of appetite may be helped by a drug called Megace.

THE MOST IMPORTANT QUESTIONS YOU CAN ASK
♦ Should I see another physician to confirm that this tumor is or is not resectable for cure?
♦ Could I benefit from an investigational therapy available at another institution?
♦ How sick will the proposed chemotherapy make me relative to its potential benefit?
♦ Can anything be done to improve the quality of my life?

HEAD AND NECK

James T. Helsper, MD, and Malin Dollinger, MD

◇

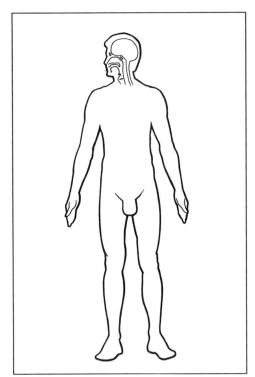

Taken together, head and neck cancers account for 5 to 10 percent of all malignancies. These cancers are more common in men by a ratio of 3 to 1 and are much more common in people over 50. They have a rather good cure rate if they are found early, evaluated adequately and treated with the best available therapy. All three main treatment methods—surgery, radiotherapy and chemotherapy—are used.

There are about 43,000 new cases in the United States each year, and about one third of head and neck cancer patients die of their disease. The use of chemotherapy (such as cisplatin + 5-fluorouracil or low-dose 5-fluorouracil continuous infusion) as an adjuvant to surgery and radiotherapy has produced a definite improvement in response rates. Active clinical trials of combined therapy are under way in an effort to provide a better cure rate in the future.

The broad category of head and neck cancers includes tumors in several areas.

♦ Lip and oral cavity. This includes the lips, tongue, the inside lining of the cheeks (buccal mucosa), the floor of the mouth, the gums (gingiva) and the hard palate.

♦ Paranasal sinuses and nasal cavity. Sinuses are found below and above the eyes and behind the nose.

♦ Salivary glands. These glands produce saliva to moisten our mouth and help us chew and swallow food.

♦ Oropharynx. This is the upper part of the throat that can be seen when you say "ahhh." It also includes the tonsils.

♦ Nasopharynx. The nasopharynx is behind the nose and above the oropharynx. It cannot be seen directly, but is viewed with a mirror or a scope.

♦ Hypopharynx. This is the lower part of the throat (pharynx) where food goes just before we swallow it.

♦ Larynx. The larynx (voice box) is in the front of the neck in the region of the Adam's apple.

♦ Metastatic squamous cell cancer to cervical (neck) lymph nodes. If a cancer that is discovered in lymph nodes in the upper part of the neck is squamous cell (or epidermoid), it is usually a metastasis from a head and neck cancer. Unless some other primary source can be found (such as lung cancer), this tumor is generally treated as a head and neck cancer. It is important to know that this type of metastatic cancer may be curable (discussed later in the chapter) (*see also* "Cancer of an Unknown Primary Site").

The most common locations for head and neck cancers—almost half of all cases—are

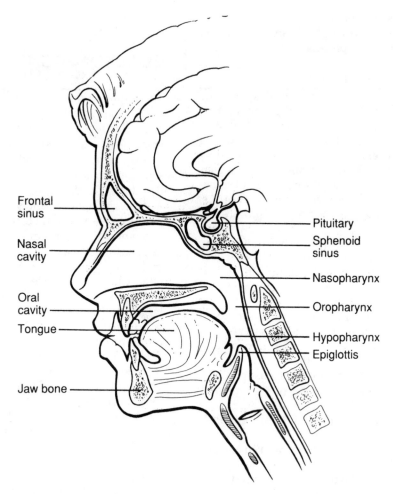

Frontal sinus
Nasal cavity
Oral cavity
Tongue
Jaw bone

Pituitary
Sphenoid sinus
Nasopharynx
Oropharynx
Hypopharynx
Epiglottis

Cross-section of head showing potential cancer sites

the mouth and throat (oral cavity and oropharynx). About a third are in the larynx.

These cancers and their treatment can have serious results. Because they tend to involve the upper digestive tract and the upper respiratory tract, these tumors can interfere with eating and breathing. Laryngeal cancer directly affects speech. Several sensory functions are located here—vision, hearing, smell and taste—and the loss or malfunction of any of them is significant.

Successful treatment must, therefore, not only include an attempt to eradicate all the cancer but also take into account:

♦ The need for adequate function—swallowing, eating, speech—after treatment.
♦ A satisfactory cosmetic result. It is as important to consider reconstruction, rehabilitation and prostheses as it is to achieve an adequate surgical removal.

Many health care workers are essential to success. In addition to the head and neck (or ear, nose and throat) surgeon, the treatment team may include the primary physician, radiation and medical oncologists, dentists, rehabilitation specialists, plastic surgeons, dieticians, pathologists, radiologists, oncology nurses and social workers. The patient and his or her family, friends and employer are all involved in the recovery process.

RISK FACTORS

The use of tobacco and/or alcohol is the most important contributing factor. Smokers and drinkers who fail to stop after treatment for a primary head and neck cancer are at significantly higher risk of developing another cancer. In fact, anyone with a head and neck cancer is somewhat more likely to develop another, although giving a drug called 13-cis-retinoic acid to such patients has decreased the chance of their developing a second primary tumor.

♦ Poor oral hygiene, poorly fitting dentures or broken teeth cause chronic irritation of oral membranes.

♦ Wood dust inhalation (furniture workers) is related to nasal cavity cancer.

♦ Betel nut chewing (India) is related to cancer of the lining of the cheek.

♦ Increased carcinoma of nasopharynx among southern Chinese (environmental, not genetic).

♦ Epstein-Barr virus (EBV) infection is associated with nasopharyngeal cancer.

♦ Chronic iron deficiency in women is associated with tongue and postcricoid carcinoma.

♦ Nickel exposure is associated with paranasal sinus cancer.

SCREENING

Screening is not generally practiced in North America. There are three approaches to early detection.

♦ Your awareness of typical signs and symptoms and your calling them to the attention of your physician.

♦ A careful examination of the head and neck by your doctor, including an examination of the larynx with the aid of a mirror (indirect laryngoscopy) or a scope.

♦ Your dentist is in an excellent position to call your attention to suspicious lesions in the mouth such as the premalignant lesion called leukoplakia (white patches). Many oral cancers are discovered by dentists.

COMMON SIGNS AND SYMPTOMS

These tumors can appear as ulcerations of the mucous membranes with hard, rolled edges, or less commonly as protruding growths that look like small mushrooms. Specific symptoms depend on the location.

♦ *Mouth and oral cavity:* a swelling or ulcer that doesn't heal.

♦ *Nose and sinuses:* pain, swelling, bloody nasal discharge, nasal obstruction, double vision or chronic sinus trouble that does not respond to antibiotics.

♦ *Salivary glands:* painless swelling and later paralysis of one side of the face.

♦ *Oropharynx:* difficulty or pain on swallowing and ear pain. May also have no symptoms.

♦ *Hypopharynx:* difficulty swallowing, ear pain and enlarged lymph nodes in the neck. May have no symptoms.

♦ *Nasopharynx:* bloody nasal discharge or nasal obstruction, decreased hearing, nerve signs (double vision, pain, hoarseness) or enlarged lymph nodes in the neck.

♦ *Larynx:* persistent hoarseness, difficulty breathing, pain.

♦ *Metastatic squamous cell cancer:* swollen, painless lymph nodes in the neck.

DIAGNOSIS

Specific tests depend on the location of the cancer.

Physical Examination

♦ Inspection of the oral and nasal cavities, using mirrors and telescopes.

♦ Examination of suspicious lesions with the fingers (palpation), as well as examination of the back of the tongue.

Blood and Other Tests

♦ Epstein-Barr (EB) virus antibody measurements may be helpful in diagnosing hidden nasopharyngeal primary cancer in patients with metastatic cancer in the cervical lymph nodes.

Imaging
♦ X-rays of the sinuses and skull.
♦ CT and MRI scans, barium esophogram, laryngogram and chest x-ray.

Endoscopy and Biopsy
♦ Biopsy of suspicious lesions.
♦ In cases of metastatic cancer in cervical lymph nodes, biopsy of apparently normal tissues in the tonsils, throat and nasopharynx may be necessary to discover the site of origin.

STAGING

Head and neck cancers are staged according to the TNM system. Accuracy of staging is especially critical, since a slight difference in the location and size of the tumor has a significant effect on the therapy chosen, the extent of surgery and the prognosis.

Accurate staging requires visual inspection, x-rays, appropriate biopsies, blood tests (such as complete blood counts and liver tests) and careful palpation and measurement of enlarged lymph nodes. The mobility of enlarged nodes should be determined since a lymph node that cannot be moved back and forth may contain cancer that has spread to adjacent tissues. Sometimes examination under anesthesia is needed to directly inspect inaccessible areas such as the larynx, nasopharynx, and oropharynx, as well as to perform necessary biopsies.

TNM STAGE GROUPING
Stage I: T1, N0, M0
Stage II: T2, N0, M0
Stage III: T3, N0, M0
           T1–3, N1, M0
Stage IV: T4, N0 or N1, M0
           Any T, N2-3, M0
           Any T, any N, M1

For most subsites there are also other TNM categories that define the tumor more precisely.

STAGING OUTLINE

Oral cavity, oropharynx (tumor can be seen directly)	Nasopharynx, hypopharynx, larynx (tumor cannot be seen directly)
Tx Tumor cannot be measured	
T0 No evidence of primary tumors	}SAME
Tis Carcinoma in situ	
T1 Tumor no larger than 3/4 in. (2 cm)	Tumor confined to one site
T2 Tumor 3/4 –1 1/2 in. (2–4 cm)	Involves more than one site at origin
T3 Tumor over 1 1/2 in. (4 cm)	Tumor extends beyond primary site
T4 Massive tumor, over 1 1/2 in. (4 cm) with extension to adjacent structures	}SAME

NX Nodes cannot be measured
N0 No involved lymph nodes
N1 Single involved node, same side, less than 1 1/4 in. (3 cm)
N2 Single involved node, same side,
    N2a one node, 1 1/4 –2 1/2 in. (3–6 cm)
    N2b multiple nodes, none over 2 1/2 in. (6 cm)
N3 Massive involved lymph nodes
    N3a a node over 2 1/2 in. (6 cm) on same side
    N3b nodes on both sides
    N3c nodes only on opposite side

LIP AND MOUTH (ORAL CAVITY)

These cancers usually arise from the floor of the mouth and the tongue. They can be treated with surgery, radiation therapy or a combination of both depending on the location and size of the tumor and whether it has spread to lymph nodes. Reconstruction and rehabilitation are essential parts of the treatment plan.

Early cancers (Stages I and II) of the lip and oral cavity are highly curable by surgery or radiation therapy, with the choice depending on the anticipated functional and cosmetic results.

Advanced cancers (Stages III and IV) are usually treated with a combination of surgery and radiotherapy. A few patients with small T3 lesions who have no involved lymph nodes larger than 3/4 in. (2 cm) might receive either surgery or radiation. Patients with these stages commonly develop recurrences near the primary tumor or metastatic disease after treatment and should be considered for clinical trials involving radiation modifiers or the use of combination chemotherapy in addition to surgery and/or radiation. Patients whose tumors grow into blood vessels have a worse prognosis.

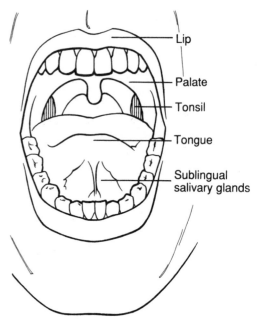

Mouth structures that may develop cancer

TREATMENT OVERVIEW

♦ If surgery is the chosen method, the tumor must be removed along with the areas in the neck where it usually first spreads, to provide a margin of safety. The chosen surgeon must be able to reconstruct the area, working with dentists who are specialists in reconstructing portions of teeth that have had to be removed to provide the best chance of cure. This helps return the patient to the most normal quality of life.

♦ If the cervical nodes are involved, all the lymph nodes on that side of the neck usually have to be removed (radical neck dissection).

♦ Radiation therapy for lip or oral cancer can be with either external beams or occasionally the implantation of radioactive seeds into the tumor site for a specified time to give a calculated dose of radiation. Either method can be used alone, but most centers use the two in combination.

♦ Surgery to remove a tumor of the tongue often requires removing a generous portion of the tongue to provide a margin of safety. Surprisingly, there may be very little effect on speech and swallowing, although if the tumor is large, a larger portion of the tongue has to be removed and speech becomes more of a problem. A speech therapist may be needed for proper rehabilitation.

♦ Cancer of the space around the teeth usually requires the removal of some of the teeth as well as the primary cancer site in the gingiva (gums). The dental prosthodontist creates a specialized plate for complete rehabilitation.

♦ Occasionally, when the cancer involves

the upper gums it may be necessary to remove a portion of the sinus. The prosthodontist is again needed for reconstruction.

♦ For larger cancers that have a lower cure rate with surgery alone, treatment combines all three methods—chemotherapy, followed by surgery, followed by radiation therapy.

TREATMENT BY LOCATION AND STAGE

STAGE I
Standard Treatment

♦ *Lip:* Surgery or radiotherapy, depending on cosmetic and functional results.

♦ *Front of tongue:* Wide local excision. For larger lesions, either surgery or radiotherapy.

♦ *Inside of cheek:* Surgery for small lesions (with skin graft, if needed) or radiotherapy for larger lesions.

♦ *Floor of mouth:* Surgery or radiotherapy.

♦ *Lower gums:* Surgery, possibly with removal of some bone and the use of a skin graft. Radiotherapy results are usually not as good as surgery.

♦ *Behind wisdom teeth (retromolar trigone):* Can usually be controlled by external radiotherapy. Alternatively, surgical removal, including part of jawbone.

♦ *Upper gums and hard palate:* Surgery, with postoperative radiation if needed.

Five-Year Survival 90 to 100 percent (lip and upper gums), 96 percent (tongue), over 90 percent (inside of cheek), 90 percent (lower gums), 88 percent (floor of mouth)

STAGE II
Standard Treatment

♦ *Lip:* Surgery alone, if simple closure is satisfactory. If surgery has to be complex, radiotherapy produces better cosmetic and functional results.

♦ *Front of tongue:* Surgery initially for smaller lesions. Additional surgery, and

sometimes radiation therapy, are used later if tumor remains or recurs. Both surgery and radiotherapy are used for tumors that are growing deeper.

♦ *Inside of cheek:* Small T2 lesions are treated with radiotherapy or surgery. Larger T2 lesions are treated with surgery, radiotherapy or both.

♦ *Floor of mouth:* For small T2 lesions, surgery if the tumor is attached to bone and radiotherapy if lesions involve the tongue. Both surgery and radiotherapy can be used for large T2 lesions. The choice depends on the expected disability from surgery. For larger lesions, radiotherapy may be used postoperatively.

♦ *Lower gums:* Small lesions treated with surgery, sometimes requiring removal of some bone as well as a skin graft. Radiotherapy has been used, but results are generally not as good as with surgery alone.

♦ *Behind wisdom teeth:* Same as Stage I.

Five-Year Survival 90 percent (lip, inside of cheek and lower gums), 70 percent (tongue and floor of mouth)

STAGE III
Standard Treatment Surgery and/or radiotherapy is used, depending on the location of the tumor. Chemotherapy before either surgery or radiotherapy (neoadjuvant) has been used to shrink large tumors and improve the possibility of successful treatment with surgery or radiation. Patients with advanced lesions should have radiotherapy to lymph nodes or surgery to remove them.

♦ *Lip:* Combination of surgery and radiotherapy. Alternatively, these patients are appropriate candidates for clinical trials.

♦ *Front of tongue:* Radiotherapy (may include implant) for less extensive lesions, and surgery with postoperative radiotherapy for more extensive lesions.

♦ *Inside of cheek:* Radical surgery alone, radiotherapy alone or both in sequence. Clinical trials involve adding chemotherapy.

♦ *Floor of mouth:* Extensive surgery or

radiotherapy (may include implant).

♦ *Lower gums:* Combined radiotherapy and radical surgery.

♦ *Behind wisdom teeth:* Surgery followed by radiotherapy. Clinical trials involve adding chemotherapy.

♦ *Upper gums:* Superficial lesions are treated with radiotherapy alone. Deep lesions also require surgery.

♦ *Hard palate:* Same as upper gums.

Five-Year Survival 50 percent (lip and inside of cheek), 50 to 60 percent (tongue), 70 percent (floor of mouth), 90 percent (lower gums), 80 percent (hard palate and upper gums)

STAGE IV
Standard Treatment Surgery and/or radiotherapy, depending on the location of the tumor. Neoadjuvant chemotherapy has been used to shrink tumors and improve the possibility of successful treatment with surgery or radiation. Patients with advanced lesions should have radiotherapy to lymph nodes or surgery to remove them.

Clinical trials involving adjuvant chemotherapy are in progress and are appropriate for all sites.

♦ *Lip:* Combined surgery and radiotherapy. Both sides of the neck have to be treated.

♦ *Front of tongue:* Extensive surgery with postoperative radiotherapy for selected patients. For very advanced lesions, radiotherapy alone for palliation.

♦ *Inside of cheek:* Radical surgery, radiotherapy or both in sequence.

♦ *Floor of mouth:* Combination of surgery and radiotherapy. If there are large (over 2 in./5 cm) fixed nodes, radiotherapy is given preoperatively.

♦ *Lower gums:* Advanced tumors are poorly controlled with surgery, radiotherapy or both.

♦ *Behind wisdom teeth:* Surgery followed by radiotherapy.

♦ *Upper gums:* Surgery and radiotherapy.

♦ *Hard palate:* Surgery and radiotherapy.

Five-Year Survival Up to 40 to 50 percent for all locations

RECURRENT CANCER

Treatment depends on the location and size of the recurrent tumor, as well as the nature of the original treatment. If radiotherapy was used initially, surgery is preferred. If surgery was used initially, radiotherapy or a combination of both may be used. Because results are poor after using the "other" treatment for a recurrence, clinical trials using chemotherapy or hyperthermia should be considered.

PARANASAL SINUS AND NASAL CAVITY

These cancers are often diagnosed late because they may have no symptoms in early stages or symptoms may resemble chronic sinusitis. They can easily spread throughout the sinus area, and cure rates are generally less than 50 percent. Local growth into vital areas is a more common cause of death than metastases.

There are six sinuses, two just below the eyes (maxillary), two above the eyes (frontal) and two in the center, behind the nose (ethmoid and sphenoid). The maxillary sinus is the one most commonly involved, and cancer there can be difficult to diagnose. It may be necessary to expose the maxillary sinus through a small opening in the mouth above the canine teeth in the upper jaw (Caldwell-Luc procedure).

TREATMENT OVERVIEW

Treatment of these tumors is very complex and requires very precise pretreatment evaluation and planning. Most patients require a combination of radiotherapy and surgery.

♦ Since lymph nodes are involved in only about 20 percent of cases, surgery or radiotherapy to the lymph nodes in the neck is used only if these nodes contain tumor.

♦ For patients who have tumors that can be removed at surgery, the surgery may be followed by radiotherapy. In some centers, all Stage II and III tumors are treated with radiotherapy before surgery.

♦ Sometimes it is necessary to surgically explore the area of the tumor to see if definitive surgery can be done. If the tumor extends to areas that would be difficult or hazardous to remove surgically, then the treatment is usually radiotherapy.

♦ The radiotherapy dosage must be quite high in all cases.

♦ If the disease recurs, chemotherapy may improve the quality of life and the length of survival.

♦ All patients are candidates for clinical trials of new therapies.

STAGE I
Standard Treatment Surgery is used for small tumors of the lower part of the maxillary sinus. If the tumor extends near the surgical margin, radiotherapy is then given.

For ethmoid sinus cancer, which is usually advanced, extensive surgery (if possible) is followed by radiotherapy. If the cancer cannot be removed, radiotherapy is used alone. Sphenoid sinus cancers are treated with radiotherapy, similar to nasopharyngeal cancers. Nasal cavity cancers are treated with either surgery or radiotherapy.

Occasionally, melanomas and some sarcomas—such as cancers of cartilage (chondrosarcomas) and bone (osteosarcomas or Ewing's sarcoma, a rare type of bone cancer)—occur in this area. Melanomas and sarcomas are surgically excised if possible.

There is also a special kind of tumor in this area called an inverting papilloma.

This is most often described as benign, but some consider it a low-grade cancer because it tends to grow aggressively and because it requires therapy similar to that for cancer. Inverting papillomas are treated with surgery, with radical additional surgery if they recur.

There is also a condition called midline granuloma. Although not classified as cancer, in some cases this is thought to represent a rare kind of lymphoma. Midline granulomas are treated with radiotherapy.

Five-Year Survival 60 to 70 percent

STAGE II
Standard Treatment
♦ *Maxillary sinus:* Surgery and high-dose radiotherapy (pre- or postoperative).

♦ *Ethmoid sinus:* Radiotherapy is generally preferred. Localized lesions can be removed surgically (radical surgery), but radiotherapy is needed afterwards.

♦ *Sphenoid sinus:* Same as nasopharyngeal tumors, using radiotherapy.

♦ *Nasal cavity:* Surgery or radiotherapy for tumors of the septum, radiotherapy elsewhere.

♦ *Inverting papilloma:* Same as Stage I. Radiotherapy may be needed if further surgery is unsuccessful.

♦ *Melanomas and sarcomas:* Surgery if possible.

♦ *Midline granuloma:* Radiotherapy.

♦ *Nasal vestibule (front part of nasal cavity):* Surgery if no deformity is expected or there is no need for reconstruction. Otherwise, radiotherapy.

Five-Year Survival 60 to 70 percent

STAGE III
Standard Treatment
♦ *Maxillary sinus:* Surgery with high-dose pre- or postoperative radiotherapy.

♦ *Ethmoid sinus:* Extensive surgery followed by radiotherapy.

♦ *Sphenoid sinus:* Radiotherapy.

♦ *Nasal cavity:* Surgery or radiotherapy alone. Usually postoperative radiotherapy is preferred.

♦ *Inverting papilloma:* Same as Stage II Radiotherapy may be needed if further surgery is unsuccessful.

♦ *Melanomas and sarcomas:* Surgery if possible, otherwise radiotherapy.

♦ *Midline granuloma:* Radiotherapy.

♦ *Nasal vestibule:* Radiation first and surgery later if needed.

Clinical trials are in progress for ethmoid sinus and nasal cavity tumors, using chemotherapy combinations in addition to surgery or radiotherapy.

Five-Year Survival 25 to 35 percent

STAGE IV

Standard Treatment Chemotherapy is given before surgery or radiotherapy in an attempt to shrink tumors and make them more treatable. This should be considered for each of the sites below except inverting papilloma and midline lethal granuloma.

♦ *Maxillary sinus:* If the tumor is extensive, surgery may not be appropriate and radiotherapy is used. Sinus drainage must be established first.

♦ *Ethmoid sinus:* Radiotherapy or extensive surgery with pre- or postoperative radiotherapy.

♦ *Sphenoid sinus:* Same as nasopharyngeal cancers.

♦ *Nasal cavity:* Surgery or radiotherapy alone or combined.

♦ *Inverting papilloma:* Surgery. Radiotherapy or radical surgery may eventually be necessary.

♦ *Melanomas and sarcomas:* Surgery if possible, but radiation and chemotherapy

should be considered.

♦ *Midline granuloma:* Radiotherapy.

♦ *Nasal vestibule:* Radiation if possible and surgery if unsuccessful.

Clinical trials for maxillary sinus, ethmoid sinus and nasal cavity tumors are evaluating chemotherapy combinations in addition to surgery or radiotherapy.

Five-Year Survival 10 to 25 percent

RECURRENT CANCER

Chemotherapy is given if there is a recurrence in the original area following surgery or radiotherapy or if there are distant metastases. Chemotherapy is promising, and may offer effective palliation, improved quality of life and improved survival for patients who respond.

♦ *Maxillary sinus:* Radiotherapy, or extensive surgery followed by radiotherapy.

♦ *Ethmoid sinus:* After limited surgery, extensive surgery, radiotherapy or both.

♦ *Sphenoid sinus:* Radiotherapy. If unsuccessful, chemotherapy.

♦ *Nasal cavity:* If it recurs after radiotherapy, extensive surgery. If it recurs after surgery, radiotherapy. If recurrent after both, then chemotherapy.

♦ *Inverting papilloma:* Same as previous stages.

♦ *Melanomas and sarcomas:* Surgery if possible and chemotherapy directed at the specific cell type.

♦ *Nasal vestibule:* If radiotherapy fails, surgery is appropriate. If surgery fails, radiotherapy or a combination of further surgery and radiotherapy. If these fail, chemotherapy may be given.

For maxillary sinus, ethmoid sinus and nasal tumors, clinical trials using chemotherapy should be considered.

SALIVARY GLANDS

There are four kinds of salivary glands. The parotid glands are in front of each ear (enlarged in mumps), the submaxillary (or submandibular) glands are just below the lower jaw bones, the sublingual glands are under the tongue, and many small, minor salivary glands line the mouth, nose and throat.

There are both benign and malignant tumors of these glands, although the term benign may be misleading. These "benign" tumors rarely if ever metastasize, but their growth can be fairly aggressive and the surgery needed to control them may resemble that needed for malignant tumors of the same gland. There have been cases in which benign salivary gland tumors have caused death by recurring and invading the tissues of the face or brain.

There are at least six kinds of malignant tumors and about the same number of benign ones. The treatment is different for each kind of tumor, so expert pathologic study is necessary.

Twenty-five percent of parotid tumors, 40 percent of submandibular tumors, 95 percent of sublingual tumors and 50 percent of minor salivary gland tumors are malignant.

The most common site of malignant tumors is in the parotid glands. The most common site of tumors of the minor salivary gland tumors is in the palate. These tumors can also occur anywhere in the mouth, the pharynx, larynx and paranasal sinusus.

Salivary gland cancers are caused mainly by the heavy use of tobacco. Increased incidence is also associated with previous radiation exposure to the head and neck. Radiotherapy was used to treat acne during the 1930s, 1940s and 1950s, with a resulting five to eight times higher risk of developing cancer of these salivary glands.

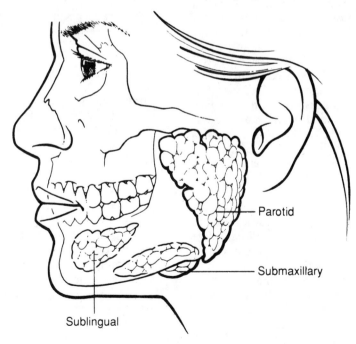

Major salivary glands

TREATMENT OVERVIEW

Early-stage, low-grade salivary gland tumors, especially tumors of the parotid gland, are usually curable by surgery. Large, bulky or high-grade tumors have a poorer prognosis and often receive postoperative radiotherapy. Tumors that cannot be completely removed surgically or that recur may be treated with radiotherapy or respond to chemotherapy.

Prognosis also depends on which gland is involved, the microscopic pattern, the grade of malignancy, the stage and whether the tumor has extended to involve the skin, lymph nodes, nerves or distant sites.

♦ Minimum therapy for low-grade malignancies of a portion of the parotid gland is a superficial parotidectomy. Great care is taken to preserve the facial nerve that goes through the middle of this gland and controls the muscles on that side of the face. This surgery is very delicate.

For other kinds of parotid tumors, a total parotidectomy is needed to obtain a safe margin around the tumor because it frequently grows microscopically far beyond where it is visible to the surgeon.

♦ Postoperative radiotherapy is being used more and more, especially for lesions that are high grade or have close margins. This seems to improve the cure rate. Fast neutron beam radiation therapy—available in a limited number of centers—has been effective in the treatment of inoperable, unresectable and recurrent tumors, and may be more effective than conventional x-ray therapy.

♦ There is no established role for chemotherapy, but it is sometimes used in special circumstances when radiation or surgery are refused, or for recurrent or unresponsive tumors.

♦ In high-grade cancer, radiation therapy is almost always added. The surgery is often more extensive and may require removal of the facial nerve.

♦ When the tumor has spread to lymph nodes in the neck, an additional operation—called a radical neck dissection—is needed to remove these nodes. One possible result is a drooped shoulder, as well as a flattening of the side of the neck. This must be considered a small price to pay to have a better chance of permanently controlling the cancer. Sometimes radiotherapy is used to treat the neck.

♦ Chemotherapy is sometimes considered when surgery or radiotherapy are refused or have already been used as much as they can be. Prospects for cure in this situation are low and prolonging life is the goal of therapy.

♦ For patients whose disease has spread beyond the neck, no curative treatment is available.

♦ There are several investigational protocols in use, including chemotherapy, radiation therapy with neutron beams, or radiation accompanied by anticancer drugs such as doxorubicin, cisplatin, carboplatin, cyclophosphamide and 5-fluorouracil.

TREATMENT BY STAGE

STAGE I
Standard Treatment
♦ For low-grade tumors, surgery alone. Radiotherapy may be an alternative if surgery would cause significant cosmetic or functional problems. Radiotherapy is also used after surgery if the margins are involved. Fast neutron beam radiotherapy may be used for tumors that have spread to lymph nodes.

♦ For high-grade tumors, surgery alone, although adjuvant radiotherapy may also be given (especially with positive surgical margins). If the tumor cannot be removed, radiotherapy may be used for palliation. If the tumor has spread to the neck lymph nodes, these nodes should be removed.

Local recurrence may be reduced by adjuvant radiotherapy. Neutron beam radiation is under clinical evaluation, and recent studies indicate that these tumors may also respond to chemotherapy.

Five-Year Survival 90 percent

STAGE II
Standard Treatment
♦ For low-grade tumors, surgery alone, with the same considerations as Stage I. Radical surgery is generally required.
♦ For high-grade tumors, same considerations as Stage I. Postoperative radiotherapy is used to reduce the local recurrence rate if the surgical margins are positive or the nerves or soft tissues of the neck are involved.

Five-Year Survival 55 percent

STAGE III
Standard Treatment
♦ For low-grade tumors, same as Stages I and II.
♦ For high-grade tumors, same considerations as Stages I and II. Chemotherapy should be considered when surgery or radiation is refused or for recurrent or unresponsive tumors.

Studies are trying to improve local control with fast neutron beam therapy, radiosensitizers and chemotherapy.

Five-Year Survival 45 percent

STAGE IV
Standard Treatment There is no curative standard therapy for this stage, in which the tumor has spread to distant sites, so consideration should be given to investigational protocols such as combination chemotherapy, conventional radiotherapy or fast neutron beam therapy.

Metastatic disease can be treated with combinations of doxorubicin, cisplatin, cyclophosphamide and 5-fluorouracil.

Five-Year Survival 10 percent

RECURRENT CANCER
The prognosis is poor regardless of the cell type or stage. Treatment depends on the specific cancer, earlier treatment, area of recurrence and the medical problems of the patient. Surgery is often the first choice, followed by radiation. Investigational treatments are appropriate and should be considered.

OROPHARYNX

The most common cancers in this area begin in the base of the tongue and the tonsils. Almost all cases of oropharyngeal cancer are related to cigarette smoking or other forms of tobacco use such as pipe smoking and tobacco chewing. Heavy alcohol consumption along with tobacco use further increases the risk. Poor oral hygiene or bad teeth can also contribute to cancer. Most oropharyngeal cancers occur in men, although as more women are smoking they now have a higher chance of developing these cancers.

TREATMENT OVERVIEW
♦ This cancer rarely spreads early in its course, but often spreads later. Should the primary site not be controlled and it recurs there, the rest of the body should be evaluated for tumor spread.
♦ The prognosis seems to decrease as the origin of the cancer is located farther back from the lips. The lips have the best prognosis, the tongue second, the area behind the wisdom teeth (retromolar trigone) third. The prognosis is poorest in the hypopharynx. Patients whose tumors grow into blood vessels have a worse prognosis.
♦ A multi-disciplinary approach provides the best chance for cure. The team usually consists of a head and neck surgeon, radiation and medical oncologists, an oral prosthodontist (a dentist experienced in

dental reconstruction). Since these tumors often extend into areas that are not easily seen (upwards into the nasopharynx and downwards into the hypopharynx), these areas have to be evaluated before treatment is started. It is often necessary to examine the patient when he or she is anesthetized, using small scopes to see and map the extent of the tumor.

♦ The risk of having a second primary cancer is as high as 15 percent, so endoscopic examinations of the nasopharynx, hypopharynx and esophagus (triple endoscopy) are done to detect other cancers.

♦ A useful maneuver with large tumors is to mark the edge with an India ink tattoo. In patients who receive radiotherapy or chemotherapy to shrink the tumor before surgery, the surgeon will be able to tell precisely where the edge of the tumor was and remove all the tissue originally involved.

♦ No single treatment program offers a clear-cut survival advantage over others. Various choices are possible and the decision will depend on a review of each case, the type and stage of the cancer, the physical and emotional condition of the patient, as well as the experience of the physicians and the facilities available.

TREATMENT BY STAGE

STAGE I
Standard Treatment The choice is determined by the anticipated functional and cosmetic results. Radiation therapy is commonly used. Surgery is equally successful. Either might be used in locations such as the tonsil, where function is expected to be normal after surgery. In areas such as the base of the tongue, radiation is preferred, since surgery would result in major functional problems. Radiation protocols using hyperfractionation (more than one treatment daily) should be considered.

Five-Year Survival 60 to 80 percent, depending on the site

STAGE II
Standard Treatment If radiation is used, the technique is individualized by a radiation oncologist experienced in treatment of tumors of this area. Radiation implants may be needed. Surgery is an alternative, and the same considerations apply as for Stage I about when surgery or radiotherapy are preferred. The same choice of hyperfractionated radiotherapy applies.

Five-Year Survival 50 percent when the tumor is in the tonsil or back of the tongue

STAGE III
Standard Treatment The preferred treatment usually combines surgery with postoperative radiotherapy. There are new surgical techniques for removal of the tumor and reconstruction. Radiation implants and hyperfractionation techniques are becoming more useful.

All patients in this stage are candidates for neoadjuvant chemotherapy trials.

Five-Year Survival 20 percent (back of the tongue) to 30 percent (tonsil)

STAGE IV
Standard Treatment As in Stage III, aggressive combined surgical and radiotherapy treatments by physicians experienced in treating this type of cancer are necessary. If the tumor can't be removed, radiotherapy is used. Chemotherapy (neoadjuvant) has been used to shrink tumors and make them easier to treat with surgery or radiation.

Clinical trials are combining chemotherapy or radiation sensitizers with radiotherapy or radiation protocols using hyperfractionation or radiation implants.

Follow-up is essential, and should be done monthly for one year, every two months for the next year, every three months the next and then every six months.

Five-Year Survival 14 percent (tonsil) to 20 percent (back of the tongue)

RECURRENT CANCER

Standard therapy is surgery (if possible) if radiotherapy was used originally. If surgery was used before, then radiotherapy is given for recurrent tumors provided it is safe to give more. If surgery was used first, additional surgery is sometimes possible.

Chemotherapy can be used in combination with surgery or radiotherapy. Chemotherapy is also used for metastatic disease or if there is a recurrence that can no longer be treated with surgery or radiation.

The same follow-up is required as for Stage IV.

SUPPORTIVE THERAPY

An essential part of the treatment is the need for rehabilitation after aggressive surgery and radiation. The patient must be motivated and total rehabilitation requires a team approach, with speech therapists, social workers, physical therapists, prosthodontists, occupational therapists and nurses all playing important roles.

Cosmetic appearance, swallowing, speech, chewing and psychological functioning have to be considered. The family is extremely important in supporting the patient during and after therapy. Some functions and appearances may be different, but the *person* is the same.

NASOPHARYNX

The nasopharynx is right behind the nose and above the oropharynx. It cannot be seen directly. It is shaped somewhat like a box. On the sides are the eustachian tubes that adjust the air pressure in our middle ears. At the top is the sphenoid sinus.

Cancers of the nasopharynx are different from other head and neck cancers in that there does not appear to be a link with alcohol and tobacco use and they occur 10 to 20 years earlier (one group in young adulthood and another between 50 and 70 years). The Epstein-Barr (EB) virus has been implicated in most patients. Blood tests available for anti-EB virus antibodies aid in diagnosis as well as screening of high-risk groups.

The most common first sign is a mass in the neck (a lymph node metastasis). At least 80 percent of patients will have some evidence of spread to these lymph nodes, some only microscopically. Other symptoms are hearing loss or signs of middle ear infection, nasal obstruction or nosebleeds, ringing in the ears, inability to equalize the air pressure between the ears, and cranial nerve problems.

Evaluation of patients includes a very careful physical examination, as well as endoscopic examinations of the nose and throat. This is the most likely primary site for the "unknown primary" cancer diagnosed in enlarged lymph nodes in the neck. Most of these cancers are the squamous cell type. The diagnosis is best made by biopsy of the primary site in the nasopharynx and *not* the enlarged neck lymph nodes. If the primary tumor is not seen and random biopsies of the nasopharynx are negative, then a needle biopsy of the enlarged lymph nodes in the neck is done.

Once the diagnosis has been made by biopsy, CT and MRI scans are essential in determining stage, for the tumor cannot be seen directly. A chest x-ray is usually done because there may be lung metastases. Liver scans and bone scans may also be needed to search for metastases. Staging is difficult to determine exactly. Most patients are probably in Stage IV at the time of diagnosis.

Various factors appear to affect prognosis, including bone involvement, the presence of pain, the length of time symptoms have been present and the location of lymph nodes involved by tumor. Patients who have evidence of Epstein-Barr virus infection (as shown by a blood test) have a poorer prognosis after treatment.

TREATMENT OVERVIEW

Small cancers of the nasopharynx are curable by radiotherapy in 80 to 90 percent of cases. Moderately advanced tumors that have not spread to the lymph nodes in the neck can be cured in 50 to 70 percent of cases. Advanced tumors, especially with extension to other structures such as bone or cranial nerves, are difficult to control.

♦ In patients with extension of tumor into the skull bones or involving cranial nerves, the use of surgery is rarely of help and is seldom attempted.

♦ Radiotherapy is used for treatment of neck metastases. Surgery is usually used only for lymph nodes that do not disappear after radiotherapy or that reappear. Radiation implants may be used in certain selected situations.

♦ Once treatment is completed, extensive follow-up is essential. This includes physical examination, x-rays and scans, blood tests, tests of thyroid and pituitary function, attention to dental and oral hygiene, jaw exercises and evaluation of vision and hearing.

STAGES I and II
Standard Treatment High-dose radiotherapy to the primary area and both sides of the neck.

Five-Year Survival 65 to 95 percent (Stage I), 50 to 65 percent (Stage II)

STAGE III
Standard Treatment Same as for Stages I and II, but surgical neck dissection may be needed if enlarged lymph nodes in the neck either do not completely disappear after radiotherapy or recur.

Neoadjuvant chemotherapy given before radiotherapy has been shown to significantly improve the response to treatment and survival in advanced nasopharyngeal cancer.

Five-Year Survival 30 to 60 percent

STAGE IV
Standard Treatment High-dose radiotherapy to the primary area and the neck. Neoadjuvant chemotherapy (before radiation) is used as in Stage III. Surgical neck dissection is done for persistent or recurrent enlarged lymph nodes.

Five-Year Survival 5 to 40 percent

RECURRENT CANCER

Selected patients may be given additional radiotherapy, both external beam and implants. Some may be candidates for surgical removal of recurrent tumors.

Metastatic disease and local recurrences not treatable by surgery or radiation may be treated with chemotherapy. Clinical trials are evaluating chemotherapy as well as interferon.

HYPOPHARYNX

The hypopharynx is below the oropharynx. It is the place the food first passes through when we swallow. There are three areas in the hypopharynx:
♦ postcricoid area (junction of pharynx and esophagus);
♦ pyriform sinus; and
♦ posterior (back) pharyngeal wall.

This area is best examined with mirrors, fingers or scopes that can be passed into the mouth. Almost all of the cancers in this area are squamous (or epidermoid) cancers arising in the mucous membranes. A few cancers are of minor salivary gland origin.

These cancers first spread by direct invasion, growing down from the surface membranes into the next layer (the submucosa), then into the muscles and finally into the tissues that surround the pharynx. Further spread is to the lymph nodes in the neck (even at this stage the cancer may still be curable), then to the lungs and elsewhere in the body (where the chance of cure is very remote).

Sometimes these cancers begin with a white plaque or coating on the membrane (leukoplakia), a premalignant condition similar to that found in the mouth, but many cancers begin without any preliminary change. Not all white patches are leukoplakia, and biopsy is necessary to rule out other causes, such as fungal infections or a disease called lichen planus.

Other cancers may occur elsewhere in the head and neck at the same time or later, so the larynx, pharynx, nasopharynx and the entire oral cavity should be searched. The esophagus should also be evaluated. CT and MRI scans are useful in establishing the extent of the disease. Since treatment will vary depending on the stage and extent of disease, it is very important to establish the stage precisely before therapy is begun.

Symptoms generally occur late and spread tends to occur early, so the survival rates for cancers in this area are lower than for other sites in the head and neck.

No single therapeutic approach offers an advantage over the others, so treatment decisions depend on a careful review of each case with attention to the stage, the physical condition, age and emotional status of the patient, the experience of the physicians and the treatment facilities available.

TREATMENT BY STAGE

STAGE I
Standard Treatment Except for rare very small T1 cancers, treatment is primarily surgery, usually followed by radiotherapy. Since early symptoms are rare, fewer than 2 percent of patients are diagnosed when their tumors are small, protrude from the surface and are treatable with radiotherapy alone.

Standard treatment is laryngopharyngectomy and neck dissection. In selected cases, only part of the larynx has to be removed and the voice can be preserved. In larger (T2) tumors, post-operative radiotherapy is used.

There are several approaches to the use of radiation therapy. Some treatment centers give it preoperatively. Others also treat an extended area of potential spread of tumor, including both sides of the neck.

Five-Year Survival 50 to 80 percent

STAGE II
Standard Treatment Therapy is similar to that for Stage I. Treatments being studied include neoadjuvant chemotherapy to shrink tumors and improve the ability to treat them with surgery or radiotherapy. Such neoadjuvant chemotherapy protocols are in common use because of the low survival rate.

Five-Year Survival 50 to 60 percent

STAGE III

Standard Treatment Treatment is complex. Extensive surgery is done, which requires reconstructive procedures using portions of the stomach or small bowel. Radiotherapy is given postoperatively. Surgical and radiotherapy methods and programs, as well as the time schedules involved, vary among treatment centers but give similar results. Patients should be managed by surgeons and radiation oncologists experienced in these complex procedures and treatments.

Patients should be considered for clinical trials evaluating adjuvant or neoadjuvant chemotherapy.

Five-Year Survival 30 to 50 percent

STAGE IV

Standard Treatment If the tumor can be removed, similar considerations and methods to those for Stage III are used. If it can't, radiotherapy is used.

Chemotherapy and radiation sensitizers with the radiotherapy are under clinical evaluation. There are also radiotherapy protocols evaluating hyperfractionation schedules (more than one treatment daily).

Careful and frequent post-treatment follow-up is essential.

Five-Year Survival 15 to 25 percent

RECURRENT CANCER

If radiotherapy was originally used, the standard treatment is surgery if it is possible. If surgery was used originally, then radiotherapy is given unless previous radiotherapy dosage precludes additional treatment. Additional surgery may be possible. Chemotherapy protocols are under clinical evaluation.

LARYNX

The larynx, or voice box, is divided into three regions. From the top down, these are:

♦ The supraglottic larynx. This includes the epiglottis (a flap that keeps food from going into the lungs), the false vocal cords, ventricles, aryepiglottic folds and arytenoids. Tumors of this area cause sore throat, painful swallowing and sometimes a change in voice quality.

♦ The glottis. This includes the true vocal cords and the anterior (front) and posterior (back) commissures. Tumors here may involve one or both vocal cords or may extend out on either side of them. Tumors are usually detected early because they cause hoarseness. Because of these early symptoms and the lack of lymphatic channels where cancer can spread, the cure rate is very good.

♦ The subglottis. This area is below the true vocal cords and extends downwards to about the first tracheal ring (cartilage ring around the trachea). Tumors here are rare.

Almost all cancers of the larynx arise from the lining membrane (mucosa) and are called squamous cell cancers. Salivary gland cancers and other types can also occur in this area.

Cancers spread by growing directly into surrounding tissues and then to lymph nodes in the neck, usually on the same side as where the tumor started. They may still be curable at this stage, but not when they have spread elsewhere.

Common symptoms can include persistent sore throat or hoarseness, difficulty in swallowing, the feeling of something in the throat, a change in voice quality and the appearance of a lump in the neck.

A complete diagnostic examination includes examination with tongue blade, mirrors and scopes, physical examination to rule out other areas of spread and determine the tolerance and precautions for therapy, x-ray barium esophogram to show if there is any distortion of the esophagus, CT or MRI scan to outline the tumor and show its extent, chest x-ray to rule out spread to the lungs and biopsy of the lesion to establish the diagnosis.

It is also usually necessary for the larynx to be examined under anesthesia with the aid of a laryngoscope. The area of cancer can be carefully examined and additional biopsies taken along the edges to establish the extent of tumor involvement.

TREATMENT OVERVIEW

Small cancers of the larynx have a good prognosis. If there is no spread to lymph nodes, the cure rate is 75 to 95 percent. Although most early lesions can be cured by radiotherapy or surgery, radiotherapy is often chosen first in an attempt to preserve a better voice. Surgery is used later if the tumor recurs. Laser excision surgery is also used, especially if the tumor is limited to one vocal cord. However, a substantial number of such patients may require additional treatment.

♦ Locally advanced lesions, especially with large involved lymph nodes, are poorly controlled by either method of treatment or by both methods used together.

♦ Intermediate-sized cancers require individual decision making about the most appropriate treatment. Factors such as the site, stage, degree of lymph node involvement and general status of the patient will influence the type of therapy chosen.

♦ Second primaries have been reported in up to a quarter of these patients.

♦ Most recurrences occur in the first two to three years, and close follow-up is essential so that cure may still be possible. Examinations as well as previously abnormal staging studies are repeated to document the progress of treatment or detect recurrence.

♦ Because of other illnesses related to smoking and alcohol use, many patients die from illnesses other than the cancer.

♦ Small localized superficial cancers can be successfully treated with radiotherapy alone, surgery alone or laser excision. Radiation tends to be used first to try to preserve the voice. There are also some surgical procedures for small cancers that preserve the voice.

♦ Recent studies of patients with advanced laryngeal cancer suggest a role for chemotherapy before radiotherapy in an attempt to preserve the larynx.

♦ Advanced cancers are often treated by a combination of surgery and radiotherapy. Because the cure rate is low, consideration should be given to clinical trials evaluating chemotherapy, hyperfractionated (several doses a day) radiotherapy, radiation sensitizers or particle beam radiotherapy.

♦ Most subglottic cancers are treated with combined surgery and radiotherapy.

TREATMENT BY STAGE

STAGE I
Standard Treatment

♦ *Supraglottis:* External beam radiotherapy alone or supraglottic laryngectomy. There are frequent problems with the functioning of the larynx after the latter procedure.

♦ *Glottis:* Radiotherapy, which provides both cure and good voice quality in most patients. Selected patients with small (T1) superficial lesions can have a portion of the vocal cord removed. Partial or sometimes total laryngectomy may be done depending on the tumor's location and size. Laser excision is under clinical evaluation.

♦ *Subglottis:* Radiotherapy alone, with surgery used for recurrence.

Five-Year Survival 75 to 95 percent

STAGE II
Standard Treatment

♦ *Supraglottis:* External beam radiation therapy is used for smaller tumors, which preserves the voice. Another option is a supraglottic laryngectomy or total laryngectomy, depending on the location of the lesion and the status of the patient. Care is needed when selecting this option to ensure adequate lung and swallowing function after surgery.

If a patient is not cured by radiation given as the primary treatment, surgery is then used in an attempt to cure. If surgery is the primary treatment, postoperative radiotherapy is used if tumor is found in surgical margins or lymph nodes in the neck.

♦ *Glottis:* Radiotherapy or surgery (partial or total laryngectomy).

♦ *Subglottis:* Radiotherapy (with voice preservation), with surgery reserved for patients whose tumors recur or those who might not have adequate follow-up evaluation.

Five-Year Survival 55 to 65 percent (supraglottis), 60 to 80 percent (glottis), 30 to 40 percent (subglottis)

STAGE III
Standard Treatment

♦ *Supraglottis:* Standard therapy is surgery with postoperative radiotherapy, but many centers are now treating some patients with external beam radiotherapy initially, depending on the tumor location and patient status. The voice is preserved in about half of these patients. If this treatment is unsuccessful, surgery is necessary.

Investigational protocols are using chemotherapy, hyperfractionated radiotherapy, radiation sensitizers, and particle beam radiotherapy.

♦ *Glottis:* Surgery with postoperative radiotherapy, if necessary for the primary site and/or positive lymph nodes. Patients who refuse or cannot tolerate surgery are given radiation therapy.

Again, many centers are treating selected patients with radiotherapy as primary treatment. Careful follow-up is vital, since surgery is needed if the tumor recurs.

♦ *Subglottis:* Laryngectomy, including also thyroidectomy and tracheoesophageal

lymph node dissection, all followed by radiotherapy. Some patients are not candidates for surgery and are treated with radiotherapy alone, but surgical treatment may still be needed if there is a recurrence. The Stage III investigational protocols described under supraglottic tumors should be considered.

Three-Year Survival 45 to 75 percent (supraglottis), 55 to 70 percent (glottis), no data for subglottis

STAGE IV
Standard Treatment

♦ *Supraglottis:* Total laryngectomy with pre- or postoperative radiotherapy. Patients who refuse surgery or who are inoperable are treated with radiotherapy. Investigational protocols as described earlier should be considered.

♦ *Glottis:* Same as for Stage III glottic cancer, except that radiation therapy is not an elective option initially, being used only in patients who refuse or cannot tolerate surgery. Investigational protocols as described earlier should be considered.

♦ *Subglottis:* Same as Stage III subglottic tumors.

Three-Year Survival 15 to 35 percent (supraglottis), 10 to 25 percent (glottis), few data for subglottis

RECURRENT CANCER

Treatment includes further surgery or investigational protocols. If patients were treated initially with surgery alone or radiotherapy alone, further surgery and/or radiotherapy may be used. Some patients may respond to chemotherapy. Patients whose tumors recur after both radiotherapy and surgery are candidates for investigational palliative chemotherapy.

SUPPORTIVE THERAPY

Patients who have had their voice box (larynx) removed need supportive treatment to help them to learn to speak again. There are three methods.

♦ One involves the use of an esophageal voice, where a patient is taught to swallow air and bring it back up and speak.

♦ An electronic larynx—a buzzer-like battery-operated unit—may be pressed against the neck while the mouth and tongue form the words.

♦ A third method uses a unit that looks like a pipe. The sound is put into the mouth and the words are fashioned with the tongue and lips.

♦ There is also a method that requires a surgical procedure (tracheoesophageal puncture) to create a connection between the airway and the esophagus to insert a voice prosthesis ("button") and breathing valve.

METASTATIC SQUAMOUS NECK CANCER WITH A HIDDEN PRIMARY SOURCE

Enlarged neck lymph nodes containing squamous cell cancer may be the first sign of cancer elsewhere in the body. Since this type of cancer always begins elsewhere and never begins in these nodes, a search is made for the primary site. If a cancer has previously been diagnosed elsewhere, it naturally is the likely source, especially if the pattern under the microscope is similar.

Sometimes the biopsy of the lymph nodes will show adenocarcinoma or lymphoma. In these cases the primary site is less likely to be in the head and neck. For enlarged nodes containing squamous carcinoma in the lower half of the neck, the primary site may be the head and neck but may also be in the esophagus, lung or genitourinary tract.

Most epidermoid carcinomas found in lymph nodes in the upper half of the neck are a result of spread from primary head and neck cancers.

Evaluation A very careful history and physical examination is necessary to try to find the primary tumor. This frequently turns up cancer in the nasopharynx, oropharynx or larynx. If a cancer originating in the head and neck is found, other organs such as the lungs, liver and bones should be evaluated. If the cancer has already spread to one of these sites, then the treatment plan is directed towards metastatic disease and not to cure of the

primary lesion (which would involve very aggressive local therapy).

Repeated examinations will sometimes find the primary tumor still at a treatable stage. A vital part of the solution to the puzzle is provided by pathologic examination of the biopsy specimen. Immunohistochemical and electron microscopic studies may be helpful. Special stains can be applied to the tissue slides to help in diagnosis. The problem is more significant in poorly differentiated tumors, since well-differentiated tumors tend to resemble the tissue of origin and the pathologist can often suggest the likely diagnosis. With poorly differentiated tumors the diagnosis is more uncertain.

Diagnosis and Staging If possible, biopsy is delayed until studies have tried to find the primary site. These studies include examination of head and neck areas directly and with mirrors and scopes. Suspicious areas are biopsied. If there are no suspicious areas, random biopsies are done of the nasopharynx, base of the tongue and the pyriform sinus on the same side as the neck lesion. If the tonsil is not present, a biopsy is done where the tonsil used to be. If the tonsil is present, it should be biopsied or removed. Sinus x-rays are often done and any abnormality is also biopsied. Other studies include MRI and CT scans.

Staging systems have been described, but of course the "T" classification has no relevance, since the primary tumor has not been found. Three-year local control and survival rates for squamous cancers involving the lymph nodes of the neck, with unknown primary tumor, following surgery and/or radiotherapy, are:

N1 (single node smaller than 1 1/2 in./3 cm, one side) ....**40 to 50 percent**
N2 (nodes 1 1/4–2 1/2 in./3–6 cm, one side) ....**38 percent**
N3 (larger nodes, either or both sides) ....**26 percent**

Treatment If a head or neck primary is found with these studies, treatment is given as outlined. If the primary is not found, the treatment is a surgical neck dissection followed by radiation therapy.

♦ If the lymph nodes in the neck are enlarged or are on both sides, radiation therapy is given first. If any lymph nodes persist after radiotherapy, then surgical lymph node dissection is done.

♦ Alternatively, many centers use radiotherapy as the first treatment for unknown primary cancer of the head and neck. External radiation may be about equally effective as neck dissection for control of neck metastases, although surgical neck dissection may be required for those tumors that persist or recur after radiotherapy.

♦ Radiation fields to treat the likely primary sources are extensive and include the nasopharynx, the base of the tongue and the pyriform sinuses.

♦ Chemotherapy may also be appropriate for the most treatable likely primary site. Follow-up is extremely important.

♦ Options under clinical evaluation include neoadjuvant chemotherapy (cisplatin + 5-fluorouracil) followed by radiation therapy. Other investigational protocols are available.

RECURRENT CANCER

If the disease progresses, recurs or relapses, the prognosis is poor. Further treatment depends on the type of cancer, earlier treatment, site of recurrence and personal factors. Patients are candidates for investigational protocols.

THE MOST IMPORTANT QUESTIONS YOU CAN ASK

♦ What is the primary site or source of my cancer?

♦ What is the stage and what organs are involved?

♦ What tests are necessary to find this out? Are they uncomfortable?

♦ Is there a choice between surgery and radiation? Should you use both? In which order?

♦ Is there a role for chemotherapy? When?

♦ What kind of functional disability might I have? Will I have trouble eating, swallowing or speaking?

♦ How will I look after the treatments? Will I have a cosmetic disability?

♦ How much experience has the surgeon and radiation oncologist had with this type of tumor, and with what results?

♦ What complications can I expect from treatment?

♦ How long does it take to recover from the treatment?

♦ How often will you examine me afterwards?

♦ When will I know I am safe?

ISLET CELL AND
OTHER PANCREATIC CARCINOMAS

Ernest H. Rosenbaum, MD, Malin Dollinger, MD, and Sean J. Mulvihill, MD

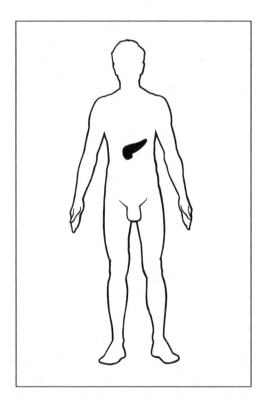

The pancreas is both an exocrine gland that produces enzymes to help digestion and an endocrine gland that produces insulin to regulate the body's metabolism of glucose. Cancer of the islet cells, or pancreatic endocrine gland, is a very uncommon tumor, making up about 5 percent of all pancreatic cancers (about 200 to 1,000 cases each year). Unlike the much more common exocrine pancreatic cancers, islet cell tumors are sometimes curable (*see* page 406).

These glandular tumors may be either functioning or non-functioning. *Func-*

tioning tumors secrete one or more hormones normally produced by the bowel endocrine cells and pancreatic islet cells. These hormones include insulin, gastrin, glucagon, vasoactive intestinal polypeptide (VIP), somatostatin, pancreatic polypeptide (PP), ACTH and others.

Most functioning tumors producing insulin are benign and are classified as adenomas. Most islet cell cancers are non-functioning, and 90 percent of these non-functioning tumors are malignant.

Types The pancreatic islet cells have many different cell types, including alpha, beta and delta cells, each of which normally produces a specific hormone or polypeptide. Overproduction of the hormone or polypeptide by the tumor produces symptoms. Islet cell tumors are named for the main type of hormone or polypeptide they produce—those that produce gastrin are called gastrinomas, those that produce insulin are insulinomas and so on.

How It Spreads Spread may be by invasion of nearby tissues or metastases via the lymph system or bloodstream.

What Causes It Unknown.

RISK FACTORS

No special group is susceptible, but it is often found in those afflicted by the familial complex of tumors known as MEN (multiple endocrine neoplasia) type-I, a genetically transmitted group of endocrine abnormalities. These people develop several kinds of islet cell tumors—54 percent have multiple gastrinomas, 21 percent develop insulinomas, 3 percent glucagonomas and 1 percent VIPomas. They also have a tendency to develop pituitary, parathyroid and adrenal gland tumors.

SCREENING

When there is a family history of MEN-I, serum studies for calcium gastrin, glucagon, insulin and VIP may be useful.

COMMON SIGNS AND SYMPTOMS

There is frequently a long delay between the initial symptoms and the diagnosis. The 90 percent of the non-functioning tumors that are malignant produce symptoms both by growing to a size where they put pressure on other tissues and by spreading to other organs.

The functioning, mainly benign islet cell tumors secrete active agents that have characteristic metabolic effects that create more symptoms than the tumor itself. When a functioning tumor becomes extremely large or metastatic, it will cause the same types of signs and symptoms as any other malignant tumor, as well as the hormonal symptoms.

♦ Gastrinomas (Zollinger-Ellison syndrome) produce an excess amount of gastrin leading to increased production of stomach acid, severe peptic ulcer disease (multiple ulcers in unusual locations such as the jejunum) and often severe diarrhea. This syndrome accounts for less than 1 percent of all people with peptic ulcers. Other symptoms include abdominal pain and extreme weight loss.

♦ Insulinomas secrete excess insulin, leading to low blood sugar (hypoglycemia). Often, the symptoms of weight loss, fatigue, weakness and hunger are attributed to psychological or neurologic disorders. Symptoms may be worse during fasting.

♦ The overproduction of glucagon by glucagonomas causes a characteristic skin rash (necrolytic migratory erythema) and a painful tongue (glossitis). Blood clots in the legs, which may travel to the lungs, have also been reported.

♦ An islet cell tumor producing VIP (vasoactive intestinal polypeptides) results in a syndrome with massive, watery diarrhea, high serum calcium and low serum potassium, chloride and blood sugar (hypoglycemia). VIPomas are characterized by secretory diarrhea (pancreatic cholera), which persists even when fasting (this tumor is also referred to as WDHA—watery diarrhea, hypokalemia achlorhydria). With severe diarrhea, up to 1 1/2 gallons (6 L) of small bowel fluid can be lost each day. Persistent diarrhea during fasting is very suspicious for VIPomas.

♦ Tumors that overproduce somatostatin cause electrolyte (mineral) abnormalities, diabetes mellitus, weight loss, malabsorption of food in the intestine (steatorrhea), loss of gastric acid (gastric achlorhydria) and occasionally gallstones.

DIAGNOSIS

Blood and Other Tests

♦ Diagnosis can be confirmed with specific hormonal assays measuring the levels of gastrin, glucagon, insulin, VIP, somatostatin or other hormones.

♦ An elevated serum gastrin level (often 10 times normal) and an elevated stomach basal acid output for those who have not had surgery should raise suspicions of the Zollinger-Ellison syndrome and its associated gastrinoma.

♦ Measurement of plasma proinsulin may be helpful for diagnosing an insulinoma.

♦ Low serum potassium levels caused by secretory diarrhea may indicate a VIPoma.

♦ Elevated levels of serum somatostatin and diabetes with severe malabsorption should suggest a somatostatin producing tumor.

Imaging

♦ Chest x-ray.

♦ Abdominal CT and MRI scans.
♦ Ultrasonography. This may be performed with a probe on the skin (transcutaneous), within the lumen of the stomach (endoscopic) or directly on the pancreas during surgery (intraoperative).
♦ Pancreatic arteriography can diagnose about 50 percent of cases, for some tumors—insulinoma, for example—are rich in blood vessels and have a tumor "blush." This method is rarely used since the advent of ultrasound and CT.

Endoscopy and Biopsy
♦ Fine needle aspiration (FNA).

STAGING

There is no acceptable staging system for islet cell cancers. They can best be categorized as localized (in one site), regional (in several sites within the pancreas) and metastatic to regional lymph nodes or to distant sites.

TREATMENT OVERVIEW

Surgery and chemotherapy are the two treatment methods used, but only surgery can cure the disease. Careful observation may be an alternative approach for some islet cell tumors. Radiotherapy is not effective.

 Surgery Surgical removal of the tumor may lead to a cure. Depending on the location of the tumor, part of the pancreas may be removed (partial pancreatectomy) or the tumor cells may be excised locally — or "shelled out"—of the head of the pancreas (enucleation). When the tumor can't be completely removed, reducing its size (debulking) may still be a helpful palliative measure, given that these tumors are slow growing.

 Chemotherapy Several biological and chemotherapy agents appear to be active against islet cell tumors. These include interferon-alpha, a synthetic somatostatin analogue called octreotide (Sandostatin), Adriamycin, Cytoxan, DTIC (dacarbazine), 5-fluorouracil (5-FU), streptozocin and etoposide (VP-16) for advanced islet cell cancer. A novel and promising treatment called chemoembolization delivers chemotherapy directly to the tumor via a catheter positioned in a suitable blood vessel. Currently this is useful for patients with tumor limited to the liver.

TREATMENT BY TYPE
GASTRINOMA
Sixty to 75 percent of gastrinomas are malignant and metastatic at the time of diagnosis. Gastrinomas usually occur in the head of the pancreas but up to one-third are found in the duodenum.

Standard Treatment The tumor should be removed if it can be precisely located by preoperative imaging studies or during surgery. Usually, small lesions can be shelled out from the pancreas without the need for removing the whole organ. Removal of a localized tumor results in a high chance of cure.

Sometimes, the tumor cannot be found. In this case, the best approach is to block the acid production from the stomach with medicines such as histamine H-2 receptor blockers or Omeprazole. This prevents the two main problems with the tumor: ulcers and diarrhea.

Cutting the acid secretion nerves to the stomach (vagotomy) and removing part of the stomach (partial gastrectomy) are not effective. If medical therapy fails to control acid secretion and ulcerations recur or diarrhea persists, a total gastrectomy is the treatment of choice.

In severe cases, primary management may include continuous stomach suction and intravenous replacement of sodium, potassium and chloride to maintain electrolyte balance. Surgery can then remove a functioning tumor when the patient is stable. Postoperative gastrin levels are used for monitoring.

Treatment for Metastatic Gastrinoma

Occasionally active drugs include doxorubicin, streptozocin, 5-FU, etoposide and Cytoxan. Chemotherapy is often reserved for patients who cannot tolerate surgery and cimetidine (Tagamet).

♦ Interferon-alpha has recently shown some effectiveness in controlling tumors and reducing symptoms.

♦ Combining chemotherapy drugs and blocking the blood supply to the liver (hepatic artery chemoembolization) may successfully treat liver metastases.

 Palliation Octreotide (Sandostatin) is a synthetic, long-acting somatostatin analogue that significantly decreases hormone secretion by tumor cells. It is extremely useful for suppressing gastrin levels and inhibiting the hypersecretion of gastric acid on a sustained basis for managing the Zollinger-Ellison syndrome. This may be helpful if Omeprazole treatment fails.

Five-Year Survival 65 percent

INSULINOMA

Insulinomas usually occur between ages 40 and 60. Ninety percent are benign and curable.

Standard Treatment Removal of the pancreatic tumor is the basic approach, depending on the size and the site (in the head of the pancreas versus the body or tail). Most of these tumors can be enucleated and formal pancreatic resection is not required. Occasionally, patients benefit from surgical removal of metastases to help reduce symptoms of increased insulin and low blood sugar.

For pancreatic tumors that can't be removed or for widespread metastatic tumors, combination chemotherapy (5-FU + streptozocin) or diazoxide or somatostatin/octreotide (Sandostatin) can be given.

 Palliation Dietary changes, including frequent small meals and increased carbohydrates, may help reduce low blood sugar (hypoglycemia). Insulin-inhibiting drugs such as diazoxide may also help. Radiation therapy is not effective. Octreotide may be used to block insulin release from the tumor.

Five-Year Survival 80 percent

GLUCAGONOMAS

These tumors are often very large by the time they are discovered.

Standard Treatment The tumor should be removed, if possible. If not, palliation of symptoms usually is possible with octreotide.

Chemotherapy with 5-FU and streptozocin may be helpful. Occasionally, partial surgical removal of the tumor will relieve symptoms.

VIPomas

Over 40 percent of these tumors are malignant. VIPomas may occur outside the pancreas, usually associated with nerves.

Standard Treatment Single lesions can be removed or a partial pancreatectomy can be done for multiple lesions in the 50 percent of patients who do not have liver metastases. Debulking tumors that can't be removed may reduce diarrhea. Prednisone may also help relieve diarrhea.

Combination chemotherapy with 5-FU + streptozocin may be given if the tumors cannot be removed.

 Palliation Octreotide (Sandostatin) is effective in reducing VIPoma symptoms, but it is not curative and often works for only a limited time. Fluids and electrolytes have to be replenished.

SOMATOSTATIN-PRODUCING TUMORS

This is a rare tumor, with fewer than 100 cases reported in the world medical literature. They are almost always malignant.

Standard Treatment Surgical removal of the tumor is the standard treatment for local disease. Combined chemotherapy with 5-FU and streptozocin is used in patients with metastases. A few patients with liver metastases benefit from liver resection or chemoembolization.

 Palliation Drugs used to relieve symptoms include the insulin-inhibiting drug diazoxide and phenoxybenzamine (Dibenzyline), an alpha-adrenergic blocking agent.

RECURRENT CANCER

Before deciding on further therapy for recurrences, the clinical situation will have to be re-evaluated. Surgery or medical therapy as indicated for metastatic disease could be considered depending on the stage, the site of recurrence, the presence of metastases and individual factors. Participation in clinical trials should also be considered.

THE MOST IMPORTANT QUESTIONS YOU CAN ASK

♦ Will the removal of my tumor reduce or eliminate my symptoms?
♦ Can medical treatment control my cancer and reduce my symptoms?
♦ Are there any cancer centers where I could go for a second opinion?

KAPOSI'S SARCOMA

Ivan J. Silverberg, MD

◇

Kaposi's sarcoma (KS) consists of characteristic skin lesions: flat to raised purple plaques. They are tumors that have a rich network of small blood vessels. Red blood cells moving slowly through these channels lose their oxygen, changing in color from red to blue. The mixture of red and blue cells gives the KS lesion its characteristic purple color.

There are several types of KS based on cause rather than appearance. The "classic" Kaposi's sarcoma is found predominantly in Mediterranean males and often also in males of Ashkenazic origin (mid-European Jews). This type of KS, described years ago, is rare.

In the 1950s a large number of KS cases were found in Africa, with the total number of cases increasing dramatically since then.

KS was later found to be a common result of altered body immunity. There are two circumstances under which this takes place. The first is in cases when direct depression of the immune system—the body's constant guard against outside threats—is part of a specific treatment, for example in kidney or other organ transplants. Powerful drugs are given to shut down the immune system so that the foreign organ will not be rejected. KS may arise after such drugs are used and will sometimes disappear when the drugs are stopped. The second circumstance is associated with AIDS (Acquired Immune Deficiency Syndrome).

Types KS lesions are divided into three groups by appearance, with much overlapping.

♦ Nodular lesions are of varying size and thickness. They are purple and will at times have a halo of brown or yellow pigment around them.

♦ Infiltrating lesions may be quite large, may be raised and grow downward beneath the skin.

♦ Lymphatic lesions may mimic other causes of swollen lymph nodes and may require a biopsy to rule out infection.

To a pathologist looking at a biopsy under the microscope, all three types of KS appear similar. Three sub-types have been identified, all of which are treated much the same. Clinically, the spindle cell variety is the slowest growing, the anaplastic is the most aggressive, and the mixed cell has a somewhat intermediate growth rate.

How It Spreads Most malignancies arise in one area, perhaps in one or a small group of cells. As the tumors grow, there comes a time when they spread either by direct invasion or through the blood or lymphatic systems. But KS often appears simultaneously in many sites. This suggests that there is a causal agent, possibly in the blood, that triggers the formation of the lesions in several areas. In this, KS bears a strong resemblance to some viral "rash" diseases, like measles and chicken pox. As the lesions grow, they fuse together, thicken and may protrude from the skin or ulcerate.

What Causes It The cause of classic, old-fashioned KS is unclear. KS as it originally occurred in Africa likewise has no clearly defined cause. Epidemic KS, occurring as a disease that defines AIDS, is thought to have a cause—the virus named HIV (human immunodeficiency virus). If given a blood test for HIV, nearly all patients with epidemic KS will show evidence of being infected.

Various ideas have been put forward to explain how the virus causes this illness. One theory is that the virus, either directly or by initiating a chain of events, causes a normal cell to become malignant. Various agents that may be involved in such a change have been identified. Yet another idea has to do with the body's T cells. Some of these cells hunt for malignant cells that develop spontaneously and kill them off before they can become established as cancers. Under this theory, the T cell is infected with the HIV virus and cannot kill the malignant cells.

With AIDS-related KS, there is also the continuing issue of whether HIV alone is responsible for the disease. Other factors have been suggested as co-producers of the illness, including drugs and other viruses. The agent most often mentioned is CMV (cytomegalovirus), but this is by no means the only one. It may also be that CMV and other agents produce substances that stimulate the growth of KS through interleukin-6 or other factors.

KS in people who have taken drugs to depress the body's immune response is thought to occur in a fashion similar to that in patients with epidemic KS.

Who Gets It Each form of this illness occurs in fairly specific groups. Classic KS is a disease of the elderly, with the average age of onset being over 70. The disease is more frequent in people of Mediterranean background and is more common in Jews, with Ashkenazic rather than the Sephardic Jews being affected. Men get classic KS 14 times more frequently than women.

The form that follows immune-suppressing drugs accounts for about 3 percent of all tumors that occur in people who have had kidney transplants, which is a very high rate of occurrence. Men get this form of the disease twice as frequently as women. The age of occurrence depends on the age when the medical treatment started.

Non-AIDS-related African KS accounts for nearly 10 percent of all cancers in central Africa. This is an illness that attacks young adults and affects about 10 males to every female. This ratio drops to three to one in children.

Epidemic AIDS-related KS occurs in all age groups. Babies of infected mothers may develop AIDS and KS, as can people who have contracted HIV from a blood transfusion received before 1985. (With current blood screening methods, the risk of contracting HIV from a contaminated unit of blood is estimated to be once for every 153,000 units of blood. There is no risk of contracting HIV by donating blood.)

Among the unexplained observations in epidemic KS is that different rates of occurrence are found in each of the groups of people with AIDS. The tumor is nearly 10 times more frequent in gay men with AIDS than in people who have AIDS because of blood transfusions, IV drug use or hemophilia. The occurrence of AIDS-related KS is decreasing in all these groups at about an equal rate, again for unknown reasons. Recent data indicate that there may be groups of people who do not acquire the disease despite repeated exposure to the virus.

AIDS-related KS occurs through transmission of the virus from the body fluids of an infected person. There is no evidence of spread through casual contact. The rate of contagion with infected blood is high; lesser rates of spread are thought to occur with other body fluids including semen, urine, vaginal fluids and (very rarely) saliva.

RISK FACTORS

Being of mid-European Jewish origin confers a risk for contracting classic KS, but this is a relativeley rare disease. There are no known risk factors for the African variant except possibly geographic origin. The type that occurs after immunosuppressive drug treatment has only the drug as a source of risk.

At Significantly Higher Risk

♦ People who share or use HIV-contaminated needles. According to multiple studies presented at the 1993 International AIDS meeting, spread can be eliminated in drug users by never sharing needles.

♦ People—both straight and gay—who have unprotected sexual contact with a person who is infected with HIV. The risk increases with the number of unprotected sexual encounters.

♦ Convincing data shows that safe sexual practices can dramatically decrease the incidence of AIDS and, therefore, of KS.

SCREENING

There are no screening tests for KS. But because of the relationship of HIV to AIDS and KS, many health care workers now recommend routine blood testing for HIV in high-risk groups. Screening for HIV is now routinely done on all blood products in the United States.

COMMON SIGNS AND SYMPTOMS

There are no general symptoms of early Kaposi's sarcoma. In the epidemic form, KS may be the first sign of AIDS. The first lesion often follows an illness of months or years. During this time the patient may have had non-specific symptoms such as fever, weight loss and sweating. Or there may have been other illnesses such as lymphoma or tuberculosis before the first KS lesion developed.

Once the disease occurs, symptoms relate to the site of involvement. Early and even more advanced skin lesions are usually only mildly uncomfortable, although painful ulcers may occur. Gastrointestinal lesions are common but rarely cause significant symptoms. Early lesions in the lung have no symptoms, but severe lung involvement will produce profound air hunger.

DIAGNOSIS

Careful physical examination of anyone suspected of having KS requires an evaluation of all organ systems. Physical findings relate to the site of involvement. The most common sign of the illness is the appearance of the characteristic Kaposi's sarcoma lesion. Lesions may be found in many locations, although the characteristic finding in classic KS is a single raised purple-red nodule or a cluster of lesions in a single area of the body, especially on the legs.

Physical Examination

♦ The skin must be carefully examined. Although the dominant lesion of classic KS is on the arms and legs, all forms of the disease can affect any area of the skin.

♦ Epidemic KS may have a peculiar appearance. Typical early lesions are flat to slightly thickened, round or slightly irregular purple spots. They are painless when they first appear and only infrequently during the course of the disease do they cause significant pain. As the disease progresses, the lesions grow, often reaching an inch or so in each direction. They also thicken.

♦ There may be different-sized spots at all stages, often growing at seemingly different rates. Many patients will have yellow-brown pigment around the purple lesions. This bruise-like appearance is due to a small amount of blood leaking into the tissue.

♦ In late stages of the disease, the plaques and nodules may grow together, occupying large areas of the skin, blocking drainage from an extremity, causing swelling, and breaking down in areas, resulting in infection.

♦ Lymph nodes may be enlarged. A biopsy is needed to distinguish KS in nodes from other causes of lymph node enlargement.

♦ Mucous membranes are often involved. In the oral cavity, the hard and soft palates are most frequently affected.

♦ The membrane covering the eye (conjunctiva) may be involved, or lesions may be seen beneath the white of the eye (sclera).

♦ Involvement of internal organs may be suspected by physical examination, but cannot be proven without further testing. The physician will look for enlargement of the liver or spleen and feel for abnormal masses.

Blood and Other Tests

♦ Only the form of KS associated with HIV has abnormal blood tests associated with it. None of the tests, however—including HIV, P-24 antigen or beta-2 microglobulin—is predictive, meaning they do not indicate that KS is about to occur, its rate of growth or the chances of its responding to treatment.

♦ Useful information can be obtained from the total lymphocyte count and the "helper/suppressor" ratio.

Imaging

♦ KS may appear on a chest x-ray but cannot be distinguished from infections or other tumors. A direct view of the lung (bronchoscopy) may be needed.

Endoscopy and Biopsy

♦ Careful rectal examination with an anoscope or proctoscope may reveal involvement.

♦ The only diagnostic test for KS is biopsy of a suspicious lesion.

STAGING

There are several systems designed to stage KS, but none is entirely satisfactory or accepted by all physicians. A representative system designed at New York University divides patients into four groups:

1. Skin lesions, locally indolent (slow growing).
2. Skin lesions, locally aggressive, with or without local lymph node involvement.
3. Skin and mucous membrane involvement, generalized, with or without lymph node involvement.
4. Deep organ involvement.

All stages are then divided into either A (no symptoms) or B (with weight loss or fever).

TREATMENT OVERVIEW

KS is not considered curable in any stage by any current treatment. Neither surgical removal of the first-detected lesion nor obtaining a complete remission of multiple sites with chemotherapy or other techniques results in cure.

Nevertheless, long-term survival does occur both with and without treatment. Survival in classic KS is usually years and sometimes decades. Some patients with AIDS-related KS are still alive 10 years into the epidemic, though most survive only a few years. Treatment decisions at this time are usually aimed at palliation.

New drugs are always being tried, however. Thought should be given to participation in clinical research programs in major medical centers and hospitals.

 Surgery Surgical biopsy for microscopic examination of a suspicious lesion is needed to confirm the diagnosis of KS. Sometimes more than one biopsy is needed. Once the diagnosis is made, biopsy of other lesions is usually not needed except in cases where a deep lesion—a lung tumor, for example—has to be evaluated.

Other than for a biopsy, surgery is not commonly used in KS treatment. Lesions in the gastrointestinal tract may uncommonly bleed or obstruct the passage of food and require surgical correction. Conventional surgery and lasers have been used to remove bulky lesions in the mouth. Removal of multiple skin lesions does little to provide any meaningful relief of symptoms.

 Radiation All forms of KS are sensitive to radiation therapy. Radiation is clearly useful for lesions that are cosmetically disturbing, painful, involve the mouth extensively, block lymphatics, bleed or protrude greatly from the skin. Response rates are quite high and treatment is usually well tolerated.

The normal tissues of the mouth, however, are very sensitive to radiation in KS related to AIDS, resulting in a poor tolerance to treatment. The surfaces of the mouth may become inflamed or ulcerated. The treatment itself is painless, but the resulting sore mouth can be quite uncomfortable during the time needed for healing, usually several days. Anesthetic mouthwashes are often advised to control pain and speed the healing.

Local radiation usually uses energy beams that do not penetrate deeply into the body. Different centers use various combinations of numbers of treatments and dose per individual treatment, ranging from one single high dose to small doses five days a week for four or five weeks. Response rates appear roughly similar with the different methods.

The use of small doses of radiation over half the body and very superficial radiation (electron beam) to the entire body over many weeks are being investigated.

 Chemotherapy Because of the small number of patients, response rates of classic KS to chemotherapy are not well known. The disease is highly responsive to Velban, with response rates in the range of 90 percent. Very little information is available on the response to other drugs, although it would be logical to assume similar responsiveness of epidemic KS to the common chemotherapy agents.

Because of the relative rarity of the condition, there are also no good data on the response of patients with KS caused by immunosuppression. African KS appears to respond in a similar way to epidemic KS.

Determining whether a lesion becomes smaller with treatment can be quite difficult. Many patients have multiple lesions that are hard to measure accurately and may not respond in the same way to therapy. Changes in a lesion's shape or color may indicate some effect of treatment but not a significant one. One concern about using very aggressive therapy is that the treatment itself might depress the immune system.

♦ Velban has been the most studied and used single agent. It is well tolerated when given intravenously weekly. In epidemic KS, response rates of about 25 percent are obtained, with rare complete responses.

♦ Oncovin, closely related to Velban, has very different side effects and a slightly lower response rate. Weekly treatment with both of these drugs combined, at a lower dosage or alternating full dosage on a weekly schedule, raises the response rate to 40 to 75 percent. Side effects are remarkably low, and some complete responses are seen.

♦ Vepesid (etoposide, VP-16), given either orally or intravenously, is an attractive drug because it is well tolerated. It is difficult to use, however, because of its potential to depress blood counts in people who may already have marginal blood counts. Where it can be used, it has a high response rate. The same general comments apply to Adriamycin, which can be used only intravenously.

♦ Daunomycin is very similar to Adriamycin chemically. When coated with fat (lipid) it appears to concentrate in and be active in KS lesions. Studies show a 70 percent response rate with low toxicity. The drug is available in Europe, with Phase III investigational studies being completed in the United States.

♦ Bleomycin is active against KS, although it appears to be more effective in combinations than as a single agent. Responses to it as a single agent appear to be short, but very little blood count depression occurs.

♦ Methotrexate is similarly active, and ways can be found to give it with little blood count depression. Its use is limited, however, because it can cause rather marked blistering of the mouth.

♦ Among the new agents being tested are drugs related to Retin-A, an anti-wrinkle drug.

Combination Chemotherapy In the early days of AIDS, combinations of chemotherapy drugs were nearly always used. They fell into disfavor because of the high death rate from drug toxicity, often resulting in infections such as pneumocystis pneumonia. With the use of newer drugs such as AZT, inhaled pentamadine and foscarnet and with combination therapy for *Mycobacterium avium* infections, combinations are being used again, with higher response rates.

Many combinations of all these agents are being studied. Current standard therapy is either of the two Velban-Oncovin programs on a weekly treatment schedule or a combination of Adriamycin, bleomycin and vincristine (Oncovin) (ABV) given every week.

Whenever possible, patients should consider participating in a clinical trial with the hope of improved response and survival. If not in a study, treatment should *always* be given by a physician experienced in using these agents.

Local Therapy KS is one of the few tumors that respond to local injections of chemotherapy. Many anticancer drugs cause intense local damage if they are accidentally injected into tissue. This undesirable side effect has been used in a positive way to treat KS skin lesions.

Diluted solutions of various drugs have been injected directly into the lesions using tiny needles. A small amount of inflammation may occur for a few days, but this is not usually painful. The lesions will often flatten and shrink so they look like freckles. They can stay this way for weeks or months before they recur.

Bleomycin, Oncovin and Velban are among the anticancer drugs used in this way. Velban is the most commonly used because of its relative cheapness and ease of use. Treatments are usually given weeks to months apart and are no more painful than any other injection would be. They will not permanently control the lesions, nor will they control lesions that have not been injected. There are no generalized side effects or bone marrow depression. These treatments are especially useful for cosmetically disturbing KS lesions, such as a lesion on the face.

 Biological Therapy Immunologic treatment of KS is mainly a study of the effects of the interferons, mainly alpha.

Other agents, especially interleukin-2, are being studied but there is not yet clear data on their effects. Patients interested in these biologic response modifiers should ask their doctors for more information.

♦ There is not much data on the effects of interferon on classic KS, but because this form of the disease does not involve an immunologic defect, responses to this agent are not likely.

♦ Drug-induced KS is often very responsive to removing whichever agent depressed the body's immune system in the first place. When this is done, regressions of the disease, often complete, frequently occur.

♦ The most information on the effects of interferon is available with respect to HIV-associated KS. Treatment produces responses independent of the site of involvement or the amount of tumor present, which is a most unusual finding in cancer treatment.

♦ Both survival and the response rate drop if there are symptoms (fever, sweating, weight loss), opportunistic infections or low T4 cell counts. In one study, 45 percent of patients with T4 cell counts over 400 responded to chemotherapy, but only 2 percent of those with T4 cell counts less than 100 responded. There is some suggestion of an increase in survival if the amount of KS decreases, but final data are not yet available.

♦ Responses are more frequent as larger doses are given, but higher doses cause unacceptable side effects much more often. Some physicians start their patients at a low dosage of interferon and gradually increase it. This appears to result in fewer side effects when the higher dosage is eventually reached, but obviously the KS takes longer to respond.

♦ Studies of interferon plus chemotherapy have failed to produce any consistent improvement over either agent used by itself.

♦ AZT has been added to interferon with some suggestion of increased effect.

♦ Because one of the most worrisome side effects of chemotherapy is the depression of white blood cell counts, with the risk of subsequent infections, it has become standard practice to give G-CSF and GM-CSF.

TREATMENT BY STAGE AND SITE

Treatment considerations for KS are different than for any other solid (non-blood origin) tumor. There are two major reasons.

♦ The first is that there is never a stage or site of origin that can be cured.

♦ The second is that there is no relationship between the stage of the tumor and the response to treatment. Starting therapy early in the disease does not appear to change either the prognosis or the overall length of survival.

For these reasons, many physicians will not treat early disease with systemic (drug) therapy. Patients with early localized disease may receive radiation to the spots or local chemotherapy injections, or their condition may be monitored without any treatment given until it is needed.

Decisions on whether, when and how to treat patients are based on a number of factors such as the rate of growth, the site of involvement, the general physical condition of the patient and the severity of symptoms.

Standard Treatment Lesions of the gastrointestinal tract (stomach, small and large intestine) are common but usually do not cause symptoms. When they do cause symptoms—such as pain, bleeding or an inability to eat a normal volume of food—either chemotherapy or local radiation may be useful.

Lung lesions have a poor prognosis. Patients find it harder and harder to get enough air. When this happens they may live only a few months. Radiation therapy to the lungs plus chemotherapy given at the same time, followed by so-called maintenance therapy, has been used with a moderate degree of success.

A recent study of the combination of bleomycin and Velban (and in some patients Adriamycin) reported substantial improvement in lung symptoms.

SUPPORTIVE THERAPY

There are many common treatment-related problems with KS—especially depression of the bone marrow (causing anemia, low white blood cell counts that make infections more likely and low platelet counts with the possibility of bleeding), hair loss and nerve damage from the medicines.

♦ Frequent checks of the blood counts help reduce the risk of serious bone marrow effects.

♦ Nerve damage will be regularly

checked, with changes in medicine as needed to minimize this problem.

♦ Tourniquets or ice caps around the scalp can reduce blood flow to the scalp during treatment, which may reduce the amount of hair loss.

♦ Patients often need emotional and psychological support. Physical appearance is an important part of self-image, and cosmetics may be needed to cover lesions (*see* Chapter 22).

♦ Pain is not common, but if it does occur pain relievers may be needed.

♦ Both common and uncommon infections will often be seen. After appropriate cultures are taken, antibiotics may be needed.

♦ Nutrition is a common problem. In patients with poor appetites, appetite stimulants such as Megace or Provera may be useful. A derivative of marijuana (Marinol) may also now be prescribed as an appetite stimulant. Some patients will lose weight even with what appears to be good intake of food, and these patients may benefit from nutritional counseling. A clinic to measure metabolic parameters and counsel patients has met with some early success.

♦ Fluid may build up in body tissues, especially the legs, because KS lesions can block drainage. Local radiation may relieve the obstruction. The use of diuretics (medicines that increase the flow of urine) under close supervision is also sometimes effective.

♦ Psychosocial aspects of the illness also have to be dealt with. Dealing with the fear of death is a continuing problem, and with the high incidence of AIDS-related KS in North America there are many problems such as job loss and job discrimination, unwarranted public fear, treatment costs and facilities and death in young people.

Help may be found from a variety of organizations devoted to these problems. In some communities the spectrum of help ranges from psychiatry/counseling to the exceedingly valuable support given in one-to-one contact through such groups as Shanti.

TREATMENT FOLLOW-UP

To discover whether the treatment is working, the physician will often measure lesions in selected areas of the body. The physical examination will also try to detect areas of trouble such as internal organ involvement. Follow-up is primarily concerned with supportive care.

RECURRENT CANCER

Because KS is not now curable, the disappearance of detectable disease (clinical remission) means only that the disease's presence cannot be demonstrated at a particular time. The question really is how long treatment should be continued once remission has been obtained.

It is often the case that patients in either complete or partial remission who discontinue treatment relapse quite rapidly. If the treatment program does not cause severe side effects and does not involve drugs that cause more damage the longer they are used, treatment should continue indefinitely, although often at a reduced frequency.

THE MOST IMPORTANT QUESTIONS YOU CAN ASK

♦ When should treatment begin?

♦ When in the disease is interferon helpful?

♦ What types of drug treatment are available?

♦ When is radiation useful?

♦ How long will treatment last?

♦ Are there any new treatments available?

♦ What supportive services and treatments are available?

KIDNEY

Alan Yagoda, MD

◇

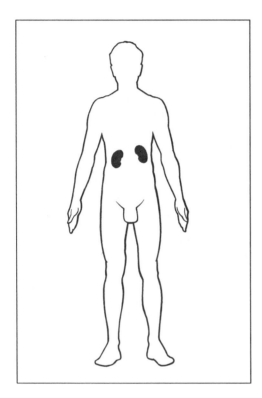

Cancer of the kidney—also called renal cell cancer, kidney adenocarcinoma or hypernephroma—accounts for about 2.5 percent of new cancers in the United States, 27,600 cases a year. Unfortunately, five-year survival rates have not changed for the past 30 years, partly because two-thirds of these cancers are not localized in the kidney when they are diagnosed. About 11,300 persons will die of kidney cancer in 1994.

Kidney tumors do not lend themselves to early diagnosis since these organs lie deep in the body between the lining of the body cavity (peritoneum) and the back muscles at the level of the last two ribs. By the time symptoms such as back pain and bloody urine are noted, the tumor is large (average size is 3 in. or 7.5 cm), has invaded lymph nodes and/or surrounding structures and is very vascular because of its ability to attract blood vessels. This increased vascularity soon leads to spread to the lungs, liver and bone. Five-year survival ranges between 50 to 80 percent for small tumors within the kidney that can be completely removed by surgery, whereas high-grade advanced disease invading lymph nodes, inferior vena cava or adjacent and distant organs has a cure rate of only 5 to 45 percent.

Renal cancer arises from the outer portion of the kidney called the parenchyma (as opposed to the renal pelvis, which briefly collects the urine, which is then carried by a tube, the ureter, to the bladder for storage before it is expelled). The parenchyma is made up of many single units called nephrons that filter water and toxic products from the blood.

Types More than 85 percent of renal cancers develop in glandular tissue (adenocarcinoma). The pure clear cell variety is seen in 25 percent of cases, the granular in 12 percent, the clear cell mixed with other more aggressive components such as granular in 50 percent and sarcomatous elements in about 10 percent. Studies using a test called flow cytometry suggest that the number of chromosomes in the tumor cells may help predict the chance for recurrence and disease-free survival. The normal two chromosomes (diploid) is favorable, while any other number (aneuploid) is less favorable. For example, two of every three low-grade (Grade 1) and low-stage tumors are diploid with less than 20 percent developing metastases and more than 80 percent surviving 5 years.

Another renal cancer, Wilms' tumor, is found exclusively in children. (*See* "Childhood Cancers.")

How It Spreads Kidney cancer cells frequently spread through the bloodstream by penetrating blood vessels within the tumor, then entering the renal vein and/or the inferior vena cava, the largest abdominal vein. Once cells have entered the bloodstream, they can lodge in the lungs, liver, brain or bone.

Cells also can directly invade the abdominal lymph nodes that drain the kidney and extend into structures surrounding the kidney (perinephric) such as fat, adrenal gland and liver. This kind of invasion is found at diagnosis in about 45 percent of cases. Invasion of the inferior vena cava is found in 10 to 15 percent of cases and of local lymph nodes in 10 to 30 percent. In over half the cases with lymph node involvement, distant metastases are found.

In over 40 percent of patients, the symptoms that cause them to seek medical attention are due to metastases.

What Causes It Risk factors are poorly defined, although the incidence is twice as high for those using tobacco (cigars, chewing tobacco, cigarettes).

RISK FACTORS

At Significantly Higher Risk
♦ This tumor is twice as frequent in men than in women, occurring mostly between the ages of 30 and 70.
♦ Those who smoke tobacco.
♦ Patients on long-term dialysis with acquired polycystic kidneys have an increased risk, as do those with the inherited disease von Hippel-Lindau syndrome.
♦ Other (but weak) risk factors include obesity in women and a high animal-fat diet, both of which suggest a hormonal imbalance.

♦ A new finding is the frequent abnormality in the chromosome 3 genes, particularly in familial renal cancers. Both genes are needed to suppress tumor formation, and absence of one gene permits tumor growth. Such findings have led to trials of gene insertion therapy.

SCREENING

Examination of the urine for blood (hematuria) is used for detecting early lesions that can be surgically removed. Ultrasound screening of the kidney, which is used in some countries, would be more accurate but is not cost-effective. Intravenous pyelography (IVP) and CT scans are used only in the diagnostic work-up to discover the cause of persistent and unexplained symptoms such as abdominal or flank pain, anemia and fever. Better screening procedures will have to await a simplified and less expensive urine or blood test using kidney cancer specific monoclonal antibodies. Such tests should soon be available.

COMMON SIGNS AND SYMPTOMS

The most common symptom is blood in the urine (hematuria), which is present in up to 65 percent of cases. Abdominal pain is found in 40 percent of patients and an abdominal mass in 35 percent. Other common symptoms include anemia, bone pain, unexplained weight loss, low-grade fever, general weakness or loss of energy and loss of appetite.

Unusual symptoms may include hypercalcemia (high blood calcium), high blood pressure, abnormal liver tests or too many red cells in the blood (polycythemia). These symptoms develop because renal tumors can produce substances that indirectly affect other organs, producing conditions called paraneoplastic syndromes.

DIAGNOSIS

Physical Examination
♦ Abdominal mass.
♦ Neck mass due to enlarged lymph node.
♦ Abdominal bruit (sound over renal artery).

Blood and Other Tests
♦ Liver function tests.
♦ Complete blood count.
♦ Blood calcium determination.
♦ Urinalysis.

Imaging
♦ Intravenous pyelogram (IVP).

♦ Ultrasound is the most sensitive test, being able to find masses as small as 3/4 in. (2 cm) in over 90 percent of cases. Sonograms can readily distinguish between the more commonly occurring benign or non-cancerous cyst and a solid tumor. When this test is combined with the intravenous pyelogram (IVP), the accuracy of a tumor diagnosis is over 90 percent. The sonogram can also be very helpful in determining whether the tumor has induced a clot in or invaded the renal vein or the inferior vena cava.

♦ CT with intravenous dye (the same dye used for intravenous pyelograms) will

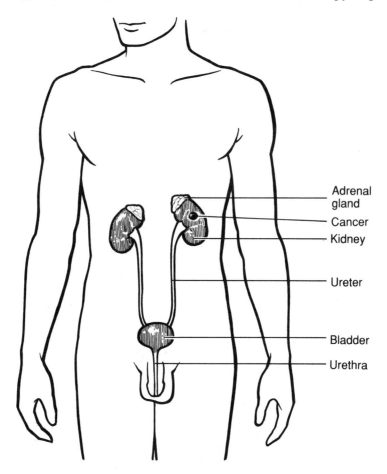

Adrenal gland
Cancer
Kidney

Ureter

Bladder
Urethra

Kidneys and adrenal glands

accurately diagnose renal tumors in 95 percent of cases and be falsely positive in fewer than 2 percent. This test may also show the tumor extension outside the kidney and can determine the extent of lymph node, liver and blood vessel involvement.

♦ MRI has replaced the inferior vena cavagram for determining more clearly the extent of blood vessel involvement and involvement of adjacent structures.

♦ Selective renal arteriography is helpful in finding small tumors and providing information that sometimes may be needed at the time of surgery about uncommon blood vessel patterns and, in selected cases, determining the possibility of a partial nephrectomy (removal of only a portion of the kidney) for small localized tumors.

♦ Other tests before surgery simply assure that there are no distant metastases. These include chest x-rays (if abnormal it may be followed by a chest CT scan), bone scans or skeletal x-rays and a liver scan (unnecessary when an abdominal CT scan is performed).

Biopsy

♦ Ultimately, the diagnosis is made either by removing the kidney (nephrectomy) or by a thin needle aspiration through the skin for cytologic slide examination. Looking for tumor cells in the urine is not useful.

TREATMENT OVERVIEW

Surgical removal of the kidney (simple nephrectomy) and the surrounding fat, adrenal gland and lymph nodes (radical nephrectomy) can lead to a cure for Stages I and II and can even cure Stage III in a few cases.

Surgery Partial nephrectomy can be performed for a tumor in patients with only one kidney or with tumors in both kidneys and for small, low-grade tumors. If

both kidneys have to be removed, long-term renal dialysis is required.

Renal transplantation can play a role for cancers in both kidneys. However, there is a risk of metastases being increased because the immune system has to be suppressed by drugs to prevent rejection of a transplanted kidney.

While there is renewed debate about the effectiveness of radical compared to simple nephrectomy in prolonging survival, no evidence exists that preoperative or postoperative radiation therapy, radiation therapy alone without surgery or renal artery embolization—clotting the arterial supply, thereby destroying both the tumor and the kidney—are beneficial in preventing metastases or increasing survival.

Adjuvant Therapy Without any effective treatment for advanced disease, there is no role for routine preoperative (neoadjuvant) or postoperative (adjuvant) therapy. Nor is there any for immunotherapy with interferon, interleukin-2 (alone or combined with lymphokine-activated killer cells), monoclonal antibodies or vaccines. Similarly, there is no role for hormone manipulation (female hormone progesterone) or chemotherapy (vinblastine). Any of the above therapies should only be given as part of an investigational randomized study.

 Radiation Although radiation therapy can control bone and brain lesions, it has not successfully prevented local tumor recurrence, nor has improvement in survival been definitely shown with radiation given before or after surgery.

 Chemotherapy The most effective standard chemotherapy drugs for metastatic disease are vinblastine and nitrosoureas—lomustine (CCNU) and carmustine (BCNU)—which produce tumor regression in only 5 to 10 percent of cases. Combination chemotherapy regimens have not yet demonstrated any superiority to single-drug therapy.

 Biological Therapy Interferon-alpha reduces tumors in 10 to 30 percent of patients, mostly those with lymph node and lung metastases. The usual dose of 6 to 9 million units—self-administered under the skin in the thigh three times weekly—should be continued for about three months before a decision is made about its effectiveness. Interferon-alpha—which is not yet licensed by the FDA for this disease despite response rates similar to interleukin-2 (IL-2)—must still be considered investigational. IL-2, with or without your own lymphokine-activated killer (LAK) or tumor-infiltrating lymphocytes (TIL), is licensed because a few patients with limited lung and lymph node metastases experienced complete disappearance of disease for more than 1 or 2 years.

IL-2 toxicity is significant, and includes nausea and fever, severe fatigue, anemia requiring blood transfusions, and congestive heart failure with fluid accumulating in the lungs and other tissues in about 40 percent of cases. Diarrhea, mouth soreness and hypotension (low blood pressure) requiring admission to an intensive care unit occur in 10 to 20 percent, yet fewer than 3 percent of patients will have a lethal reaction to high doses. Low-dose continuous infusion, now being tried, seems to be as effective and less toxic.

Investigational regimens are combining different interferons with cytotoxic chemotherapy, tumor necrosis factor and IL-2. Some early studies have reported responses in 30 percent of cases, although no combination has been definately proven superior to interferon-alpha or IL-2 alone.

Vaccines are being explored but are as yet of unproven benefit. Monoclonal antibodies, either given alone or with cytotoxic, biological or radioactive drugs attached to the antibody, are now being used in clinical trials and may well be a more promising treatment method. The use of these monoclonal antibodies is being investigated for both diagnosis and treatment. Lastly, you should inquire about participating in the innovative experimental gene insertion trials.

TREATMENT BY STAGE

STAGE I
TNM T1, N0, M0
T2, N0, M0
In Robson's staging system, Stage I means the tumor is confined within the renal capsule and is either less than 3/4 in. (2 cm) (T1) or more than 3/4 in. (2 cm) (T2) and with no lymph node or distant metastases.

About one-third of cases present with Stage I disease, many of which are Grade I (very well-differentiated) to Grade II (moderately well-differentiated). Almost one-third of Stage I cases are found to have micrometastases or microscopic disease after surgery.

Standard Treatment Simple or radical nephrectomy. It can be partial in selected cases, for low-grade small masses less than 1 1/4 in. (3 cm) in the cortex or outer area of the kidney, for tumors within one kidney and for tumors in both kidneys.

As long as tumor-free surgical margins are obtained, partial nephrectomy can be performed either with the kidney in place but isolated from the normal blood supply or by using an *ex vivo* technique, in which the kidney is removed from the body (so-called bench surgery). Bench surgery is needed for tumors in the middle portion of the normal kidney. After excision of the tumor, the remaining normal kidney is autotransplanted back into an appropriate area.

Radical nephrectomy involves tying the renal artery and vein, removing the surrounding fibrous layer (called Gerota's fascia) and thereby completely excising the kidney, the surrounding fat, the adrenal gland, regional lymph nodes and the ureter.

A new surgical advance is removal of a kidney tumor by laparoscopic surgery. A small camera video system, suction instruments and electrosurgical instruments are inserted into the abdomen through small incisions. The whole kidney and lymph nodes are removed in a plastic sac. Although this technique is only for highly selected patients, it is much less invasive, since the whole abdomen is not opened. This permits a shortened hospital stay with more rapid convalescence and causes less patient discomfort.

Five-Year Survival 60 to 80 percent

Investigational None.

STAGE II
TNM T3a, N0, M0
The tumor invades the surrounding fat or adrenal gland.

About 10 percent of cases are diagnosed in Stage II, and one-third of those patients will have micrometastases found at the time of surgery.

Standard Treatment Radical nephrectomy or, in selected cases, a simple nephrectomy.

Five-Year Survival 50 to 65 percent

Investigational Postoperative interferon and IL-2 are being evaluated.

STAGE III
TNM T3b, N1–3, M0
The tumor invades the renal vein (T3b, N0, M0), the inferior vena cava (T3b) or regional lymph nodes (T3b, N1–3, M0).

Approximately 25 to 35 percent of cases are found in Stage III, 60 percent of whom will have micrometastases found at the time of surgery.

Standard Treatment Radical nephrectomy.

Five-Year Survival 30 to 45 percent

Investigational Same as for Stage II.

STAGE IV
TNM T4, N3–4, M1
The tumor invades adjacent organs (T4), nearby lymph nodes (N4) or has distant metastases (M1).

Approximately 30 percent of cases are diagnosed in Stage IV, with 10 percent having a low-grade and more than 60 percent a high-grade tumor.

Standard Treatment The role for radical nephrectomy is debatable, since most patients die from metastatic disease. In the past it was thought that removing the primary cancerous kidney would cause the metastases to shrink. But spontaneous shrinkage of tumors has been documented in only 2 percent of cases at best, so the era of treatment of metastases by radical nephrectomy following embolization is over.

Nephrectomy is again being considered, however, to debulk (reduce) the tumor volume in order to make immunological treatment more effective for remaining disease. Nephrectomy for Stage IV cases should only be considered when part of an investigational study or for severe hemorrhage.

Five-Year Survival 5 percent

Investigational
♦ Participation in an experimental protocol, as outlined for Stage II, would be very appropriate.

TREATMENT FOLLOW-UP
♦ Regular physical examinations.
♦ Blood chemistry panel (includes alkaline phosphatase, which may signify bone or liver metastases if elevated).
♦ Chest x-rays (every 3 months) and

abdominal CT scan (every 3 to 6 months).

♦ Bone scan (and specific bone x-rays) if bone pain is present or serum alkaline phosphatase is elevated.

♦ Selected x-rays or imaging studies for specific areas (brain CT or MRI for persistent headaches; spine MRI for back pain with leg weakness or nerve symptoms).

RECURRENT CANCER

New investigational treatments should be explored before starting standard therapy, particularly monoclonal antibodies and gene insertion therapy. The results with currently used standard cytotoxic agents—vinblastine and a nitrosourea such as lomustine or carmustine—as well as currently used immunological agents (interferon) are very limited.

THE MOST IMPORTANT QUESTIONS YOU CAN ASK

♦ Has my cancer spread?

♦ What is the chance for cure with surgery?

♦ Can laparoscopic surgery be performed?

♦ What are the complications of surgery?

♦ Is there any role for other treatments such as chemotherapy?

♦ Is there a role for biological therapy with interferon, IL-2 or other agents?

♦ What is the status of gene insertion therapy and of monoclonal antibodies?

LEUKEMIA
Timothy S. Gee, MD

◇

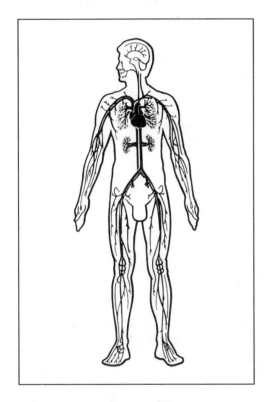

Leukemia is a cancer of the cells in the blood. It usually involves the various forms and stages of the white blood cells, although on rare occasions it may involve red blood cells and platelets.

Leukemia is often thought of as primarily a childhood disease, but it strikes many more adults than children. Adults account for 25,000 of the estimated 28,600 new cases expected in the United States in 1994. Acute leukemia is the most common childhood malignancy. The incidence of leukemia has not changed dramatically over the past 50 years, but survival rates for some forms of the disease have improved, especially in children, with the development of new types of treatment and chemotherapy agents. With acute lymphocytic leukemia in adults, for example, the five-year survival has increased from 4 percent in the early 1960s to about 50 percent today. More than half of the children who develop acute lymphocytic leukemia are alive five years after diagnosis, the majority being considered cured.

Types The many different forms of leukemia are generally divided into acute or chronic and then classified according to the cell type involved. There are two major types of white blood cells—granulocytic (myeloid) and non-granulocytic (lymphoid). Under a microscope, myeloid cells contain particles (granules), lymphoid cells generally do not. The diagnosis may be confirmed by new techniques for identifying certain biological markers and chromosomal characteristics.

♦ *Acute* An acute leukemia is associated with early (precursor) white blood cells called blast forms that do not become mature. These abnormal cells interfere with the production of the more mature cells normally seen in the bone marrow and blood, with the result that the normal cells are generally diminished or not seen at all. Because of the decreased number of normal cells, symptoms may include anemia, easy bruising, bleeding and sometimes infections. Without treatment, people with acute leukemia have an average survival of three to five months after diagnosis.

♦ *Chronic* Chronic leukemia usually involves the white blood cells, although the red blood cells may rarely be involved. Unlike acute leukemia, the leukemic cell clone involved in chronic leukemia does show all stages of maturation, with only a few blast forms. But even though they appear normal, the cells are abnormal. They do not function like normal cells. The white cells, for example, are not able to help fight infection. Because the bone marrow shows normal-appearing maturing cells, the diagnosis is made on the basis of the clinical picture, blood counts, the predominance of a particular cell line, genetic characteristics and the presence of certain proteins on the cell surface (cell surface markers).

The disease is controlled easily with medication or may not even need medication in its early stages. Average survival is measured in years rather than months.

How It Spreads Because it is a cancer of the blood, leukemia is found wherever blood travels. It is most commonly found in the bone marrow, spleen, liver and lymph nodes. In extremely rare cases, leukemia may first appear as a single localized mass of leukemia cells (chloroma) in the breasts, ovaries, testicles or brain. There may also be skin involvement by leukemic cells.

What Causes It There is no known cause. There are, however, known oncogenes in leukemia cells that may be associated with some types of the disease. Some forms of leukemia are associated with exposure to a retroviral infection such as HTLV-1. Certain abnormalities in the chromosomes are also associated with specific types of leukemia.

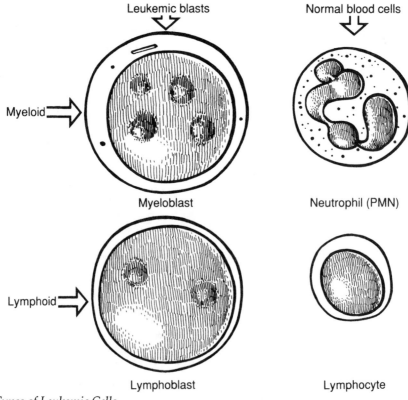

Two Types of Leukemic Cells

RISK FACTORS

At Slightly Higher Risk
♦ Men are slightly more likely than women to develop leukemia, and whites are more likely than blacks.
♦ People who have been exposed to prolonged or significant doses of radiation have a higher risk of developing leukemia.
♦ Prolonged exposure to toxic organic chemical compounds may be associated with increased risk.

COMMON SIGNS AND SYMPTOMS

A significant proportion of people with leukemia are completely free of symptoms and are diagnosed on a routine physical examination. The doctor may find an enlarged lymph node or an enlarged liver or spleen. Then again, the physical examination may be completely normal, but the routine blood test is abnormal.

People who do have symptoms commonly complain about generalized weakness, fevers, frequent infections, anemia or easy bruising or bleeding. Bleeding may be from the gums or nose or there may be blood in the stool or urine. Some people may have enlarged lymph glands, abdominal fullness or pain from enlargement of the liver or spleen. Less commonly, there may be complaints of headaches, fevers, skin rash or breast masses.

DIAGNOSIS

The initial diagnostic work-up—and treatment—of adults with acute leukemia can be carried out in many community medical centers, but children with acute leukemia should usually be evaluated in a pediatric cancer center because of the sophisticated testing required.

Physical Examination
♦ Enlarged lymph nodes.

♦ Swollen gums.
♦ Enlarged liver and spleen.
♦ Bruises or a small pinpoint red rash (petechiae) on the skin.

Blood and Other Tests
♦ A complete blood count (CBC) usually is abnormal, but on rare occasions may be normal.

Endoscopy and Biopsy
♦ The definitive test is a bone marrow aspiration and biopsy. The aspiration is performed by putting a needle into the breastbone (sternum) or pelvic bone under local anesthesia.
♦ A marrow biopsy may also be required. It is performed in the same fashion as an aspirate but with a larger, specialized needle.
♦ Additional amounts of marrow may be withdrawn for more specialized tests, such as chromosomal or DNA analysis.

STAGING

There is no staging system for leukemias, except for the chronic lymphocytic form (CLL). With CLL there are several staging classifications, the most frequently used being the RAI and the International. Both systems are based on the presence or absence of enlarged lymph nodes, liver or spleen and, most important, on the degree of anemia or low platelet counts.

Staging in the RAI system varies from Stage 0 to Stage IV, with average survivals ranging from over 12 years in the early stage to about a year in the late. Average survivals are comparable in the International classifications of A, B and C.

The RAI system has been modified by grouping Stage I as a low-risk group, Stage II as an intermediate-risk and Stage III and IV combined as a high-risk group. This offers a comparable grouping of average survival to the International classification of A, B and C groups.

TREATMENT OVERVIEW

Leukemia is treated mainly with chemotherapy, although radiotherapy and biological therapy can play a part with some forms of the disease. Surgery has no role. The goals of therapy are to relieve symptoms and obtain a remission. Remission is the condition in which leukemia is no longer detected and the marrow is normal again.

Bone Marrow Transplantation The utility or usefulness of this procedure must be decided on an individual basis. In some cases, bone marrow transplantation is used in acute myelogenous leukemia during the period of first remission, and in acute lymphoblastic leukemia as "salvage" therapy on relapse (*see* Chapter 12). There are two forms of marrow transplantation.

♦ Autologous transplantation uses the patient's own marrow. The marrow is collected while the patient is in remission, and it is often treated with chemotherapy agents or monoclonal antibodies before being given back. This is an effort to eliminate the few leukemic cells that might still be present but are undetectable.

♦ An allogeneic bone marrow transplant uses marrow from a normal donor, preferably a brother or sister who has the same tissue types. If a sibling is not available, a search of national and international tissue banks could be made for a non-related normal donor.

A bone marrow transplant requires four to six weeks in a hospital and the cost is currently about $150,000 to $250,000. Not all hospitals are able to perform the procedure but it is becoming more widely accepted.

The risk of dying is higher for an allogeneic marrow transplant than for an autologous transplant. Part of the reason is the potential of a graft-versus-host reaction. Some allogeneic transplants are performed with removal of the T-lymphocytes, the immunologic cells that bring about a graft-versus-host reaction. As technologies improve, the morbidity and mortality of allogeneic and autologous transplants continue to decrease. The current tendency is to investigate the use of either allogeneic or autologous marrow transplants earlier rather than later in the disease. It is apparent now that first remission transplants may offer better long-term results than with chemotherapy alone. The only exception to this is in patients with acute lymphoblastic leukemias where the results with chemotherapy alone and transplant are very similar. In this group of patients, it is still reasonable to consider a transplant during the second remission or early in the first relapse.

PRELEUKEMIA (MYELODYSPLASTIC SYNDROME)

Preleukemia is a form of early leukemia that in most if not all cases will progress into an acute leukemia in a few months to a year.

A significant number of people with this syndrome will have a chromosomal abnormality associated with the disease. The syndrome is often found in patients who have had chemotherapy or radiation therapy for some other malignancy. Exposure to toxic organic chemicals or radiation may also be possible causative agents associated with myelodysplasia. Perhaps because of the possible association of toxic chemicals and/or radiation, approximately half of the patients with myelodysplastic syndrome will have a detectable chromosomal abnormality in the leukemic cells.

Like other types of leukemias, a definitive diagnosis is generally made by evaluating a bone marrow sample. Treatment is often not urgently necessary—not within hours or days of a diagnosis. Some patients with preleukemia may be followed closely by their physicians without treatment for weeks or months, with blood transfusions given at two- to four-week intervals if necessary.

In almost all cases, however, the disease will eventually progress to a point where treatment with chemotherapeutic agents should be started. The progression will be signaled by physical deterioration, an increase in the white blood cell counts, lowering of platelet counts and/or progressive anemia.

It is not yet known whether there is any significant difference in survival between people treated immediately after diagnosis and those who defer their treatment until there is a clinical indication.

Standard Treatment Treatment depends on the overall goal at a given point in the course of the disease. Approaches include:

♦ *Palliative* Treatment is intended to control the disease, not necessarily to eradicate it or bring about a remission. This is particularly true when the white blood count rises. At that point, in addition to palliative blood transfusions, the white blood count may be controlled by Hydrea (hydroxyurea), an oral chemotherapy agent. Other agents such as Thioguanine (6-thioguanine) and Myleran (busulfan) may also be used. Eventually, in spite of these palliative attempts, the disease will break through. There is no remission or cure for patients on palliative treatment.

♦ *Chemo-modulation* This concept of therapy involves an attempt to "differentiate" the leukemia cells to a more normal stage of development in the hopes that they may behave more like normal cells in growth pattern and function.

The treatment commonly involves the use of a standard chemotherapy agent—Cytosar (cytosine arabinoside)—in low doses given by a 24-hour intravenous infusion or daily injections for 10 to 14 days. This has been temporarily helpful in 20 to 30 percent of cases, but the disease eventually progresses.

♦ *Investigational* Treatment with other, more experimental, agents can also try to "push" the leukemic cells in the direction of normal cells in appearance and function. Investigative agents now being evaluated include growth factors or cytokines such as G-CSF (granulocyte colony stimulating factor), a new synthetic chemical agent called HMBA (hexamethylene bisacetamide), IL-3 (interleukin-3) or vitamin A analogues (retinoic acid). It is too soon to know how effective these innovative treatments are.

♦ *Intensive chemotherapy* When the preleukemic stage becomes similar to an acute leukemia—in other words, it becomes a more aggressive form with survival a matter of months—standard therapy is similar to that described for acute leukemia.

♦ *Bone Marrow Transplantation* Even though bone marrow transplantation has been available for the past 15 years, it is still a new type of management. In several large studies on allogeneic marrow transplantations for young patients with myelodysplastic syndrome, there seems to be some indication that approximately half the patients may obtain a long-term disease-free survival. This is still an investigational treatment.

ACUTE LEUKEMIAS

There are two major subdivisions in adult acute leukemias, with the identification of the various forms based on the appearance of the cells and on studies of various biological and cell surface markers. Chromosome analysis often helps to identify the type of leukemia involved.

◆ Eighty percent of adult patients have an acute myeloid (AML) form. AML is divided into many subtypes such as acute myelogenous or myeloblastic, acute monocytic or monoblastic (AMOL), acute myelomonocytic (AMML), acute promyelocytic (APL) or, less commonly, erythroleukemia. With the exception of APL, there are minimal differences in the prognosis and treatment response for each of the subtypes. Therapy is similar for all of them. Patients with acute promyelocytic leukemia have a better response to a differentiating agent, all-trans-retinoic acid (ATRA), in combination with standard chemotherapy.

◆ Twenty percent of adult patients have acute lymphoblastic leukemia (ALL), which is similar to the childhood form of leukemia. The treatment for ALL is generally different than for AML, because the lymphoblasts respond to a larger variety of chemical agents and also because ALL occurs in a younger population.

The probability of a long-term remission is better for ALL, with one exception. People with ALL cells that have a specific chromosome abnormality (the "Philadelphia chromosome") have a prognosis similar to patients with AML.

Adult patients with ALL, like children with ALL, are at risk of their leukemia eventually involving the central nervous system—the brain and spinal cord. Both treatment and prognosis are influenced by this potential complication.

AML and ALL patients are susceptible to the development of localized areas of leukemia involvement. These may show up as skin rashes or lumps in the breasts, testicles or ovaries. The prognosis is worse when these localized areas of leukemia appear.

Treatment Overview The goal of treatment is to obtain a complete and long-term remission. Anything short of that offers no substantial survival benefit. Treatment is divided into two phases:

◆ Induction. This is the attempt to attain a remission, meaning that the bone marrow appears normal.

◆ Consolidation. This involves giving the same or different treatment, even when someone appears to be in remission, because of the suspected or assumed presence of residual disease that cannot be detected but that may cause a later relapse.

Some patients may receive a third phase called maintenance treatment to prolong the remission. Maintenance treatment is more commonly associated with the treatment of ALL than AML.

Survival Remission rates are inversely related to age. The response rate decreases as the patient's age increases, and age is directly related to increased risk for complications and death during the induction phase of treatment. On average:

◆ Patients with AML have a 60 to 70 percent probability of having a remission. Twenty percent of those who do attain a remission can expect to survive three years or more with a possibility of being cured, with chemotherapy alone.

◆ Patients with ALL have an 80 to 90 percent probability of achieving a remission, with 35 to 45 percent surviving five or more years, again with a possibility of being cured, with chemotherapy alone.

ACUTE MYELOBLASTIC LEUKEMIA (AML)

Standard Treatment Standard treatment includes two drugs, Idamycin (idarubicin) and Cytosar (cytosine arabinoside). These are commonly given intravenously, Idamycin for three days and Cytosar for five to seven days.

These drugs may cause significant nausea and vomiting, so patients are also given drugs such as Benadryl, Compazine, Vistaril, Reglan, Ativan and Zofran.

The chemotherapy drugs will kill normal and leukemic cells equally, so the most significant side effect besides nausea and vomiting is a temporary reduction of normal white blood cells and platelets. The deficiency of white cells means a loss of normal defenses against bacterial and fungal organisms, leaving the patient open for infections. Low platelets mean that the patient may bruise or bleed easily. All patients should be closely watched in the hospital until this effect is over.

Supportive treatment during this period includes blood and platelet transfusions and intravenous antibiotic treatment. Because of the intensive supportive treatment required, therapy for AML is given in the hospital, with the duration of hospitalization ranging from four to six weeks.

Investigational
♦ Different combinations of chemotherapy agents such as mitoxantrone and etoposide, amsacrine (AMSA) and higher doses of Cytosar alone or carboplatinum and Cytosar are being evaluated. The use of purine nucleotides such as 2-chlorodeoxyadenosine (2-CdA) is also under investigation for patients with acute myeloblastic leukemia. All combinations have the common side effects of bone marrow suppression with resulting low white blood cell and platelet counts. The benefits of treatment with these newer combinations are not yet clear.
♦ Treatment with growth factors such as GM-CSF (granulocyte/macrophage colony stimulating factor) or G-CSF (granulocyte colony stimulating factor), or differentiation agents such as HMBA, or all-*trans*-retinoic acid (ATRA) is also being evaluated. Patients with acute promyelocytic leukemia seem to have additional benefits with the use of ATRA in combination with standard chemotherapy. It is hoped that treatment with these agents will be less toxic and more effective than current chemotherapy programs.
♦ Another new concept in therapy involves using specific antibodies. These are proteins that bind to leukemia cells and not to normal cells. The antibodies can carry some cell killing agent such as ricin or radioactive isotopes directly to the leukemia cells, letting the agent kill the leukemia cells while sparing the normal white blood cells and platelets. In this way, complications such as infection and bleeding may be avoided. Results on this type of treatment will be available in the next few years.

ACUTE LYMPHOBLASTIC LEUKEMIA (ALL)
Children with ALL have a better long-term survival than adult patients. There are many possible reasons for this difference. Twenty percent of adult patients have a chromosomal marker, the Philadelphia chromosome, which signifies a more difficult form of leukemia to treat. However, adult patients may still have a significant response. A bone marrow transplant may be considered in first remission in adults with Philadelphia-chromosome-positive ALL.

Standard Treatment ALL patients have a higher response rate to chemotherapy than do patients with AML and more drugs are available to treat this form of the disease. Drugs commonly used for induction treatment include vincristine (Oncovin), prednisone, idarubicin (Idamycin) or doxorubicin (Adriamycin), L-asparaginase, Cytoxan and Cytosar.

Again, treatment includes an induction and consolidation phase, and generally a maintenance phase for one to two years. Because of the known risk of central nervous system leukemia (leukemic meningitis), patients are also treated with chemotherapy (usually methotrexate) via a spinal tap or an Ommaya reservoir surgically implanted under the scalp or by radiation therapy to the head in an effort to prevent this complication. As with AML treatment, most patients will be in the hospital when treatment is started.

Investigational

♦ Because of the availability of the growth factor such as G-CSF, more intensive combinations of chemotherapy are being given initially in hopes of increasing the number of patients obtaining long-term disease-free survival.

♦ The use of monoclonal antibodies continues to be investigated.

♦ Bone marrow transplantation.

CHRONIC LEUKEMIA

Like acute leukemia, there are two major categories based on cell appearance, histochemical stains and biological markers. Because chronic leukemias involve cells that are either mature or become mature, these cells may have a normal appearance.

The two major types of chronic leukemia are chronic myelogenous leukemia (CML) and chronic lymphocytic leukemia (CLL). They are easily distinguished under the microscope.

♦ CLL involves mature lymphocytes, cells that differ from the cells in CML in size, nuclear pattern and generally by the absence of cellular particles. The diagnosis of CLL can be confirmed by cell surface marker studies. These studies can be particularly helpful because sometimes appearance alone may not distinguish between CLL and lymphoma that happen to involve the blood and/or bone marrow.

♦ The CML cells are larger and appear normal. Chromosome studies on CML cells are sometimes needed to tell the difference between a person with CML and preleukemia (myelodysplastic syndrome) or even someone with a normal elevation in peripheral blood counts because of an infection. The more sensitive DNA analysis of the CML cells may be used to confirm a diagnosis. In 80 to 90 percent of CML patients, the chromosomal and DNA abnormality will confirm the presence of the (abnormal) Philadelphia chromosome.

Most people with CML and CLL have a high white blood cell count but may have few or no symptoms. A good number of these cases are diagnosed on a routine blood test performed as part of a routine or pre-employment physical examination. A doctor may find an enlarged spleen in someone with CML, and enlarged lymph nodes, with or without an enlarged spleen, in those with CLL.

CHRONIC LYMPHOCYTIC LEUKEMIA (CLL)

The decision on whether or when to treat patients with CLL depends on many factors, including the stage of disease. Because CLL is not curable and because it generally occurs in older people without symptoms and often progresses slowly, it is usually treated in a conservative fashion.

Standard Treatment In the early stages, most patients do not require any treatment. In a typical case, the white blood cell count is very high but there are no symptoms. Management ranges from periodic observation by the physician (with treatment of infection, bleeding or immunologic complications as they occur) to standard chemotherapy.

In moderate to advanced disease—RAI intermediate and high-risk or International B and C—observation without treatment may still be the plan if there are no symptoms and the CLL does not progress.

If therapy is indicated because of symptoms or signs—enlarging lymph nodes or spleen or adversely changing blood counts—the conventional treatment is chemotherapy with medications taken by mouth such as Leukeran and Cytoxan, singly or in combination with a steroid preparation like prednisone.

On uncommon occasions when there is one single site of lymph node enlargement, radiation to the site is appropriate. The use of total (generalized) lymph node irradiation for CLL is no longer used as conventional treatment.

Investigational Patients with newly diagnosed CLL or early stage CLL are generally not candidates for investigational treatments.

♦ Chemotherapy agents are constantly being developed. Fludarabine is now thought to be a most useful drug; patients with CLL obtained complete and partial responses of 70 to 80 percent in some studies. The long-term results of Fludarabine therapy are not yet known. Fludarabine is also being used in combination with more standard drugs such as Cytoxan (cyclophosphamide).

♦ Cytokines and biologic response modifiers such as monoclonal antibodies, interferon-alpha and 2′-deoxycoformycin are being evaluated.

CHRONIC MYELOGENOUS LEUKEMIA (CML)

This chronic leukemia affects the myeloid cell line rather than the lymphocytes. The disease usually affects people in their fifth and sixth decades of life, but may occur even in infants.

The average survival for people with CML is 42 to 45 months with current therapies. About 60 to 70 percent of CML patients with the Philadelphia chromosome abnormality will progress into an acute or blastic phase. Without change in treatment at this stage, the average survival is four or five months.

Interferon-alpha, a biologic protein given by injection first daily then several times a week, has been shown in CML patients to effectively control white blood counts and decrease the size of the spleen. It has also been effective in reducing the number of leukemia cells with the Philadelphia chromosome in the marrow for a short period (months to one or two years). It has been shown to produce an improved survival in patients who respond.

The only possible chance for a prolonged survival or possible cure is the use of an allogeneic bone marrow transplant while the disease is in the chronic phase. With such a transplant soon after diagnosis, there will perhaps be a 25 to 40 percent chance for a longer survival. Once the disease is in the blastic phase, even with intensive treatment similar to the treatment for acute leukemia there is only about a 20 percent response rate at best, with the duration of the response generally less than a year.

Since no standard treatment offers a cure, prevents the blastic phase from occurring or prolongs the average survival, all newly diagnosed patients should be considered for an allogeneic marrow transplant and for clinical trials of new therapeutic approaches.

Standard Treatment Most CML patients have unusually high white blood cell counts, so the initial standard therapy tries to lower the counts toward more normal levels. There are two ways of doing this:

♦ Chemotherapy is the most common method, with either Hydrea or Myleran taken as an oral medication. Both are effective and offer excellent control over a prolonged period. Myleran is longer acting and has the potential of overdosage unless the blood counts are followed closely. It also has the potential long-term side effect of causing lung complications. Hydrea also has to be monitored closely by the physician. It is a much shorter acting drug so the problem of overdosage is less. Hydrea has no known complications after long-term use, so it is now more in favor as the chemotherapy agent for CML.

Along with these drugs, patients with CML who have unusually high counts will be placed on Zyloprim (allopurinol). This drug prevents high levels of uric acid that can be caused by the rapid killing of the leukemia cells. A high level of uric acid may cause problems such as kidney stones or impaired kidney function.

♦ The other method is called leukopheresis. This is effective, but generally only as a short-term means of control in patients with very high white blood cell counts.

Leukopheresis involves using a mechanical centrifuge machine to remove the white blood cells. To perform this procedure, a large needle is placed in a vein in each arm. The needles are attached to a catheter, which allows the blood from one arm to run into the centrifuge. There the white cells are separated out and the remaining blood cells and plasma are returned through the other arm. The procedure takes two to three hours.

The white blood count will stay lowered for a few days to a few weeks before the procedure has to be repeated. Obviously, this is not an acceptable method for controlling the disease over a long time. But it may be useful over a brief period, especially if the white blood count is very high, which is associated with risks of brain complications (strokes) as well as respiratory and vascular complications.

Further therapy may involve the removal of the spleen if it is enlarged, causing symptoms and not responding to chemotherapy. In rare cases, the spleen may be removed to improve the abnormally low counts of other normal blood cells caused by the removal of these cells by the enlarged spleen.

Investigational
♦ For patients with unusually high platelet counts (over 1 million/cmm.) and unable to be controlled with the standard palliative chemotherapy, the drug Anagrelide seems to be useful.

Bone Marrow Transplantation All patients under 50 should be tissue-typed along with their immediate family members to determine if there is a relative who could be a marrow donor. If there is, then an allogeneic marrow transplant should be considered. In some institutions patients under 60 would still be considered for marrow transplantation.

The current consensus is that a marrow transplant should be performed within two years of diagnosis. Transplants further from diagnosis have been performed, but preliminary results have not been as good as when transplants were performed earlier in the course of the disease.

Again, marrow transplantation is the only treatment that offers the chance of a cure to CML patients. There is a 20 percent probability that a transplant patient may die during or shortly after the transplant from a variety of problems—infections, graft rejection, graft-versus-host (GVH) problems, lung complications and bleeding. Patients who survive the procedure are also susceptible to a recurrence of the disease.

MISCELLANEOUS LEUKEMIAS

This is a group of leukemias rarely seen in adults. They either do not belong to the usual classification of acute and chronic leukemias or are unusual variations of the forms already described.

HAIRY CELL LEUKEMIA
This is a moderately rare leukemia that is more like a chronic than an acute leukemia.

The diagnosis is usually made by reviewing the bone marrow and blood smear and finding a specific lymphoid cell, a cell that uniquely describes this leukemia. Some special blood stains and antibodies help confirm the diagnosis made on the marrow. The tartrate resistant acid phosphatase (TRAP) stain, for example, is diagnostic for hairy cell leukemia.

People who get this leukemia are usually elderly and go to their doctor with symptoms of weakness and/or after finding a lump in their abdomen, which is an enlarged spleen. Blood counts are abnormal. Usually the white count is low and in some cases the counts of red cells and platelets are also low.

This disease is rarely cured and about 10 percent of patients may not need treatment for years. Patients may have prolonged survival with treatment.

Standard Treatment Before 1985, the recommended standard treatment was quite limited. The surgical removal of the spleen relieved symptoms and improved the blood counts in over 60 percent of the patients. But about half of those who did show improvement from the splenectomy would again get the same symptoms. The best long-term response to a splenectomy is found in patients with a very enlarged spleen.

Now there is an effective form of treatment in addition to or instead of removing the spleen. 2-chlorodeoxyadenosine (2-CdA) has shown it to be an extremely useful drug, offering complete remission in 70 to 80 percent of patients. The 2-CdA is administered in a one-week intravenous treatment. Although there are often long-term responses, it is too early to know if such responses will result in cure.

Interferon-alpha is still an effective drug in patients with this disease. However, because of the availability of 2-CdA administered over one week versus the continued application of interferon-alpha by injections as well as the somewhat unpleasant side effects, most physicians and patients prefer the use of 2-CdA.

2-deoxycoformycin (Pentostatin) also is effective in hairy cell leukemia and is generally given intravenously every other week for three to six months, offering approximately a 50 percent response.

PROLYMPHOCYTIC LEUKEMIA

It is difficult to distinguish this rare leukemia from chronic lymphocytic leukemia and some types of lymphoma.

Like hairy cell leukemia, the diagnosis is made by examining the cells in blood and bone marrow samples. Even the most current technologic methods find it difficult to specifically identify lymphocytic cells as to their placement in the diagnosis of CLL or lymphoma.

The clinical course is moderately aggressive with enlarging spleens, lymph nodes and progressive blood count change.

Standard Treatment Chemotherapy with the drugs used in the treatment of CLL or lymphoma.

MEGAKARYOCYTIC, BASOPHILIC AND EOSINOPHILIC LEUKEMIA

These extremely rare leukemias are probably associated with the blastic phase of chronic myelogenous leukemia.

Because they are so rare, there is no standard treatment. People with these forms of the disease are managed like those who have acute non-lymphoblastic leukemia.

The prognosis and survival rates with these leukemias are very poor.

THE MOST IMPORTANT QUESTIONS YOU CAN ASK

♦ What is the prognosis for my type of leukemia?

♦ Is treatment necessary immediately? If not, when will it be necessary and how do you decide when to start?

♦ What type of treatment is needed and what are the chances of a response?

♦ How long will the treatment continue?

♦ What are the risks and complications?

♦ Are any investigational treatments available?

♦ Should the treatment be done at the local community hospital or should it be directed or done at a major specialty institution?

LIVER

Alan P. Venook, MD

◇

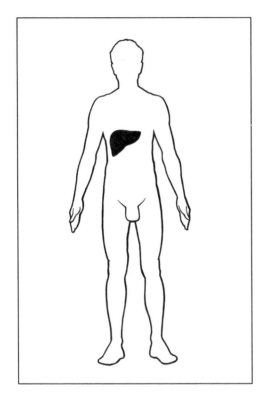

cancer within it causes major metabolic problems. The treatment now available for advanced liver cancer is not particularly effective, and the principal goal of therapy is to relieve the symptoms related to the disease.

Types The most common type of cancer originating in the liver itself—referred to as primary liver cancer—develops in liver cells and is called hepatocellular carcinoma. Rarely, tumors arise from blood vessels in the liver (hemangioendothelioma), other glands in the liver (adenocarcinoma) or connective tissue in the liver (sarcoma, angiosarcoma). An unusual type of hepatocellular carcinoma called fibrolamellar tends to occur in young women. Tumors that develop in the bile ducts are called cholangiocarcinomas (*see* "Bile Duct").

Most commonly, cancer in the liver has spread there from another organ and is therefore a type of metastatic cancer (*see* "Metastatic Cancer").

How It Spreads Liver cancers can spread to other areas through either the lymph system or the blood. Most often the cancer first moves into the lymph nodes in the region of the liver (porta hepatis), then goes to other lymph nodes or into the lung or bones. Tumor cells can also spread into the abdominal cavity, causing the accumulation of fluid (ascites) or masses elsewhere in the abdomen (*see* page 406).

What Causes It Hepatocellular carcinoma most often develops in damaged livers. Long-standing infection with either the hepatitis B or hepatitis C virus often pre-

Primary liver cancer—also called hepatocellular carcinoma or hepatoma—may be the most common cancer worldwide. It occurs with great frequency in Asia and Africa, but is relatively uncommon in the United States. About 8,000 cases are diagnosed yearly in the U.S., although immigration patterns are changing the rates at which primary liver cancer is seen in this country.

Partly because it is so uncommon here, liver cancer is generally not suspected and is at an advanced stage by the time it is diagnosed. Because the liver plays a vital role in removing toxins from the blood,

cedes it and is therefore seen as a significant risk factor.

Cirrhosis of the liver (from, for example, a viral infection, alcohol, toxin exposure or a genetic defect of metabolism) also increases the likelihood of hepatocellular carcinoma, presumably because of chronic inflammation in the liver. In fact, an estimated 5 percent of all people with cirrhosis of the liver will eventually develop liver cancer. Fifty to 80 percent of all people with liver cancer have cirrhosis.

Certain chemicals are associated with increased liver cancer, and a link has been established with a plant fungus (aflatoxin) that is ingested with the normal diet in a region in Africa. Oral steroid use may also increase the risk.

RISK FACTORS

At Significantly Higher Risk
♦ Worldwide, men are twice as likely as women to develop liver cancer.
♦ Chronic hepatitis B and/or hepatitis C virus infection, with or without cirrhosis of the liver. The usual route of transmission of hepatitis B and C is through blood transfusions or drug needles. Because hepatitis B virus may also be transmitted by a mother to her offspring during pregnancy or childbirth or may be transmitted between partners during sexual intercourse, it is not unusual for members of the same family to develop liver cancer after becoming infected with hepatitis B.
♦ Cirrhosis of the liver from any cause—alcohol damage or inborn errors of metabolism such as hemochromatosis or enzyme deficiencies.
♦ Exposure to aflatoxin, a fungus contaminant found in the soil in Africa.
♦ Exposure to the fumes of vinyl chloride or to Thorotrast (a contrast material no longer used for radiologic procedures) is associated with an increased risk of angiosarcoma of the liver and hepatocellular carcinoma.

At Slightly Higher Risk
♦ Anabolic steroid use, as by weightlifters and other athletes, is known to increase the risk of benign liver tumors and may cause an increase in liver cancer.
♦ Estrogen therapy, such as oral contraceptives, may increase the risk, although this has not been proven.

SCREENING

People with known chronic hepatitis and/or cirrhosis of the liver may benefit from the use of screening tests to try to find the cancer before it has spread beyond the liver. Thorough screening includes frequent monitoring of serum alpha-fetoprotein (a product found in the blood of 50 to 70 percent of all hepatocellular carcinoma patients in the U.S. and more commonly worldwide) and ultrasound of the liver. These tests are not useful for identifying primary liver tumors other than hepatocellular carcinoma.

Although these screening methods may be useful in Asia and Africa, where liver cancer is very common, they are not routinely used in North America because of this cancer's rarity. Screening of hepatitis B virus-infected Asian and African immigrants to the U.S. may be beneficial.

COMMON SIGNS AND SYMPTOMS

Common symptoms include bloating, abdominal pain, fever, weight loss, decreased appetite and nausea. But because liver cancer is so rare, its symptoms are usually attributed to more common, benign conditions. Frequently, the diagnosis of cancer is not considered until these symptoms persist or until a person develops an enlarging abdominal mass or fluid in the abdomen. Jaundice (the skin turning yellow) and swelling in the legs are usually associated with more advanced tumors. Sometimes, people with liver cancer feel entirely well.

DIAGNOSIS

Physical Examination
There are no findings specific only to liver cancer on physical examination. Findings may include the following, all of which may have other explanations:

♦ Fever.
♦ Enlarged liver and spleen.
♦ Enlarged, hard lymph nodes.
♦ Swelling of the abdomen from fluid (ascites).
♦ Jaundice (the skin turning yellow).
♦ Swelling of the legs (edema).

Blood and Other Tests
♦ A complete blood count may be normal or may show a decrease (anemia) or increase in red blood cells.
♦ Routine liver function studies—blood tests measuring serum bilirubin and liver enzymes—may be abnormal, but can be entirely normal even in advanced stages of primary liver cancer.
♦ Prothrombin Time and Partial Thromboplastin Time (PT and PTT) tests of clotting—usually done if a liver problem is suspected—may be abnormal.
♦ The serum alpha-fetoprotein (AFP) is elevated in 50 to 70 percent of people in the U.S. with primary liver cancer. It may also be elevated in people with germ cell cancer, gastric cancer or cirrhosis of the liver or in pregnant women.

Imaging
♦ Abdominal ultrasound can evaluate the density of the liver if there is a suspicion of a mass. It can reveal the presence of fluid in the abdomen and is particularly useful for distinguishing a solid mass from a non-cancerous accumulation of fluid within the liver (benign cyst).
♦ A CT scan is useful for determining the extent of a tumor within the liver and evaluating the possible extension of tumorous tissue into lymph nodes or to other structures within the abdomen.
♦ Magnetic resonance imaging (MRI) may be helpful in determining if the liver cancer can be surgically removed by revealing whether the tumor involves both lobes of the liver or is invading blood vessels. Usually, MRI is not necessary because the CT scan provides essentially the same information.
♦ An x-ray involving the injection of dye into the artery going to the liver (arteriography) is necessary before any attempts are made to remove the tumor, since the surgeon needs to know exactly what the blood supply of the tumor is in order to remove it.
♦ If surgery is being considered, a chest x-ray should be done. If the cancer has spread to the lungs or any other organ, surgery should be reconsidered.

Endoscopy and Biopsy
♦ Biopsy, either by fine needle aspiration (FNA) or with a regular needle, is almost always necessary. This procedure can be done through the skin without significant danger. Because of the variation in the tumor cells of different types of cancer, the biopsy sample can be used to distinguish between a primary liver cancer or a cancer that has spread from another organ. Occasionally, if the AFP is extremely high and the tumor very large, a biopsy may not be necessary.

STAGING
Although a TNM staging system exists for hepatocellular carcinoma, for purposes of deciding about therapeutic options, there are only three stages—localized resectable, localized unresectable and advanced disease.

TREATMENT OVERVIEW
Surgery is the only way to cure primary liver cancer, so the goal of the diagnostic work-up is to discover if all the cancerous tissue can be removed. This is often not possible, either because the tumor has already spread beyond the liver or because

the liver is too damaged and removal of liver tissue would leave a person without enough liver function to survive.

Chemotherapy and radiation therapy are occasionally helpful in relieving symptoms. Primary liver cancer may progress rapidly, but these and other measures can be taken to maintain the quality of life. Newer treatments, such as more effective chemotherapy or liver transplantation, may someday allow the surgical removal of cancers now felt to be inoperable.

Surgery Surgery can cure liver cancer if the entire tumor can be removed. The liver has two distinct lobes—right and left—and a tumor confined to one lobe can often be removed even if the patient has cirrhosis of the liver. If cirrhosis is only minimally or not at all present, a tumor involving parts of both lobes of the liver can be removed with an extensive operation (trisegmentectomy). This surgery is potentially dangerous, however, and people with poor liver function may not survive it.

Liver transplantation may be considered for someone whose cancer has not yet spread and who cannot tolerate the removal of part of the liver because of underlying liver disease or the size of the tumor. So far, this approach has been beneficial only in people with the fibrolamellar variant. Even if patients with hepatocellular carcinoma have no evidence of metastases, the tumor almost always redevelops after transplantation, perhaps because of the suppression of the immune system that allows the transplanted liver to function. Rarely, cancer is not found in the liver until after a person has had a transplant for another reason. Such patients may be cured because the cancer is in an earlier stage.

The presence of tumor anywhere else in the body—lung, bone or lymph nodes, for example—means that removal of the liver tumor alone will not bring about a cure. If the disease has already metasta-sized, removing part of a liver tumor is not considered beneficial because of the side effects of surgery, including a long recuperative period.

◆ **Investigational** A new surgical technique called cryosurgery involves freezing the tumor tissue by placing a cold probe directly into it. A tumor that cannot be removed because it is too close to blood vessels or because of extensive underlying liver disease may be "killed" by this technique. The effectiveness of this therapy is being evaluated.

Chemotherapy Chemotherapy may result in tumor shrinkage, but this does not necessarily prolong survival. The standard drug, Adriamycin, may shrink tumors in 15 to 20 percent of patients and seems to help some. But the side effects of this drug, including nausea, vomiting and hair loss, may leave patients in a worse condition even if the tumor shrinks. Other drugs that may decrease the tumor size are 5-fluorouracil, mitomycin-C, etoposide and mitoxantrone, although these have similar side effects to Adriamycin.

These drugs seem to shrink tumors more successfully when administered directly into the liver via the hepatic artery. Although tumors within the liver regress in about 50 percent of patients, the therapy is difficult to give and is extremely toxic to an already damaged liver. Because few patients feel better after such therapy and because distant metastases nearly always develop, it is generally not advisable to surgically implant an infusion device into the hepatic artery.

◆ **Investigational** There is substantial experience in Asia and at some institutions in the U.S. with a process called chemoembolization. This involves administering a combination of chemotherapy and colloid particles directly into the liver tumor via its main (hepatic) artery.

Generally, it is performed as a single treatment and does not require surgery or prolonged bed rest. Preliminary results show that tumors will shrink in about 50 percent of patients, although prolonged survival has not been proven.

There may also be a role for chemoembolization before the surgical removal of the liver tumor, since significant shrinkage may enable the removal of a previously unresectable tumor. This has not yet been proven, however.

 Radiation The usefulness of radiation is limited in liver cancer because it is extremely damaging to non-cancerous liver tissue. It is sometimes used to treat the liver area after a tumor has been removed, although this has not been shown to be of definite benefit. The principal role for radiation is the management of painful liver masses or metastases.

♦ **Investigational** The combination of external beam radiation, chemotherapy and a unique antitumor monoclonal antibody has been shown recently to benefit some patients with otherwise unresectable cancer. The effectiveness of this combination is still not certain. Institutions studying this therapy are best equipped to perform it.

TREATMENT BY STAGE

LOCALIZED RESECTABLE
The tumor is confined to a portion of the liver that allows for its complete surgical removal. The tumor may be localized to either the right or the left lobe of the liver or possibly involve the right lobe and only a portion of the left lobe.

Standard Treatment Surgery is the standard therapy but depends on the relative health of the remaining underlying liver, since a person with cirrhosis of the liver may not be able to tolerate the removal of

one-half or two-thirds of the liver tissue. Surgery also depends on the presence of a clear zone between the tumor and the neighboring blood vessels. Only a small percentage of people are candidates for surgery and, unfortunately, the majority experience a tumor recurrence.

Five-Year Survival 10 to 30 percent

Investigational
♦ The role for chemotherapy after surgery is unknown. Although Adriamycin is often recommended, no systematic studies have been done to see if it increases the chances of cure.
♦ Similarly, radiation is often applied to the liver area after surgery but has never been proven to be beneficial in such patients.

LOCALIZED UNRESECTABLE
Despite being a localized mass, the tumor may be unresectable because crucial blood vessel structures are involved or because the liver is impaired.

Standard Treatment There is no standard therapy, so patients should be considered for clinical trials.

Two-Year Survival Less than 5 percent

Investigational
♦ Liver transplantation may be attempted in patients who are deemed unresectable because of poor liver function and whose tumors are not intertwined with blood vessels in the abdomen. This seems to be of benefit in patients with the fibrolamellar variant. Preliminary data suggests that some patients with typical liver cancer may benefit from liver transplantation, but only if those patients are carefully selected and receive other treatment directed against the cancer.
♦ Cryosurgery holds some promise to allow the removal of otherwise unre-

sectable tumors, but the technique is done only by a few specialized physicians.

♦ Radiation and an antibody that identifies and attacks liver tumor cells (the polyclonal antiferritin antibody) may allow some patients to be treated surgically, as might chemoembolization.

ADVANCED DISEASE

The tumor involves all lobes of the liver and/or has spread to involve other organs such as the lungs, intra-abdominal lymph nodes or bone.

Standard Treatment No standard therapy is known to prolong survival. The usual approach is a trial of single-agent chemotherapy such as Adriamycin or 5-fluorouracil. Radiation to the tumor along with intravenous chemotherapy may relieve the pain of large liver masses, and radiation to painful bone or other metastases may also be appropriate.

Two-Year Survival Less than 5 percent

Investigational
♦ Combination chemotherapy or new drugs may prove to be better treatment than those currently available. These would best be administered in a clinical trial, rather than using random combinations.
♦ Chemoembolization may improve symptoms even if there is metastatic disease.
♦ Newer drugs, including Taxol and interferon, are being studied.

TREATING OTHER PRIMARY LIVER TUMORS

The approach taken with other primary liver tumors is generally the same as for hepatocellular carcinoma. Patients with these other tumors are more likely to be candidates for surgery because they usually do not have underlying liver disease.

ANGIOSARCOMA AND HEMANGIOENDOTHELIOMA

These diseases are less predictable than hepatocellular carcinoma and survival is variable.

♦ They may not have spread at the time of diagnosis and surgery should be considered.
♦ As in hepatocellular carcinoma, no systematic study of adjuvant chemotherapy or radiotherapy has been done.
♦ Localized unresectable disease may respond to the same intravenous chemotherapy used for sarcomas and the tumors may occasionally shrink enough to allow the surgeon to remove them completely.
♦ Advanced disease is approached in the same way as a sarcoma.

ADENOCARCINOMA

This type of tumor is approached in the same way as hepatocellular carcinoma. Its prognosis is similar.

SUPPORTIVE THERAPY

♦ Pain relievers are sometimes called for in liberal doses. Narcotics may have excessive side effects because they are metabolized by the liver, which may not be functioning properly.
♦ Non-steroidal anti-inflammatory drugs may be surprisingly effective even against the severe pain associated with liver cancer.
♦ Frequent small meals may be necessary to provide enough nutrition, since an enlarged liver might reduce the capacity of the stomach.
♦ The loss of appetite that frequently accompanies liver cancer may be relieved with a medication called Megace.
♦ The use of water pills to relieve fluid in the abdomen or legs may cause significant imbalance in kidney function and can create major problems if not carefully monitored.
♦ Nausea should be adequately treated with standard medications, including suppositories.
♦ Sleep disturbances are common. Most

sleeping pills are metabolized by the liver, however, so they should be used carefully.

TREATMENT FOLLOW-UP

Careful follow-up is important after the removal of localized liver cancer because patients are at risk for a second occurrence as well as tumor metastases. Such follow-up should include:

♦ Serum alpha-fetoprotein (AFP) every two to three months. A rising AFP suggests tumor recurrence, which might still be curable with further surgery.

♦ CT scans should be done every two to three months for the first year after surgery. Tumors are most likely to grow again within the first year and they may still be curable if caught in the early stages.

♦ The liver function of patients with underlying cirrhosis or hepatitis has to be closely monitored, since it may deteriorate after surgery.

THE MOST IMPORTANT QUESTIONS YOU CAN ASK

♦ Should I see another physician to confirm that this tumor can or cannot be removed for cure?

♦ Could I benefit from an investigational therapy available at another institution?

♦ How sick will the proposed chemotherapy or radiation treatment make me relative to the potential benefit?

♦ Should any tests be done on my spouse or children to see if they are at risk for developing this cancer?

♦ Is a liver transplant an option for me?

LUNG: NON-SMALL CELL

Alan B. Glassberg, MD, and Patricia Cornett, MD

◇

Lung cancer is the second most common cancer and the number one cause of cancer death. Although there has always been a higher incidence in men, the incidence in women has risen rapidly in recent years. In fact, lung cancer has now surpassed breast cancer as the number-one cancer killer of women. It has long been the number-one cancer killer of men.

An estimated 172,000 people will develop lung cancer in the U.S. in 1994, and about 153,000 people will die of it. This is especially unfortunate because it is one of the most preventable cancers. The cause is well known. Before tobacco use became popular, lung cancer was a rare disease. Furthermore, it has been estimated that if all tobacco were removed from the earth, the number of all cancers would fall by 17 percent.

There are two general types of lung cancer—small cell and non-small cell. The non-small cell variety is much more common, accounting for 75 percent of all lung cancer cases. Although some of these tumors can be cured by surgery, the overall five-year survival for people with this kind of cancer is only 10 percent. There has been no improvement in the survival rate in decades, which is a reflection of both the lack of a satisfactory screening test that could detect it in the early stages and, up to the present time, the lack of truly effective treatment with clear survival benefits.

Types Non-small cell cancer contains at least three distinct types—squamous cell, large cell and adenocarcinoma—but the treatment of all three is generally similar. Squamous cell carcinoma is the most common type, but for reasons not understood adenocarcinoma is increasing in frequency.

Squamous cell (epidermoid) carcinoma of the lung is the microscopic type most frequently related to smoking. This type is also more commonly associated with spread of the tumor to distant sites (metastasis), but surgical removal of the tumor along with the nearby lymph nodes more often produces a cure than in other types.

Adenocarcinoma of the lung accounts for 30 percent of all lung cancer cases. It is more common in women and is the most frequent type seen in non-smokers, although it occurs in smokers as well. It is more likely than other types to be in the peripheral portions of the lung (near the edge) and therefore may invade the lining of the chest and produce fluid in the chest cavity more commonly than in other types.

Large cell carcinoma of the lung is more commonly associated with spread of the tumor to the brain.

How It Spreads Non-small cell cancer can spread by the lymphatic system and through the blood. It can also directly invade to involve the center of the chest (mediastinum), the lining of the chest, the ribs or, if it is in the top part of the lung, the nerves and blood vessels leading into the arm. When this kind of cancer enters the bloodstream, it can spread to distant sites such as the liver, bones, brain and other places in the lung.

What Causes It Cigarette smoking has been a major factor in the development of both small cell and non-small cell lung cancers. The increase in cigarette smoking by men in the 1920s, apparently related to increased cigarette advertising about that time, was followed in the 1940s by a dramatic increase in the incidence of lung cancer in men. The marked increase in cigarette smoking by women in the 1940s, perhaps because it became more socially acceptable during the war, was unfortunately followed 20 years later by a similar increase in the incidence of lung cancer among women.

Lung tissue affected by the connective tissue disease scleroderma may be associated with bronchoalveolar carcinoma. Lung cancer may predispose a person to a higher incidence of developing another lung cancer later. Lung cancer may also occur at sites of old scars in the lung resulting from an infection (tuberculosis, for example) or injury (scar carcinoma).

RISK FACTORS

At Significantly Higher Risk
◆ Cigarette smokers.
◆ The male to female ratio remains 4 to 1. Peak incidence occurs between ages 50 and 60, with less than a 1 percent incidence under the age of 30 and about a 10 percent incidence in people over 70.
◆ Workers exposed to industrial substances such as asbestos, nickel, chromium compounds and chloromethyl ether, especially those who smoke.

At Slightly Higher Risk
◆ Patients with previous or pre-existing lung disease.
◆ Former smokers.
◆ People exposed to second-hand smoke over many years.
◆ People exposed to radon.

SCREENING

Lung cancer is very difficult to detect at an early stage. Tests such as the examination of sputum (phlegm) for malignant cells and regular chest x-rays have not proved to be beneficial. Cancer may be detected earlier in cigarette smokers, however, by regular chest x-rays.

COMMON SIGNS AND SYMPTOMS

A new or changing cough, sometimes containing blood, is a common symptom, along with hoarseness and shortness of breath or increased shortness of breath during exertion. There may also be an increase in the amount of sputum, recurrent episodes of lung infection (sometimes in the same lobe of the lung as the cancer), weight loss and swelling of the face or arms.

If the tumor has spread or metastasized, the symptoms can include severe headaches, double vision, and pain in bones, the chest, abdomen, neck and down the arms.

DIAGNOSIS

Physical Examination
◆ Lymph node enlargement in the neck or in the region above the collarbones.
◆ Enlarged liver or another mass in the abdomen.
◆ Signs of a mass in one lung such as decreased breath sounds, noises in the lung that are not usually present, or areas of dullness when the chest is tapped with the fingers.

Blood and Other Tests
◆ Sputum examination for malignant cells.

Imaging
◆ If a chest x-ray shows an abnormality, this does not establish a diagnosis until some tissue is obtained and examined under the microscope.
◆ CT scans of the chest and often the liver and adrenal glands.
◆ Sometimes CT or MRI scans of the brain.

Endoscopy and Biopsy
◆ Fiber-optic bronchoscopy with brushing

or biopsy.

♦ Mediastinoscopy with biopsies. In this procedure, a small incision is made at the base of the neck and a long thin tube called a mediastinoscope is inserted down to the lymph nodes in the middle of the chest. Tissue can be obtained through this instrument, and the procedure is safe and easy.

♦ Needle aspiration of a mass in the chest, often with CT guidance.

♦ Removal and analysis of fluid in the chest to detect tumor cells.

♦ Pleural (chest lining) biopsy.

♦ Lymph node biopsy.

♦ Bone biopsy.

♦ Liver biopsy.

♦ Biopsy of a nodule during surgery.

♦ DNA analysis. With the advent of genetic probe studies, certain genes appear to be more frequent in patients who develop lung cancer. Patients with amplification of the k-*ras* oncogene, for example, have a much worse prognosis. There may come a time when we can have our genes analyzed and be made aware of our risks, not only for lung cancer but for other cancers as well.

STAGING

Once a diagnosis of a malignant tumor is made, further staging studies are carried out because the stage of disease determines prognosis and the selection of treatment.

Stage is based on a combination of clinical findings (physical examination, chest x-ray and lab studies) and pathologic findings (biopsy). The stages are now commonly defined according to the TNM classification.

TREATMENT OVERVIEW

 Surgery Surgical treatment—removal of the tumor—remains the mainstay of curative treatment for non-small cell lung cancer. This will involve removing a lobe of the lung or, if appropriate, a wedge resection of the tumor. Sometimes the entire lung has to be removed.

 Radiation If surgery is not considered feasible either because of the patient's condition or because the lymph nodes are so involved that surgery could not remove all the cancer, then radiation therapy can be used as the primary treatment.

 Chemotherapy The role of chemotherapy has not yet been completely defined, although it has been found to be more successful since the advent of platinum compounds. Up through Stage II disease, the response rate has been reported to be in excess of 50 percent. In Stage IV disease, the response rate is lower.

When a platinum drug is combined with drugs such as vinblastine, vindesine or etoposide, response rates of about 30 percent have been observed in Stage IV cancer. Although there is no evidence of major survival improvement by the use of these agents in Stage IV disease, they may give palliative benefit by reducing the size of the tumors and relieving the symptoms. Recent trials using a cisplatin-based regimen showed a four- to five-month improvement in average survival. This exciting work has suggested that chemotherapy might be used earlier in treatment in hopes of improving survival.

Neoadjuvant Chemotherapy and Radiation New protocols to explore curative strategies in lung cancer include using chemotherapy, radiation therapy or both before surgery to try to convert some patients from an inoperable stage to one where the tumor can be removed. Examples are the use of cancer chemotherapy initially in Stage IIIB lung cancer patients. Several studies have indicated that this approach may be beneficial, although it is too early to make any definite claims about this technique.

In view of the poor survival rate in Stage IIIA lung cancer, similar studies have been carried out using chemotherapy and radiation therapy before surgery in patients who are potentially operable. Again, preliminary results are providing optimism about the future management of locally advanced lung cancer.

 Laser Therapy Laser bronchoscopy with light-sensitizers has been an interesting experimental technique to try to open the airways when they are blocked by a tumor (*see* Chapter 9).

Bone Marrow Transplantation A general principle of chemotherapy has been to increase the dose to increase the destruction of tumor cells. Generally, the amount of chemotherapy that can be given is limited by the effect of the drugs on the bone marrow. If these effects could be overcome, higher dosages could be given.

Accordingly, autologous bone marrow transplantation is being investigated. In this technique, bone marrow is removed from the patient and stored while very high doses of chemotherapy are administered. This could be lethal but the patient is "rescued" by reinfusion of his or her own bone marrow, which then grows back. It is not yet known whether this will result in longer survival.

TREATMENT BY STAGE

STAGE I
TNM T1–2, N0, M0
The tumor can be removed surgically and has not spread to involve the lymph nodes.

Standard Treatment If possible, the lobe of the involved lung with the tumor in place is removed along with the nearby lymph nodes. Sometimes the entire lung on one side needs to be removed to insure that all of the tumor is resected.

In patients with a small (T1) tumor, or

in patients with impaired lung function, only a wedge resection, which removes the tumor with a small amount of surrounding tissue, is done.

In those patients with severe lung or heart disease who cannot tolerate surgery, radiation therapy is sometimes used.

Five-Year Survival 30 to 80 percent

STAGE II
TNM T1–2, N1, M0
The tumor has spread to the hilar nodes.

Standard Treatment This stage is likewise treated with surgery. Once again, patients unable to withstand this kind of rigorous surgery may be candidates for radiation therapy with intent to cure.

Five-Year Survival 10 to 35 percent

Investigational
♦ Trials are exploring the use of radiation therapy and/or chemotherapy before surgery to see if the cure rate can be improved.

STAGE IIIA
TNM T1–2, N2, M0 or T3, N0–2, M0
Stage III is divided into IIIA and IIIB. Both show involvement of nodes in the center of the chest, but Stage IIIA tumors may be removed under certain circumstances.

Standard Treatment These tumors are treated mainly with radiation therapy, surgery or both, depending on the clinical circumstances.

Although most patients do not completely respond to radiation therapy alone, 5 to 10 percent do experience long-term survival benefit.

Radiation therapy is frequently given after surgery. Although there is no evidence that this improves survival, there can be a decrease in recurrences at the original tumor site.

Patients whose tumors invade the chest

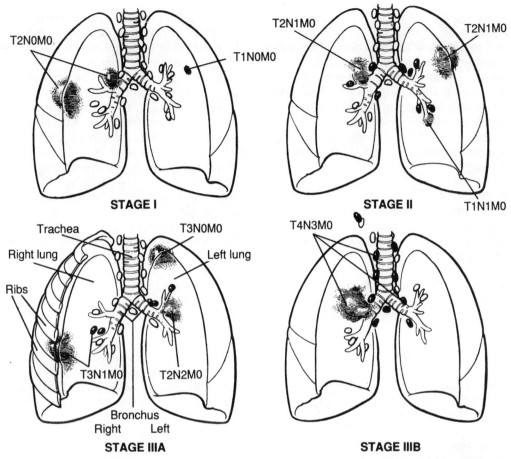

Stages of lung cancer, showing size and location of primary cancer, and lymph nodal involvement
Credit: Based on drawings in *Contemporary Internal Medicine* Sept. 1990.

wall can sometimes be treated with surgery, which may involve the removal of some of the chest wall, including ribs. Radiation therapy is often used along with surgery.

Some patents with extensive metastatic disease in the center of the chest may develop what is called the superior vena cava syndrome, in which the great vessels in the chest are compressed by the tumor. When this involves the large vein that returns blood to the heart, the blood gets backed up into the tissues of the neck, head and arms. This is an urgent situation and patients should be given prompt radiation therapy.

A special situation under Stage III is called a superior sulcus tumor, which involves cancers in the top of the lung that invade local nerves and cause pain in the arm. These tumors seem to have a reduced potential for distant metastases, so local radiation therapy is possible for cure. Surgery is frequently used after radiation.

Five-Year Survival 10 to 15 percent

Investigational
♦ Adjuvant chemotherapy must still be considered investigational, but it can provide a slight increase in disease-free sur-

vival and a trend toward improved overall survival.

♦ Treatment with radiation or chemotherapy or both before surgery has been used on an investigational basis. Preliminary results suggest that there may be benefit by combining all three treatments in selected cases. Newer trials are giving cisplatin with etoposide or other agents together with radiation, followed by surgery.

STAGE IIIB
TNM Any T, N3, M0 or T4, any N, M0
The tumor cannot be removed because of technical reasons or because there would be no benefit to the patient.

Standard Treatment These tumors are best managed with radiation therapy. Surgery usually has no benefit at this stage.

Five-Year Survival Less than 5 percent

Investigational
♦ Trials are examining the effectiveness of chemotherapy and/or radiation therapy before surgery. These treatments have occasionally converted some patients to an operable stage, but it is too soon to know if using this aggressive approach will increase the rate of cure.

STAGE IV
TNM Any T, any N, M1
The cancer has spread to distant sites.

Standard Treatment Metastatic disease cannot be cured by surgery, so treatment for this stage is directed toward relieving symptoms with either radiation therapy or chemotherapy.

Radiation may relieve local symptoms such as tracheal, esophageal or bronchial compression, bone or brain metastases, pain, vocal cord paralysis, coughing blood (hemoptysis) or superior vena cava syndrome. Patients without symptoms should be kept under close observation. Sometimes treatment may appropriately be deferred until symptoms or signs of a progressive tumor develop.

Chemotherapy with, for example, a platinum compound combined with drugs such as vinblastine, vindesine, etoposide or mitomycin-C has response rates of about 30 percent in Stage IV cases. Although there has been no evidence of major survival improvement with these agents, they may give palliative benefit by reducing the size of the tumors and relieving symptoms.

Recent trials using a cisplatin-based regimen of chemotherapy showed some survival benefit and give hope for more benefit in the future. Combinations currently in use include: cisplatin + etoposide, carboplatin + etoposide, cisplatin + mitomycin-C + vinblastine and cisplatin + etoposide + ifosfamide.

Other potentially useful adjuncts to the treatment of advanced lung cancer include feeding gastrostomies when the esophagus is obstructed by the cancer and the use of lasers to open up an airway obstructed by a tumor mass.

Adjuvant or neoadjuvant protocols may be useful.

Five-Year Survival Less than 5 percent

Investigational
♦ New drugs that may be effective include Taxol, CPT-11, topotecan and navelbine.

SUPPORTIVE THERAPY

The importance of supportive therapy in the treatment of lung cancer cannot be overemphasized.
♦ Quite clearly, malnutrition results in a bad outcome in patients with lung cancer. Patients must be served a palatable meal and attempts must be made to work with patients to determine food likes and dislikes.
♦ Pain control is of critical importance,

and the tools to achieve control are available even for the most advanced cases. These include the use of pain-relieving (analgesic) drugs such as non-steroidal anti-inflammatory agents, mild narcotics, strong narcotics, continuous narcotics and narcotics delivered into the spinal canal (epidural). Pain control can generally be achieved without interfering with mental competence.

♦ Nausea can be controlled with a variety of drugs (*see* Chapter 17).

♦ Physical therapy will help maintain muscle strength to keep life as normal as possible.

Maintaining the Quality of Life In the management of lung cancer (as well as all other malignancies), it is critical that the patient maintain as high a quality of life as possible. Patients must feel that they are contributing members of society. Certainly, this keeps them in a happier mental frame.

Being with family and friends, going out to meals and movies and participating in enjoyable recreational events are all important parts of maintaining lifestyle. Family members and physicians should try to provide as much of this as possible. With the services now available, it is usually possible to maintain these goals.

However, when the time comes that patients are no longer able to participate in such activities, we must all be sensible enough to ensure comfort by whatever methods we can. Even if mental ability has been compromised in order to relieve the pain, pain control should come first and remain all-important. Comfort care is the key phrase at this stage of life.

TREATMENT FOLLOW-UP

People who have lung cancer have to be followed carefully by their physicians, generally being examined every one to three months during the first two years, for that is when the risk of relapse is greatest.

♦ Chest x-ray every three to four months in the absence of symptoms.

♦ Chest x-rays more often should symptoms occur.

♦ Blood chemistry tests every three to four months.

♦ Physical examination of the chest, lymph nodes and abdomen.

♦ Neurologic examination.

♦ After two years, follow-up every six months with x-rays and blood surveillance.

Patients should, of course, see their physician if any unusual symptoms occur.

RECURRENT CANCER

See treatment for Stage IV disease.

THE MOST IMPORTANT QUESTIONS YOU CAN ASK

♦ What is the stage of my disease and what is my prognosis?

♦ What is the role of surgery and what is the chance of it curing me?

♦ What is the role of radiation therapy?

♦ How sick will I be on chemotherapy and can we control the sickness?

♦ If chemotherapy cannot cure my cancer, why should I expose myself to its side effects and toxicities?

♦ What is the chance that I will die from this tumor? How much time am I likely to have?

LUNG: SMALL CELL

Alan B. Glassberg, MD, and Patricia Cornett, MD

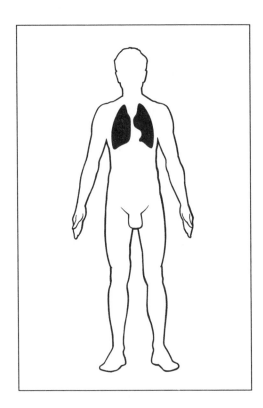

In 1994, there will be 172,000 new cases of lung cancer in the United States. Small cell lung cancer accounts for about a quarter of all lung cancer cases. Also called oat cell carcinoma of the lung, it has the most rapid clinical course of any type of lung cancer, with average survival from diagnosis of only several months without treatment. Compared with other types of lung cancer, small cell carcinoma has a greater tendency to have spread widely by the time of diagnosis, but is more responsive to treatment with chemotherapy and radiation than are the other types of lung cancer.

Seventy percent of patients with small cell carcinoma of the lung have distant metastases at the time of diagnosis. With modern staging procedures, the areas of spread can be discovered in two-thirds of these patients.

Small cell cancer is not always confined to the lung. Occasionally it may occur in other organs such as the esophagus or cervix and sometimes may occur without the primary site of origin being identified. The management of these tumors will be addressed in chapters concerning those organs; chemotherapy remains the fundamental basic treatment.

Types There are several types of small cell lung cancer, defined by the tumor's appearance under the microscope. These include small cell, mixed small cell/large cell and combined small cell. It is unclear whether these types of tumor have different prognoses.

This tumor arises from what are called neuroendocrine cells and is known as an APUD (amine precursor uptake decarboxylation) tumor. Under the electron microscope, hormone-producing (neurosecretory) granules can be seen. These tumors, therefore, can abnormally produce hormones and cause what have been known as paraneoplastic syndromes. For example, if the tumor produces too much cortisone, the condition is called Cushing's syndrome. If antidiuretic hormone (ADH) is produced, water is retained in the body and the apparent salt (sodium) level decreases. Each of these paraneoplastic syndromes produces its own signs and symptoms.

How It Spreads Small cell lung cancer can spread via lymphatic vessels to the lymph nodes in the center of the lung (hilar nodes), the center of the chest (mediastinal nodes), in the neck and above the collarbone (supraclavicular nodes), and in the abdominal cavity. It is likely to spread through the bloodstream to the liver, lungs, brain and bone.

What Causes It Cigarette smoking has been a major factor in the development of both small cell and non-small cell lung cancers. The increase in cigarette smoking by men in the 1920s, apparently related to increased cigarette advertising about that time, was followed in the 1940s by a dramatic increase in the incidence of lung cancer in men. The marked increase in cigarette smoking by women in the 1940s, perhaps because it became more socially acceptable during the war, was unfortunately followed 20 years later by a similar increase in the incidence of lung cancer among women. It has been estimated that if all tobacco disappeared from the earth, 17 percent of all cancers would also disappear. The attempt to discontinue cigarette smoking remains one of the most crucial medical issues in our society.

Lung cancer may predispose a person to a higher risk of developing another lung cancer later.

RISK FACTORS

There are no specific environmental or genetic factors known except those discussed in the section on non-small cell lung cancer.

At Significantly Higher Risk
♦ Cigarette smokers.
♦ Workers exposed to industrial substances such as asbestos, nickel, chromium compounds and chloromethyl ether and/or air pollutants.

SCREENING

There is no good screening test for this kind of cancer.

COMMON SIGNS AND SYMPTOMS

As with non-small cell cancer, a new or changing cough, sometimes containing blood, is a common symptom, along with hoarseness and shortness of breath or increased shortness of breath on exertion. There may also be an increase in the amount of sputum, recurrent episodes of lung infection (sometimes in the same lobe of the lung as the cancer), weight loss and swelling of the face or arms.

If the tumor has metastasized, the symptoms can include severe headaches, double vision, and pain in the bones, chest, abdomen, neck and down the arms.

One point that needs to be emphasized is that this disease is usually widespread at the time of diagnosis.

DIAGNOSIS

The diagnosis of small cell lung cancer is usually apparent by routine microscopy. Other techniques that may be useful in selected cases, particularly when the diagnosis is in doubt, include electron microscopy, which detects the small cell cancer's neuroendocrine granules, and immunocytochemical stains, which can detect certain markers characteristic for small cell cancer. Newer techniques, still investigational, include examining the tumor DNA for chromosome abnormalities, overexpression of oncogenes and deletion of tumor suppressor genes.

Blood and Other Tests
♦ Chemistry profile.
♦ Sputum (phlegm) examination.
♦ Removal of fluid from the chest and examination of it for malignant cells.

Imaging
♦ Chest x-ray.
♦ CT scan of the chest and abdomen.
♦ MRI or CT scan of the brain.
♦ Bone scan.

Endoscopy and Biopsy
♦ Fiber-optic bronchoscopy with brushings or biopsy.
♦ Mediastinoscopy with biopsies. In this safe and easy procedure, a small incision is made at the base of the neck and a long thin tube called a mediastinoscope is inserted down to the lymph nodes in the middle of the chest. Tissue can be removed through this instrument for analysis.
♦ Needle biopsy through the chest wall, under local anesthetic and often under CT guidance.
♦ Biopsies of the chest lining, lymph nodes, bone and liver.

STAGING
The detailed staging techniques and classifications used for non-small cell lung cancer are not commonly used for small cell lung cancer. Instead, the staging system focuses on whether disease is limited or extensive. The stage of the tumor (limited vs. extensive) will determine the prognosis and may affect the choice of treatment.

The staging procedures commonly used to document distant metastases include bone marrow examination, CT scans of the brain and liver and radionuclide bone scans. MRI scans can also be used to evaluate the brain and bones.

Limited-stage means that tumor is confined to the side of the chest where it originated, the mediastinum and the supraclavicular nodes. This area can be encompassed within a tolerable radiotherapy port. There is no universally accepted definition of "limited-stage." Patients with fluid around the lung (pleural effusion), massive or multiple pulmonary tumor masses on the same side and enlarged supraclavicular nodes on the opposite side have been both included in and excluded from "limited-stage" by various treatment centers.

Extensive-stage disease means that tumor is too widespread to be included within the definition of limited-stage disease. (*See* next page.)

TREATMENT OVERVIEW
At the time of diagnosis, about one-third of patients with small cell lung carcinoma will have limited-stage disease. Most people who survive at least two years without a recurrence of the cancer come from this group. In limited disease, average survival of 10 to 16 months is a reasonable expectation with current treatments. The small proportion of patients with limited disease who can undergo surgery have an even better prognosis.

With extensive-stage disease, the prognosis is worse. Average survival is 6 to 12 months with current treatments. There is long-term disease-free survival in some patients, so treatment is certainly recommended. Patients who achieve a complete response to treatment (the tumor appears to go away completely) have the best overall survival.

In small cell lung cancer, 10 to 20 percent of patients may achieve long-term remissions with aggressive combined radiation and chemotherapy. Most of the improvement in survival has been the result of treatments discovered by clinical trials.

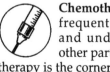

Surgery Removing the primary tumor produces little benefit with this type of cancer, although a very small number of patients might possibly benefit from surgery followed by adjuvant chemotherapy. This is an option only for those whose lung function is adequate and whose tumor is confined to the lung where it started or to the lung and the hilar lymph nodes on the same side.

Chemotherapy Because of the frequent presence of hidden and undetectable spread to other parts of the body, chemotherapy is the cornerstone of treatment for small cell lung cancer, since it also treats tumors too small to detect. Once remission is achieved, there is no evidence that maintenance therapy is beneficial. There is little evidence that more than six months of treatment is of value.

 Radiation Doses in the range of 4,000 to 5,000 cGy or more are needed to control chest tumors effectively. If radiation therapy is given with combination chemotherapy, there are higher response rates and better survival than when radiation therapy is given alone. Radiation therapy plus combination chemotherapy is also superior to chemotherapy alone for controlling the primary chest tumor, but there is no evidence that this approach provides better control for metastatic disease.

Studies have shown some survival benefit when combined therapy is given, especially in limited disease, so long as radiation therapy does not result in a delay of the administration of proper doses of chemotherapy. There are increased side effects with combined programs, and some treatment-related mortality because of lung and bone marrow toxicities.

Some patients have a tumor mass in the center of the chest that presses on the large vein draining blood from the head and arms (the superior vena cava). This pressure causes a fluid backup, resulting in swelling of the face and arms and sometimes even the brain. If this superior vena cava syndrome is present, combination chemotherapy alone can be given or radiation therapy given with it.

Because of the high frequency of brain metastases in small cell lung cancer, especially in patients with prolonged survival, prophylactic radiation of the head has been used by many physicians. This reduces the frequency of subsequent brain metastases, especially in patients with complete responses to therapy, but has not been shown to influence survival. There may be late complications of this type of treatment, with significant neurologic, mental and thinking deficits in some long-term survivors who were given high daily dose fractionation. It may be preferable to give smaller doses each day.

It must also be emphasized that many treatment centers do not recommend the use of prophylactic brain irradiation because there has not been ample proof of a survival benefit and there is a valid concern about the neurologic side effects of the treatment. If necessary, radiation therapy can be given when the brain metastases are demonstrated to occur.

TREATMENT BY STAGE

LIMITED STAGE

Standard Treatment Limited-stage small cell lung cancer is highly responsive to treatment with combination chemotherapy. Multiple drugs are clearly superior to single-agent treatment. Current programs give objective response rates (the tumor gets smaller) of 80 to 90 percent, with complete response rates (the tumor disappears) of 45 to 75 percent. Radiation therapy given with the chemotherapy may improve the survival rate.

As noted, a small minority of limited-stage patients without evidence of tumor in the mediastinum might benefit from surgery followed by adjuvant chemotherapy.

Two-Year Survival 15 percent

EXTENSIVE STAGE

Standard Treatment Extensive-stage small cell lung cancer patients are given chemotherapy in much the same fashion as those with limited-stage disease. Current programs result in response rates of 70 to 85 percent and complete response rates of 20 to 30 percent.

Commonly used combination chemotherapy regimens include CAV (cyclophosphamide + Adriamycin + vincristine), CAVP16 (cyclophosphamide + Adriamycin + etoposide) and VPP (cisplatin + etoposide).

There is no pressing need to include chest irradiation with combination chemotherapy, but radiotherapy may relieve symptoms caused by the primary tumor or metastatic disease. For example, symptoms from brain metastases and pain from bone metastases can be promptly relieved with radiation.

If the superior vena cava syndrome is present, chest irradiation may result in a very rapid initial response.

Two-Year Survival 2 percent

TREATMENT FOLLOW-UP

After treatment is completed, patients should be seen every one or two months for at least two years. Visits can then be spread out, perhaps every four months for two years and every six months for another two years.

During the first two years, follow-up should include:

♦ Physical examination of the lungs, chest wall, lymph nodes and abdomen.

♦ Chest x-ray every three to four months, or more frequently if indicated.

♦ Blood chemistry tests every three to four months.

♦ Neurologic examination.

RECURRENT CANCER

If small cell lung cancer recurs, the prognosis is very poor regardless of stage or treatment. The expected average survival is two to three months, so a patient should be considered for either palliative therapy or participation in clinical trials.

♦ Palliative therapy could include chemotherapy agents that have not yet been used or radiation therapy for bone metastases or when otherwise appropriate.

♦ Other palliative treatments include measures for pain relief and orthopedic aids.

THE MOST IMPORTANT QUESTIONS YOU CAN ASK

♦ What is the stage of my disease and what is my prognosis?

♦ How sick will I be on chemotherapy and what can be done to control the side effects?

♦ If chemotherapy cannot cure my cancer, why should I expose myself to its side effects and toxicities?

♦ What is the chance that I will die from this tumor? How much time am I likely to have?

♦ Are there investigational protocols for which I may be eligible?

LYMPHOMA: AIDS-ASSOCIATED

Alexandra M. Levine, MD

◇

Lymphoma is not one disease, but rather consists of about 20 different types of tumors. In general, lymphoma is a cancer of a type of white blood cell called the lymphocyte, an extremely important cell in the immune system. In lymphoma, the lymphocytes start to grow for no known reason and continue to grow and expand, seemingly unable to stop. The result is enlargement of lymph glands or other organs in which lymphocytes normally grow and the development of "lumps and bumps" on the body. Dysfunction of various organs may also develop as the abnormal lymphocytes grow, taking up so much space that normal cells don't have room to function.

Types The lymphomas occurring in people infected with the human immunodeficiency virus (HIV) are high-grade, B cell lymphomas. These are tumors that grow very rapidly. They usually consist of either small non-cleaved lymphoma (also called Burkitt's lymphoma) or immunoblastic lymphoma.

What Causes It It is not known why some HIV-infected patients develop lymphoma, while most do not.

Who Gets It All people with HIV infection are at increased risk for developing lymphoma. Lymphoma is an initial AIDS-defining condition in about 3 percent of patients with HIV disease, and the incidence increases in time. The chance of developing lymphoma is about 20 percent approximately three years after a diagnosis of AIDS.

SCREENING

There is no way to screen for this disease and no reason to do so, unless there are certain symptoms or findings that suggest lymphoma.

COMMON SIGNS AND SYMPTOMS

People with lymphoma usually develop abnormal lumps or bumps. This could be an enlarged lymph gland or an enlarged lump almost anywhere in the body, including the jaw, the stomach cavity, the skin, the liver or elsewhere.

If lymphoma first starts in the stomach or intestines, the first symptom might be belly pain or a bloating or enlargement of the abdominal area. If lymphoma first begins in the bone marrow (the factory where all blood cells are made), the initial symptom might be bone pain or anemia (lowering of the red blood cell count, causing weakness and fatigue).

Aside from tumor masses, "systemic B symptoms" may develop as the first manifestation of disease. These include persistent fever, drenching night sweats (so that the bed linens have to be changed several times each night) and/or the loss of more than 10 percent of the normal body weight.

DIAGNOSIS

The diagnosis of lymphoma can be made only after biopsy. The biopsy is taken from the specific area of abnormality, such as an enlarged lymph gland or other mass.

STAGING

Several tests are performed to determine the precise extent of lymphoma before starting treatment. This staging work-up usually includes a CT scan of the chest, abdomen and pelvis, a gallium scan, a bone marrow biopsy and a spinal tap to see if there are lymphoma cells floating in the spinal fluid surrounding the brain and spinal cord. If there are symptoms or other evidence suggesting involvement of the bones, stomach or other specific areas, tests such as x-rays may be done.

TREATMENT OVERVIEW

Several factors affect the prognosis and, therefore, the decisions about treatment. Factors associated with poorer prognosis include a history of AIDS before the diagnosis of lymphoma, T4 cells less than 200, a low performance status (the patient is weak and debilitated instead of vigorous and strong), involvement of the bone marrow (stage IV lymphoma) and the presence of primary central nervous system lymphoma, in which the only place the lymphoma is found is in the brain.

Having lymphoma in the body and also lymphoma cells in the spinal fluid is not a bad prognostic sign, provided that the spinal fluid is treated for involvement.

Very intensive regimens of multi-agent chemotherapy have traditionally been used for patients with lymphoma not associated with AIDS. But those with AIDS-related lymphoma may be treated more effectively and safely with low dosages of chemotherapy drugs. These are given along with additional chemotherapy into the spinal fluid to prevent relapse in this important site. If complete remission is achieved—in other words, all evidence of the disease disappears, with a return to a state of well being—no further maintenance therapy or other treatment is given.

 Chemotherapy Multiple chemotherapy drugs are given, usually once each month, for four to six months.

♦ One commonly used regimen is a low-dose modification of M-BACOD, consisting of methotrexate, bleomycin, Adriamycin, Cytoxan, Oncovin and Decadron.

♦ CHOP—Cytoxan, Adriamycin, Oncovin and prednisone—is also commonly used.

These agents are given by vein during the first day of each monthly cycle. During the first month of therapy, spinal taps are repeated once a week for four weeks. Specific chemotherapy drugs such as cytosine arabinoside (Ara-C) or methotrexate are injected directly into the spinal fluid to prevent relapse in this site.

 Radiation If the brain is involved by lymphoma, radiation therapy will also be given. But for all practical purposes, there is no such thing as localizing AIDS-related lymphoma. All patients must receive multi-agent chemotherapy in order to achieve cure. Local radiation therapy alone is not expected to be effective in the long run.

SUPPORTIVE THERAPY

Many forms of supportive therapy can be given to someone with AIDS-related lymphoma undergoing chemotherapy.

♦ Medicines to prevent nausea and vomiting should be given routinely. Zofran, a new and extremely effective anti-nausea medicine, is given by vein just before the chemotherapy. Zofran or other anti-nausea medications should also be given for use on an outpatient basis.

♦ Neupogen (G-CSF) is an important new medicine that can limit the decrease of normal white blood cells caused by chemotherapy. When the level of these normal white blood cells (granulocytes or polys) is lowered by chemotherapy, patients are at an increased risk for developing serious, even life-threatening infection. Patients can inject themselves with Neupogen under the skin, similar to an insulin injection.

The G-CSF is begun on the day following chemotherapy and is continued until the white blood cells have fully recovered (about 10 days). G-CSF can prevent serious infection, decrease the number of days spent in the hospital for infections and decrease the need for antibiotics, which can be very expensive.

♦ If the red blood cell count becomes low because of the chemotherapy, erythropoietin (EPO or Procrit) can be given three times a week by injection under the skin, similar to G-CSF. This will increase the bone marrow's production of red blood cells and improve or resolve the anemia possibly caused by the chemotherapy.

♦ Medication to prevent *Pneumocystis carinii* pneumonia (PCP) is mandatory during and for at least three months after chemotherapy, regardless of the T4 count.

Psychological Support There is a close relationship between mind and body, and it is very important for people with AIDS-related lymphoma to maintain their "fight" and will to live. A positive attitude helps them work *with* the chemotherapy in attempting to cure the lymphoma.

Anything that can be done to maintain this fighting attitude is useful. This might include meditation, prayer, participation in support groups, acupuncture, exercises, talking to a psychologist, psychiatrist, family members or friends and other such endeavors.

TREATMENT FOLLOW-UP

A CT scan is repeated after about two to four months of chemotherapy to be sure that all the sites of lymphoma have responded well to the chemotherapy. When complete remission is documented on the scan, an additional two cycles of chemotherapy will be given in an attempt to prevent the lymphoma from coming back.

When chemotherapy has been stopped, follow-up includes visits to the physician once each month or more frequently, depending on other illnesses or conditions.

♦ Routine blood tests are obtained, including a chemistry panel and a complete blood count (CBC).

♦ An elevation of the LDH is an important indication that the lymphoma might have relapsed, so this test should be routinely ordered during follow-up.

♦ A physical exam should also be performed once each month and a careful history taken to see if any new symptoms have developed.

♦ The CT scan should be repeated in six months and yearly thereafter. A CT scan should also be repeated if any new symptoms or findings on physical exam develop or if the LDH becomes elevated.

THE MOST IMPORTANT QUESTIONS YOU CAN ASK

♦ Have you treated other patients with AIDS-related lymphoma?

♦ What specific type of lymphoma do I have and what is its extent in my body?

♦ What regimen of chemotherapy will be used?

♦ Will you use G-CSF?

♦ Will you let me participate in my own care in terms of sharing my lab values, test results and so forth with me?

LYMPHOMA: HODGKIN'S DISEASE

Sandra J. Horning, MD, and Russell Hardy, MD

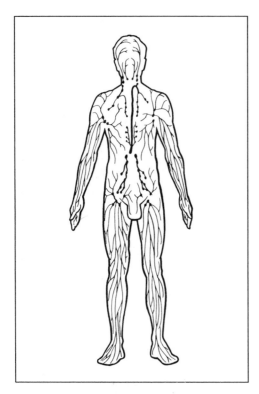

Hodgkin's disease—also called Hodgkin's lymphoma—is a cancer of the lymphoid system. It has special historical interest because it was the first malignancy of the lymphoid system to be described. The first cases were reported in 1832 by British physician Thomas Hodgkin, who recognized that this disorder was distinct from other causes of enlarged lymph nodes such as tuberculosis or other infectious diseases. Hodgkin's lymphoma has characteristic features that distinguish it from all the other cancers of the lymphoid system, and so these other cancers have come to be collectively referred to as non-Hodgkin's lymphomas.

Hodgkin's disease (HD) is an uncommon malignancy. Hodgkin's and non-Hodgkin's lymphomas combined account for 6 percent of newly diagnosed cancers each year, with HD accounting for only 15 percent of all lymphomas. In 1994, about 7,900 new cases of HD will be diagnosed in the U.S. out of a total of 1.2 million new cases of cancer. Despite the relatively low incidence, it is an important disease because it afflicts adolescents and young adults and because it has a substantial cure rate. Treatment is approached with much optimism.

The systematic approach to the pathologic diagnosis, staging, treatment strategies and clinical trials that have been developed for Hodgkin's disease over the past 30 years serves as a model for all modern cancer therapy. These methods transformed an almost always fatal disease into one of the most curable cancers. With so many cases being cured, attention has recently turned toward the complications of therapy and issues of "survivorship." Here again, HD is leading the way in treatment design and evaluation.

Types The malignant cell characteristic of Hodgkin's disease is known as the Reed-Sternberg cell, named after the two pathologists who first described it. One feature unique to Hodgkin's disease among other cancers is that the "tumors" contain very few cancer cells. In most cases, the affected lymph nodes contain mixtures of mostly normal and less frequent malignant cells. It is believed that the collections of normal cells and scar tissue within affected lymph nodes represent a host response to the tumor cells. Occasionally it can be very difficult or impossible to locate a single diagnostic Reed-Sternberg cell, but Reed-Sternberg "variants" or atypical large cells are regularly identified in HD tissues.

Like the non-Hodgkin's lymphomas, Hodgkin's is divided into sub-types according to the appearance of the affected lymph nodes under the microscope. In the commonly used scheme called the Rye classification, there are four major categories based on the types and arrangements of malignant and non-malignant cells and on associated pathologic features. Each sub-type is associated with characteristic age groups, sex and stages of the disease, but because of the overall success of therapy, sub-type generally has less prognostic importance in HD than in the non-Hodgkin's lymphomas.

RYE CLASSIFICATION

Nodular sclerosis (NS) The affected lymph node has nodules of normal lymphocytes and other "reactive" cells, together with Reed-Sternberg cells, separated by bands of scar-like tissue. This is the most common type of HD and is the only type more common in women than in men. It is usually found as a limited-stage disease involving the lymph nodes of the lower neck, above the collarbones and within the chest in adolescents and young adults. This type is unusual in people over age 50.

Lymphocyte predominant (LP) The affected lymph nodes are composed largely of reactive lymphocytes. The malignant cells have a "popcorn" appearance, distinct from Reed-Sternberg cells (which are rare in this sub-type). The cells may be arrayed in a nodular or diffuse pattern. This type is most common in people under 35 and affects men more frequently than women. The disease is most often in

limited stage when it is discovered and patients rarely have symptoms at the time of diagnosis. Recent information has linked the nodular variety to the B cell of the immune system, similar to most non-Hodgkin's lymphomas. Some pathologists and clinicians feel this sub-type should be reclassified as a non-Hodgkin's lymphoma.

Mixed cellularity (MC) The affected lymph node contains a mixture of inflammatory cells in addition to abundant Reed-Sternberg cells. Adults with this type are often older and have widespread disease at the time of diagnosis.

Lymphocyte depletion (LD) This is the least common variant and is usually discovered in an advanced stage. Two forms have been described. One has abundant scar-like tissue (fibrosis) with sparse lymphocytes and Reed-Sternberg cells. The other has sheets of malignant cells of different sizes and shapes. It is important to distinguish this sub-type from non-Hodgkin's lymphoma.

How It Spreads One of the unique features of Hodgkin's disease is its pattern of spread. As a rule, HD progresses in an orderly fashion from one lymph node group to the next group on the same side (ipsilateral) or the opposite side (contralateral). Non-Hodgkin's lymphomas, by contrast, are often widespread at diagnosis.

The most characteristic pattern of HD spread is extension of the disease from the lymph nodes in the neck (cervical) to the nodes above the collarbones (supraclavicular), then to the nodes under the arms (axillary) and within the chest (mediastinal and hilar). Although there are different patterns, it is unusual to find areas that have been "skipped," meaning that no apparent disease is found at a site where it would be expected by the rule of orderly progression.

Hodgkin's disease often involves the

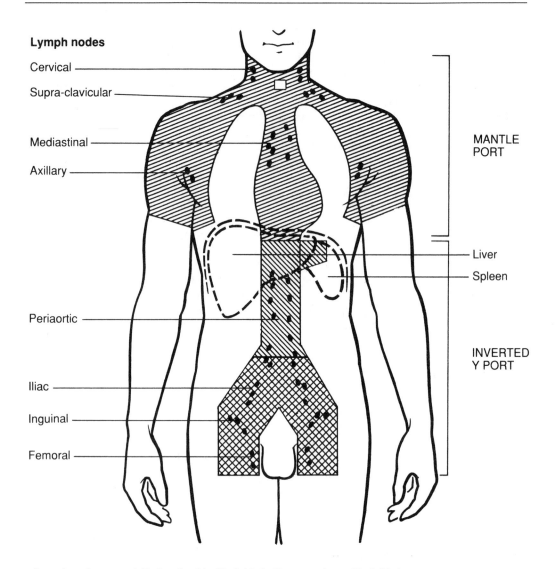

Lymph nodes

Cervical

Supra-clavicular

Mediastinal

Axillary

Periaortic

Iliac

Inguinal

Femoral

MANTLE
PORT

Liver

Spleen

INVERTED
Y PORT

Lymph nodes potentially involved in Hodgkin's disease and non-Hodgkin's lymphomas, and radiotherapy fields

spleen and may spread to the liver, bone and bone marrow. Involvement of the central nervous system is extremely rare.

What Causes It Unknown. There is a theory that HD is the rare result, possibly determined by genetics, of an infection acquired in late adolescence or early adult-hood. Family clusters have been reported and several viruses have been suggested as the cause, but no genetic or infectious basis for the disease has been proved.

RISK FACTORS

In developed countries there are two peaks of incidence of Hodgkin's disease, the first in young adults (ages 15 to 35) and the second after age 50. Men are affected slightly more commonly than women.

The frequency of the various sub-types depends on age. At the National Cancer Institute, where the majority of patients are young, nodular sclerosis accounts for 70 percent of cases and lymphocyte predominant for 15 percent. Mixed cellularity and lymphocyte depletion are more common in the elderly, in socioeconomically underdeveloped areas and in people with AIDS.

There are no clearly established risk factors for Hodgkin's disease, although in the United States there is some increased risk with small family size, higher education and higher socioeconomic position. Brothers and sisters of people with Hodgkin's disease have an incidence seven times higher than in the general population. Sophisticated studies are in progress to explore the genetics of Hodgkin's disease.

SCREENING

There are no known effective ways to screen for Hodgkin's disease other than a physical examination and a chest x-ray when an enlarged lymph node is found.

COMMON SIGNS AND SYMPTOMS

People who develop Hodgkin's disease often see their physicians because of the persistent swelling of painless lymph nodes in the neck or underarms. The swollen nodes may be the only sign of disease or they may be accompanied by unexplained fevers, chills, night sweats, weight loss or itching.

Young people with limited disease usually feel entirely well, but occasionally have symptoms such as itching. Cough, shortness of breath or chest discomfort can be the first symptoms of HD in the chest, although it is not unusual for a mass to be detected on a chest x-ray done for totally unrelated reasons. Less commonly, Hodgkin's disease in the abdomen may be signaled by an enlarged spleen or enlarged groin lymph nodes. These are much more likely to be signs of non-Hodgkin's lymphoma than of HD, however.

DIAGNOSIS

Physical Examination

♦ Enlarged lymph nodes in the neck, above the clavicles, under the arms or in the groin.
♦ Skin breakdown from scratching (excoriation) over most of the body because of itching.
♦ Fluid around the lungs (pleural effusion).
♦ Liver or spleen enlargement.
♦ Abdominal mass.
♦ Areas of bony tenderness.

Blood and Other Tests

♦ Complete blood count, including erythrocyte (red cell) sedimentation rate.
♦ Blood chemistries, including serum copper. These may be abnormal because of the tumor or because of the involvement of bone, the kidneys or liver.

Imaging

♦ Chest x-ray may show masses within the chest, direct involvement of the lung or a pleural effusion.
♦ CT scan of the chest, abdomen and pelvis to look for enlarged lymph nodes or the involvement of the liver or spleen.
♦ Lymphangiogram, which uses a contrast dye injected into the feet to highlight the lymphatic system. The dye will stay within the pelvic and abdominal lymph nodes for many months or years, during which the disease can be followed by simple x-rays of the abdomen.
♦ Bone x-rays and/or bone scan if there are tender bony areas.
♦ After injection of the isotope gallium, scanning may reveal "hot spots" indicating areas of HD.

Endoscopy and Biopsy
♦ Bone marrow biopsy to look for the presence of Hodgkin's disease.
♦ Biopsy of an enlarged lymph node.
♦ Surgical exploration of the abdomen (laparotomy) with removal of the spleen (splenectomy) may be needed to evaluate any hidden disease that could influence the choice of treatment.

STAGING

The stage is identified through a careful history, physical exam and laboratory and x-ray studies including a lymphangiogram. For those patients whose treatment decision requires it, exploratory abdominal surgery (staging laparotomy) may also be done.

The classification used for staging Hodgkin's disease is known as the Ann Arbor Staging System.

Stage I Involvement of a single lymph node region (Stage I) or localized involvement of a single organ or site other than lymph nodes (IE).

Stage II Involvement of two or more lymph node regions on the same side of the diaphragm (either above or below the breathing muscle separating the chest from the abdomen) (Stage II) or localized involvement of a single associated organ or site other than lymph nodes (extralymphatic) and its nearby lymph nodes, with or without other lymph node regions on the same side of the diaphragm (IIE).

Stage III Involvement of lymph node regions on both sides of the diaphragm (Stage III) that may also be accompanied by localized involvement of an extralymphatic organ or site (IIIE), involvement of the spleen (IIIS) or both (IIIS+E).

Stage IV Widespread involvement of one or more sites other than lymph nodes, with or without associated lymph node involvement, or isolated extralymphatic organ involvement with distant lymph node involvement.

Each stage may be further sub-divided into A or B according to the presence or absence of general symptoms. "A" means the absence of "B" symptoms, which include any of: unexplained fevers over 38°C (100.4°F), drenching night sweats or the unexplained loss of at least 10 percent of body weight.

TREATMENT OVERVIEW

About 75 percent of all newly diagnosed people with Hodgkin's disease can be cured with current radiotherapy and combination chemotherapy.

The most important factors for determining the prognosis and outlining treatment plans are the stage of disease, the presence or absence of symptoms and the presence of large masses. Other factors include the patient's age, the extent of splenic disease found during a laparotomy, the extent of abdominal lymph node involvement and the results of a laboratory test measuring the erythrocyte (red cell) sedimentation rate.

 Radiation Radiation therapy is considered the treatment of choice for those with favorable localized disease—Stage I and Stage II, with no large masses and no symptoms.

 Chemotherapy For all other patients, chemotherapy is required. Combined radiation and chemotherapy is commonly used for large individual tumor masses, so-called bulky disease. Even patients who have recurrent disease after initial treatment with radiation have an excellent chance for a prolonged disease-free survival with combination chemotherapy. Patients with recurrent disease after chemotherapy have a less favorable prognosis, but long remissions have been reported after more chemotherapy or intensive chemotherapy and radiation therapy followed by bone marrow transplantation.

Investigational The leading clinical investigations in early-stage Hodgkin's disease are designed to decrease the toxicity of treatment without reducing the overall excellent results.

More effective therapy is needed for patients with very extensive disease and better chemotherapy programs are needed for the elderly. The use of hematopoietic growth factors is likely to improve treatment for both (*see* Chapter 8). Current studies will eventually define the best use of intensive chemotherapy, radiation therapy and bone marrow transplantation.

TREATMENT BY STAGE

STAGE IA and IIA "FAVORABLE"
The disease is classified as favorable if there are no large masses.

Standard Treatment Traditionally, patients have exploratory abdominal surgery (a staging laparotomy) to evaluate the spleen, liver and abdominal lymph nodes. This might be avoided when there is little likelihood of disease below the diaphragm, as is the case with disease that appears only in the chest (no lymph nodes), with high neck disease of the nodular sclerosis or lymphocyte predominant sub-types and with young women with Stage I disease. Fewer laparotomies are being performed because of the ability to better predict occult subdiaphragmatic disease and acceptance of a slightly higher risk of relapse.

The standard treatment is radiation to the chest, the lymph nodes in the neck and underarm, and the deep abdominal lymph nodes.

Investigational alternatives include involved field radiation plus mild chemotherapy and combination chemotherapy

such as ABVD (Adriamycin + bleomycin + vinblastine + dacarbazine [DTIC]), VBM (velban + bleomycin + methotrexate), and NOVP (Novantrone + Oncovin + vinblastine + prednisone).

Five-Year Survival About 90 percent

STAGE IB and IIB "FAVORABLE"
Standard Treatment If radiotherapy alone is to be considered, a staging laparotomy is essential. Sub-total or total lymphoid irradiation is favored in some centers, particularly those with modern radiotherapy equipment and extensive experience.

Combination chemotherapy programs commonly used include:

MOPP (mechlorethamine [nitrogen mustard] + vincristine + procarbazine + prednisone), ABVD, a MOPP-ABV hybrid (without dacarbazine) and alternating cycles of MOPP and ABVD.

An alternative therapy in laparotomy-staged patients is involved field radiation plus mild chemotherapy.

Five-Year Survival 75 to 90 percent

STAGE IA or IB and IIA or IIB "UNFAVORABLE"
The disease is classified as unfavorable if there is a large mass.

Standard Treatment Staging laparotomy is not indicated.

Combination chemotherapy such as those mentioned before in combination with radiation therapy to the involved field is the standard treatment.

Five-Year Survival 75 to 90 percent

Alternative Chemotherapy A number of MOPP-like chemotherapy combinations have been studied, either alone or together with radiotherapy. These include: PAVe (procarbazine + Alkeran [melphalan] + velban [vinblastine]), ChlVPP (chlorambucil + vinblastine + procarbazine + prednisone), and MVPP (mechlorethamine + vinblastine + procarbazine + prednisone) in selected older patients to avoid the possibility of vincristine nerve toxicity.

Investigational
♦ Stanford V (Mustard + Adriamycin + vinblastine + Oncovin + bleomycin + etoposide [VP-16] + prednisone).

STAGE IIIA
Standard Treatment The treatment for Stage IIIA patients is controversial. For laparotomy-staged IIIA patients with limited splenic disease (fewer than five nodules), total lymphoid irradiation alone may be considered in centers specializing in radiotherapy.

For patients staged clinically (on the basis of physical examination, x-rays and laboratory tests) or patients pathologically staged with more than five splenic nodules, combination chemotherapy such as MOPP, ABVD, MOPP alternating with ABVD or the MOPP-ABV hybrid should be used.

For patients with Stage IIIA disease with bulky masses, both chemotherapy and irradiation are recommended.

Five-Year Survival 65 to 85 percent

Investigational
♦ New chemotherapy combinations, alone or together with radiotherapy.

STAGE IIIB and STAGE IV
Standard Treatment Combination chemotherapy with MOPP, ABVD, the MOPP-ABV hybrid and MOPP alternated with ABVD. Recent studies have demonstrated the superiority of ABVD alone or in combination with MOPP over MOPP alone. The alternating and hybrid regimens were of equal efficacy in two clinical trials.

Radiation therapy may be added to sites of bulky disease.

Five-Year Survival 60 to 80 percent

Investigational
♦ New chemotherapy combinations, alone or with radiotherapy.

TREATMENT FOLLOW-UP

All patients must be followed up at regular intervals with a physical examination, blood counts and radiological studies. This is particularly important because of the young age of the population and the ability to cure patients with secondary therapy.
♦ For patients treated with limited radiation after clinical staging alone, annual abdominal CT scans are recommended. Sites of previous bulky disease should receive particular attention.
♦ All patients receiving radiation therapy to the thyroid should have annual thyroid function tests. In a significant percentage of patients, thyroid function may become low (hypothyroid) because of radiation treatments, requiring the taking of thyroid hormone.
♦ Surveillance is needed to be on the lookout for secondary malignancy, solid tumors in patients treated with irradiation and acute leukemia in patients treated with MOPP (*see* "Complications of Therapy").

Complications of Therapy These may be divided into acute and chronic. Acute toxicities for the various chemotherapy drugs are well described and should be discussed before treatment. Acute toxicities of radiation therapy depend on which area of the body is irradiated.

Now that the cure rate for Hodgkin's disease is so high and so many patients are alive many years after treatment, the late complications of therapy are receiving more attention. These include:
♦ Nearly universal sterility in males and infertility and premature menopause in women over age 25 who receive the equivalent of six cycles of MOPP. These effects appear to be largely irreversible. But children born to parents treated for Hodgkin's disease by any of the standard

treatments have had normal birth weights and no increased incidence of birth defects.

♦ MOPP is also associated with an increased risk—between 1 and 5 percent—of acute leukemia, which is most common about four years after treatment and is no longer appreciated by 10 years. The risk of leukemia may be increased by the use of MOPP after splenectomy.

♦ Non-Hodgkin's lymphomas are increased in HD patients treated by any method.

♦ Patients receiving radiotherapy are at increased risk of developing a second malignancy in the irradiated tissues, particularly skin cancer, breast cancer, stomach cancer, soft tissue and bone cancer and lung cancer. Any patient who is irradiated would be very wise to stop smoking, since the incidence of lung cancer is strongly related to tobacco use.

♦ There are theoretical concerns with the use of ABVD in that bleomycin may be toxic to the lungs and doxorubicin is associated with cardiac toxicity. Both of these effects depend on the dose used and are also affected by the combined use of radiotherapy.

RECURRENT CANCER

Combination chemotherapy with the outlined programs is used for patients who were initially treated with radiotherapy alone.

Cancer that recurs more than one year after chemotherapy has been given as the initial treatment may be treated with either the same chemotherapy program, an alternative combination high-dose chemotherapy or chemotherapy and radiation therapy followed by bone marrow transplantation.

Progression on initial treatment with chemotherapy or relapse during the first year after chemotherapy may be treated with high-dose chemotherapy or chemotherapy and radiation therapy (depending on the earlier treatment) followed by bone marrow transplantation.

THE MOST IMPORTANT QUESTIONS YOU CAN ASK

♦ What is my stage? Is it favorable or unfavorable?

♦ Do I need to have a laparotomy for staging?

♦ Should I have treatment with radiation only, chemotherapy only or both? Why?

♦ What side effects can I expect from the treatment and how can they be minimized?

♦ Will this treatment make me sterile (or infertile)?

♦ What is my risk of future malignancy?

♦ If the Hodgkin's disease recurs, what therapy will be required and what are my chances for cure? Should bone marrow transplantation be considered?

LYMPHOMAS: NON-HODGKIN'S

Russell Hardy, MD, and Sandra J. Horning, MD

◇

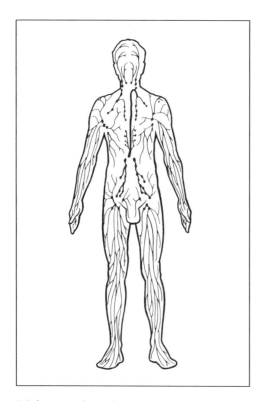

Malignant lymphomas are cancers that arise from the lymphoid system, the complex network of cells and channels that runs throughout the body as a basic part of the immune system. Normally, the cells of the lymphoid system, lymphocytes, are either arranged in clusters—called lymph nodes or lymph glands—or they circulate through the bloodstream and the lymphatic channels to all the tissues of the body except the brain.

Cancers that develop within the lymphoid system—malignant lymphomas—may be found wherever normal lymphocytes go. They may occur in an isolated lymph node, a group of lymph nodes, in organs such as the stomach or intestine, the sinuses, bone, skin or any combination of these sites.

About 45,000 new cases of malignant lymphoma and lymphocytic leukemia (a lymphoid cancer that primarily involves the blood and bone marrow) will occur in 1994 in the United States. They are the seventh most common cause of cancer deaths. The increase in the incidence of non-Hodgkin's lymphoma between 1973 and 1987 was larger than the increase during that period for any other major cancer except melanoma and lung cancer.

Although lymphoma refers to any cancer of the lymphoid system, malignant lymphomas actually represent a variety of cancers ranging from slow-growing chronic diseases to rapidly progressive, acute diseases that may be life-threatening if appropriate therapy is not begun quickly. Cancer of the lymphoid system was first described by British physician Thomas Hodgkin, in 1832. The form he described behaves in a very predictable way and has come to be called Hodgkin's disease. Despite their diversity, all of the other malignant lymphomas are referred to as non-Hodgkin's lymphomas (NHL).

Types There are two main types of cells in the lymphoid system—B cells, which make antibodies in response to infection, and T cells, which are responsible for the regulation of the immune system. Both B cell and T cell lymphomas occur, but the vast majority of lymphomas in the U.S. are of B cell origin.

Whatever the origin, the features that

best predict the prognosis and guide decisions about therapy are the size, shape and pattern of the lymphocytes as seen under the microscope. Malignant lymphocytes may be small and round or angulated (cleaved). Others may be large. Combinations of small and large cells may also be seen. Intermediate-sized lymphocytes with rapidly dividing cells are characteristic of aggressive (high-grade) lymphomas.

Within normal lymph nodes there are microscopic clusters (follicles) of specialized lymphocytes. In some malignant lymphomas, the lymphocytes arrange themselves in a similar pattern that is called fol-

licular or nodular. Small cell and follicular lymphomas typically have a chronic course with an average survival of 6 to 12 years. In the more aggressive lymphomas, the normal appearance of the lymph node is lost by diffuse involvement of tumor cells, which are usually moderate-sized or large.

A variety of systems have been used to classify NHL sub-types according to their microscopic appearance and the behavior of the disease. The Rappaport classification is an older scheme still commonly used. More recently, an international group of pathologists and clinicians developed a Working Formulation to establish

International Working Formulation	Rappaport Classification
Low-Grade	
Small lymphocytic, consistent with chronic lymphocytic leukemia	Diffuse lymphocytic, well-differentiated
Follicular, predominantly small cleaved cell	Nodular lymphocytic, poorly differentiated
Follicular mixed, small cleaved and large cell	Nodular mixed, lymphocytic and histiocytic
Intermediate-Grade	
Follicular, predominantly large cell	Nodular histiocytic
Diffuse, small cleaved cell	Diffuse lymphocytic, poorly differentiated
Diffuse mixed, small and large cell	Diffuse mixed, lymphocytic and histiocytic
Diffuse large cell (cleaved or non-cleaved)	Diffuse histiocytic
High-Grade	
Immunoblastic, diffuse large cell	Diffuse histiocytic
Lymphoblastic (convoluted or non-convoluted)	Diffuse lymphoblastic
Small non-cleaved cell, Burkitt's or non-Burkitt's	Diffuse undifferentiated, Burkitt's or non-Burkitt's

a common terminology. This defined 10 major sub-types categorized as low-, intermediate- or high-grade. These terms relate to the relative malignant potential characterized by a growth rate that may be low (slow), high (rapid) or intermediate (moderately rapid).

How It Spreads Since lymphocytes normally travel throughout the body via the blood and the lymphatic system, malignant lymphomas can either start in or spread to virtually any organ.

A lymphoma may arise in a single lymph node or organ and stay there even when a large mass is present, or many different sites may be involved at the time of diagnosis. Low-grade lymphomas most often involve lymph nodes, bone marrow and the spleen when they are diagnosed. Intermediate- and high-grade lymphomas are most commonly found in lymph nodes, but about one-third of cases primarily involve organs separate from lymph nodes and are called extranodal.

What Causes It The immune system is so complex and dynamic that there are many opportunities for errors in regulation. Many lymphomas are thought to result from such errors or "accidents," which are statistically more probable when the immune system is continually stimulated.

Chronic disorders of the immune system or the chronic administration of drugs to suppress the immune system (such as those used after an organ transplant) predispose a person to lymphoma. Exposure to radiation increases the risk too.

Several types of viruses have been linked. The Epstein-Barr virus, which causes infectious mononucleosis, is associated with African Burkitt's lymphoma. A T cell virus related to the HIV virus associated with AIDS has been linked to an aggressive T cell lymphoma found in Japan, the Caribbean and the southeastern United States.

The mechanism common to each of these appears to be a significant alteration in the normal regulation of the immune system.

RISK FACTORS

At Significantly Higher Risk

♦ The incidence of lymphoma increases with age and is more common in men that in women. Most occur in people who were previously healthy.

♦ Occupational exposure in the flour and agricultural industries has been reported to increase the risk of developing certain types of intermediate- and high-grade lymphoma.

♦ People with congenital or acquired abnormalities of their immune systems or who take medicine to suppress their immune systems have a higher incidence of lymphoma.

♦ There is an increased incidence of intermediate- and high-grade lymphomas in people infected with the HIV virus for four or more years is markedly increasing.

♦ Exposure to radiation or chemotherapy.

SCREENING

There are no known effective ways to screen for lymphoma.

COMMON SIGNS AND SYMPTOMS

People with lymphoma most often seek medical attention because of one or more enlarged lymph nodes. Sometimes these have developed in association with a variety of non-specific symptoms such as fatigue, fevers, chills, night sweats, decreased appetite and weight loss.

But many people are found to have lymphoma when they see their doctors about a variety of symptoms related to the site and extent of tumor involvement. People may develop shortness of breath or cough because of chest disease; abdominal pain or fullness because of an abdominal mass; ulcers, or bleeding or a change in bowel habits because of stomach or intestinal involvement. There can also be nasal stuffiness or sore throat or difficulty swallowing because of a lymphoma involving the sinus, upper airway or throat. If the brain is involved, there may be headaches, changes in vision or seizures. If the bone marrow is involved, there may be recurrent or persistent infections, bleeding or profound fatigue.

Disease outside the lymphatic system is more common in intermediate- and high-grade lymphomas.

DIAGNOSIS

Physical Examination
♦ Enlarged lymph nodes in the neck, under the arms or in the groin.
♦ Swelling in the area of the tonsils, throat or upper airway.
♦ Fluid around the lungs (pleural effusion).
♦ Liver or spleen enlargement.
♦ Abdominal mass.
♦ Soft tissue swelling.
♦ Tenderness when pressure is applied to areas of the skeleton.
♦ Neurologic findings such as numbness or muscle weakness.

Blood and Other Tests
♦ Complete blood count may show circulating lymphoma cells or other blood abnormalities because of lymphoma in the bone marrow.
♦ Blood chemistries may be abnormal because of the tumor or because of the involvement of bone, lungs, the liver or the kidneys.
♦ HIV test.

Imaging
♦ Chest x-ray may show masses within the center of the chest (mediastinum or hilum), involvement of the lungs or fluid around the heart or lungs.
♦ CT scan of the chest, abdomen and

pelvis may show enlargement of lymph nodes, spleen or liver or the involvement of the lungs or other organs.

There are also several optional imaging methods, including:
♦ Lymphangiogram, which uses a contrast dye injected into the feet to highlight the pelvic and abdominal lymph nodes. The dye will stay in the lymph nodes for many months or years, during which the disease can be followed by a simple x-ray of the abdomen.
♦ A spinal tap or CT or MRI scan of the brain may be done if central nervous system involvement is suspected. MRI may allow more accurate assessment of the tumor, particularly in the spinal cord and vertebrae.
♦ An imaging scan using the radioactive isotope gallium may show "hot spots" in areas of lymphoma.

Endoscopy and Biopsy
♦ Diagnosis is usually made in a lymph node, but a biopsy of other involved tissues (extralymphatic) may be performed.
♦ Bone marrow biopsy may detect the presence of lymphoma, in which case further studies will be done to identify the type.

STAGING

The staging system used for non-Hodgkin's lymphomas is the Ann Arbor convention developed for the staging and treatment (primarily with radiation) of Hodgkin's disease.

Sometimes a distinction has been made between "clinical" and "pathologic" staging. Clinical staging describes the apparent stage of the disease as determined by physical examination, x-rays and blood tests. Pathologic staging has generally involved exploratory abdominal surgery (laparotomy) to assess lymph nodes, the liver and spleen for lymphoma. Laparotomy cannot now be recommended for staging of NHL. Strictly speaking, biopsy of the bone marrow is pathologic staging, but the procedure is commonly included as part of clinical staging.

Stage I Involvement of a single lymph node region (Stage I) or localized involvement of a single organ or site other than lymph nodes (IE).

Stage II Involvement of two or more lymph node regions on the same side of the diaphragm (either above or below the breathing muscle separating the chest from the abdomen) (Stage II) or localized involvement of a single associated organ or site other than lymph nodes (extralymphatic) and its regional lymph nodes, with or without other lymph node regions on the same side of the diaphragm (IIE).

Stage III Involvement of lymph node regions on both sides of the diaphragm (Stage III) that may also be accompanied by localized involvement of an extralymphatic organ or site (IIIE), involvement of the spleen (IIIS) or both (IIIS+E).

Stage IV Widespread involvement of one or more extralymphatic sites, with or without associated lymph node involvement, or isolated extralymphatic organ involvement with distant lymph node involvement.

Each stage may be further sub-divided into A or B according to the presence or absence of general symptoms. "A" means the absence of "B" symptoms, which include any of: unexplained fevers over 38°C (100.4°F), drenching night sweats or the unexplained loss of more than 10 percent of body weight.

TREATMENT OVERVIEW BY GRADE

The microscopic appearance and the stage of the lymphoma are the most important factors in determining both the prognosis and the appropriate thera-

py. Other factors affecting the prognosis for a particular person include age, general physical condition, the presence of "B" symptoms, abnormal laboratory tests, the presence of large masses and the number of extralymphatic sites.

With greater understanding of the biology of NHL, other factors have recently been recognized—biologic parameters such as determination of growth fraction or genetic changes—that can be related to the clinical outcome of the disease. It is expected that these will play a greater role in deciding on treatment in the future.

Low-Grade Although low-grade lymphomas grow slowly and respond readily to chemotherapy, they almost invariably return and are generally regarded as incurable cancers.

It is usual for the low-grade lymphomas to be widespread at the time of diagnosis, including involvement in the bone marrow. Despite this, the average survival of people with these lymphomas is 6 to 12 years.

The long-term outcome of the disease has not been favorably affected by the use of immediate chemotherapy in patients who have no symptoms, so close observation alone may be the initial therapy of choice, particularly in patients over age 60. Single agent or combination chemotherapy or radiation therapy may be required when the disease progresses or begins to cause symptoms.

Because of the apparent inability to cure low-grade lymphoma patients, it is important that patients with this diagnosis are presented with the opportunity to participate in clinical trials designed to test new strategies or new agents with the goal of improving the prognosis for low-grade lymphoma.

Patients with limited (Stages I and II) disease provide the exception. They may have prolonged responses to radiation therapy.

It is well known that low-grade lymphomas may transform into more aggressive lymphomas. Therapy appropriate for the more aggressive cancer is required at that time.

Intermediate- and High-Grade These lymphomas are curable. Combination chemotherapy is almost always necessary for successful treatment.

Chemotherapy alone or abbreviated chemotherapy and radiation cure 70 to 80 percent of patients with limited (Stages I and II) intermediate-grade lymphoma. Advanced (Stages III and IV) disease can be eradicated in about 50 percent of patients. Recently, an international collaboration resulted in an index that is useful in assessing prognosis. The five factors identified—age, stage, performance status (general well-being), a blood chemistry measurement called lactate dehydrogenase, and the number of extralymphatic sites—allow a more precise assessment of prognosis.

♦ Patients with B cell immunoblastic lymphoma respond in a manner similar to those with intermediate-grade large cell lymphoma. Several recent reports indicate that T cell lymphomas may be somewhat less favorable for cure.

♦ The intermediate sub-types follicular large cell and diffuse small cleaved cell lymphoma are less common and less well characterized. Some physicians suggest that they should be treated more like the low-grade lymphomas, but others favor an aggressive approach.

♦ Lymphoblastic lymphoma is a high-grade malignancy treated with an intensive drug program similar to that used for acute leukemia, including treatment of the central nervous system.

♦ The small non-cleaved cell lymphomas, including Burkitt's lymphoma, are rapidly progressive neoplasms that are exquisitely sensitive to chemotherapy.

For each of these high-grade malignancies there is a 40 to 50 percent cure rate with conventional therapy. Limited stage and other favorable high-grade lymphomas have a high rate of cure, but more effective treatment approaches are needed for patients with the greatest tumor burden.

Because of medical problems that may occur when treatment is started, patients with extensive lymphoblastic lymphoma or Burkitt's lymphoma should receive their initial chemotherapy treatment in the hospital.

Unclassified Lymphomas With more experienced morphologic assessment and the use of ever-increasing numbers of reagents for laboratory analysis, several "new" lymphomas have been recognized. These include the mucosa-associated lymphomas (MALT) and monocytoid B-cell lymphomas, both of which are considered low-grade. Diffuse intermediate lymphocytic lymphoma, also known as mantle cell lymphoma, is more difficult to classify. Although these lymphomas generally recur after therapy, like the low-grade lymphomas, the average survival time may be shorter than other low-grade lymphomas.

TREATMENT BY GRADE AND STAGE
LOW-GRADE LYMPHOMA
STAGE I and STAGE II
Standard Treatment Radiation therapy is the standard treatment, particularly for patients under the age of 40. While total lymphoid irradiation has been associated with longer disease-free survival, there is no overall survival benefit over regional or limited irradiation.

STAGE III and STAGE IV
Standard Treatment The best treatment for advanced-stage disease remains controversial. Options include:
♦ No initial treatment, with close observation for patients who have no symptoms.
♦ Single-drug therapy, most often oral chlorambucil or Cytoxan.

♦ Combination chemotherapy with CVP (Cytoxan + Oncovin + prednisone), (C)MOPP (Cytoxan + Oncovin + procarbazine + prednisone) or CHOP (Cytoxan + Adriamycin + Oncovin + prednisone).

Five-Year Survival 90 percent for Stages I and II, 80 percent for Stages III and IV

Investigational
♦ A variety of biologic agents have been used, most notably interferon-alpha. This is a modest antitumor agent when used alone and is being studied in combination with chemotherapy or as an adjuvant to chemotherapy in an attempt to prolong remission.
♦ Monoclonal antibodies directed against specific surface markers or more general B cell markers have been used alone, tagged with a radioisotope, combined with a toxin or used in a combined approach with chemotherapy and interferon.
♦ Selected research institutions are investigating the efficacy of high-dose chemotherapy and fractionated total-body radiation and bone marrow transplantation.

Therapy for Relapsed Disease The treatment used initially is often successful when used again after a relapse in the low-grade lymphomas. Fludarabine and 2-chlorodeoxyadenosine (2-CdA), two newer agents, have been shown to produce significant responses in previously treated patients. High-dose chemoradiotherapy and bone marrow transplantation are under investigation. Radiotherapy may be useful to reduce bulky or painful disease sites. Any of the investigational treatments may also be used.

INTERMEDIATE-GRADE LYMPHOMAS
FAVORABLE STAGES I AND II
Limited-stage lymphomas are generally considered favorable if the disease is not bulky (usually less than 4 in./10 cm in diameter), the serum lactate dehydrogenase (LDH) is normal, the general well-being is good and there are no "B" symptoms.

Standard Treatment Treatment options for favorable Stages I and II include:
♦ Chemotherapy alone with CHOP (Cytoxan + Adriamycin + Oncovin + prednisone).
♦ Abbreviated combination chemotherapy plus limited radiation therapy.
♦ Primary radiation therapy to the site of disease in selected Stage I cases, particularly in patients with minimal disease who cannot tolerate chemotherapy.

Five-Year Survival 80 to 90 percent for Stage I, 70 to 80 percent for Stage II

Investigational Because initial therapy is so successful, the goals of investigational efforts are reducing the toxicity of treatment and trying to predict which patients are most likely to fail primary therapy and therefore need other treatment approaches.

UNFAVORABLE STAGES I AND II, STAGE III AND STAGE IV
Standard Treatment Combination chemotherapy, with programs such as:
♦ CHOP (Cytoxan + Adriamycin + Oncovin + prednisone).
♦ m-BACOD (high-dose methotrexate + bleomycin + Adriamycin + Cytoxan + Oncovin + dexamethasone).
♦ ProMACE-CYTABOM (prednisone + high-dose methotrexate + Adriamycin + Cytoxan + etoposide [VP-16] + cytosine arabinoside + bleomycin + Oncovin).
♦ MACOP-B (methotrexate with leucovorin rescue + Adriamycin + Cytoxan + Oncovin + prednisone + bleomycin).

Five-Year Survival About 40 to 50 percent, although the prognosis for patients varies depending on the prognostic factors listed in "Treatment Overview by Grade."

Investigational Because patients with multiple risk factors have a poor prognosis, participation in an investigational program should be considered. Most investigational efforts have the goal of increasing the intensity of treatment by using hematopoietic growth factors or bone marrow transplantation. Modulation of multi-drug resistance is also under investigation.

Therapy for Relapsed Disease A number of chemotherapy combinations have demonstrated antitumor activity. These include:
♦ MINE (mesna + ifosfamide + Novantrone + etoposide [VP-16])
♦ CHAD/DHAP (cisplatin + cytosine arabinoside [Ara-C] + dexamethasone)
♦ ESHAP (etoposide [VP-16] + Solumedrol + cytosine arabinoside [Ara-C] + cisplatin)
♦ CEPP (Cytoxan + etoposide [VP-16] + procarbazine + prednisone).
♦ Because secondary chemotherapy has generally failed to provide a cure, many patients under age 55 have been given high-dose chemotherapy alone or with radiation followed by a bone marrow transplant with moderate success (approximately 20 percent long-term disease-free survival). An international clinical trial is testing the benefit of autologous marrow transplant compared with secondary chemotherapy.

HIGH-GRADE LYMPHOMAS
LYMPHOBLASTIC LYMPHOMA
Standard Treatment Multi-agent chemotherapy, primarily with Cytoxan, Adriamycin, Oncovin and prednisone, is given together with central nervous system prophylactic therapy.

Patients with extensive disease—usually Stage IV on the basis of bone marrow and/or central nervous system involve-

ment—and a high serum lactate dehydrogenase (LDH) have generally done poorly with conventional therapy. Early use of intensive chemotherapy and radiation followed by bone marrow transplantation is being evaluated.

Five-Year Survival 80 percent for limited disease, 20 percent for extensive disease with bone marrow and central nervous system involvement

Investigational
♦ Intensified treatment for high-risk patients is being investigated. One strategy is early use of bone marrow transplantation.

Therapy for Relapsed Disease Secondary chemotherapy and bone marrow transplantation at relapse have some antitumor activity but have most often failed to cure this rapidly fatal condition.

SMALL NON-CLEAVED CELL LYMPHOMA (BURKITT'S/ NON-BURKITT'S)
Standard Treatment The management of this lymphoma is similar to that of lymphoblastic lymphoma. Multi-agent chemotherapy, based upon high-dose Cytoxan, frequently incorporates methotrexate, Oncovin, prednisone and Adriamycin together with central nervous system prophylactic therapy.

Patients with extensive disease—usually Stage IV on the basis of bone marrow and especially central nervous system involvement—and a high serum lactate dehydrogenase (LDH) have generally fared poorly with chemotherapy.

More intensive treatment programs used successfully in pediatric cases, with or without bone marrow transplantation, are under investigation.

Survival data, investigational approaches and therapy for relapsed disease are essentially the same as for lymphoblastic lymphoma.

AIDS-ASSOCIATED LYMPHOMAS

Intermediate- and high-grade lymphomas are being seen increasingly in HIV-infected patients. These tumors can be highly aggressive. The management of these patients is often challenging because their immune systems are already compromised by the HIV infection. These patients can be extremely sensitive to the bone marrow suppressive effects of chemotherapy and are more likely to develop infectious complications than other lymphoma patients. The "best" chemotherapeutic regimen has yet to be identified, but a number of centers are investigating modified versions of regimens similar to those used for the other intermediate- and high-grade lymphomas. Infectious prophylaxis and hematopoietic growth factors are incorporated in the treatment regimen. HIV-related lymphomas more often primarily involve the central nervous system. In addition to the prognostic factors described earlier, immunocompetence as assessed by quantification of T cells and previous manifestations of AIDS have prognostic significance. (*See also* "Lymphoma: AIDS-Associated.")

TREATMENT FOLLOW-UP

Follow-up varies considerably, depending on the initial grade of lymphoma and the treatment.

♦ Patients with low-grade lymphoma require life-long follow-up because of the strong likelihood that the disease will recur and/or will transform into a higher-grade malignancy.

♦ Some forms of intermediate-grade lymphoma, particularly diffuse small cleaved cell and follicular large cell lymphoma, may also relapse over long periods.

♦ Recurrence of intermediate-grade diffuse large cell and mixed lymphomas or high-grade lymphomas usually occurs within three years after treatment. Relapse is rarely hard to find, given the rapid growth characteristics of these lymphomas. All patients should be seen at regular intervals for physical examination, complete blood counts and radiologic studies. Newer biologic markers of minimal disease may be used in the future.

THE MOST IMPORTANT QUESTIONS YOU CAN ASK

♦ What is my prognosis? What is the likelihood of cure?

♦ If the standard treatment won't cure me, are there any investigational treatments I should consider?

♦ What side effects can I expect from the treatment and how can they be minimized?

♦ If I have a low-grade lymphoma, what are the risks and benefits of immediate treatment as opposed to no initial therapy?

♦ If I have recurrent (relapsed) lymphoma, should bone marrow transplantation be considered?

MELANOMA
Malcolm S. Mitchell, MD

◇

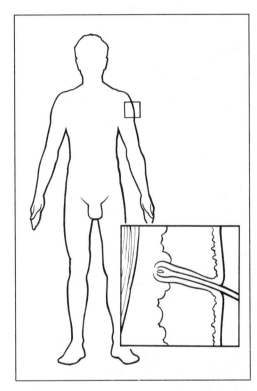

Most skin cancers are not generally considered very dangerous, since they are easily cured by surgery or medicines applied to the skin. The malignant mole called melanoma—which means black tumor—is a notable exception. Not only is melanoma the most malignant of all skin cancers, it is among the most malignant of *all* cancers.

Melanoma can spread to nearly every organ and tissue in the body and can lead to death within a year after it recurs in distant sites. Although it is very rare for a mother's tumor to spread to her fetus, melanomas lead the list among those tumors that do spread in this way.

Melanoma is also one of the most common tumors to spread to the brain and spinal cord.

Melanoma is not yet among the most common cancers, but its incidence is rising faster worldwide than any other. In the United States alone, more than 32,000 cases are expected during 1994.

Yet amidst all these bleak aspects there are some very encouraging ones. When melanoma first appears as a malignant mole of the skin or eye—and occasionally on the gums, in the vagina or in the anus—it is often curable by limited surgery. This points up the importance of recognizing the early signs of melanoma and bringing them to the attention of a physician so that an experienced dermatologist, surgeon or oncologist can become involved. In addition, several advances in biological treatment have prolonged useful survival, even at advanced stages of the disease.

Once the melanoma has penetrated deeply into the skin and has reached the lymphatic and blood vessels in the second level of the skin (the dermis), it is difficult to cure, but a long period of quiescence may still be achieved by surgery.

Types There is only one type of malignant cell composing all melanomas—the malignant pigment-producing cell called a melanocyte—but there are a few variants distinguished by their shapes, such as cuboidal or spindle-shaped. The behavior of each is generally similar in skin melanomas, although in eye melanomas the shape determines the behavior to a significant degree.

All melanocytes have pigment granules in them even when the cells are not black or dark brown. In all cases, they have the enzymes necessary to produce melanin, the black pigment. When melanomas spread, they often do not produce pigment and are said to be amelanotic, but the degree of malignancy of both amelanotic or melanotic melanomas seems to be the same.

Melanomas are most commonly found on the skin, but 10 percent arise in the eye. The most common variants in the skin are called the superficial spreading melanoma and the nodular melanoma, terms that describe the pattern of enlargement.

Melanomas can arise in somewhat unusual locations, such as under the nail of a finger or toe or on the mucosa lining the inside of the mouth, vagina or anus. Primary melanomas have also been found on the pigmented tissue covering the brain (the meninges). It is important not to confuse melanomas under the nail with fungal infections, although that mistake is sometimes made at the beginning of the disease.

Melanomas of the eye occur in the colored regions at the front (the iris), just behind the iris in the structure controlling the shape of the lens (the ciliary body) and in the pigmented layer (the choroid) covering the eyeball behind the retina.

How It Spreads There are two phases of growth of melanomas—the radial (outward on the surface of the skin) and the vertical (deeply into the layers of the skin). Sometimes, superficial spreading melanomas can remain in a radial growth phase for over a year. Nodular melanomas grow vertically soon after their appearance. Detection in a biologically early phase is, therefore, more likely with superficial spreading melanomas, but these tumors do eventually enter a vertical growth phase. When they do, they are as dangerous as nodular melanomas.

Most eye melanomas grow very slowly. They may be observed by ophthalmologists for 5 to 10 years with little increase in size. The eye melanomas composed of spindle-shaped cells (called spindle A and spindle B) are almost non-malignant in their behavior, with almost all patients surviving more than 10 years after the tumor is detected. Other varieties, composed of cells shaped more like skin cells (epithelioid) are much more malignant.

Melanomas can also spread through the lymphatic system and the blood to just about every organ in the body, with the lungs and liver being the most common sites.

What Causes It Intermittent episodes of intense sun exposure causing sunburns rather than tanning is more commonly associated with melanoma than the sort of chronic exposure to sunlight associated with more benign skin cancers. Typically, office workers or schoolchildren who spend hours on the beach on weekends, rather than farmers, dockworkers or sailors who work in the sun daily, are liable to develop melanomas.

There is no conclusive evidence to support an association with hormones, although anecdotes continue to surface that suggest at least some women are highly susceptible to developing melanoma or recurrent melanoma when they are pregnant or have taken oral contraceptives. Individual patients have had a striking history of recurrences and rapid progression of disease related to pregnancy. Taking oral contraceptives, which contain mostly progestational agents, has also been associated with an increased incidence of superficial spreading melanomas.

RISK FACTORS

Caucasians living in tropical or sub-tropical climates, such as the American Southwest, equatorial Africa, Hawaii or Australia, have the highest incidence. Obviously, exposure to ultraviolet light, particularly that leading to sunburn, is strongly suspected as a cause.

There are about 15 cases among each 100,000 Caucasians in California or Arizona, while 30 cases are found per 100,000 Caucasians in Hawaii and Australia. Blacks, brown-skinned people and Orientals in the same regions have a much lower incidence.

Even in the Northeast, the incidence is more than 10 per 100,000, up from 8 per 100,000 10 to 15 years ago. Melanoma is becoming a major concern in countries of the Northern hemisphere such as Sweden, Finland and England, where the incidence is increasing for reasons that are not entirely clear.

Melanoma is most common in people in their forties to sixties and is rare before puberty. An increasing number of young adults with primary melanomas are being seen, however; many of them had episodes of intense sunburn in their childhood. A tumor known as clear cell sarcoma, arising in the soft tissues such as muscle or the tissue under the skin, is made up of the same type of malignant melanocytes as adult melanomas. Children and adults can have this form.

Eye melanomas are most common in fair-skinned people living in sunny climates, suggesting that dark glasses

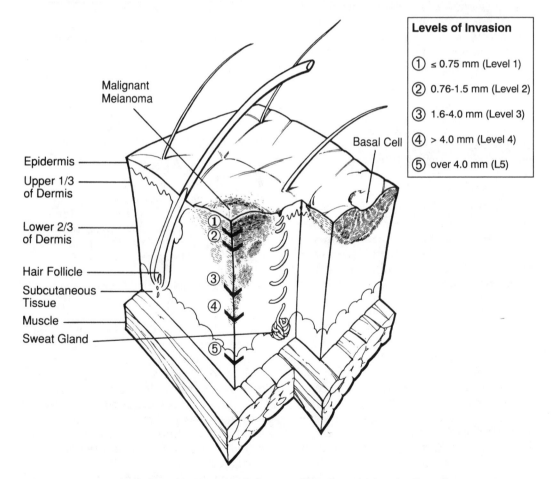

Levels of Invasion

① ≤ 0.75 mm (Level 1)

② 0.76-1.5 mm (Level 2)

③ 1.6-4.0 mm (Level 3)

④ > 4.0 mm (Level 4)

⑤ over 4.0 mm (L5)

Malignant Melanoma

Basal Cell

Epidermis

Upper 1/3 of Dermis

Lower 2/3 of Dermis

Hair Follicle

Subcutaneous Tissue

Muscle

Sweat Gland

Layers of skin, showing a malignant melanoma and a basal cell carcinoma

completely blocking ultraviolet rays should be worn by blue-eyed people when out in bright sunlight.

♦ Among Caucasians, red-haired people with very fair complexions are at the highest risk, followed by blond, blue-eyed people.

♦ Primary melanomas can occur even in dark-skinned people on the palms and soles, under the skin and in the membranes lining the mouth, rectum and anus.

♦ White people with a large number of moles are at increased risk. Those with sporadic dysplastic nevi—unusual moles that under the microscope have features resembling melanoma—are probably not at increased risk of developing melanoma from those nevi. People with a strong family history, however (familial dysplastic nevus syndrome), have an increased tendency to develop melanoma.

SCREENING

There is no effective screening procedure, but because melanoma arises on the skin or in the eye its presence is usually obvious to anyone aware of its features.

COMMON SIGNS AND SYMPTOMS

Cure requires early diagnosis and appropriate surgery. Family practitioners, internists and patients themselves must recognize the early-warning signs that ordinarily occur in sequence: *darkening* of an existing mole, an *increase* in its size, *irregularity* of margins and *elevation* of the lesion. The American Cancer Society's often quoted sign of bleeding is one of the later signs of the disease.

Further changes in the color of the mole, such as depigmentation of a portion of it or a reddish or bluish tinge, may also occur. Bleeding usually occurs after some minor injury sometime after these changes become apparent. Itching is common, as is scaling or crusting of the lesion. Occasionally, an entirely new pigmented spot appears.

It should be emphasized that most pigmented spots are not melanomas. Chronic inflammatory conditions, benign fibrous tumors (fibromas) and basal cell carcinomas—one of the most common low-malignancy skin tumors—are sometimes pigmented. Benign tumors can also bleed after being irritated by underwear or after shaving. It is nevertheless better to bring any suspicious changes to the attention of a doctor. It is far better to risk being thought a hypochondriac than to run the risk of letting a melanoma get out of hand.

DIAGNOSIS

Blood and Other Tests

♦ There are no blood tests available for screening or confirming the diagnosis of primary melanomas.

♦ Tumor-associated antigens shed by the tumor are now being looked at as possible markers in the bloodstream, but results are inconclusive. Carcinoembryonic antigen (CEA), which is found in several cancers, is not found in melanomas.

Endoscopy and Biopsy

♦ An adequate—in other words, an excisional—biopsy is necessary for diagnosis. Examination of the tumor under the microscope reveals characteristic melanoma cells, which are typically plump and usually contain dustlike grains of melanin pigment. The malignant melanocytes are seen to migrate into the dermis to various depths, where they are found singly, in small groups or in large aggregations. Immunological staining procedures with special antibody-carrying dyes are now available to confirm the diagnosis in cases that do not appear typical.

♦ Shave biopsies are not recommended. They do not allow the depth of invasion into the skin to be determined, and this needs to be known to help predict whether the patient will be cured or has a risk of recurrence.

♦ Cauterization or freezing should never be done. These procedures destroy the superficial part of the melanoma, making diagnosis and staging impossible. They also leave tumor cells in deeper locations at the site, which could later give rise to seeding of other parts of the body.

♦ Eye melanomas are not biopsied to avoid damage to sight. The appearance of eye melanomas is so characteristic that experienced ophthalmologists have no difficulty in making an accurate diagnosis in almost all cases.

STAGING

Skin Melanomas

Several systems are used to stage skin melanomas. The depth of invasion is the best predictor of outcome. One classification categorizes primary melanomas into five levels of invasion that a pathologist can easily recognize under the microscope (Clark's levels).

♦ Level 1 is melanoma at the place of origin, in the basal layer of the epidermis at the epidermal-dermal junction, where the outer and underlying layers of the skin meet.

♦ Level 2 is extension to the upper third of the dermis, the papillary dermis.

♦ Level 3 melanoma extends to the border of the papillary and reticular dermis.

♦ Level 4 involves the reticular dermis.

♦ Level 5 invades subcutaneous tissue, such as fat.

Level 1 melanomas are almost always curable by surgical removal of the lesion. Levels 4 and 5 recur in over 85 percent of cases. Level 3 melanomas recur in perhaps 60 percent of patients.

Another classification system (Breslow level) using the exact measurement of the thickness of the tumor under the microscope has recently been introduced and is used together with the other system.

Melanomas less than 0.75 mm are usually considered highly curable by surgery alone, although some people with such "thin" lesions have had recurrences. Tumors 0.76 mm to 1.5 mm are considered to have a moderately deep invasion and

have a worse prognosis than thin lesions. Melanomas 1.6 mm or more are very deep, particularly those over 4 mm.

While no exact relationship exists between the two classification schemes, an approximate correlation can be made between levels and thicknesses.

It is prudent to consider any lesion deeper than 0.75 mm potentially recurrent and, therefore, dangerous. Close contact with the surgeon or a medical oncologist for follow-up examinations and scans is required in these circumstances.

The presence of the tumor in regional lymph nodes draining the site of the primary tumor—such as the lymph nodes in the armpit draining a melanoma of the forearm—is another sign of a poor prognosis. Lymph nodes usually provide an immunological barrier against the tumor. When they are filled with tumor, they have obviously lost the battle and cancer cells have usually passed beyond them into the blood and traveled to distant organs. Over 80 percent of patients with involved nodes have a recurrence elsewhere.

AJCC Staging

Another system in common use is the American Joint Commission on Cancer (AJCC) staging system, which lumps levels and sites of tumor into convenient smaller categories. Table 1 shows the stages, as modified in 1988.

Eye Melanomas

Melanomas of the eye are classified by direct observation and ultrasound measurements into small, medium and large tumors, based on their diameter and elevation.

♦ Small tumors have a better prognosis and are often followed without removal to see how fast they are growing.

♦ Medium tumors are often followed, but there is some debate about whether this is the best course of action.

♦ Large melanomas are usually treated early, but if they are not significantly

TABLE 1: Stage Grouping for Melanoma: American Joint Commission on Cancer

Stage	Criteria
IA	Localized melanoma ≤ 0.75 mm or level 2* (T1, N0, M0)
IB	Localized melanoma 0.76 mm to 1.5 mm or level 3* (T2, N0, M0)
IIA	Localized melanoma > 1.6 mm to 4 mm or level 4* (T3, N0, M0)
IIB	Localized melanoma > 4 mm or level 5* (T4, N0, M0)
III	Limited nodal metastases involving only one regional lymph node basin (area), or fewer than 5 intransit metastases but without nodal metastases (any T, N1, M0)
IV	Advanced regional metastases (any T, N2, M0) or any patient with distant metastases (any T, any N, M1 or M2)

* When the thickness and level of invasion criteria do not coincide with a T classification, thickness should take precedence.

impairing vision they can also be watched for a time.

If the rules that govern skin melanomas are correct, any size of eye tumor carries a significant hazard of permitting the tumor to reach the bloodstream (the eye has few lymph vessels). Since the ocular melanoma appears to be much more slow growing than skin melanoma and usually occurs in elderly people, however, it does not have the same degree of risk.

The appearance of eye melanoma cells under the microscope is also an indicator of outcome. Spindle-shaped cells are less malignant and patients almost always live 15 years. Melanoma cells resembling skin cells (epithelioid) are more malignant, with 34 percent of patients living 5 years and 28 percent 15 years. Survival is a little better for melanomas in which spindle cells are mixed with epithelioid cells (46 percent and 41 percent, 5- and 15-year survivals respectively).

In general, small melanomas of the spindle cell type are almost entirely benign and the patient may never have widespread disease or require treatment of any kind.

♦ Melanomas arising from the colored portion at the front of the eye (the iris) are usually noted very early and frequently contain spindle cells.

♦ Large melanomas of the epithelioid variety require treatment soon after discovery. Despite treatment, there is spread to a different part of the body—often the liver—in 65 percent of all patients.

TREATMENT OVERVIEW

 Surgery The removal of the tumor, along with sufficient margins of normal skin, is the only curative treatment for all but the most advanced stages of disease. Nearby lymph nodes may also be removed if they are involved. Surgical removal of a single brain metastasis is also very useful to control the tumor in a later stage.

Chemotherapy Single-drug chemotherapy is effective in no more than 20 percent of patients with advanced disease. Recent reports suggest that drug combinations can cause responses—more than 50 percent shrinkage of all tumor masses for at least four weeks—in 40 to 64 percent of cases. The percentage of complete remissions is low and the duration of response is still fairly short, but the increased percentage of responses is encouraging.

High-dose chemotherapy with drugs such as Thiotepa or melphalan, followed by replacement of the patient's own stored bone marrow—autologous bone marrow transplantation—has similar high response rates, but the short duration of remission (four months) does not yet justify the considerable risk of mortality (15 to 25 percent). (*See also* Chapter 11.)

 Radiation Radiation therapy can help shrink isolated large lesions, particularly nodules under the skin, or relieve pain, but high individual doses of at least 500 cGy are usually required to overcome the resistance of melanoma cells to radiation. Somewhat lower radiation doses (300 to 400 cGy) are used for brain metastases. A new method of focused radiation (stereotactic radiotherapy) is now replacing neurosurgery in some centers for treatment of one or a low number of small brain metastases.

Hyperthermia in conjunction with radiation may improve local control of large lesions.

 Biological Therapy Stimulating the immune system with biological response modifiers to reject the tumor has already shown some degree of success, sometimes with less severe side effects than chemotherapy.

Giving moderate doses of interferon-alpha three times a week under the skin (subcutaneously) has resulted in about a 20 percent response rate. Major advantages include self-administration by the patient or family members, minor side effects (controllable fever, chills and fatigue) and availability. The high cost of interferon-alpha is a drawback, but the two major companies that manufacture it both offer cost-assistance programs for those suffering financially because of the treatment.

Various doses of a new biological substance called interleukin-2 (IL-2) has had responses in approximately 25 percent of patients. Remarkable degrees of shrinkage have been observed in the liver (usually a very difficult site to treat), as well as in the lungs, lymph nodes, skin, bone and adrenal glands.

It is not necessary to receive so-called LAK cells (IL-2 or lymphokine-activated killer cells) or very high dose IL-2 to achieve this response rate. IL-2 can also be given subcutaneously in lower dosage, which allows patients to administer it to themselves, and also has fewer side effects.

Active specific immunotherapy (melanoma vaccines) has also shown considerable promise in treating advanced melanoma and theoretically should be even more effective in early stages of the disease. About 20 percent of patients have had partial or complete remissions with the most successful of the melanoma vaccines. Patients who have a clinical response have an improved survival rate, even with residual disease.

There are no side effects from the vaccine except for some short-term soreness at the site of injections and, possibly, painful lumps after a long series of treatments. This makes it one of the easiest cancer treatments to tolerate. Melanoma and kidney cancer appear to be unusually sensitive to biological therapy, and a great variety of emerging biological agents and approaches will be tried first in these two diseases.

Adjuvant Therapy The removal of draining lymph nodes as a preventive (prophylactic) measure in patients without clinically enlarged lymph nodes has not been proved to improve the cure rate but still has its advocates among surgeons. The issue is being studied by university surgeons in an international trial nearing completion.

Several trials are addressing the issue of whether biological response modifiers such as tumor vaccines, interferons or interleukins that have proved useful in Stage IV disease can help prevent recurrence when used after surgery for Stage II and III disease.

There is suggestive evidence that some tumor vaccines can prolong disease-free survival, and more definite results should be forthcoming from several trials within the next few years.

Investigational Several new treatment methods have shown some promise in treating melanoma.

♦ Highly specific antibodies engineered in the test tube (monoclonal antibodies) to act against surface components of melanoma cells are being evaluated. Antibodies by themselves have not been too effective, but when used as carriers for killer molecules—radioactive isotopes, strong chemotherapeutic drugs, enzymes or toxins—good effects have been achieved in animals. Trials in humans have already shown that antibodies have "homed" to the tumor and can show its location accurately on radioisotope scanning (*see* Chapter 8).

♦ There are 12 interleukins, several of which are now being tested on humans. Other combinations include interferons and interleukins together or in sequence.

♦ High-dose chemotherapy, with single drugs or in combinations, followed by autologous bone marrow transfusion, has had too many dangerous side effects associated with the drugs in current trials and too short a duration of response. The general approach, however, is very promising. Even now the rate of response is in

the order of 60 percent.

♦ Several groups, including one at the National Cancer Institute, have begun investigating immunotherapy with tumor-infiltrating lymphocytes (TIL) or cloned killer and helper T cells. This form of "adoptive" immunotherapy involves removing blood cells from the patient, stimulating and multiplying them, then returning them, usually with IL-2. Insertion of genes for cytokines, such as IL-2, TNF or GM-CSF, into irradiated tumor cells (for vaccines) or T cells (for adoptive immunotherapy) is being tried to make vaccines more effective or to increase the number and lifespan of the transferred T cells in the body. This "gene therapy," particularly as applied to tumor vaccines, may be a way of boosting the immune system beyond what the weak tumor antigens can do by themselves. Whether it is better than current methods of boosting immunity with less glamorous approaches, such as by mixing vaccines with bacterial substances, remains to be seen.

SKIN MELANOMAS
STAGE I

Standard Treatment Surgery with a wide excision of normal tissue, and a skin graft if necessary, is preferred except when the lesion is on the face. A margin of at least 1/2 in. (1 cm) and preferably 1 1/4 in. (3 cm) away from the edges of the tumor is usually maintained on cosmetically less important areas such as the back.

Five-Year Survival 80 to 100 percent

STAGE II
Standard Treatment Surgery, as for Stage I.

Five-Year Survival Up to 65 percent

STAGE III
Standard Treatment For deep melanomas without palpable lymph nodes, surgery as for Stage I is the standard pro-

cedure. If the melanoma was called Stage III because of an enlarged lymph node, that node should be removed. The radical removal of all draining lymph nodes at the site is highly controversial and cannot be routinely recommended.

Five-Year Survival 20 to 50 percent

STAGE IV

Standard Treatment Systemic therapy using immunological or chemotherapy agents or regional therapy with radiation (*see* "Treatment Overview").

Five-Year Survival Less than 10 percent

EYE MELANOMAS

Standard Treatment Small tumors are usually followed closely by direct observation by an ophthalmologist, who uses a slit lamp and ultrasound or CT scanning to chart the exact diameter and height of the lesions. If they become large, they can be treated in the same way as medium and large melanomas.

Such medium and large melanomas are treated either by removing the eye (enucleation) or by applying radioactive plaques.

If the melanoma extends outside the eye to the surrounding bone, the prognosis is very poor. Surgical treatment combined with radiation therapy is usually given, but there is no solid evidence that this intensive therapy alters the bad outcome.

If the eye melanoma spreads to other parts of the body, it is usually handled in the same way as widespread skin melanoma, even though the tumors arising in the two locations may not be completely similar.

Investigational

♦ Immunological treatment found to be effective against skin melanomas may be studied against medium and large primary eye melanomas within the next few years. It would be a major advance if at least partial sight could be preserved by arresting tumor growth by immunological means.

TREATMENT FOLLOW-UP

Melanoma can involve so many parts of the body that any new symptom should be reported to the doctor.

♦ Since the liver and the lung are common sites for tumor cells to lodge and grow after traveling through the bloodstream, these organs should be watched carefully at three-month intervals after removal of the primary melanoma and more often during treatment of disseminated disease.

♦ Liver function tests (especially LDH and alkaline phosphatase) should be done.

♦ CT scans of the abdomen with contrast material injected to show the liver should be done every six months. MRI or ultrasound examinations of the abdomen are good alternatives. MRI is better than CT for evaluating the pelvis.

♦ A chest CT scan is preferable to a chest x-ray and can be performed at the same time as an abdominal scan, but a chest x-ray can suffice as a screening tool in patients with no known lung metastases. Expense and exposure to radiation are major problems with frequent CT scans, even though the scans' ability to detect lesions is far better than with routine x-rays.

♦ Lumps under the skin, usually colorless or reddish-purple and occasionally black if *in* the skin, can be felt and seen by patients, often during a bath. Lymph nodes under the arms or in the groin can also be felt and/or seen.

♦ Brain involvement causing neurologic symptoms is becoming more common as therapy improves for disease elsewhere in the body and patients live long enough to allow the slow-growing brain metastases to enlarge. Early, single brain metastases can be effectively controlled by surgery or stereotactic radiation. Therefore MRI scans (or, less desirably, a CT scan) of the brain should be performed at least semi-annually or at the first sign of headaches or changes in mental ability, vision, muscle strength, sensation or balance.

RECURRENT CANCER
Similar to Stage IV.

SUPPORTIVE TREATMENT
Melanoma usually has remarkably few debilitating effects on the system. Patients feel and look good through most of their disease.

Unless the tumor is in a place where it can cause symptoms because of its size—such as pressing on a nerve and causing pain, or causing headaches if it is in the brain—melanoma is not generally associated with severe symptoms. This is in sharp contrast to cancers such as those of the head and neck or the bowel, where patients may lose their appetite and become thin fairly early in the course of their disease. Patients should do everything they feel like doing, without fear of adversely affecting their disease. Modern treatments are designed to permit and encourage a full and active life.

♦ Low-or non-impact aerobic exercise, such as swimming or walking, can be pursued by all patients who feel good. More active exertion is often possible so long as there are no bad results, such as damage to the bones.

♦ Good, balanced nutrition is helpful, which means whole grains, lean meats and complex carbohydrates. Fad diets should be avoided, as they often lack essential nutrients. Many patients who are doing well are convinced that their use of high doses of some vitamin or extract is causing their response, although most are also receiving conventional treatments such as immunotherapy or chemotherapy.

♦ As in any cancer, psychological support is essential to a good outcome. An upbeat attitude is an important element. Support groups emphasizing psychological adjustment and channeling of mental strength into overcoming the tumor, often with visualization techniques, are increasing in popularity and perform a valuable function. See the list of support groups in "Resources" at the back of the book. While no one can yet explain it, there is little doubt that people who believe they will do well in fact do better than those who give up hope when they learn they have cancer. Mental attitude alone cannot do everything, but without a positive outlook even an objective remission of disease cannot make a patient truly better.

OTHER ISSUES
Melanoma is such a variable disease that someone who is diagnosed should not feel totally disheartened. Long disease-free intervals are often achieved after the deep primary tumors are removed, and early melanomas are usually curable. If the disease comes back in a lymph node, it can be removed surgically. If it comes back elsewhere, such as in the lungs or liver, a variety of treatments are available. Some of the most exciting developments in immunotherapy are occurring in the treatment of melanoma, where prolonged survivals of several years are becoming fairly common.

It is important for all patients to know that there is now good news to replace the old bad news, when there was very little anyone could do about widespread disease.

Check any information you may gain from reading about the disease with an oncologist who knows about melanoma. Above all, don't let your relatives, neighbors or friends tell you all they "know" about melanoma.

THE MOST IMPORTANT QUESTIONS YOU CAN ASK

♦ What are the alternatives to the plan you are suggesting?

♦ Can you arrange a second opinion about the surgery you are proposing?

♦ What is the response rate and duration of response of the therapy you are proposing, and do you think they justify the side effects I may have?

♦ Are there investigational treatments available anywhere in the country? Can you help me find out about them?

MESOTHELIOMA

Malin Dollinger, MD, and Ernest H. Rosenbaum, MD

◇

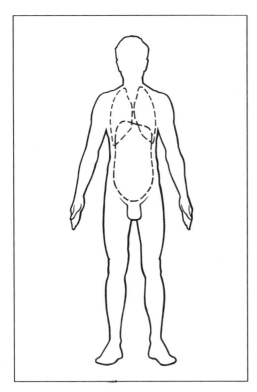

Mesothelioma is a malignant tumor in the lining of the chest and abdominal cavities. It is a rare form of cancer, with about 2,000 cases diagnosed in the United States each year. Most people who develop this cancer have a history of exposure to the widely found carcinogen asbestos.

Malignant mesothelioma is usually not curable, although some surgical cures have been reported in a very few patients with very localized tumors. Most patients, however, have widespread disease at the time of diagnosis, with chest pain and a buildup of fluid within the cavity involved—chest or abdominal—that causes shortness of breath or abdominal swelling. Treatment at this stage, which may involve removing the fluid and the tumor, is usually directed toward relieving these symptoms.

Types Malignant mesothelioma is a sarcoma that can have both fibrous and epithelial elements. Epithelial cancers that develop in the tissues that cover the surface or line internal organs are carcinomas, so the epithelial form of mesothelioma is sometimes confused with adenocarcinomas of the lung or metastatic carcinomas. Epithelial mesotheliomas seem to have a better prognosis than other types.

How It Spreads Mesotheliomas start in the membranes lining the chest (pleural cavity) or the membranes of the abdominal cavity (the peritoneum). They can extend within and beyond the cavity of origin and metastasize to other organs such as the lungs, the chest wall and abdominal organs such as the bowel.

What Causes It Inhalation of asbestos fibers is a primary cause. About 70,000 tons of asbestos are used in the United States each year, in cement, brake linings, roof shingles, insulation, flooring products and packing materials. Asbestos has also been found as a contaminant in talc, which is also associated with ovarian cancer. Many urban water reservoirs contain asbestos-like fibers and most public and private buildings contain asbestos. Only recently has the strong association between asbestos exposure and malignancy been recognized and appropriate industrial and health standards for exposure been put into effect.

It is sometimes difficult to prove the relationship between asbestos exposure and the development of mesothelioma. The risk of developing the disease begins about 15 years after the first exposure and increases each year up to 40 to 45 years after the first exposure. It is estimated that about 8 million people living in the United States have been occupationally exposed to asbestos over the last half century during the mining and milling of the mineral and during various manufacturing processes.

RISK FACTORS

At Significantly Higher Risk
Anyone exposed to asbestos fibers, even for a few months, particularly:
◆ Miners and millers in contact with asbestos.
◆ Producers of asbestos products.
◆ Laborers who install plumbing, boilers and heating equipment in ships, factories and homes.
◆ Workers who are near the material but do not handle it directly (carpenters, electricians and shipyard welders, for example).
◆ Heating and construction tradespeople.
◆ People living near asbestos mines have an increased chance of developing asbestosis, the associated scarring of the lung, as well as mesothelioma.
◆ Inhabitants of the Anatoli region of Turkey, where zeolite is found in the soil and in homes.

At Somewhat Higher Risk
◆ Spouses and children of asbestos workers presumably because of asbestos fibers brought home in the hair and on clothing.
◆ Demolition workers and workers who repair structures that contain asbestos.
◆ Although smoking greatly increases the risk of lung cancer in asbestos workers, it does not increase the risk of mesothelioma.

SCREENING

Regular chest x-rays are essential to follow the course of people with any significant asbestos exposure, although the scar tissue and shadows related to asbestosis that are seen on the x-rays will be chronic and may progress slowly over the years even without the development of malignant mesothelioma. The tumor may not appear on a chest x-ray as a single mass with sharp edges, so rather than depend on x-rays as a screening method, the best procedure is to biopsy any suspicious area for a possible malignancy.

COMMON SIGNS AND SYMPTOMS

Patients with mesothelioma may have shadows on their chest x-rays related to asbestosis, though the development of chest pain, significant shortness of breath and especially fluid around one lung or in the abdomen should suggest a diagnosis of mesothelioma. People with peritoneal mesothelioma usually have signs of advanced disease, including an abdominal mass, pain, fluid in the abdomen (ascites) and weight loss.

If the tumor has extended to the ribs, bones, nerves and the superior vena cava, common symptoms include pain, trouble swallowing, nerve compression syndromes or swelling of the neck or face.

Involvement of the the membrane around the heart (pericardium) may cause heart rhythm disturbances. Tumors in the lining of the abdominal cavity (peritoneum) may extend to produce bowel obstruction. Fever, clotting abnormalities, thrombophlebitis and anemia have also been seen in a large number of patients with peritoneal mesothelioma.

DIAGNOSIS

Careful questioning about the history of asbestos exposure should focus on the period 20 to 50 years before diagnosis and include possible exposure to household contacts. Because asbestos is so widespread, a brief exposure may have been forgotten.

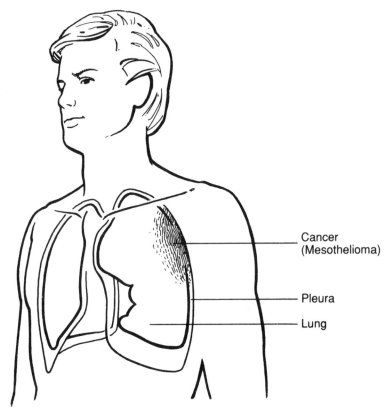

Chest membranes that may be involved with mesothelioma

Physical Examination
♦ Swelling of the neck and face.
♦ Abdominal mass.

Blood and Other Tests
♦ Lung function tests usually show a smaller amount of normal lung tissue available for breathing.
♦ A test for elevated levels of the carcinoembryonic antigen (CEA) in the blood may help distinguish an adenocarcinoma from mesothelioma, with a markedly elevated level suggesting an adenocarcinoma. This distinction may be important, for adenocarcinoma of the lung can be much more treatable than mesothelioma.
♦ Patients with peritoneal mesothelioma may have elevated platelet counts and clotting abnormalities.

♦ Laboratory studies are not particularly helpful.

Imaging
♦ CT scan to assess the extent of disease and to assist decision-making on therapy.
♦ Chest x-rays will often reveal thickening of the pleural membranes in half the patients with peritoneal mesothelioma.

Endoscopy and Biopsy
♦ If mesothelioma is suspected, attempts at a diagnostic biopsy should be made. Sometimes fluid removed during a chest "tap" (thoracentesis) may be examined for tumor cells in a way similar to a Pap test. A needle biopsy may also be done.
♦ Most cases require an open surgical biopsy, since needle biopsies seldom

produce enough diagnostic material. Since a simple biopsy done with a surgical incision into the chest under general anesthesia (thoracotomy) may make it technically difficult to remove the tumor later, the surgeon doing the biopsy should be prepared to do the definitive surgical treatment if that seems appropriate.

♦ The usual examination of the biopsied tissue under the microscope will often prove that the tissue is malignant but may not distinguish adenocarcinoma of the lung from mesothelioma. So a specimen is often processed by special methods—electron microscopy and special stains—to help document the type of tumor.

♦ Cytology of the sputum either coughed up by the patient or obtained through a bronchoscopy may document a bronchogenic adenocarcinoma, which may not be visible on routine chest x-rays.

♦ Patients with peritoneal mesothelioma eventually have exploratory surgery of the abdomen (laparotomy), with an open directed biopsy. Sometimes a simpler procedure, peritonoscopy, may yield enough tissue for diagnosis. An adequate biopsy is essential, since peritoneal mesothelioma can be confused with adenocarcinomas arising in other tissues, especially the ovary.

STAGING

There are a number of different staging systems for malignant mesothelioma, including a TNM system. All list four stages of tumor from very localized to metastatic, but no one system is universally agreed upon. The PDQ classification into localized and advanced disease seems most appropriate for decision-making.

There is no satisfactory staging system for peritoneal mesothelioma, although the tumor is usually confined to the abdomen. Since metastasis is rare, extensive staging studies outside the abdomen may not be necessary. CT scans will usually adequately define the extent of tumor.

TREATMENT OVERVIEW

Surgery is the only treatment method that can lead to a cure, but only people with very early stage disease—a small minority of patients—have long-term survival. Mesothelioma is usually incurable, so treatment efforts are designed to control the accumulation of fluids (effusion) as well as pain and other symptoms.

There is a large number of clinical trials investigating aggressive radiation therapy and chemotherapy programs.

 Chemotherapy Extensive attempts have been made to discover chemotherapeutic agents that have some effectiveness against this tumor. Many drugs have been tested, but only a few have modest activity. Doxorubicin, cyclophosphamide and cisplatin are active, and so are 5-azacytidine, 5-fluorouracil and high-dose methotrexate with leucovorin rescue.

Response rates to combinations of chemotherapy drugs may be higher. Recent studies evaluating combinations containing doxorubicin indicate that this drug may be an important part of all combinations.

 Radiation The usefulness of radiation therapy is difficult to define. The natural history of these tumors varies and interpretation of the effects after treatment is difficult, both because of chronic shadows on the chest x-ray before and after treatment and because so few patients have been treated with this method. Early research did suggest some benefit from radiation therapy.

One problem is that usually one entire side of the chest is at risk for tumor and has to be treated. It may be difficult to administer a dose of radiation high enough to control tumor growth without risking toxic effects to adjacent structures including the heart, the stomach, intestines, liver and kidneys.

The radiation therapy physician must also be careful in giving radiation to the area of the heart. This is even more of a problem after surgery to remove the left lung, with the resulting shift of the heart toward the left side of the chest. Sophisticated radiation methods have to be used with this cancer, which may involve electron beam treatments as well as the usual external radiation therapy.

Combined Therapy There has been a lot of interest in combined treatments, especially with radiation therapy being used as an adjuvant to surgery. This has also included the use of adjuvant intraoperative radiotherapy (IORT). New cooperative studies are evaluating various chemotherapeutic agents such as radiation sensitizers, especially doxorubicin.

Very recent research has also involved the preliminary use of chemotherapy, followed by surgery if the disease responded.

TREATMENT BY STAGE

LOCALIZED MALIGNANT MESOTHELIOMA

Localized mesotheliomas are either solitary tumors or tumors that have spread within the cavity involved (intracavitary) but are confined to the serosal sufaces where they started.

Standard Treatment Occasional patients with this stage of disease can be cured by aggressive surgery. A solitary tumor can be completely removed along with adjacent structures to ensure wide margins of cancer-free tissue.

Standard surgery for intracavitary mesothelioma will also involve the removal of portions of the lung and diaphragm in selected patients. Some surgeons favor more extensive operations to include whatever tissue is necessary to remove all visible tumor as long as this doesn't interfere with the functioning of the remaining organs.

To relieve the symptoms of disease, collections of fluid in the cavity (effusions) are drained. A chemical irritant can then be introduced into the chest to make the layers of the membranes adhere to one another. This may prevent further fluid accumulations.

Radiotherapy is also sometimes given to the lung involved to eliminate blood flow in the area and improve breathing.

Five-Year Survival Unusual. Average survival for localized chest disease is about 16 months.

Investigational
♦ Chemotherapy within the chest cavity (intracavitary) after aggressive surgery.
♦ Clinical trials of new chemotherapeutic agents and radiotherapy techniques.

ADVANCED MALIGNANT MESOTHELIOMA

In this stage, the tumor has spread beyond the cavity of origin, with metastasis outside the serosal surface. This extension can include the lung, the chest wall, as well as abdominal organs such as the bowel.

Standard Treatment In some patients, surgical removal of the tumor may be done as a palliative measure. Radiation therapy may also be given in an attempt to control the growth of the malignancy and reduce symptoms in the lung.

As for localized disease, chemical irritants are used to control collections of fluid caused by irritation from the tumor. The fluid is drained beforehand and the chemical irritants introduced through a chest tube.

Five-Year Survival Less than 10 percent—the average survival is about 5 months.

Investigational Same as for localized disease.

PERITONEAL MESOTHELIOMA

Standard Treatment Therapy for peritoneal mesothelioma is difficult, especially as it is usually widespread by the time it is diagnosed. Removal of the tumors for cure is rarely possible and the role of surgery is generally confined to relief of bowel obstruction, relief of ascites by placing shunts for drainage or the palliative removal of large tumors.

Radiation therapy has often been used, but its role has not yet been defined. Since the entire abdomen is at risk, all of the abdominal organs will also be affected by radiation. To protect the liver, kidney, bowel and spinal cord, the dose has to be lower than would be desirable for tumor control.

Although radiation may not be effective in most patients with large, bulky tumors because of the problems posed by an adequate dose, there may be some benefit from lower doses—in the range of 3,000 cGy—if most of the tumor has been successfully removed and only small amounts remain.

The use of chemotherapy for peritoneal mesothelioma has lately focused on the use of chemotherapy given via a catheter directly into the abdominal cavity (intraperitoneal). This permits a much higher concentration of drug to be delivered to the area of the tumor. Intraperitoneal cisplatin, with special measures to neutralize the drug's toxic effects in the body, resulted in a significant complete response rate in one study, but unfortunately many of these patients relapsed after treatment.

Survival Beyond one year is unusual.

Investigational

♦ Because present treatment programs for advanced mesothelioma usually do not have a major impact on the disease, we strongly recommend participation in clinical trials of new forms of therapy.

♦ Important studies are currently under way with combined treatment therapy, using, for example, surgery and chemotherapy (cyclophosphamide + doxorubicin + dacarbazine) in combination with abdominal radiotherapy.

♦ Another current trial involves the removal of larger tumor nodules, followed by intraperitoneal chemotherapy with cisplatin and doxorubicin and a "second-look" operation to determine response. Radiotherapy is given if there has been complete control of the tumor and more chemotherapy is given before the radiation treatment if there is any residual disease left. The preliminary results of this combined program did produce a very significant response rate with acceptable toxicity.

TREATMENT FOLLOW-UP

Mesotheliomas usually progress rapidly and frequent follow-up evaluations are needed.

♦ A physical examination every six to twelve weeks.
♦ Chest or abdominal x-rays or CT scans every three to six months.
♦ Blood counts and chemistry panel every three to six months.
♦ Lung function tests, depending on symptoms.

THE MOST IMPORTANT QUESTIONS YOU CAN ASK

♦ Should I stop smoking?
♦ What can surgery accomplish?
♦ Should radiation be used?
♦ Is there any role for chemotherapy?
♦ How long can I live with this tumor?

METASTATIC CANCER

Alan P. Venook, MD

◇

When a cancer spreads (metastasizes) from its original site to another area of the body, it is termed metastatic cancer. Virtually all cancers have the potential to spread this way. Whether metastases do develop depends on the complex interaction of many tumor cell factors, most of which are not completely understood.

The treatment of metastatic cance depends on where the cancer started. When breast cancer spreads to the lungs, for example, it remains a breast cancer and the treatment is determined by the tumor's origin within the breast, not by the fact that it is now in the lung. About 5 percent of the time, metastases are discovered but the primary tumor cannot be identified. The treatment of these metastases is dictated by their location rather than their origin (*see* "Cancer of an Unknown Primary Site").

Although the presence of metastases generally implies a poor prognosis, some metastatic cancers can be cured with conventional therapy.

Types Virtually all cancers can develop metastases.

How It Spreads Metastases spread in three ways—by local extension from the tumor to the surrounding tissues, through the bloodstream to distant sites or through the lymphatic system to neighboring or distant lymph nodes. Each kind of cancer may have a typical route of spread. The most likely sites of metastases for each tumor are listed in the individual tumor chapters.

What Causes It The characteristics of each tumor are different, and it is not known what factors make the metastasis develop in particular places.

COMMON SIGNS AND SYMPTOMS

Many patients have no or minimal symptoms related to the tumor, and their metastases are found during a routine medical evaluation. If there are symptoms, they depend on the site involved.

◆ Brain metastases may cause headaches, dizziness, blurred vision, nausea or other symptoms related to the nervous system.

◆ Bone metastases may be evident because of pain, although they frequently cause no symptoms. The first sign of a bone metastasis may be when the affected bone breaks, often after a minor injury or no injury at all.

◆ Lung metastases may cause a non-productive cough, or a cough producing bloody sputum, chest pain or shortness of breath.

◆ Liver metastases may cause weight loss, fevers, nausea, loss of appetite, abdominal pain, fluid in the abdomen or jaundice (the skin turning yellow).

DIAGNOSIS

Physical Examination

There are no specific findings for metastatic cancer on physical examination. But there may be:

◆ fever
◆ tenderness of the bones
◆ tumors under the skin
◆ enlarged liver and spleen
◆ enlarged, hard lymph nodes
◆ fluid in the abdomen (ascites)
◆ jaundice (the skin turning yellow)
◆ swelling of the legs (edema)

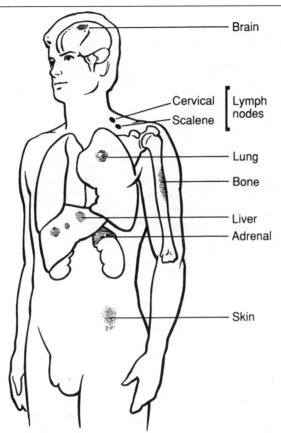

Brain

Cervical — Lymph
Scalene — nodes

Lung

Bone

Liver
Adrenal

Skin

Areas of Potential Cancer Metastases

Blood and Other Tests

♦ Routine liver function studies—blood tests looking at serum bilirubin and liver enzymes—may be abnormal. They can, however, be completely normal even in advanced stages of metastatic cancer.

♦ There may be serum blood tests that are abnormal. Metastatic colon cancer, for example, may be associated with an elevated carcinoembryonic antigen (CEA), testicular cancer with a high alpha-feto-protein (AFP) and/or elevated HCG and ovarian cancer with an elevated CA-125. But not all tumors have specific serum markers.

Imaging

♦ Abdominal ultrasound is one way to evaluate the abdomen if a mass is suspect-

ed. It can reveal the presence of fluid in the abdomen and is particularly useful for distinguishing a solid mass from a non-cancerous accumulation of fluid within the pelvis or liver (benign cyst).

♦ A bone scan will identify most tumor spread to the bones. It involves the injection of a special contrast agent into a vein, followed by whole-body imaging by a special camera. The image produced is a miniaturized skeleton that may show abnormal areas. But abnormal findings on a bone scan almost always have to be evaluated further with plain x-rays of the suspicious area.

♦ A CT scan is useful for determining the extent of a tumor within the head, chest or abdomen and for evaluating the possible spread of tumorous tissue into lymph nodes or other structures in the abdomen.

♦ Magnetic resonance imaging (MRI) may help determine if the cancer can be surgically removed, but it is usually not necessary.

♦ If metastases have been found on biopsy, a chest x-ray should be done because the lungs are a very common site of metastases.

Endoscopy and Biopsy

♦ A biopsy, either with a fine needle (FNA) or regular needle, is often necessary. This procedure can be done through the skin without significant danger. The biopsy sample can be used to distinguish between types of malignancy because the tumor cells of different cancers have characteristic features under the microscope.

TREATMENT BY TYPE

Treatment of metastatic cancer primarily depends on the original site of the cancer, so for specific treatment recommendations refer to the chapters dealing with the primary cancers. In some clinical situations, however, metastases may be treated in specific ways.

BRAIN METASTASES

The treatment of brain metastases depends on many factors such as the tumor of origin, the number and location of lesions within the brain and the extent of cancer in places other than the brain.

Standard Treatment Most patients are placed on steroids (Decadron) to relieve significant brain swelling that can cause severe symptoms. Many patients will also take an antiseizure medicine (Dilantin), since seizures are a common complication.

Patients with brain metastases from lymphoma, leukemia or small cell cancer should generally be given radiation therapy to the entire brain, although these tumors may also be treated with systemic chemotherapy.

The standard approach with brain metastases of any other origin is to decide if the tumor can be removed. A CT scan or an MRI should be done to discover whether there is more than one tumor and to define the specific site in the brain where the tumor or tumors are located.

♦ If there is only one tumor and the patient's overall condition is good, surgical removal of the metastasis may be attempted, although factors such as location within the brain, the duration since the primary cancer was treated and the presence of metastases elsewhere in the body have to be considered. This approach gives the best short-term and long-term palliation. After the tumor is removed, radiation therapy is given to the entire brain.

♦ In patients with more than one brain metastasis, surgery is not usually an option and radiation is delivered to the entire brain.

Investigational

♦ A method of biopsying or removing tumors called stereotaxic surgery is being studied. This allows for access to the brain tissue without causing extensive side effects (*see* "Brain Tumors: Adult").

♦ An alternative to conventional surgery on a single or a small number of brain metastases is the "gamma knife." This is a type of radiation treatment delivered by a machine that focuses multiple radiation beams directly at the offending area. This technique is offered in certain centers in the United States.

LUNG METASTASES

Metastases to the lung are common for many types of cancer. Patients may have no symptoms or they may have symptoms such as shortness of breath or coughing up blood.

Standard Treatment Lung metastases are generally treated with chemotherapy directed against the primary tumor type. But occasionally tumors metastasize to form a single deposit in the lungs. The likeliest primary tumor to do this is a sarcoma, although it may occur with almost any primary cancer.

If the CT scan and MRI suggest that the tumor is isolated, it may be surgically removed without causing significant loss of lung function. In fact, sarcomas may metastasize slowly enough that as many as three or four discrete tumors can be removed. This aggressive approach should be considered in any patient with a solitary lung metastasis, although most of the time the presence of other systemic tumors is likely to limit any gains from surgery.

One problem caused by metastases to the lung and the tissue lining the lung (pleura) is the accumulation of fluid within the chest. This may make the lung collapse, creating breathing difficulties. The fluid can be removed through a needle or through a larger tube inserted through the skin into the chest cavity. After the fluid is removed, an irritant such as doxycycline or bleomycin may be injected into the cavity to cause scarring of the tissues and prevent the reaccumulation of fluid.

If a metastatic tumor causes bleeding into the lungs, a patient may begin coughing up blood. Radiation therapy directed precisely at the tumor may alleviate the problem. If that cannot be done, it may be possible to stop the bleeding by injecting a special material into a blood vessel in the lung. This requires a specific radiologic technique but occasionally is very effective.

BONE METASTASES
Bone metastases may be discovered on a routine x-ray or bone scan or may be found because of pain, swelling or a fracture of the weakened bone.

Standard Treatment Bone metastases that don't produce symptoms and involve bones that are not weight-bearing (weight-bearing bones include the hip, upper leg, and shoulder) may be treated with the chemotherapy appropriate for the primary tumor.

Bone metastases that cause symptoms can also be treated with systemic therapy, although to take this approach depends on the type of cancer and the likelihood of getting much benefit from the treatment. If the tumor is not likely to respond to chemotherapy or if the bone involved is a weight-bearing one, the best option is to give radiation focused only on the involved area. The symptomatic relief is usually rapid and complete. Each bone can tolerate only a limited amount of radiation, although radiation can often be used to treat many different sites of tumor involvement.

If the bone metastases become apparent because of a fracture, the management issues are complicated. Surgery may be required to repair the bone and should be done if it is a weight-bearing bone. Fractured ribs, on the other hand, are not treated with a cast or immobilization. All such fractures should be treated with radiation therapy as well.

Bone metastases to the spine are a particular concern because a fractured vertebra can result in the loss of function of the limbs or bowel and bladder. Tumors in these bones, therefore, may need to be treated even though they are not weight-bearing bones and even when there are no symptoms.

LIVER METASTASES
Treatment of liver metastases depends on the organ where the cancer originated.

Standard Treatment For most metastatic tumors to the liver, systemic chemotherapy directed at the tumor type should be offered. But metastases from some cancers may be approached in a different way.

Occasionally, metastases to the liver are localized in one part of the liver or exist as solitary masses. Such tumors may be surgically removed with a possibility of achieving a cure, particularly with metastases from colon and kidney cancers or sarcoma. Generally, no more than four tumors should be removed from the liver, however. Removing more than four metastases rarely results in a cure and exposes the patient to significant surgical risks.

Liver metastases from colon cancer may be treated with combination chemotherapy, but because of the particular biological properties of some colon cancers, patients may develop liver metastases without ever having other sites of tumor involvement. Patients with such limited cancer may benefit from chemotherapy infused directly into the liver. Delivered by an implanted pump connected to the hepatic artery, this therapy takes advantage of the liver's ability to metabolize some drugs, meaning that the tumor may be exposed to high concentrations of chemotherapy while the rest of the body is spared the side effects.

This approach initially requires surgery for the implantation of the pump and the removal of the gall bladder, but the rest of the therapy can be done on an outpatient basis. The treatment causes tumor regression more often than standard chemotherapy.

Investigational

♦ New combinations of chemotherapy drugs may improve results for patients with colon cancer metastases, both to the liver and elsewhere. Such treatments are being studied for systemic treatment as well as for treatment to the liver.

♦ A treatment called chemoembolization involves administering a combination of chemotherapy and colloid particles directly into the liver tumor via its main (hepatic) artery. The procedure is performed by a radiologist and does not require surgery or prolonged bedrest. It is very effective for primary tumors, but it is much less effective for metastases.

♦ Cryosurgery—cold surgery—holds out some promise of allowing the removal of some otherwise unresectable tumors. So far, this technique is performed only by a few specialized physicians.

♦ Liver transplantation can be performed. But it should almost never be done for patients with metastatic tumors in the liver, for it can be assumed that the cancer will spread to other organs.

SUPPORTIVE THERAPY

♦ Pain relievers are sometimes called for in liberal doses. Narcotics may have excessive side effects, however, because they are metabolized by the liver, which may not be functioning properly.

♦ Non-steroidal anti-inflammatory drugs may be effective even against the severe pain associated with metastatic cancer.

♦ The loss of appetite that often accompanies metastatic cancer may be relieved with a medication called Megace.

♦ The use of water pills to alleviate fluid in the abdomen or legs may cause a significant imbalance in kidney function, creating major problems if their use is not carefully monitored.

♦ Nausea can be adequately treated with standard medications, including suppositories.

♦ Sleep disturbances are common, but sleeping pills (sedatives) should be used carefully, since most are metabolized by the liver.

TREATMENT FOLLOW-UP

Careful follow-up is necessary after treatment of metastases. Depending upon the organs involved, diagnostic tests will be done to identify new areas of tumor involvement that may cause problems and to look for tumor recurrences.

THE MOST IMPORTANT QUESTIONS YOU CAN ASK

♦ Should I see another physician to confirm that my metastatic tumor is being treated in the right way?

♦ Could I benefit from an investigational therapy available at another institution?

♦ How sick will the proposed chemotherapy make me relative to its potential benefit?

♦ How sure are you that you know the primary source of my cancer?

MULTIPLE MYELOMA

Robert A. Kyle, MD

◇

Multiple myeloma is a cancer of the plasma cell, a type of B lymphocyte responsible for producing antibodies that take part in the immune response. A treatable but rarely curable disease, multiple myeloma—also called plasma cell myeloma, myelomatosis or Kahler's disease—is characterized by the overgrowth of malignant plasma cells, mostly in the bone marrow. Although multiple myeloma usually involves the bones, it must be distinguished from cancers that begin in another organ such as the breast or lung and then spread to the bones.

Multiple myeloma is an uncommon malignancy, making up only 1 percent of all cases of cancer. In a population of 1 million people, only 40 cases would be found each year. There have been reports that the incidence of myeloma has increased two- to threefold during the past 40 years, but careful studies from the United States and Europe suggest that the incidence has not truly changed. The apparent increase is most likely due to more and better medical facilities and diagnostic techniques.

Types Ninety percent of multiple myeloma cases involve the bone marrow. There are several types, each with its distinctive features and each producing a variety of diagnostic findings and symptoms:

♦ Patients with smoldering multiple myeloma (SMM) have enough myeloma cells in the bone marrow and a large amount of an abnormal protein (monoclonal or M-protein) in the blood to indicate multiple myeloma, but they do not have the anemia, kidney failure or skeletal lesions that are also characteristic of the disease. There are no symptoms.

♦ Patients with plasma cell leukemia have large numbers of plasma cells circulating in the blood. Plasma cell leukemia may be the first feature of multiple myeloma leading to a diagnosis or it may occur late in its course after a resistance to chemotherapy has developed.

♦ With non-secretory myeloma, patients have abnormal plasma cells in the bone marrow and frequently have holes (lytic lesions) in the skeleton, but no abnormal protein is detectable in the blood or urine.

♦ Osteosclerotic myeloma (POEMS syndrome) patients usually have pain, burning, numbness and weakness produced by the involvement of nerves by the disease (polyneuropathy). The liver and spleen are often enlarged; there may be a darkening of the skin and increased growth of body hair. The breasts may become enlarged and the testicles smaller. Bone x-rays usually reveal dense (sclerotic) areas in the bone. Anemia, kidney failure and fractures are rare with this type.

♦ Solitary plasmacytoma (solitary myeloma of bone) means there is a single plasma cell tumor in the bone. X-rays of the bones show no other lytic lesions and the bone marrow is normal. Characteristically, the patients have no abnormal M-protein in the blood or urine. This tumor should be treated with high doses of radiation to the lesion, but about 60 percent of patients will develop multiple myeloma within 10 years.

♦ Extramedullary plasmacytoma is a tumor consisting of myeloma cells but occurs *outside* the bone marrow. The most commonly involved area is the back of the nose and throat (nasopharynx), and the sinuses may also be involved.

Eighty percent of cases involve the upper respiratory area.

Extramedullary plasmacytomas may also involve the stomach, small bowel, colon, urinary bladder, thyroid, breast or the brain. Examination of the bone marrow is normal, and the patients have no lytic bone lesions or M-protein in the blood or urine. If an abnormal protein is present, it should disappear after treatment. Diagnosis of a plasmacytoma is made after a biopsy of the tumor. It is treated with large doses of radiation therapy. Most patients are cured, but the disease may recur in a nearby area. The development of typical multiple myeloma is uncommon.

What Causes It The cause is not known, although exposure to radiation may be a factor in some cases. Survivors of the atomic bomb explosions in Japan had an increased incidence of multiple myeloma.

There is little evidence that chemicals cause myeloma in humans, although some reports have linked multiple myeloma with benzene or asbestos. An increased risk of multiple myeloma has been recognized in farmers in several countries and has been noted in rubber workers, furniture workers and those exposed to pesticides. The number of cases is small, however, and more information is needed to confirm this association.

There have been reports of two or more family members with multiple myeloma, but the genetic influence is minimal. There is no evidence that allergies, chronic infections or other immune-stimulating conditions play a role.

RISK FACTORS

At Significantly Higher Risk
♦ Multiple myeloma occurs in older people. The average age is 60 to 65 years; 3 percent are under 40.
♦ Its incidence in African-Americans is twice that in caucasians.

SCREENING

Screening is of no value in a healthy person because anyone with multiple myeloma should not be treated unless there are symptoms or serious laboratory abnormalities. Many patients are found to have an M-protein in their blood during a routine examination, but if there is no other evidence of multiple myeloma these patients are considered to have a benign condition called monoclonal gammopathy of undetermined significance (MGUS).

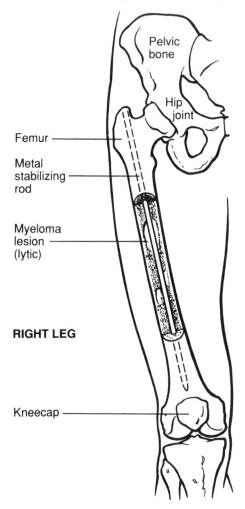

Bone with lytic myeloma lesion and stabilizing rod

COMMON SIGNS AND SYMPTOMS

At the time of diagnosis, more than two-thirds of people with multiple myeloma have bone pain, typically in the back or chest and less often in the arms and legs. The pain is usually made worse by movement and does not occur at night except after a change in position. Patients may lose several inches in height because of the collapse of vertebrae.

Weakness and fatigue are common and are often associated with anemia. Fever is rare, and when it occurs it is usually from an infection. Occasionally, there may be bleeding from the nose and gums or easy bruising. The initial symptoms may be from an acute infection, most often pneumonia, though meningitis or bloodstream infections may also occur. There may also be symptoms of elevated serum calcium (*see* "Supportive Care").

DIAGNOSIS

There are minimal criteria for the diagnosis of multiple myeloma. There must be at least 10 percent abnormal plasma cells in the bone marrow or proof of an extramedullary plasmacytoma *plus* the usual clinical features of multiple myeloma *and* at least one of the following abnormalities:
♦ an M-protein in the blood (usually greater than 3 gm/dL)
♦ an M-protein in the urine (Bence Jones protein)
♦ osteolytic lesions.

Connective tissue diseases (such as rheumatoid arthritis, polymyositis or scleroderma), chronic infections, metastatic cancer, lymphoma and leukemia may resemble some of the characteristics of multiple myeloma.

The diagnosis must differentiate those with true multiple myeloma from those with monoclonal gammopathy of undetermined significance (MGUS) and smoldering multiple myeloma (SMM), since people with these conditions should be observed indefinitely and not given therapy unless they develop features of multiple myeloma.

Physical Examination
♦ Physical findings are often general and non-specific. Pallor (paleness) is the most common physical finding.
♦ The liver can be felt in about one-fifth of patients; the spleen is rarely felt.
♦ There may be tumors outside the bone marrow (extramedullary plasmacytomas).

Blood and Other Tests
♦ A complete blood count (CBC) reveals anemia in two-thirds of patients.
♦ An increased total serum protein may be one of the first clues to the presence of an M-protein. An elevated serum calcium occurs in about 30 percent of patients. The level of serum creatinine (a measure of kidney function) is abnormal in more than one-fourth of patients at diagnosis. The serum beta-2 microglobulin level is helpful in prognosis.
♦ Serum protein electrophoresis shows an M-protein "spike" in 80 percent of patients. Immunoelectrophoresis or immunofixation is necessary to determine the type of M-protein. The amount of M-protein is measured by serum protein electrophoresis or by the measurement of IgG or IgA, the two major types of M-protein found in multiple myeloma.
♦ Ninety-nine percent of patients with multiple myeloma will have an M-protein in the blood or in the urine. If the level of M-protein in the blood is high or if the patient has blurred vision or bleeding, determining the viscosity (thickness) of the serum is necessary. Measuring of the M-protein in the serum and urine is a good way to determine whether the disease is getting worse or is responding to chemotherapy. The level of the M-protein is a direct measure of the tumor mass.
♦ A 24-hour urine specimen is essential. The total protein is determined and elec-

trophoresis is performed, making it possible to measure the amount of monoclonal light chain (of kappa or lambda origin). This is called Bence Jones protein and should be detected by immunologic techniques.

♦ Bone marrow examination is essential for diagnosis, allowing the physician to determine the number of plasma cells (myeloma cells) in the marrow and their appearance. It also provides a measure of normal red cell, white cell and platelet production.

Imaging

♦ X-rays of the skull, the entire spine, pelvis, upper legs and upper arms are necessary to detect lytic lesions, bone thinning (osteoporosis) or fractures. Skeletal abnormalities occur in 75 percent of patients at diagnosis.

♦ Bone scans with technetium-99 can be done but are not as effective as conventional x-rays for detecting lesions and are not recommended.

♦ CT or MRI scans may be helpful when the patient has skeletal pain and negative x-rays.

Serum protein electrophoresis (SPEP) pattern in multiple myeloma.
Note the M-protein spike

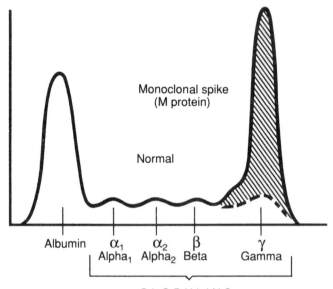

STAGING

A clinical staging system based on a combination of laboratory findings that correlate with the myeloma cell mass has often been used. Patients are generally separated into those with low-cell mass (Stage I), high-cell mass (Stage III) and those whose cell mass is between Stages I and III (Stage II). A further classification divides patients according to whether they are "A" (kidney function test is normal or only slightly elevated, with a creatinine less than 2.0 mg/dL) or "B" (the serum creatinine is equal to or greater than 2.0 mg/dL). The plasma cell labeling index (measurement of the rate of growth of the myeloma cells) and the β_2-microglobulin (β_2-M) level are more helpful prognostic factors than the staging system.

TREATMENT OVERVIEW

Multiple myeloma involves all of the red bone marrow and is widespread when the diagnosis is made. Consequently, there is no adjuvant or neoadjuvant treatment and no therapy for metastatic disease.

Not all patients who meet the minimal criteria for diagnosis of multiple myeloma should be treated. Because the disease is not curable and therapy causes potential side effects and involves cost, treatment should be delayed until there is evidence of progression, symptoms appear or treatment is needed to prevent complications.

When symptoms do develop, chemotherapy is the preferred treatment.

 Chemotherapy The major controversy in chemotherapy is whether treatment should be with a single alkylating agent such as melphalan (Alkeran) together with prednisone or a combination of alkylating agents.

Melphalan + prednisone is given daily by mouth for four to seven days every four to six weeks. This produces an objective response in 50 to 60 percent of patients. The dosage of melphalan must be changed depending upon the white cell count and platelet count, with the dosage increased to the point that some decrease in the white count or platelets occurs three weeks after the start of each cycle of therapy.

Many combinations of chemotherapy drugs—including melphalan, cyclophosphamide, carmustine (BCNU), vincristine, doxorubicin (Adriamycin) and prednisone—produce an objective response in about 70 percent of patients. But the average survival of those treated with the single alkylating agent (melphalan) and those receiving multiple alkylating agents is about the same—two to three years.

Chemotherapy should be continued until the patient responds and is in a stable (plateau) state. This usually requires one to two years of therapy. Treatment with alkylating agents should not be given after reaching the plateau state because they may damage the bone marrow, resulting in a myelodysplastic syndrome or acute leukemia. Alpha$_2$-interferon (alpha$_2$-IFN) will prolong the plateau state, but the overall survival is probably the same as for those to whom no maintenance therapy is given. The dosage of alpha$_2$-IFN must be altered so that the side effects do not interfere with the patient's well-being. Patients must be followed closely, however, and chemotherapy must be started again when there is a relapse. Most patients will again respond to the same treatment that they received initially.

Radiation The use of radiation therapy should be limited to those patients with disabling pain who have a local process that has not responded to chemotherapy. The use of Tylenol with codeine or other narcotics can usually control the pain. This approach is preferred to local radiation because pain frequently recurs in another site anyway and local radiation does not benefit anyone with generalized disease.

Investigational Chemotherapy

♦ A combination of alkylating agents (vincristine + BCNU + melphalan + cyclophosphamide + prednisone [VBMCP]) in alternating cycles with alpha$_2$-interferon (alpha$_2$-IFN) produced better-quality responses and prolongation of survival in a pilot study, but this must be confirmed in a prospective study.

♦ Myeloma cells frequently become resistant to chemotherapy. One such mechanism is characterized by the expression of glycoprotein P-170. Various agents such as verapamil or cyclosporine have been used to reverse this resistance, but only modest success has been achieved.

♦ Growth factors such as granulocyte colony-stimulating factor (G-CSF) or granulocyte macrophage colony-stimulating factor (GM-CSF) to shorten the duration of neutropenia (neutrophils fight infection) may be helpful after high-dose chemotherapy.

Bone Marrow Transplantation This approach is an alternative for the therapy of multiple myeloma. There are two major approaches: allogeneic or autologous. There is no evidence that either is curative and most patients will suffer a relapse.

♦ With allogeneic transplantation, bone marrow is given from a matched donor following high-dose chemotherapy and total body irradiation. The mortality is high (20–25 percent within the first three months) and the patient often suffers from a peculiar form of rejection called graft-versus-host disease, in which the transplanted marrow attacks the host tissue. This procedure is also possible only for people under 55, which greatly limits its use in multiple myeloma. Only 5 to 10 percent of multiple myeloma patients can have an allogeneic bone marrow transplantation because of their age and the lack of a matched donor.

♦ Autologous transplantation—in which bone marrow or peripheral blood stem cells are removed from a patient before high-dose radiation or chemotherapy and then returned—is applicable for more patients because the age limit is higher (approximately 65 years) and a matched donor is unnecessary. The mortality rate for autologous transplantation is less than 10 percent.

But there are two major problems with autologous transplantation for patients with multiple myeloma. First, it is difficult to destroy all the myeloma cells from the bone marrow even with high doses of chemotherapy and radiation. Second, it is difficult to remove the malignant myeloma cells from the bone marrow or blood before reinfusion. Using chemotherapy or monoclonal antibodies directed against myeloma cells (or both monoclonal antibodies and chemotherapy) may be helpful but is not yet practical.

SUPPORTIVE CARE

Multiple myeloma produces many complications that require close medical attention and management.

♦ *Hypercalcemia* (elevated blood calcium level) This occurs in almost one-third of all patients and should be suspected if symptoms such as loss of appetite, nausea, vomiting, excessive thirst, increased urine, constipation, weakness, change in mental alertness or confusion develop. Treatment is urgent because kidney failure is common. Therapy with intravenous fluids and prednisone is usually effective, but if it isn't there are a variety of other effective agents such as the diphosphonates.

♦ *Infections* Bacterial infections may occur and must be diagnosed and treated promptly with appropriate antibiotics. All patients should receive pneumococcal vaccine and influenza immunizations. Prophylactic penicillin or intravenous gamma globulin should be considered for those with serious recurrent bacterial infections.

♦ *Pain* Bone pain should be treated with analgesics or narcotics. People with multiple myeloma have to be as active as possible because confinement to bed increases the bone loss. Patients should do all they can to avoid falling because a fall can result in multiple fractures. The use of an intramedullary rod in the long bones of the arm or leg should be considered when a large hole (lytic lesion) is seen on x-ray. The rod will stabilize the bone and prevent fractures. Radiation therapy to relieve pain may not be necessary for someone who is beginning chemotherapy.

♦ *Kidney Failure* Increased fluid intake is necessary for patients with Bence Jones protein in the urine. They should drink enough fluids so that they produce approximately 3 quarts (3 L) of urine daily. Patients with acute kidney failure must be treated promptly with appropriate fluids and electrolytes. An artificial kidney (hemodialysis) may be necessary. In some cases, removing large amounts of plasma from the blood (plasmapheresis) may be helpful in acute kidney failure.

♦ *Hyperviscosity* This condition of "thick blood" is characterized by bleeding from the nose or gums, blurred vision, dizziness, shortness of breath or mental confusion. It can be treated effectively with plasmapheresis.

♦ *Muscle Weakness* People with multiple myeloma may develop weakness or paralysis of their legs and have difficulty urinating or controlling their bowels. If this happens, a myeloma tumor pressing on the spinal cord is a possibility and can be diagnosed with a CT or MRI scan or myelography. The tumor can be treated effectively with radiation therapy.

♦ *Emotional Support* Anyone with multiple myeloma needs substantial and continuing emotional support. The approach must be positive, emphasizing the potential benefits of therapy. It is reassuring to know that some patients survive for 10 years or more. It is vital that the physician caring for patients with multiple myeloma has the interest and capacity to deal with an incurable disease over a span of years with assurance, sympathy and resourcefulness and that patients can sense the doctor's confidence.

TREATMENT FOLLOW-UP

♦ Complete blood count (CBC) every three weeks after each cycle of therapy and before each treatment course.
♦ Calcium and creatinine measured every 6 to 12 weeks.
♦ Serum protein electrophoresis every 6 to 12 weeks.
♦ Electrophoresis of a 24-hour urine specimen every 6 to 12 weeks if an M-protein was found at the time of diagnosis.
♦ Metastatic bone survey every six months or x-rays of bones in the event of new pain.
♦ Bone marrow examination to confirm remission or relapse.

RECURRENT (AND RESISTANT) CANCER

About one-third of all patients treated initially with chemotherapy will not obtain an objective response. And almost all patients with multiple myeloma who do respond to chemotherapy will eventually relapse if they do not die of some other disease in the meantime.

The decision about further treatment after a relapse has to take a number of factors into account, including prior treatment, where the recurrence occurs and personal considerations.
♦ If the relapse occurs after the initial therapy has been stopped, therapy with the same melphalan-prednisone or multiple alkylating agent treatments is beneficial in a majority of patients.
♦ If the relapse occurs while melphalan and prednisone therapy is being used, a combination called VBAP (vincristine + BCNU + Adriamycin + prednisone) will be of some benefit to 40 percent of patients.
♦ If a patient has already received these agents or does not respond to VBAP, a combination of vincristine + Adriamycin + dexamethasone (VAD) can be given.
♦ If a patient is resistant to all of these agents or if the blood counts are low, a trial of high-dose prednisone or methylprednisolone may be beneficial.

THE MOST IMPORTANT QUESTIONS YOU CAN ASK

♦ Should I be treated now or should therapy be delayed until I have symptoms?
♦ Should I receive single or multiple alkylating agents?
♦ Should I get a second opinion?
♦ When should chemotherapy be discontinued?
♦ Should I receive an autologous or allogeneic bone marrow transplant?

OVARY

Jeffrey L. Stern, MD

◇

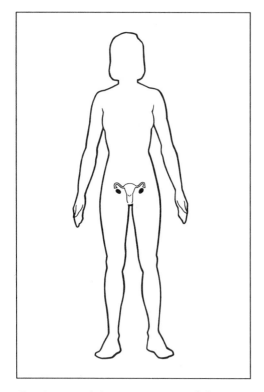

Carcinoma of the ovary is one of the most common gynecologic malignancies. In many cases, it is curable when found early, but because it does not cause any symptoms in its early stages most women have widespread disease at the time of diagnosis. Partly because of this, the mortality rate from ovarian cancer exceeds that for all other gynecologic malignancies combined. It is the fourth most frequent cause of cancer death in women in the United States. About one in every 70 women will develop cancer of the ovary and one in every 100 women will die from it. The American Cancer Society estimates that there will be 22,000 cases of ovarian

cancer diagnosed in 1994 with approximately 13,300 deaths.

Types The most common form of ovarian cancer arises from the cells covering the surface of the ovary and is known as epithelial carcinoma. There are five major types of this carcinoma—serous, mucinous, endometrioid, clear cell and undifferentiated. Epithelial carcinomas are further divided into grades, according to how virulent they appear on microscopic examination.

Tumors of low malignant potential, also known as borderline tumors, are the most well-differentiated malignancy (Grade 0) and account for 15 percent of all epithelial carcinomas of the ovary. The other three grades are well-differentiated (Grade 1), moderately differentiated (Grade 2) and poorly differentiated (Grade 3). Well-differentiated tumors have a better prognosis than poorly differentiated tumors. Clear cell carcinoma and especially undifferentiated carcinoma have a poorer prognosis than the other cell types.

The two other major kinds of ovarian cancer—germ cell tumors, which arise from the eggs, and ovarian stromal tumors, which arise from supportive tissue—are relatively uncommon and account for less than 10 percent of all ovarian malignancies (*see* "Ovarian Germ Cell Tumors").

How It Spreads Ovarian cancer spreads early by shedding malignant cells into the abdominal cavity. The cells implant on the lining of the abdominal cavity (peritoneum) and can grow on the surface of the liver, the fatty tissue attached to the stomach and large intestine (omentum), the small and large intestines, the bladder and the diaphragm.

Disease on the diaphragm may at times result in impaired drainage of fluid from the abdominal cavity, resulting, for some women, in a large collection of abdominal fluid known as ascites. The cancer cells can occasionally cross the diaphragm and spread to the surface of the lungs and chest cavity, resulting in a collection of fluid around the lungs known as a pleural effusion.

Ovarian cancer may also spread to the pelvic, aortic, groin and neck lymph nodes (*see* figure page 348).

What Causes It Unknown.

RISK FACTORS

There is a much higher incidence of ovarian cancer in industrialized countries. Some researchers have implicated talcum powder, which until recently contained asbestos, as a possible cause. Ovarian cancer can occur in any age group, but it is most common in postmenopausal women. Not ovulating—by having children, breastfeeding, using birth control pills or having a condition that interferes with ovulation such as polycystic ovaries—has been shown to offer protection against developing cancer. There may also be a genetic predisposition to this cancer. There are rare families in which several members of the same or different generation develop ovarian cancer. This is known as hereditary ovarian cancer syndrome. It generally affects women in their mid-forties. There may be up to a 50 percent risk of developing ovarian cancer in their lifetime. It can also be inherited through the male side of the family. This syndrome occurs in less than 3 percent of all women who have a positive family history of ovarian cancer. Approximately 7 percent of all women with ovarian cancer do not seem to have a genetic disposition but have a positive family history.

Ninety percent of these women have only one other family member with ovarian cancer.

Suggested management in women with a family history for ovarian cancer is as follows: Removal of both ovaries after childbearing or very close follow-up (CA-125 and pelvic ultrasound) for those women who have hereditary ovarian cancer syndrome. If there is a family history of only one relative with ovarian cancer, prophylactic removal of the ovaries is not recommended. When there are two to three relatives who have a history of ovarian cancer, then it is usually very difficult, if not impossible, to determine whether an individual has ovarian cancer syndrome or just a strong positive family history. In these women, prophylactic removal of the ovaries is controversial, and management is individualized. Close follow-up with serum CA-125 and pelvic ultrasound is strongly recommended, however.

SCREENING

There are no diagnostic methods accurate enough to be used for routine screening of women without symptoms. Nonetheless, it is recommended that all women have an annual pelvic and rectal examination since an ovarian mass can occasionally be detected. A Pap smear will detect ovarian cancer in only 10 percent of women with the disease. Recent studies have shown that a serum tumor marker known as CA-125 is elevated in 80 percent of women with epithelial ovarian cancer. Unfortunately, this test is not accurate enough for screening all women for ovarian cancer. Approximately 2 percent of normal women will have an elevated CA-125 (normal is less than 35). Approximately 1 percent of normal women will have a CA-125 greater than 65. Because of the small incidence of a false-positive test, screening all women with CA-125 has not been recommended. A great deal of research is taking place exploring the use of CA-125 as well as other tumor markers for screening. Tumor markers are, however, useful for assessing response to therapy.

A pelvic ultrasound examination may become a part of the routine annual gynecologic examination in the future. This can be done using a minimally uncomfortable vaginal probe. It is used to examine the ovaries as well as the uterus. When used in combination with CA-125, it is fairly accurate in detecting ovarian neoplasms.

COMMON SIGNS AND SYMPTOMS

Many women with early stages of ovarian carcinoma have no symptoms. The unfortunate result is that two-thirds of all women with ovarian carcinoma have advanced disease at the time of diagnosis.

Many women have vague, non-specific abdominal symptoms including pain, pelvic pressure, low back discomfort, mild nausea, feeling full early when eating, constipation and gas. Some women have abnormal uterine bleeding. Although some cases are diagnosed during a routine gynecologic examination, many women are diagnosed only when they have developed abdominal distension because of ascites.

Advanced ovarian cancer often results in blockage of the intestines, causing severe nausea, vomiting, pain and weight loss.

DIAGNOSIS

Physical Examination
♦ A careful pelvic exam is performed with attention to the ovaries, uterus, bladder and rectum.
♦ The neck, groin and underarms (axilla) are examined for enlarged lymph nodes.
♦ The lungs are carefully examined for excess fluid.
♦ The abdomen is examined for the presence of an enlarged liver, a mass or ascites.

Blood and Other Tests
♦ Complete blood count (CBC).
♦ Serum liver and kidney function tests.
♦ Serum CA-125.

Imaging
♦ Abdominal and pelvic CT or MRI scans.
♦ X-rays of the upper gastrointestinal tract (UGI series) may occasionally be done.
♦ Intravenous pyelogram (occasionally).
♦ Barium enema.

Endoscopy and Biopsy
♦ A definitive diagnosis requires microscopic examination of part or all of the involved ovary or any other suspicious abdominal mass. Cystic ovarian tumors that are less than 2 1/2 in. (6 cm) in diameter occurring in premenopausal woman are usually benign cysts.

Surgical evaluation should be strongly considered for any mass in a postmenopausal woman, masses that are larger than 2 1/2 in. (6 cm) in diameter, masses persisting longer than one menstrual cycle and masses that are suspicious on imaging of the pelvis.

STAGING

Ovarian carcinoma is staged at surgery. Stages are usually defined according to the classification system devised by FIGO (International Federation of Gynecology and Obstetricians). The TNM system corresponds to the stages accepted by FIGO.

Stage I Cancer is confined to one or both ovaries.

♦ **Ia** Cancer is limited to one ovary. There is no ascites and no tumor on the surface of the ovary and the surface of the tumor is unruptured.

♦ **Ib** The cancer is limited to both ovaries. There is no ascites and no tumor on the surface of either ovary and the surfaces of the tumors are unruptured.

♦ **Ic** The cancer is either Stage Ia or Ib and one or more of the following applies: there is tumor on the surface of one or both ovaries, at least one of the tumors has ruptured, ascites is present or the abdominal washings contain malignant cells.

Five-Year Survival 60 to 100 percent, depending on the histologic type, grade and sub-stage.

Stage II The tumor involves one or both ovaries with extension to other pelvic structures.

♦ **IIa** There is extension of the cancer or metastases to the uterus and/or fallopian tubes.

♦ **IIb** There is extension to the bladder or rectum.

♦ **IIc** The cancer is either stage IIa or IIb and one or more of the following applies: there is tumor on the surface of one or both ovaries, at least one of the tumors has ruptured, the ascites contains malignant cells or the washings from the abdominal cavity contain malignant cells.

Five-Year Survival About 60 percent

Stage III The tumor involves one or both ovaries with tumor implants confined to the abdominal cavity but outside the pelvis, or there is cancer in the pelvic, para-aortic or groin lymph nodes (*see* figure page 348).

♦ **IIIa** The tumor is grossly limited to the pelvis and the lymph nodes are negative, but there is biopsy-proven microscopic cancer on the intra-abdominal (peritoneal) surfaces.

♦ **IIIb** The tumor involves one or both ovaries and there are tumor implants on the peritoneal surfaces less than 3/4 in. (2 cm) in diameter. The lymph nodes are negative.

♦ **IIIc** The tumor involves one or both ovaries, there are tumor implants on the surface of the abdominal cavity greater than 3/4 in. (2 cm) in diameter or there is cancer in the pelvic, para-aortic or groin lymph nodes.

Five-Year Survival About 20 percent

Stage IV Growth involves one or both ovaries. There are distant metastases to the liver or lungs, or there are malignant cells in the excess fluid accumulated around the lungs.

Five-Year Survival 10 percent

TREATMENT OVERVIEW

Surgery In women with early-stage cancer, one or both ovaries are usually removed (with or without removal of the uterus) and meticulous surgical staging is performed. This involves washings from the abdominal cavity to detect malignant cells, selective sampling of pelvic and aortic lymph nodes and meticulous inspection of the abdominal cavity surfaces with biopsy of any suspicious lesion and removal of the fatty tissue attached to the stomach and large intestines (omentectomy) and multiple, random biopsies of the lining of the abdominal cavity including the surfaces of the diaphragms.

In women with advanced cancer, surgical removal of as much tumor as possible, also called tumor debulking, is standard therapy. If possible, the uterus, both fallopian tubes, both ovaries, the omentum and as much of the grossly visible cancer as possible is removed.

Recent studies have shown that 25 to 35 percent of women with ovarian carcinoma will require intestinal or urologic surgery to obtain optimal tumor debulking (defined as leaving behind no tumor implant greater than 3/4 in. (2 cm) in diameter). A permanent colostomy may occasionally be necessary but is rare in women who have had a preoperative bowel prep—a cleansing of the intestines with enemas and laxatives and administration of oral antibiotics.

To decide if further treatment is required, second-look abdominal surgery is often performed after six cycles of chemotherapy in women without evidence of persistent cancer (*see* "Treatment Follow-up"). In advanced recurrent cancer, surgery is sometimes required to relieve intestinal obstruction.

Complications of surgery can include infection, bleeding and injury to the bladder, rectum or ureter causing a leak, although this is rare. There may be blood clots in the legs, which can occasionally dislodge and travel to the lungs (pulmonary embolism).

 Chemotherapy In most cases chemotherapy is begun one to two weeks after surgery. The standard regimen includes cis-

platin or carboplatin + Cytoxan, or cisplatin + Taxol given intravenously every three to four weeks as tolerated for at least six cycles. Forty to 80 percent of patients can be expected to respond. The response rate depends to a large degree on the amount of cancer remaining after surgery, with those who have an optimal tumor debulking having a better response rate.

Carboplatin is now being used more often than cisplatin because it can sometimes be given on an outpatient basis. It causes less kidney damage, hearing loss, nausea and vomiting and peripheral nerve damage (manifested by muscle weakness and numbness or tingling). Unfortunately, it does have more bone marrow toxicity than cisplatin. Cisplatin + Cytoxan and carboplatin + Cytoxan appear to have equal response rates. Cisplatin + Taxol may have a slightly higher response rate.

Over the past several years, a technique known as intraperitoneal (intra-abdominal)

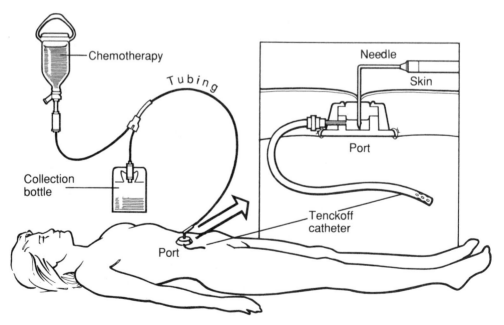

Intraperitoneal Chemotherapy for Ovarian Cancer

chemotherapy has been developed to deliver the chemotherapy directly into the abdominal cavity. This procedure requires surgery to place a port and its attached catheter beneath the skin. The catheter is brought through the abdominal wall and placed directly into the abdominal cavity. The cancer drugs are then given via a needle directly into the subcutaneous port. Complications can include infection, malfunction of the catheter and occasionally intestinal blockage.

Intraperitoneal chemotherapy is generally given monthly for six months. Although preliminary results are encouraging, it has been tested in a small number of women who have been followed only for a short time, so it is still considered investigational. Large trials are now under way to compare the effectiveness of intraperitoneal versus intravenous chemotherapy.

Chemotherapy can cause hair loss, nausea and vomiting, infection or bleeding because of bone marrow toxicity, and damage to the heart, kidneys, nerves and liver.

 Radiation There is some evidence that external beam radiation therapy is as effective as chemotherapy for patients with early stages of ovarian carcinoma who have no visible cancer remaining after their operation.

Sometimes radiation therapy is used for microscopic recurrent ovarian cancer or cancer that has not responded well to chemotherapy. Radiation may be given only to the pelvis or, more typically, to the entire abdomen (usually five days each week for four to five weeks), which results in a better survival rate. Complications and side effects can be considerable and can include diarrhea, nausea and vomiting, bleeding from the bladder or rectum, vaginal scarring, intestinal obstruction, or leaks (fistulas) in the urinary or intestinal tracts.

Radioactive phosphate inserted directly into the abdominal cavity is sometimes given to women who have no visible cancer or less than 1 mm of residual disease after surgery.

TREATMENT BY STAGE

STAGE Ia
Standard Treatment Therapy depends primarily on the age of the patient and the grade of the cancer.

For borderline, well-differentiated tumors (Grade 1) in women who want to preserve their reproductive function, standard therapy includes removal of the cancerous ovary and the adjacent fallopian tube (the other, apparently healthy ovary should be biopsied, however), partial removal of the omentum and biopsies of the pelvic and para-aortic lymph nodes.

For postmenopausal women and those who do not want to preserve their reproductive function, standard therapy includes a total hysterectomy, removal of both fallopian tubes and ovaries and careful surgical staging. Women with Stage Ia borderline or Grade 1 carcinoma are usually cured with surgery alone.

Standard therapy for Grade 2 or 3 tumors is total hysterectomy, removal of both tubes and both ovaries, meticulous surgical staging and six monthly cycles of combination chemotherapy, usually with cisplatin or carboplatin + Cytoxan or cisplatin + Taxol. Other therapies that are sometimes recommended are total abdominal and pelvic radiation or intra-abdominal administration of radioactive phosphate (P^{32}).

Investigational
♦ A Gynecologic Oncology Group trial is comparing intra-abdominal radioactive phosphate given once with giving six cycles (once every three weeks) of intravenous cisplatin + Cytoxan for women with poorly differentiated (Grades 2–3) tumors.
♦ Intra-abdominal chemotherapy with agents such as cisplatin or carboplatin or etoposide.

STAGE Ib

Standard Treatment A total hysterectomy, removal of both tubes and ovaries and meticulous surgical staging is performed. Women with tumors of low malignant potential or Grade 1 carcinomas may not require further treatment.

Women with Grade 2 or 3 cancers usually receive postoperative combination chemotherapy (usually carboplatin or cisplatin + Cytoxan or cisplatin + Taxol given every three weeks as tolerated for a total of six cycles), whole abdominal and pelvic radiation therapy or intra-abdominal radioactive phosphate.

Investigational Same as Stage Ia.

STAGE Ic

Standard Treatment Hysterectomy, removal of both fallopian tubes and ovaries, partial omentectomy and biopsy of the pelvic and para-aortic lymph nodes is done. Careful inspection of the remaining intra-abdominal surfaces is vital. Suspicious lesions should be biopsied, and washings of the abdominal cavity should be taken to check for malignant cells.

In the absence of progressive disease, standard therapy after surgery includes six courses of cisplatin or carboplatin + Cytoxan, or cisplatin + Taxol.

Investigational
♦ Intra-abdominal cisplatin or carboplatin or etoposide with or without other anticancer drugs.
♦ Intra-abdominal radioactive phosphate.
♦ Whole-abdomen and pelvic radiation therapy.

STAGE IIa

Standard Treatment The surgical procedure is the same as for Stage Ic, again with biopsy of any suspicious lesions and washings of the abdominal cavity to check for malignant cells.

If all tumor implants are less than 3/4 in. (2 cm) in diameter after surgery, combination chemotherapy including cisplatin or carboplatin + Cytoxan is given to the majority of patients for six cycles (one course every three weeks).

Whole-abdomen and pelvic radiation may be given if the residual disease is less than 1/4 in. (0.5 cm) in diameter. Intra-abdominal radioactive phosphorus can be given if the residual disease is less than 1 mm in diameter.

If there is residual cancer greater than 3/4 in. (2 cm) in diameter, intravenous chemotherapy is used exclusively. There are several commonly used combinations—CT (cisplatin + Taxol), CP (Cytoxan + cisplatin or Cytoxan + carboplatin), CAP (Cytoxan + Adriamycin + cisplatin), AP (Adriamycin + cisplatin) and CHAD (Cytoxan + hexamethylmelamine + Adriamycin + cisplatin).

Investigational
♦ One-time intra-abdominal administration of radioactive phosphate versus six cycles of intravenous cisplatin + Cytoxan.
♦ Intra-abdominal carboplatin, cisplatin or etoposide with or without other anticancer drugs.

STAGES IIb, IIc, IIIa, IIIb, IIIc, IV

Standard Treatment In women with advanced ovarian carcinoma, standard therapy involves removing as much of the tumor as possible as well as the uterus, both fallopian tubes and ovaries and the omentum. Biopsies from the pelvic and para-aortic nodes are also performed.

If there is optimal residual disease after surgery—no tumor implant greater than 3/4 in. (2 cm) in diameter—combination chemotherapy including cisplatin + Taxol (CT) and cisplatin or carboplatin + Cytoxan is given for six cycles (one course every three weeks).

Total abdominal and pelvic radiation may be given, but only if the residual disease is less than 1/4 in. (0.5 cm) in diameter. Intra-abdominal radioactive phosphate may be given only if the residual disease is less than 1 mm in diameter.

If there is residual cancer larger than

3/4 in. (2 cm) in diameter or metastases outside the abdominal cavity, intravenous chemotherapy is used exclusively. The commonly used combinations are the same as used for Stage IIa, namely CT, CP, CAP, AP and CHAD.

Investigational Many investigational protocols are being used in the treatment of ovarian cancer:

♦ Intra-abdominal administration of single agents such as interferon-alpha, cisplatin, carboplatin, Ara-C, bleomycin, mitoxantrone, 5-fluorouracil (5-FU) and etoposide.

♦ Intra-abdominal melphalan + Ara-C, carboplatin + etoposide (VP-16), monoclonal antibodies to ovarian carcinoma cells and cisplatin + etoposide with thiosulfate.

♦ Continuous infusion of intravenous 5-FU.

♦ Intravenous fludarabine, hexamethylmelamine or cisplatin + 5-FU + VP-16.

♦ Intravenous carboplatin + ifosfamide.

♦ Intravenous Taxol with other drugs.

♦ Intravenous cisplatin + Cytoxan + hyperfractionated (twice daily) abdominal radiotherapy.

♦ Sodium thiosulfate, which has been shown to protect kidney function as well as lessen the bone marrow complications of cisplatin chemotherapy.

♦ High-dose intravenous carboplatin + etoposide with autologous (self-donated) bone marrow transplant.

♦ High-dosage Cytoxan + cisplatin plus chest and abdominal radiation followed by autologous bone marrow transplant.

♦ High-dose carboplatin + ifosfamide + Mesna with autologous bone marrow transplant.

♦ Intravenous Thiotepa with autologous bone marrow transplant.

♦ Immunotherapy with interleukin-2 or interleukin-2–activated mononuclear cells.

♦ Leuprolide acetate (Lupron) in women with low malignant potential tumors.

♦ Tamoxifen.

♦ Megace.

♦ Taxol, a plant product with significant activity in ovarian cancer, is being actively studied.

TREATMENT FOLLOW-UP

Follow-up is generally performed every three months for the first two years after treatment.

♦ The neck, lungs, abdomen and pelvis are carefully examined at each visit.

♦ The serum CA-125 level is followed closely and is sometimes the first indication of recurrent cancer.

♦ Abdominal and pelvic CT or MRI scans may be done, but their routine use has not been shown to be effective in the absence of symptoms.

Second-Look Surgery If after six cycles of chemotherapy there is no evidence of progressive disease—as determined by physical examination, the serum CA-125 level and pelvic and abdominal CT scans—then second-look exploratory abdominal surgery may be performed. Although it is sometimes considered the standard of care, there has been no proven survival benefit of this procedure. It is, however, the most reliable way of determining whether any cancer is left after treatment. Any residual cancer can also be removed.

If no cancer is found during the second-look operation, a thorough procedure requires taking peritoneal washings and biopsies from any adhesions or 20 to 30 random biopsies. These include the surfaces of the bladder, pelvis, pelvic sidewalls, diaphragm and the pelvic and aortic lymph nodes if not sampled previously. If any of the omentum is still present, it is also removed. An appendectomy is usually done as well. Traditionally, if the second-look operation and microscopic examination of all the biopsies reveal no cancer, no further treatment is required.

In the hands of a gynecologic oncologist, approximately 25 to 30 percent of the women who have sub-optimal disease at the second-look surgery (any tumor nodule greater than 3/4 in./2 cm in diameter) will undergo an optimal surgical debulking. An intra-abdominal catheter for intraperitoneal chemotherapy can also be placed during the operation.

Prognosis The prognosis primarily depends on the stage, grade and type of carcinoma as well as on the amount of residual disease after the initial surgery.

Women who have Stage II, III or IV Grade 1 carcinoma and a negative second-look procedure have an excellent prognosis. Women with Grade 2 or 3 cancers and a negative second-look also have a good prognosis, but have a significant risk for developing recurrent disease. It is estimated that 30 to 50 percent of women with Grade 3 cancer will develop a recurrence within five years even after a negative second-look. As a result, many gynecologic oncologists recommend giving additional treatment—intravenous or intraperitoneal chemotherapy, radioactive phosphorus or whole-abdomen radiation—after the second look.

For women who have microscopic disease at their second-look procedure, the prognosis is not as good and is partially dependent upon the grade of the cancer. These women are treated with more intravenous combination chemotherapy, intra-abdominal chemotherapy or whole-abdomen radiation.

Women with bulky residual cancer (implants greater than 3/4 in./2 cm) after a second-look procedure have a poor prognosis despite treatment with second-line chemotherapy.

RECURRENT CANCER

Women whose cancer returns are sometimes candidates for exploratory surgery for further aggressive tumor debulking.

Postoperative therapy varies and may include intravenous chemotherapy, intra-abdominal chemotherapy or whole-abdomen radiation therapy. In most cases treatment is only palliative.

Numerous combinations of chemotherapy have been used with some benefit, including various combinations and doses of cisplatin + Taxol, Cytoxan, hexamethylmelamine, 5-fluorouracil, ifosfamide and Cytoxan, Adriamycin, carboplatin and Alkeran (melphalan).

THE MOST IMPORTANT QUESTIONS YOU CAN ASK

♦ What qualifications do you have for treating cancer? Will a gynecologic oncologist be involved in my care?
♦ What is the cell type, grade and stage of my cancer?
♦ How much cancer remained after surgery?
♦ What is the benefit of second-look surgery?
♦ What is the reason for the type of therapy you recommended after surgery?
♦ Is there a medical oncologist and radiation oncologist available for consultation?

OVARIAN GERM CELL TUMORS

Jeffrey L. Stern, MD

◇

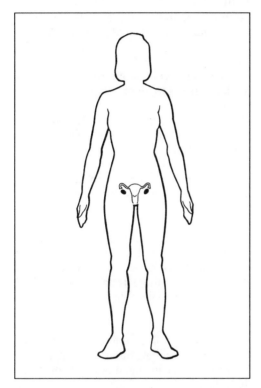

Germ cell tumors account for approximately 5 percent of all ovarian malignancies. They almost always occur in women of reproductive age and are frequently found in women in their teens or twenties. Many types of germ cell tumors are extremely aggressive, fast-growing malignancies. In the past they were often fatal within one or two years even though frequently confined to one ovary at the time of diagnosis. With surgery and modern multi-agent chemotherapy, the cure rate is higher.

Types There are six main cell types: dysgerminoma, endodermal sinus tumor, embryonal carcinoma, choriocarcinoma, immature teratoma and mixed germ cell tumors.

There are also rare cell types such as struma ovarii, carcinoid and malignant transformation of a benign dermoid.

How It Spreads Ovarian germ cell tumors can spread directly to the adjacent pelvic organs and through the lymph system to the pelvic, aortic, chest (mediastinal), groin and neck lymph nodes. They may also spread to the surfaces of the abdominal cavity and to distant organs such as the liver, lungs and brain. (*See* page 348.)

What Causes It The cause is not clear.

RISK FACTORS

At Significantly Higher Risk
♦ Premenopausal women.

At Slightly Higher Risk
♦ Women with abnormal (dysgenetic) ovaries usually containing male chromosomes.

SCREENING

No definitive screening method is available, except for a routine annual pelvic, abdominal and rectal examination.

COMMON SIGNS AND SYMPTOMS

These tumors often do not cause any symptoms. Some women, however, will have a rapidly enlarging pelvic or abdominal mass and vague pain in the lower abdomen. Other women can experience acute abdominal symptoms, including pain and shock.

DIAGNOSIS

Physical Examination
♦ In addition to a careful pelvic exam, a general physical examination should pay particular attention to the lymph nodes above the collarbone, the axillae and the groin.
♦ An abdominal examination may find an enlarged liver, a mass or masses or excessive fluid (ascites).

Blood and Other Tests
♦ Serum beta human chorionic gonadotropin (βHCG) is elevated in choriocarcinoma.
♦ Serum alpha-fetoprotein (AFP) is elevated in endodermal sinus tumors.
♦ Serum lactate dehydrogenase (LDH) is elevated in dysgerminoma.
♦ One or more of the tumor markers—serum βHCG, AFP and LDH—may be elevated in mixed germ cell tumors.

Imaging
♦ Abdominal and pelvic CT scan.
♦ Chest x-ray.

Endoscopy and Biopsy
♦ The definitive diagnosis is made on histologic evaluation of the removed ovary.

STAGING

The International Federation of Gynecology and Obstetricians (FIGO) staging classification for malignant epithelial carcinomas of the ovaries is also used for staging malignant germ cell tumors of the ovary. Germ cell tumors of the ovary are surgically staged.

Stage I
Cancer is confined to one or both ovaries.

♦ **Ia** Cancer is limited to one ovary. There is no tumor on the surface of the ovary, the surface of the tumor is unruptured and there is no ascites.

♦ **Ib** Growth is limited to both ovaries.

There is no tumor on the surface of either ovary, the surfaces of the tumors are unruptured and there is no ascites.

♦ **Ic** The tumor is either Stage Ia or Ib, but there is tumor on the surface of one or both ovaries, at least one of the tumors has ruptured, ascites is present or the abdominal washings contain malignant cells.

Stage II
The cancer involves one or both ovaries with extension to other pelvic structures.

♦ **IIa** There is extension of the tumor or metastases to the uterus and/or the fallopian tubes.

♦ **IIb** There is extension to other pelvic organs such as the bladder or rectum.

♦ **IIc** The cancer is either stage IIa or IIb, but there is tumor on the surface of one or both ovaries, at least one of the tumors has ruptured, there is ascites with malignant cells or the washings from the abdominal cavity contain malignant cells.

Stage III
The tumor involves one or both ovaries with tumor present outside the pelvis or there is cancer in the abdominal or groin lymph nodes.

♦ **IIIa** The tumor is grossly limited to the pelvis, but there is microscopic cancer involving the abdominal cavity (peritoneal) surfaces. The lymph nodes are negative.

♦ **IIIb** The tumor involves one or both ovaries, there are tumor implants on the peritoneal surfaces less than 3/4 in. (2 cm) in diameter. The lymph nodes are negative.

♦ **IIIc** The tumor involves one or both ovaries, there are tumor implants on the surface of the abdominal cavity greater than 3/4 in. (2 cm) in diameter or there is cancer in the pelvic, para-aortic or groin lymph nodes.

Stage IV
There are distant metastases to the liver or lungs or there are malignant cells present in the fluid accumulated in the chest cavity.

TREATMENT OVERVIEW

 Surgery Surgical removal of the involved ovary or ovaries and removal of as much of the grossly visible tumor as possible is performed in all cases. If there is no spread beyond the ovaries, treatment will involve meticulous surgical staging, including sampling of the pelvic and para-aortic lymph nodes, washings of the abdominal cavity to look for malignant cells and careful inspection of the abdominal surfaces with multiple, random biopsies from the diaphragms and surfaces of the abdominal cavity. An omentectomy (removal of fatty tissue attached to the stomach and large intestine) will also be performed.

The cell type of the tumor is an extremely important factor in determining the prognosis and the appropriate therapy after surgery.

 Chemotherapy Women with a tumor confined to one ovary (Stage I) or with a well-differentiated (Grade 1) immature teratoma or dysgerminoma do not require postoperative chemotherapy. All others are usually treated with multi-drug chemotherapy.

Until recently, external radiation therapy to the abdomen and pelvis (1,500 to 3,000 cGy with a 1,500 cGy boost to the para-aortic region given in divided doses daily over five to six weeks) was standard therapy for dysgerminomas, but chemotherapy is now used more often to preserve fertility.

Women with other malignant germ cell tumors are treated with chemotherapy after surgery because radiation therapy is ineffective. The most commonly used chemotherapeutic drug regimen includes cisplatin, bleomycin and etoposide given monthly for three courses.

Second-Look Surgery In those women with Stage II, III or occasionally IV disease who have no evidence of persistent cancer after chemotherapy, "second-look" exploratory abdominal surgery is performed to see if they are truly disease-free.

Second-look surgery is not usually performed on correctly staged women with well-differentiated immature teratomas, Stage Ia and Ib dysgerminomas or other Stage I germ cell tumors who had elevated alpha-fetoprotein, βHCG or LDH levels before treatment that returned to normal with chemotherapy.

Women who have bulky disease after chemotherapy may occasionally benefit from a tumor debulking at a second surgery.

TREATMENT BY STAGE AND CELL TYPE

DYSGERMINOMAS
STAGE Ia
Standard Treatment The involved ovary and fallopian tube and a wedge biopsy of the opposite, normal-appearing ovary and meticulous surgical staging is performed in women who want to preserve their fertility. Women with Stage Ia disease require no further treatment.

About 20 percent of women will have microscopic disease in the opposite, apparently normal ovary (Stage Ib). For women who do not desire more children or who are approaching menopause, a hysterectomy and removal of both tubes and both ovaries is performed.

Investigational None.

STAGE Ib
Standard Treatment Women with this

stage of disease are usually treated with three courses of cisplatin, bleomycin and etoposide or whole-abdominal radiation therapy after hysterectomy, removal of both fallopian tubes and ovaries and meticulous surgical staging.

Investigational
♦ Combinations of chemotherapy including carboplatin and ifosfamide.

STAGE Ic
Standard Treatment After surgery most gynecologic oncologists recommend three courses of cisplatin, bleomycin and etoposide or whole-abdomen radiation.

Investigational Same as Stage Ib.

STAGES II, III and IV
Standard Treatment Depending on the extent and location of disease, standard therapy includes a hysterectomy, removal of both tubes and both ovaries, aggressive tumor debulking and three courses of cisplatin, bleomycin and etoposide.

If the opposite ovary and the uterus are normal, they can be preserved in women who want to maintain their reproductive capacity. Whole-abdomen radiation may be given to those women who fail to respond to chemotherapy or who are not interested in preserving their reproductive function.

Investigational Same as Stage Ib.

NON-DYSGERMINOMATOUS GERM CELL TUMORS
These include endodermal sinus tumors, embryonal carcinoma, immature teratoma, choriocarcinoma and mixed germ cell tumors.

STAGE I
Standard Treatment Removal of the affected tube and ovary is generally all that is required since these tumors rarely occur in both ovaries.

Postoperative chemotherapy including cisplatin, bleomycin and etoposide is given to all patients for four courses with the exception of Grade 1 (well-differentiated) immature teratomas.

Vincristine, actinomycin-D and Cytoxan may be used in women who develop progressive disease.

Investigational
♦ Other combinations of chemotherapy, including carboplatin and ifosfamide, are currently under investigation.

STAGES II, III and IV
Standard Treatment Depending on the extent and location of disease, a hysterectomy, bilateral removal of the tubes and ovaries, and aggressive tumor debulking. If the opposite ovary and uterus are normal, they can be preserved in women who want to maintain their reproductive function. Four courses of chemotherapy including cisplatin, bleomycin and etoposide are given after surgery.

Investigational
♦ Experimental therapy for advanced non-dysgerminomatous germ cell tumors include combinations of other chemotherapeutic drugs such as carboplatin and ifosfamide.

FIVE-YEAR SURVIVAL RATES
The five-year survival rate for Stages Ia and Ib dysgerminomas and Grade 1 immature teratomas is over 95 percent. Even Stage III dysgerminomas have approximately an 80 percent survival rate.

The survival rate for the other stages of dysgerminomas and other histologic types of germ cell tumors are not as well established. But over the past 10 years there has been a marked improvement in prognosis since the advent of cisplatin-based chemotherapy regimens.

Survival rates for women with Stages I and II non-dysgerminomatous germ cell tumors are greater than 90 percent. Even women with Stage III and IV disease have survival rates estimated to be greater than 75 percent.

TREATMENT FOLLOW-UP

All women with germ cell tumors need careful follow-up every three months for the first two years after treatment.

♦ Follow-up should include a careful physical examination and serum βHCG, alpha-fetoprotein and LDH levels (depending on which was elevated before therapy).

♦ Occasionally, radiologic studies such as an abdominal and pelvic CT or MRI scan are performed as required.

RECURRENT CANCER

Germ cell tumors may recur in the pelvis, the abdominal cavity, liver, lungs and lymph nodes. Symptoms may include pelvic or abdominal pain, nausea, vomiting, abdominal swelling, weight loss and chronic cough.

♦ Women with recurrent cancer usually undergo an exploratory laparotomy with aggressive surgical debulking of the tumor.

♦ Women with recurrent dysgerminoma who did not receive radiation therapy previously can be treated with pelvic radiation up to a dose of 3,000 to 5,000 cGy over four to five weeks and whole-abdomen radiation therapy, up to 1,500 cGy, with a boost of up to 1,500 cGy to the para-aortic area over several weeks.

♦ Women with recurrent dysgerminoma who were initially treated with radiation therapy are treated with combination chemotherapy such as cisplatin + etoposide + bleomycin, cisplatin + ifosfamide + etoposide, vincristine + actinomycin-D + Cytoxan or carboplatin + ifosfamide.

♦ Women with non-dysgerminomatous tumors are generally treated with chemotherapy after surgery, as radiation is not effective for these tumors. The chemotherapeutic drugs of choice are cisplatin + etoposide + bleomycin, cisplatin + ifosfamide + etoposide or ifosfamide, vinblastine or vincristine + actinomycin-D + Cytoxan, or carboplatin + ifosfamide.

THE MOST IMPORTANT QUESTIONS YOU CAN ASK

♦ What qualifications do you have for treating cancer? Will a specialist in gynecologic oncology be involved in my care?

♦ What kind of germ cell tumor do I have?

♦ What stage is it?

♦ Will I still be able to have children?

♦ Will I need chemotherapy?

♦ Do I need a second-look operation?

PANCREAS

Ernest H. Rosenbaum, MD, and Malin Dollinger, MD

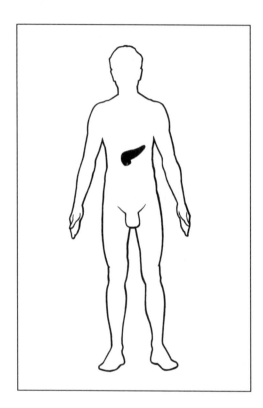

Pancreatic cancer is a common malignancy that is treatable if diagnosed early but is rarely curable. Diagnosis is usually not possible until symptoms appear and by that time the cancer is often well advanced. Because the pancreas is a deep organ resting close to the backbone and involving vital structures, and because tumors often produce few early symptoms, this cancer is not easily diagnosed at a possibly curable stage. Only rarely can pancreatic cancers be removed surgically.

Pancreatic cancer is the fifth most common cause of cancer deaths in the United States. In 1994, there will be 27,000 new cases and 25,900 deaths. For unknown reasons, the number of cases is increasing every year, especially in industrialized countries.

Types Ninety percent of pancreatic cancers are adenocarcinomas. These develop in the exocrine glands that produce enzymes that travel through the pancreatic duct to the small intestine to aid digestion. Adenosquamous, undifferentiated, small cell carcinomas, cystadenocarcinomas, and lymphomas are rare. The other cancers of the pancreas develop in the pancreatic endocrine or islet glands, which produce hormones such as insulin that are released directly into the bloodstream (*see* "Islet Cell and Other Pancreatic Carcinomas").

How It Spreads Two-thirds of pancreatic cancers are located in the head of the organ (right side), one-third in the body and tail (left side). (*See* page 406.) Tumor cells may spread to adjacent structures by direct extension and/or lymphatic metastasis to the small intestine (duodenum), bile duct, stomach, spleen, colon and lymph nodes (regional, celiac and supraclavicular). The most common sites for distant metastases are the liver, peritoneum (by lymphatic spread) and lungs (by spread through the bloodstream).

What Causes It It is not definitely known what causes pancreatic cancer, although age is a factor. There also may be racial or dietary factors. Smoking increases the risk of developing pancreatic cancer threefold. Concerns have been raised about the role of coffee, but there is *no* proof of an association.

RISK FACTORS

At Significantly Higher Risk
♦ Rare before age 40, the incidence peaks around age 60.
♦ Smokers of over two packs a day.
♦ Over 10 years' exposure to chemicals, particularly petroleum compounds and solvents.
♦ Sufferers of chronic inflammation of the pancreas (chronic pancreatitis).

At Slightly Higher Risk
♦ Some association with alcohol consumption.
♦ History of diabetes, particularly in women.
♦ Men outnumber women by a ratio of three-to-one.

SCREENING

No effective screening methods are available.

COMMON SIGNS AND SYMPTOMS

The most common symptom is pain in the upper abdomen, indicating celiac lymph node involvement (in more than 90 percent of cases). There may also be loss of appetite, nausea and vomiting, constipation (50 percent of patients), weight loss (early feeling of fullness is usual in 50 percent of cases), diarrhea, bloating, belching and hiccups. Other symptoms include itching skin, swollen legs, sleeping problems and fatigue.

Other symptoms vary according to the location of the cancer:
♦ Progressive jaundice, often painless (66 percent), can be a sign of cancer in the head of the pancreas.
♦ Itching (pruritis) due to bile duct obstruction.
♦ Diarrhea and swollen legs or mild diabetes may also develop.

There are few symptoms of cancer in the tail of the pancreas until the tumor is a large, often baseball-sized, mass.

DIAGNOSIS

Physical Examination
♦ Jaundice.
♦ Abdominal masses.
♦ Enlarged gallbladder—50 percent of cases (carcinoma of head of pancreas).
♦ Enlarged liver (hepatomegaly).
♦ Abdominal fluid (ascites).
♦ Enlarged lymph nodes.
♦ Phlebitis (swollen legs).

Blood and Other Tests
♦ Complete blood count (CBC) and platelet count.
♦ The carcinoembryonic antigen (CEA) is elevated in 50 percent of cases.
♦ CA 19-9 is elevated in 70 to 80 percent of pancreatic cancer cases and is a better test than the CEA because it is 87 percent specific. (In many cases of pancreatic cancer, both the CEA and the CA 19-9 are elevated.)
♦ Serum bilirubin is elevated in patients with bile duct obstruction.
♦ Serum alkaline phosphatase will be elevated if there are liver or bone metastases or if there is bile duct obstruction.
♦ Stools should be examined for hidden blood. The color may be abnormal. If they are white or clay-colored, the bile duct is obstructed.

Imaging
♦ Abdominal ultrasound. Ultrasound is also used at surgery to locate the exact borders of the tumor.
♦ CT scans may not detect small tumors but may identify pancreatic masses, liver metastases, enlarged lymph nodes and fluid in the abdomen (ascites).
♦ MRI may complement the CT scan.
♦ PET (Positron Emission Tomography) imaging is an experimental method for diagnosis and evaluation for liver metastases.

Endoscopy and Biopsy
♦ ERCP (endoscopic retrograde cholan-

giopancreatography) involves placing a gastroscope into the stomach and inserting a tube into the opening of the pancreatic duct.

♦ For a definite diagnosis, a biopsy is essential. Tissue can be drawn out with a fine needle (FNA) inserted into the tumor using CT guidance (diagnostic in 80 percent of cases). This will be necessary to differentiate pancreatic cancer from benign pancreatitis or pseudocyst, islet cell carcinoma or lymphoma.

Tests to Surrounding Organs

♦ Upper gastrointestinal tract x-rays (UGI series) may be done to examine the duodenum (the portion of the small intestine that surrounds the pancreas) to look for abnormalities.

♦ A needle may be inserted into the liver to discover obstructions in the bile duct (percutaneous transhepatic cholangiogram).

♦ Liver biopsy to confirm metastases, if indicated.

Ninety percent of cases can be diagnosed with abdominal ultrasound, CT scans, ERCP and a positive CA 19-9.

STAGING

The staging system for pancreatic cancer is still evolving. However, staging has limited value because treatment, regardless of stage, has had little influence on survival. Knowing the location of the cancer in the head, body or tail of the pancreas will help determine if surgery is feasible.

TREATMENT OVERVIEW

Surgery Surgery is rarely curative but can be used for palliation, improving survival and the quality of life. The radical surgical approach (pancreaticoduodenal resection) depends on whether the tumor is in the head, body or tail of the pancreas.

Cure may be achieved when the tumor is truly localized, but this stage is diagnosed in fewer than 20 percent of cases. Radical surgery (the Whipple procedure) is more feasible when the tumor is small (less than 3/4 in./2 cm), no lymph nodes are involved and there is no extension of the cancer beyond the "capsule" of the pancreas (a rare situation).

Surgery may also be advantageously used to bypass any obstruction of the biliary or gastrointestinal tract. In addition, before surgery pancreatic cancer cannot be differentiated from other cancers involving bile ducts. Overall, surgery results in only about 5 percent survival after five years, although about 22 percent are alive five years after radical surgery (Whipple procedure).

Investigational treatment for Stage I to III (locally advanced) cancers, using 5-FU and radiotherapy before surgery, has shown preliminary results of increased resectability and palliation, but further study is needed.

Radiation Sometimes when the tumor cannot be removed surgically, radiation can play a palliative role after surgery. The risks of radiotherapy can be reduced with proper treatment planning.

The risks of damage to the kidneys, spleen, liver, spinal cord and the bowel surrounding the pancreas can be minimized by careful treatment planning. Combination radiotherapy and chemotherapy (5-fluorouracil or 5-fluorouracil + cisplatin) may offer a longer survival and palliation with decreased pain.

Intraoperative radiotherapy (IORT) and interstitial I-125 radioactive implants have helped local tumor control but have not increased survival.

Chemotherapy No major palliative role for chemotherapy has been proven. The most commonly used drugs are 5-fluorouracil (5-FU), Adriamycin, mitomycin-C and streptozocin. 5-fluorouracil has had the best response but in no more than 20 percent of patients.

Various combinations such as FAM (5-FU + Adriamycin + mitomycin-C), SMF (streptozocin + mitomycin-C + 5-FU, 5-FU + platinol, and 5-FU + leucovorin + mitomycin-C + dipyridamole) may increase survival a few months and have had a good response in selected cases, but there is little proof that combination therapy is superior to 5-FU alone.

Some investigational protocols have added interferon or PALA to 5-FU and leucovorin, but the results are about the same. Better treatment needs to be developed.

 Palliation Although surgery and radiation therapy will not improve survival, both may improve the quality of life. A biliary tract obstructed by a tumor at the head of the pancreas can by bypassed (with surgery or a stent), an obstruction of the stomach outlet can be relieved, and pain control can be improved dramatically.

Other palliative measures include pain control using analgesics, celiac and splanchnic nerve blocks, spinal morphine, antiemetics to control nausea or vomiting, and nutritional support with diets and replacement of pancreatic enzymes. (*See* Chapter 18.)

TREATMENT BY STAGE

STAGE I
TNM T1 or T2, N0, M0
The cancer is confined to the pancreas or has directly spread to involve the adjacent small intestine, the bile duct or tissues surrounding the pancreas.

Standard Treatment Stage I cancer is treatable by surgery and is occasionally curable. Radical surgery—the Whipple procedure (pancreaticoduodenal resection)—is the standard treatment for cancer of the head of the pancreas or the opening of the pancreatic duct, although very few patients are eligible for total resection (80

to 90 percent have lymph node involvement at the time of diagnosis, and 70 percent have liver metastases).

A radical pancreatic resection, removing the head or all of the pancreas is very difficult surgery. Five to 30 percent of patients may not survive the operation. Fluid leaks at the connection to the small bowel (jejunum) and bleeding are the major postoperative problems.

Postsurgical local radiotherapy and 5-FU may improve survival. About 40 percent of patients treated with such combined therapy may be alive at two years, representing a twofold increase in survival. (Metallic clips are inserted during surgery to help localize the tumor for radiotherapy.)

Removing cancer involving the tail of the pancreas is uncommon because tumors in the tail are usually large and far advanced before diagnosis.

Three-Year Survival 15 percent

Investigational
♦ Radiation given during the operation—intraoperative radiotherapy (IORT)—is being evaluated.
♦ Some trials of split course radiotherapy of 4,000 to 6,000 cGy over six to eight weeks have shown one-year survival of 34 percent and five-year survival of 20 percent
♦ Brachytherapy—implanting irradiating seeds of radon or boron—is under clinical evaluation at a few centers. Results so far have not been promising.
♦ Postoperative large-field radiation with 5-FU chemotherapy is also being evaluated and it appears that this combination improves survival. Side effects include diarrhea, inflammation of the intestinal lining and liver toxicity.

 Palliation Eighty percent of pancreatic cancer patients have jaundice caused by an obstruction. A surgically created bypass from the gall bladder or the common bile duct to the intestine may be helpful.

STAGE II
TNM T3, N0, M0
The cancer has directly spread to involve adjacent organs such as the stomach, spleen or colon.

Standard Treatment Surgical bypass procedures can be carried out as a palliative measure (*see* Stage I) and neurosurgical procedures such as blocking the nerves from the stomach and pancreas (celiac ganglion nerve blocks) may relieve much of the pain.

Combined radiation and chemotherapy may be helpful. Radiation therapy alone may relieve symptoms, but clinical trials should be considered, since survival is not significantly increased with radiotherapy alone.

If the patient is jaundiced, the bile ducts can be drained through the skin (transhepatic percutaneous biliary bypass). Alternatively, a drainage tube can be placed inside the small bowel by means of a gastroscope (endoscopic stent placement).

Investigational
♦ Radiation therapy with radiosensitizers.
♦ Intraoperative radiotherapy (IORT) and implantation of radioactive seeds (brachytherapy) are sometimes combined, with and without chemotherapy for resectable or unresectable tumors.
♦ Postoperative radiation therapy plus 5-FU in resected patients.

Three-Year Survival 2 percent

STAGE III
TNM Any T, N1, M0
The cancer has spread to the regional lymph nodes.

Standard Treatment There is no reliably curative treatment and no proven adju-

vant therapy. The standard palliative treatment options for Stage II and/or clinical trials should be considered.

Three-Year Survival 2 percent

Investigational
♦ Surgery plus radiation therapy with radiosensitizers.
♦ Intraoperative radiotherapy with and without resection.
♦ Particle beam radiation therapy if a special research facility is available.

STAGE IV
TNM Any T, any N, M1
The cancer has spread to distant sites, most commonly the liver or lungs.

Standard Treatment Palliative surgical bypass, bile drainage procedures (see Stage II description).
♦ Chemotherapy (*see* Stages II and III) and pain-relieving procedures are standard treatments. Clinical chemotherapy trials should be considered.
♦ Combination chemotherapy with SMF (streptozocin + mitomycin-C + 5-fluorouracil), which has a 30 to 45 percent response rate, FAM (5-fluorouracil + Adriamycin + mitomycin-C) or 5-fluorouracil + leucovorin.

Three-Year Survival Less than 1 percent

SUPPORTIVE THERAPY

Nutrition Malnutrition is a common problem because of loss of appetite, diarrhea, poor fat absorption and the loss of bile salts because of bile drainage diversions or bile duct obstruction. Fat-soluble vitamin deficiencies (A, D, E, K) may also occur.
♦ Frequent feedings, use of digestive replacement enzymes (pancreatin, Viokase) and antinausea drugs will be needed.
♦ Low-fat food or supplements (medium-chain triglycerides) may help provide pro-

teins and calories.

♦ Gastric and jejunal tube feeding or intravenous hyperalimentation can help reduce malnutrition.

Pain Control This often becomes a major problem, but morphine or narcotics can help. If these are not effective, celiac nerve blocks or the infusion of morphine by vein or the spinal canal can help control pain in a majority of patients.

RECURRENT CANCER

The three major signs of recurrent pancreatic cancer are increased pain, jaundice and fluid in the abdomen (ascites).

Recurrent cancer can be treated with palliative surgical or radiation therapy.

♦ Chemotherapy may produce tumor regression. Treatment options are the same as for Stages II, III and IV—5-FU, FAM, SMF, 5-FU + leucovorin and PALA + 5-FU. (PALA is an investigational drug that increases the antitumor activity of 5-FU.)

THE MOST IMPORTANT QUESTIONS YOU CAN ASK

♦ Will diet help my treatments?

♦ What are the limiting factors for a surgical cure of pancreatic cancer?

♦ Are there any new chemotherapy treatments?

♦ How can using chemotherapy and radiation together help improve the chance for cure?

PARATHYROID

Malin Dollinger, MD, and Orlo H. Clark, MD

◇

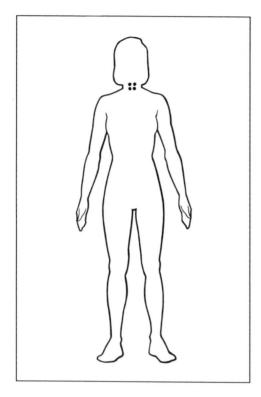

The parathyroid glands are usually located in the neck, two on each side of the thyroid gland (*see* figure page 617).

Parathyroid cancer is a rare and sometimes curable endocrine gland cancer. Though not all these tumors are functioning, those that are produce increased amounts of parathyroid hormone (parathormone), which leads to a marked elevation in blood calcium level (hypercalcemia). It is usually the signs and symptoms of elevated calcium that lead to the diagnosis.

Benign tumors of the parathyroid (adenomas) and an overgrowth of parathyroid tissue (hyperplasia) are much more common (99 percent) than malignant tumors (1 percent). These also produce parathyroid hormone and elevated blood calcium levels, so it is sometimes difficult to know at surgery if the tumor is benign or malignant. This distinction is extremely important because the treatment of a malignant parathyroid tumor requires not only removal of the tumor but removal of the thyroid gland on that side. Adjacent muscles and tissues are also removed if they are affected by cancer.

Recognition by the surgeon that the tumor is malignant rather than benign and performing the appropriate surgery, including removal of the lymph nodes, is important for good results. Malignancy is more likely if there is a very high serum calcium, a palpable or hard mass in the neck or hoarseness due to paralysis of the vocal cords on the same side.

Because this tumor usually grows slowly and because the main clinical problem is usually the effects of the elevated calcium levels, palliative reduction or debulking of the primary tumor or metastases is recommended. This may lower the blood calcium level, which is difficult to treat any other way.

Types Parathyroid carcinomas are tumors with chief cell, oxyphil, clear cell and mixed cell types.

How It Spreads Parathyroid tumors can spread directly to adjacent tissues, as well as through the lymphatic system to nearby lymph nodes and via the bloodstream to distant sites, usually the lung, bones and liver.

What Causes It Increased incidence following exposure to low-dose therapeutic radiation or in families with familial hyperparathyroidism or MEN 1.

RISK FACTORS

There are no known risk factors for parathyroid carcinoma, although benign tumors of the parathyroids (adenoma) occur more often if there has been previous radiation to the head and neck. Parathyroid tumors also occur in association with tumors of the adrenal and thyroid glands (multiple endocrine neoplasia—MEN).

SCREENING

Specific screening for this type of cancer is generally not done, because parathyroid cancer is so rare. Benign parathyroid disease is common, however, occurring in about 100,000 patients annually in the United States. Methods to search for parathyroid tumors, whether benign or malignant, include measuring the serum calcium levels—commonly performed as part of a chemistry panel—as well as examining the thyroid region for suspicious masses during routine physical examinations.

COMMON SIGNS AND SYMPTOMS

Symptoms are due to the elevated calcium or to the mass in the neck.

Symptoms usually include fatigue, muscle weakness, nausea and vomiting, kidney stones or other kidney disease, peptic ulcer and inflamation of the pancreas (pancreatitis) or hoarseness.

DIAGNOSIS

The diagnosis of overactive parathyroids is characterized by a combination of an elevated level of serum calcium plus an elevated level of serum parathyroid hormone.

Diagnosis usually is made easily by documenting an increased two-site parathyroid hormone (PTH) level in a patient with elevated levels of blood and urine calcium. Only a very rare nonparathyroid malignant tumor in such patients secretes pure parathyroid hormone. Most secrete parathyroid hormone-related peptide, and this substance does not cross-react with the new parathyroid hormone assays.

Physical Examination
♦ Mass in the neck. Benign tumors rarely have a mass in the neck.
♦ Vocal cords may be paralyzed on one side, causing hoarseness.

Blood and Other Tests
♦ The normal serum calcium level is 8.5 to 10.5 mg/dl and the level in benign tumors averages 11.0 mg/dl but most parathyroid cancers have levels over 14 mg/dl.
♦ Intact or two-site PTH levels increased.
♦ Urinary cyclic AMP levels are elevated in almost all patients.
♦ Sometimes the presence and location of a primary parathyroid tumor can be confirmed by placing a catheter into the veins draining the parathyroids or metastatic deposits. Blood samples are then taken from each site and serum parathyroid hormone levels are determined.

Imaging
♦ Reabsorption of bone on x-ray, or osteopenia (loss of bone) by bone density tests.
♦ Localization tests can be done before surgery. These include Sestamibi, CT, or MRI scans of the neck and mediastinum.
♦ Localization tests are especially helpful in patients with persistent or recurrent disease, or in patients who have had previous thyroid surgery.

STAGING

There are only two stages for parathyroid cancer. One stage is localized, meaning that the disease is confined to the parathyroid with or without invasion of adjacent tissues. The other is metastatic, in which the cancer may have spread to regional lymph nodes and/or to distant sites such as the lung, bones and liver.

TREATMENT OVERVIEW

The problem with these tumors is not predominantly the tumor itself, which grows rather slowly, but the marked elevation in calcium levels, which produces a condition (hypercalcemia) that is difficult to control medically and may eventually be fatal.

For this reason, aggressive surgical removal of bulk disease or metastatic disease has been recommended. Unfortunately, this type of surgery is not always possible, because of widespread metastasis. Better results are obtained when a surgeon experienced with hyperparathyroidism is involved.

A variety of medical means can inhibit the the action of parathyroid hormone and to improve the hypercalcemia, including the use of calcitonin, mithramycin or diphosphonates.

TREATMENT BY STAGE

LOCALIZED
Standard Treatment Localized parathyroid cancer is treated with removal of the tumor and the thyroid gland on the same side. Adjacent muscles and other tissues are included if they appear to be involved. The laryngeal nerve occasionally must be removed, which may result in hoarseness. Local recurrence is common, however, and may require repeat surgery.

Five-Year Survival About 50 percent

Investigational
♦ Clinical trials are evaluating combinations of surgery and radiation therapy, as well as radiation therapy alone.

METASTATIC
Standard Treatment For metastatic parathyroid cancer, an operation is performed similar to that for localized parathyroid cancer, with removal of adjacent neck muscles and regional lymph nodes if they are involved.

An attempt is made to remove as much tumor as possible to eliminate the source of excess parathyroid hormone, hypercalcemia and related metabolic problems.

Five-Year Survival 30 percent

Investigational
♦ As for localized cancer, clinical protocols are studying combinations of surgery and radiation therapy, as well as radiation therapy alone for metastatic parathyroid cancer.
♦ A few patients with metastatic parathyroid cancer have been treated with chemotherapy combinations, including the active agent dacarbazine (DTIC), as well as that agent combined with 5-fluorouracil and cyclophosphamide. There are no current adjuvant treatment protocols for this tumor.

TREATMENT FOLLOW-UP

♦ Physical examination of the neck and determinations of blood calcium and parathyroid hormone levels are the most appropriate methods of follow-up.
♦ Appropriate x-ray studies and scans are useful for patients with metastases.

RECURRENT CANCER

The treatment of recurrent parathyroid cancer is generally surgical removal of the primary tumor—with or without removing the lymph nodes—or debulking the tumor to reduce the production of parathormone. Under investigation are the combinations of surgery with radiation therapy, radiation therapy alone, as well as chemotherapy.

THE MOST IMPORTANT QUESTIONS YOU CAN ASK

♦ If you are not sure at surgery whether this is benign or malignant, how will you decide what kind of surgery to do?
♦ Is a frozen section reliable in helping to decide if the tumor is benign or malignant?
♦ Would radiation therapy be helpful along with surgery?

PENIS

Norman R. Zinner, MD, MS

◇

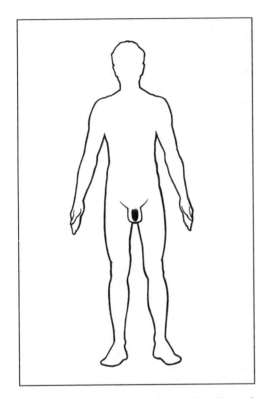

Cancer of the penis is rare in the United States, affecting only one or two men in 100,000. It is almost never seen in those who have been circumcised as babies, which is a major argument in favor of newborn circumcision. It can occur anywhere along the penile shaft, but most are on the foreskin or head (glans). It is usually a slow-growing cancer and is curable if discovered early. Unfortunately, some men do not seek medical attention until after it has spread.

Types Nearly all penile malignancies are cancers of the skin, the most common being squamous cell carcinoma similar to squa-

mous cell carcinomas on other parts of the skin such as the face or hands. Some penile cancers are melanomas, which appear as blue-brown flat growths and tend to spread more rapidly and more widely. Occasionally, the deep tissues of the penis develop cancer, typically sarcomas.

How It Spreads The tumor spreads gradually, becoming larger in the area of the skin where it first develops. Ultimately, it spreads to deep tissues inside the body of the penis and to lymph nodes in the groin (inguinal area) or pelvis. When the cancer is in the penis itself (local) and involves no more than a few nearby inguinal lymph nodes, it can be cured, but cure rates fall rapidly once it spreads to the pelvic lymph nodes.

What Causes It This is one of the few cancers where the cause is fairly well known. Men who are circumcised at birth (a common practice among whites in the United States) almost never get cancer of the penis. If circumcision is performed at puberty, the incidence of cancer is slightly higher, and men who are circumcised as adults are not protected and experience the same incidence of penile cancer as men who are never circumcised at all.

Cancer of the penis is, in a sense, a disease of poor hygiene. It is believed that the decaying cells of the undersurface of the foreskin (smegma) produce irritation leading to cancer. In addition, there may be a relationship between venereal warts (condyloma acuminata) and penile cancer. Recent studies have demonstrated an association between certain types of the virus that causes condylomata (human papilloma virus types 16 and 18) and penile cancer in about one man in three who have penile cancer. These human papilloma virus (HPV) types are also found in women who have cancer in the uterine cervix. It has also been shown that cancer of the uterine cervix may be higher in the sexual partners of men who are not circumcised. This is of special importance to female sexual partners of uncircumcised men and of men with HPV infections because the women often develop cancer of the cervix when exposed to the viruses that produce female warts, even if the men do not have a cancerous change in their warts.

RISK FACTORS

The cancer is one of later years, being rare before age 25 and typically occurring after age 50. The highest incidence is among uncircumcised men, especially those who cannot pull back their foreskins and clean them. In the United States, the highest incidence is among Afro-Americans.

SCREENING

There are no blood tests to screen for cancer of the penis. All uncircumsised men should examine the foreskin and head of the penis monthly. It is essential that they be able to retract the foreskin to be able to see all the tissue on its undersurface.

COMMON SIGNS AND SYMPTOMS

The most common finding is a painless sore on the foreskin or glans that won't heal. If the man cannot retract the foreskin the cancer may not be discovered until it grows large and appears as a cauliflower-like mass growing from beneath the pouch of the foreskin. If left alone, it will usually become inflamed and often infected. This may produce a foul odor and discomfort. It can also lead to enlargement of inguinal lymph nodes. Penile cancer rarely interferes with urination.

DIAGNOSIS

Physical Examination
♦ The main physical finding is a sore or rash on the penis that may be inflamed. It will erode and destroy the penis if not treated early.
♦ There may be swelling in the groin from inflamed lymph nodes or from nodes involved with cancer.

Imaging
♦ CT scan, chest x-ray and bone, liver and lymph node scans (lymphangiogram) are used to discover if there is spread once a cancer is confirmed on biopsy.

Endoscopy and Biopsy
♦ A biopsy is the main diagnostic test.

TREATMENT OVERVIEW

The tumor size and degree of spread locally and to other sites (stage) determines treatment options.
♦ If the tumor is small and local, it can be treated surgically, chemically or with radiation or laser without major damage to the appearance or function of the penis.
♦ If it has penetrated the deeper penile tissues or if it is large, surgery is the preferred treatment for most men. Radiation is an option, but results are less certain.
♦ If the tumor has spread to lymph nodes, surgery or radiation are used.
♦ Chemotherapy is of little value in extensive carcinoma of the penis.

TREATMENT BY STAGE: SQUAMOUS CELL CARCINOMA

CARCINOMA IN SITU
This tumor appears either as a reddish, velvety rash (erythroplasia of Queyrat) or as small, crusty bumps (Bowen's disease).

Standard Treatment These tumors are best treated with 5-fluorouracil cream applied locally twice daily for four to five weeks. If this is not successful, the local lesions can be treated with laser or removed surgically. Usually, there is little or no disfigurement, but this depends upon the size and location of the growth.

Five-Year Survival 100 percent

STAGE I

The cancer is limited to the foreskin or head of the penis and does not invade the deep layers beneath the skin.

Standard Treatment An extensive circumcision may be all that is necessary if the cancer is small and limited to the foreskin. If it is large or on the glans, surgical removal of the tumor with a wide margin may be acceptable, but partial amputation is usually needed. The remaining penile stump can be remarkably serviceable for urination and sexual intercourse, but partial amputation is disfiguring and most younger men find the emotional trauma hard to take. The main advantage of surgery is that it usually results in a cure. Because of the high incidence of microscopic metastases to inguinal lymph nodes, surgery to remove these nodes is under evaluation.

Radiation therapy, administered by external beam or with radiation implants, may preserve the entire penis. But recurrence rates are high and the urine canal often becomes very narrow. If this happens, surgical amputation can then be done.

Five-Year Survival 100 percent

STAGE II

The cancer is locally invasive but has not spread to the groin (inguinal) lymph nodes.

Standard Treatment Partial or complete amputation of the penis (penectomy) depending upon the location of the cancer. If the tumor is at the tip of the penis, a partial penectomy can be done. If it develops closer to the root of the penile shaft or

has spread, a total penectomy is usually needed. Cure rates are excellent for Stage II penile cancers treated surgically.

The decision to remove all of the penis depends on whether enough of a stump can be left to allow the man to have sexual intercourse and to urinate while standing without voiding in uncontrolled directions. Penile reconstruction or the construction of a new penis is possible with plastic surgery.

Radiation therapy can be tried in younger men and those who refuse surgery, but rates of recurrence and urethral strictures are high. If radiation fails, surgery can usually be accomplished with excellent results.

Five-Year Survival 88 percent

STAGE III

These cancers have spread to inguinal or pelvic lymph nodes, and cure rates are poor.

Standard Treatment Stage III disease is suspected when there is swelling of the inguinal lymph nodes, but this swelling can be misleading. Sometimes the lymph nodes are enlarged not because of cancer but because of an infection or inflammation. To find out if this is the case, the tumor is first treated in the same way as Stage II tumors.

If the nodes are involved with infection or inflammation, the swelling will usually subside four to six weeks after the cancer is surgically removed from the penis. The lymph nodes will no longer be felt through the skin.

If the lymph nodes can still be felt through the skin four to six weeks after surgery, some of the inguinal lymph nodes can be biopsied and examined. If they are found to contain cancer, all of the nodes of the groin and pelvis are removed.

If the patient is treated with radiation therapy rather than by surgery, the swollen inguinal lymph nodes will usually not disappear within the four-to-six-week period of observation.

Five-Year Survival 75 percent

STAGE IV
The cancer has spread to distant sites.

Standard Treatment There is no standard treatment for cure. Treatment is directed at the control of symptoms by selected radiation, surgery or experimental chemotherapy protocols.

Five-Year Survival Less than 5 percent

TREATING VENEREAL WARTS

Occasionally, venereal warts (malignant transformation of condyloma acuminata) become cancerous. Since they are also known to cause cancer in the female partners of men with some types of these warts even if the men do not have cancer them-

selves, all venereal warts should be treated. Treatment methods include:
♦ applying a liquid chemical (podophyllin) directly to the area,
♦ applying supercooled liquid gases (cryotherapy),
♦ charring (fulguration),
♦ vaporization by a laser,
♦ surgical removal, or
♦ intradermal interferon-alpha.
   If there is any suspicion of malignancy, warts should be removed surgically and examined under the microscope.

THE MOST IMPORTANT QUESTIONS YOU CAN ASK

♦ Is surgery necessary, and how extensive must it be? Are you going to remove my lymph nodes? Which ones and when?
♦ Can radiation work for me?
♦ What is the relationship between my cancer and venereal warts?
♦ Might my tumor be transmitted sexually?
♦ Should my female sexual partner be tested for HPV?

PITUITARY

Malin Dollinger, MD, Ernest H. Rosenbaum, MD, and Orlo H. Clark, MD

◇

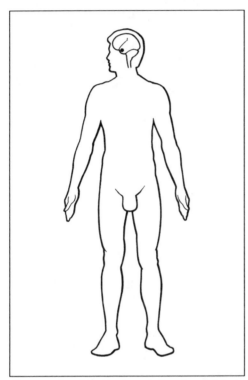

Tumors in the pituitary gland, which is located at the base of the brain (*see* page 300), are benign (adenomas) and curable over 90 percent of the time. But these tumors can become large enough to damage nearby nerves and brain tissue, sometimes permanently. By pressing on the nerves to the eyes, a pituitary tumor can cause progressive vision loss and even blindness. In some cases, the tumor compresses the pituitary gland, preventing it from producing the normal amount of hormones. Hypothyroidism, adrenal insufficiency and a deficiency in growth hormone can result.

Types Many pituitary adenomas produce excess hormones, causing significant symptoms. The increased production of growth hormone can produce a disease called acromegaly. Excess prolactin can cause impotence in men and the loss of menstrual periods and breast secretion in women. Excess ACTH (adrenocorticotropic hormone) can result in Cushing's disease. Some tumors, such as chromophobe adenomas, are non-functional but may lead to hormone deficiency by compressing the normal pituitary.

How It Spreads Since most pituitary tumors are benign, they do not spread like cancerous tumors. They may, however, cause erosion of the sella turcica, the bony structure surrounding the pituitary.

What Causes It There is no known cause, although the use of birth control pills may be a contributing factor in some cases.

COMMON SIGNS AND SYMPTOMS

Early symptoms depend on which hormone is involved. As the tumor grows, headaches may occur, and sight may deteriorate, starting with loss of peripheral vision.

DIAGNOSIS

Blood and Other Tests
♦ Sensitive radioimmunoassays for any hormone suspected of overproduction.

Imaging
♦ CT and MRI scans of the brain. MRI is the more sensitive study.
♦ X-rays of the skull may show destruction of the sella turcica.

TREATMENT OVERVIEW

Treatment depends on the type of tumor and whether it has grown beyond the area of the pituitary gland.

Tumors that produce hormones are treated with surgery or radiation, with the surgical approach—a transsphenoidal hypophysectomy—usually the treatment chosen for tumors that have not grown outside the bony cavity. Larger tumors, usually non-functioning adenomas, need additional treatment with radiation.

Prolactin-secreting tumors may stabilize and improve with time. People with these tumors usually benefit from treatment with bromocriptine.

Tumors that produce growth hormone and ACTH usually grow slowly. With any of the pituitary tumors, however, surgery is called for immediately if vision starts to deteriorate rapidly.

TREATMENT BY TYPE

ACTH-PRODUCING TUMORS
(Cushing's disease)

Standard Treatment Surgery, radiation therapy, a combination of both or Mitotane or Ketoconozol plus radiation.

Investigational
♦ Heavy-particle radiation.

PROLACTIN-PRODUCING TUMORS
Standard Treatment Surgical removal of the tumor, radiation, bromocriptine or combinations of these treatments. Bromocriptine has been of considerable benefit in reducing symptoms. A new drug, CV205-502, has been successful in patients who have failed to respond to bromocriptine.

Investigational
♦ Heavy-particle radiation.

GROWTH HORMONE–
PRODUCING TUMORS
Standard Treatment Surgery, radiation therapy, bromocriptine or somatostatin.

Which treatment is chosen depends on the size and extent of the tumor and on how urgent it is to eliminate the excess hormone production.

NON-FUNCTIONING TUMORS
Standard Treatment These tumors, usually chromophobe adenomas, are treated with surgery and radiation. The choice depends on how big the tumor is, how fast it is growing and its effect on adjacent pituitary tissue or other structures.

The surgical and radiotherapy techniques used to treat these tumors are very complex and sophisticated. Neurosurgeons and radiation oncologists experienced in treating them are best able to judge which method is preferable.

TREATMENT FOLLOW-UP

The intensity and schedule of follow-up depends on the amount of damage done to adjacent tissues before or during treatment and on whether the tumor was completely removed during surgery.
♦ An endocrinologist will usually be involved in follow-up after surgery, since hormone deficiency (ACTH, FSH, LH, TSH, sex hormones and cortisol) may occur and replacement hormones may be needed.
♦ Follow-up CT or MRI scans may be useful.
♦ Hormone levels may be measured periodically if a hormone-producing tumor was treated.

THE MOST IMPORTANT QUESTIONS YOU CAN ASK
♦ Is my tumor producing extra hormones?
♦ Is surgery or radiation the best treatment for my type of tumor and why?
♦ What is the probability that the treatment will eliminate the tumor?
♦ What are the risks, complications and side effects of treatment?
♦ Will I have to take hormones after surgery and, if so, for how long?
♦ What are the chances that my vision will improve?

PROSTATE

Norman R. Zinner, MD, MS

◇

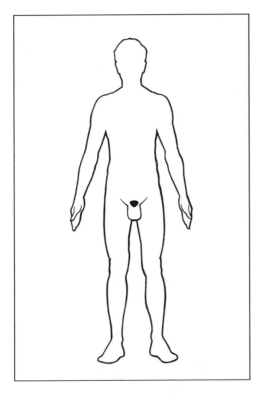

Cancer of the prostate is the most common cancer in American men, overtaking both lung cancer and cancer of the colon and rectum during the 1980s. Since this is usually a disease of men over 65, the increase appears to be due to the aging of the population. The American Cancer Society estimates that over 200,000 men will contract the disease in 1994 and about 38,000 will die from it. It is the second leading cause of cancer death in men. Prostate cancer is not related to the problem of an enlarged prostate in most older men, a condition called benign prostatic hyperplasia (BPH).

If the disease is to be cured it has to be discovered before it spreads beyond the prostate gland. Unfortunately, only about one-half of newly diagnosed patients fall into this category. New understanding of the importance of a specific blood test, prostate-specific antigen (PSA), in the early detection of prostate cancer, coupled with advances in ultrasound imaging and increased public awareness of the need for early discovery, may eventually improve the chances for a cure of this disease. But even then, the benefit is uncertain. Most men with prostate cancer will die from other illnesses never knowing they had the problem.

Types Nearly all prostate cancer arises from the glands of the prostate. Glandular cancer (adenocarcinoma) accounts for 95 percent of all prostate cancer cases. Over half of these cancers develop from the rear (posterior) portion of the prostate that lies closest to the rectum, which is why rectal examination is useful to detect the tumor.

Other types are rare. Most, including leiomyosarcoma and rhabdomyosarcoma, arise from supporting or connective tissues within or around the prostate. Others develop in the ducts within the prostate. Tumors can also spread to the prostate from other locations such as the bladder or adrenal gland.

Some types are not actually cancer but have characteristics that appear precancerous. These are called prostatic intraepithelial neoplasia (PIN), a term referring to cell growths that are almost active cancers or may soon become cancer. Men with PIN have to be observed closely and have periodic biopsies.

How It Spreads Prostatic cancers spread

through the lymphatic system to pelvic lymph nodes and through the bloodstream to bones and other tissues. The earliest spread is usually detected in lymph nodes in the pelvis near the prostate. Other areas of spread are to lymph nodes around the arteries and veins leading to the legs and pelvic organs and to bones in the spine, legs, arms and hips. Ultimately, it can reach almost any organ in the body. The tumor may also spread directly through the prostate to surrounding tissues or may grow inward, blocking the flow of urine.

What Causes It The exact cause isn't known, but hormones play a role. Any man who had his testicles removed before he reached puberty—and so did not get to produce the male hormone testosterone— will rarely develop prostate cancer. The use of hormones such as steroids by athletes or cortisone for certain diseases, however, will not cause the problem.

Some people have recently speculated that foods high in fat may play a role, but this is far from certain. Genetic factors are suspected, since prostate cancer patients with relatives who also have prostate cancer are up to three times more likely to die of their disease than those patients who do not have relatives with prostate cancer.

We know a great deal more about what does not cause it. There is no conclusive evidence that one can get cancer of the prostate from "too much sex," masturbation, infection of the prostate or benign prostatic hyperplasia (BPH). Prostatic stones or infection have no proven influence.

RISK FACTORS

There is speculation about a relationship

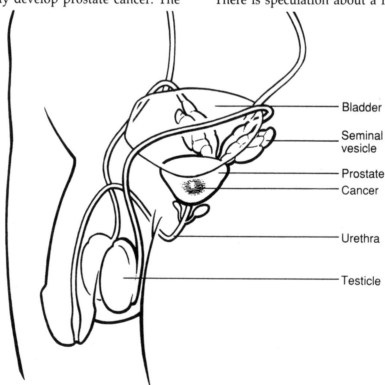

The prostate gland and associated pelvic organs

Bladder

Seminal vesicle

Prostate

Cancer

Urethra

Testicle

between prostatic cancer and industrial cancer-causing agents such as cadmium. No relationship has been shown between prostate cancer and smoking, use of alcohol, disease patterns, circumcision, weight, height, blood group, hair distribution, sexual activity or benign prostatic hyperplasia.

Is Vasectomy A Risk Factor? One in five men over 35 has a vasectomy. The recent publicity concerning a possible association between vasectomy and prostate cancer and the large number of men who have had vasectomies has caused the National Institutes of Health to convene a special panel of experts to review all information and to make recommendations to the American public. Participants at this meeting (held in March 1993) concluded that "all contraceptive methods carry risks as well as benefits. When making decisions about contraception, each individual or couple must be informed of, and weigh the various risks and benefits in light of their particular circumstances and the risks associated with pregnancy. Vasectomy is a highly effective method of family planning with low surgical risks.

"Because the results of research on the relationship between vasectomy and prostate cancer are inconsistent, and the associations that have been found are weak, there is not sufficient basis for recommending a change in clinical and public health practice at this time. Therefore, the panel recommended the following:
♦ Providers should continue to offer vasectomy and perform the procedure.
♦ Vasectomy reversal is not warranted to prevent prostate cancer.
♦ Screening for prostate cancer should not be any different for men who have had a vasectomy than for those who have not."

There are no known ways to protect against the development of prostatic cancer.

At Significantly Higher Risk
♦ The probability of having the disease increases with age. Men under 50 have less than one chance in a hundred of getting prostate cancer while about half of all men over 80 will have it.
♦ The risk is twice as high in blacks than in whites and is lowest for Asians. Jews have the lowest mortality rate from prostatic cancer, blacks the highest.
♦ The United States death rate is high compared with other countries. The urban rate is slightly higher than the rural rate.

SCREENING

Both a digital rectal examination and a prostate-specific antigen (PSA) blood level are recommended annually for men over 50. If a father, brother or uncle has had prostate cancer, these annual tests should be started at age 40. These tests may detect cancer of the prostate before it has spread.

The digital rectal examination is useful because the prostate gland's location within the rectum makes it easy to feel. The cancer often produces a lump or an irregularity which can be felt, and about one suspicious area in three will prove to be malignant.

PSA is often elevated when cancer is present. Since PSA will usually rise as tumors grow, measuring it is a good way to monitor the course of cancer once it is found. Its role in screening is less clear because it can also be elevated in benign disease or normal with cancer. Accordingly, efforts to adopt PSA as a routine screening test have led to controversy. On the one hand, since half the prostate cancers now detected have spread by the time they are discovered, it may be useful to find them earlier, before they have spread. On the other hand, while screening will probably detect many more prostate cancers earlier, research has not yet shown that such men will be less likely to die from their disease than unscreened men who are found to have prostate cancer during usual visits to their physician. Also, while screening may lead to treatment that may reduce prostate cancer death rates, it may also lead to unnecessary treatments in the thousands of men who might otherwise lead normal lives because they would not need treatment at all. Many untreated men with cancer found by screening might probably die from causes other than prostate cancer without ever realizing cancer was growing within them. For the foreseeable future, it would seem best for men 50 and over to undergo annual PSA and digital rectal check-ups.

Ultrasound, a method to image the prostate, works much like radar. It is painless and does not involve radiation. At present, its value in screening is not promising. Its main role is to confirm results of a digital examination, to locate tumors in patients who have elevated PSA levels and to guide needle biopsies.

COMMON SIGNS AND SYMPTOMS

When symptoms occur, they can be local or generalized. Local symptoms include painful or frequent urination, a sudden decrease in the size and force of the urinary stream or blood in the urine. Generalized symptoms relate to spread to bone and include pain in the back, hips, thighs or shoulders. There is weight loss and fatigue as the tumor progresses. Prostate cancer is seldom curable once symptoms develop, which is the best argument for early detection through screening.

DIAGNOSIS

Physical Examination
♦ The main finding is a lump or irregularity in the prostate, which can be felt with the examining finger. The prostate may seem enlarged but can also be normal size.

Stages of prostate cancer

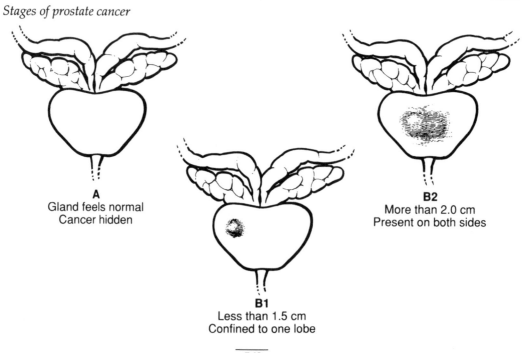

A
Gland feels normal
Cancer hidden

B1
Less than 1.5 cm
Confined to one lobe

B2
More than 2.0 cm
Present on both sides

Blood and Other Tests

♦ Blood chemistry tests to measure prostate-specific antigen and prostatic acid phosphatase, which can become elevated in prostatic cancer.

♦ Urinalysis to detect evidence of bleeding or infection in the urine.

♦ A complete blood count may show anemia if the tumor has invaded the bone marrow.

♦ A serum chemistry profile looks at 15 to 20 chemistry tests measuring liver and bone enzymes, kidney function and other studies.

Imaging

♦ Transrectal ultrasound to view the prostate and direct a biopsy needle into the tumor.

♦ X-rays of the abdomen, pelvis, kidneys and bladder to see if the tumor has spread to these structures.

♦ Intravenous pyelogram (IVP) of the urinary system (kidneys, ureters and bladder).

♦ Chest x-ray.

♦ Abdominal and pelvic CT or MRI scans.

Endoscopy and Biopsy

♦ A transrectal needle biopsy is the removal of a small piece of the tumor for examination by a pathologist. Its accuracy can often be increased by guiding the needle with ultrasound.

♦ Cystoscopy (passage of a small tube through the urinary canal) will provide a different view of the prostate and allow the doctor to move the prostate while it is being examined with a finger in the rectum. In this way, the lump can be felt from a variety of angles and it can be discovered whether the lump has become attached to adjacent tissues.

♦ Flow cytometry and nuclear shape analysis are tests to evaluate the characteristics of the prostate cells removed by biopsy. Cancer cells are less uniform than normal ones.

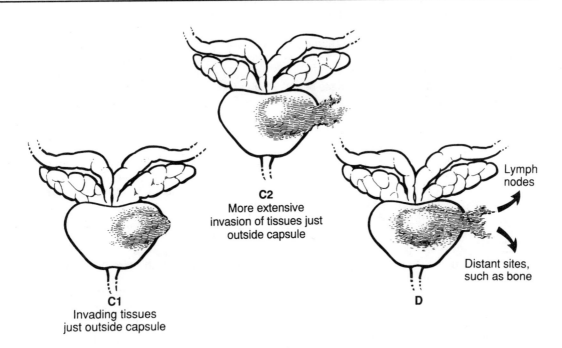

C2
More extensive
invasion of tissues just
outside capsule

C1
Invading tissues
just outside capsule

Lymph
nodes

Distant sites,
such as bone

D

STAGING/GRADING

Stages of prostate cancer are divided into A, B, C and D according to the degree of spread. Slower-growing cancer cells take longer to spread, and the grade of the tumor cells—how aggressive they are—is described by the Gleason grading system, which categorizes prostate cell growth and behavior. The Gleason rating, which is between 1 and 10, represents a total score of two parts. One part is given to the predominant cell type and the second part is given to the most aggressive cell type. These two scores are added to become the Gleason rating. Tumors rated 2 to 4 are generally slow growing and are less likely to be life-threatening. Tumors rated 8 to 10 are the more dangerous ones.

TREATMENT OVERVIEW

Treatment options depend on the tumor's stage (its size and degree of spread to other sites) and grade (the aggressiveness of the particular tumor cells). If the cancer can be caught while still confined to the prostate it can be cured. If it has spread, it can be treated but not cured. If it is low grade it is less likely to have spread than if it is high grade.

Surgery and radiation therapy are the treatments of choice if the tumor is going to be cured. The decision depends on the patient's age, medical condition and personal desires. Therapy with hormones, removal of the testicles (orchiectomy) and chemotherapy may relieve symptoms of advanced disease but will not produce a cure.

 Surgery Surgical removal of the prostate and the seminal vesicles—a radical prostatectomy—is the only certain way to remove all of the cancerous gland. This will lead to a cure if the cancer is confined to the prostate.

The surgeon will often sample lymph nodes—in a procedure called a pelvic lymphadenectomy—during the operation but before the prostate is removed. If the lymph nodes are positive for cancer, the prostate will usually not be removed, for there will be little benefit for the patient and there may be significant side effects.

The newest procedure for lymph node sampling is called laparoscopic lymphadenectomy. A long telescope (laparoscope) is inserted through a tiny opening in the abdomen and is used to observe and guide the sampling of pelvic lymph nodes to see if they contain cancer. If the lymph nodes contain cancer, most surgeons would not perform a radical prostatectomy, because the side effects and disadvantages would outweigh the potential gains. The decision to use radiotherapy may also be influenced by the findings of this procedure. This sampling procedure also creates the option for other definitive surgical procedures that are easier on the patient and that may have fewer side effects. If the lymph nodes are positive for cancer, the prostate will usually not be removed, for there will be little benefit for the patient.

The usefulness of laparoscopic pelvic lymph node sampling when done as a separate procedure is still being debated. Current recommendations include patients with clinically localized disease (Stage A or B) with a poorly differentiated tumor and a PSA of more than 30. Patients who are to have a radical prostatectomy can undergo laparoscopic lymph node sampling immediately before the perineal procedure. Many patients who are to have radiation therapy are also excellent candidates for laparoscopic lymph node sampling.

The removal of the prostate can be accomplished by an incision in the abdomen (the retropubic approach) or by an incision between the scrotum and anus (the perineal approach). The retropubic approach offers the ability to perform lymph node sampling and prostate removal in one step. Time spent in the operating room is usually less than for the perineal approach. Transfusions are often required and there is moderate pain from the abdominal incision. The perineal approach can be performed without lymph node sampling if the PSA and Gleason grade are low. More typically, it is performed in conjunction with a laparoscopic lymph node sampling. Its main advantages are less pain, less blood loss (fewer transfusions) and a shorter hospital stay.

Radical prostatectomy by either method will result in severe incontinence (leaking of urine) in about 5 percent of patients and slight loss of urine in about half of patients. The operations are complex and as with any major surgical procedure there can be wound breakdown and infection. Nearly everyone survives the operation. Newer techniques permit the majority of younger men to preserve their sexual ability, but it is lost in most men over 70. Both urine loss and impotence can be treated.

 Radiation Radiation therapy can be given by external beam or implantation of radioactive seeds into the tumor. External beam radiation usually takes about six weeks. It has the advantage of avoiding an incision, but sometimes it may not kill all the cancer cells. If so, the tumor may grow back, although it can take ten to fifteen years to return. The risks and complications of external beam radiation therapy are equivalent in number to those of surgery, but there are differences in the nature of specific problems. Six weeks of radiation can cause moderate and sometimes considerable fatigue. Severe rectal pains with diarrhea and spasms (radiation proctitis) and severe bladder urgency, frequency and pain on urination (radiation cystitis) can also occur. These can be permanent. Loss of urine (incontinence) and impotence occur nearly as often as they do with a radical prostatectomy. As well, external beam radiation may not kill all

the cancer cells.

Interstitial radiation is administered by inserting pellets or ribbons of radiation-emitting material directly into the prostate. This can be done by open surgery or via needles inserted through the skin. The main advantage of this therapy is that the radiation dosage is concentrated to the tumor and does not harm normal tissues. There is also less radiation cystitis and proctitis. If the pellets or ribbons are inserted at open surgery, the surgeon can at the same time sample the lymph nodes to see if the tumor has spread (although the use of laparoscopic sampling may make open surgery less common).

The disadvantages of interstitial radiation are that the pellets or ribbons may not be placed evenly in the tumor and areas can be missed. Also, all the cancer cells may not be killed and the tumor may recur. Interstitial radiation can also rarely produce erosion into the rectum causing urine to pass into the rectum, and stool into the bladder.

Radiation therapy is also used to relieve symptoms. Radiation to bone for local control of pain, for example, can often produce dramatic relief.

Cryosurgery Freezing of the prostate using a liquid nitrogen probe is a new technique being studied to control prostate cancer. It has the theoretical advantages of a rapid effect, little pain and potential eradication of the cancer. However, at this time, it is experimental, since its effectiveness and its side effects are not yet established.

Surgery vs Radiation There is controversy about the relative benefits of surgical treatment versus radiation therapy. Most data suggest that surgery produces the greater likelihood of avoiding tumor recurrence, since radiation may not kill all the cancer cells and injured ones may recover and grow back. Not all experts agree.

If life expectancy is the sole issue, surgery and radiation therapy produce about the same results for the first 5 to 10 years. After that time, surgery is somewhat better.

Observation Recent studies have shown that watchful waiting (without any treatment) produces a 10-year survival rate, which is almost equivalent to that experienced by patients treated more aggressively with surgery or radiation therapy. Much of the decision to observe or treat aggressively depends upon personal factors such as a man's peace of mind and his anticipated quality of life if one or the other approach is taken. In general, the best candidates for aggressive therapy are men with slow-growing cancers who are in good health and younger than 70. Men 80 or older are best treated by watchful waiting. Men between 70 and 80 must be evaluated for quality of life factors, personal choice, aggressiveness of tumor and general state of health. There are no clear universal guidelines that establish the best approach for a given individual.

Hormonal Therapy When the prostate cancer can no longer be cured with surgery or radiation or when the patient is not a candidate for these methods perhaps because of other illness, hormonal therapy is used to slow the growth of the tumor and reduce symptoms. It is not a cure, but results can be very good. The idea behind this treatment is that the male hormone testosterone helps prostate tumor cells thrive. Depriving the tumor cells of this hormone will often retard the tumor's growth.

Hormonal therapy can be given by removing the testicles (the body's main source of male hormone) or by giving other hormones or chemicals to shut down the body's production of testosterone or counteract its effects. Patients receiving hormonal therapy often experience dramatic relief of symptoms, which can sometimes last for years. But ultimately, the tumor returns.

All the methods used to manipulate the male hormone system will cause men to lose their desire for sex. They may also produce hot flashes.

♦ Removing the testicles (orchiectomy) is a simple surgical procedure that can be done under local or general anesthesia in an outpatient department. Once this is done there is no need for further hormonal therapy. Some men find this procedure undesirable, but the effect is the same as for other hormonal treatments. The scrotum, the sac containing the testicles, is left in place, so the outward appearance is little changed.

♦ Giving men the female hormone estrogen will shut down the gland in the brain (pituitary) that stimulates the testicles to make testosterone. The effect of estrogens on prostate cancer is similar to the effect of orchiectomy, but the female hormone can cause breast development and breast tenderness, although this can usually be prevented by first giving a small dose of radiotherapy to the breast area. Estrogens can also be associated with an increased incidence of heart disease. The pills must be taken daily for life.

♦ Newer hormones such as leuprolide (Lupron) or Goserelin (Zoladex) have much the same effect as orchiectomy or estrogen therapy but are less likely to produce the breast enlargement or heart problems experienced with estrogens. These hormones are expensive and are administered by monthly injections for life.

♦ There are hormonal agents (antiandrogens) that bind to the prostate cell and prevent testosterone from helping it thrive. Flutamide is one such antiandrogen being used in addition to other forms of hormonal therapy. It does not produce a cure, and there may be undesirable side effects, but some studies have indicated that in selected patients it can prolong life about six months longer than if it was not used. And there are non-hormonal chemical agents such as ketoconazole that reduce male hormone levels and mimic the effect of orchiectomy.

 Chemotherapy When orchiectomy or hormonal therapy fail, chemotherapy may be used in advanced stages, but results are poor.

TREATMENT BY STAGE

STAGE A

These tumors are hidden from usual clinical observation. They cannot be felt and are typically found in tissue samples taken after the prostate has been removed because of a benign obstructive disease or when biopsies are taken after ultrasound shows something suspicious.

STAGE A-1

The tumor is limited to less than 5 percent of the prostate tissue removed at surgery and is low grade.

Standard Treatment Most men do not require treatment for this stage of tumor. It is slow growing and will rarely cause symptoms. Fewer than 2 percent will have unsuspected spread to lymph nodes when the tumor is discovered.

Men under 60 may consider radical prostatectomy or external beam radiation therapy because their longer life expectancy will give the slow-growing tumor a greater time to produce symptoms.

STAGE A-2

The tumor extends to more than 5 percent of the tissue removed at surgery and is usually medium to high grade. It is a dangerous tumor, and 34 percent of patients have unexpected spread to lymph nodes when the tumor is found.

Standard Treatment Removal of the pelvic lymph nodes, followed by radical prostatectomy during the same operation

if the lymph nodes are found to be negative. If the tumor location and tissue conditions permit, nerve-sparing methods may be used to preserve sexual ability.

Postoperative radiation therapy should be considered if the tumor is found to invade or penetrate the prostate capsule or if serum PSA levels remain elevated three weeks after surgery.

♦ External beam radiation therapy using the linear accelerator.

♦ Careful observation or hormonal therapy may be acceptable in patients with other serious medical problems that might indicate a short life expectancy or an inability to withstand the stress of surgery or radiation.

Five-Year Survival 60 percent

Investigational
♦ Interstitial radiation with I-125 inserted at open surgery, often with removal of the pelvic lymph nodes. With ultrasound guidance, the isotope can also be inserted without an open incision.

♦ Lymph node sampling without open surgery (laparoscopic lymphadenectomy).

♦ Therapeutic trials using newer isotopes such as iridium-191 and palladium are under way.

♦ Neutron beam radiation therapy is also undergoing evaluation.

STAGE B

Stage B tumors are palpable lumps that are confined to the prostate and do not penetrate the prostate capsule. The size and grade of the tumor determine the possibility for cure.

STAGE B-1

The tumor is less than 5/8 in. (1.5 cm), does not invade the capsule and is limited to one lobe of the prostate. Approximately 15 to 20 percent of patients have unsuspected lymph nodes with cancer when the lump is discovered, which is why pelvic lymph node sampling is required before the prostate is removed.

Standard Treatment Same as Stage A-2.

Five-Year Survival 75 percent

Investigational Same as Stage A-2.

STAGE B-2
The tumor is larger than 3/4 in. (2 cm) and involves more than one lobe of the prostate. It does not invade the capsule. Thirty-four percent of patients have unexpected spread to lymph nodes at the time the tumor is found.

Standard Treatment Same as Stage A-2.

Five-Year Survival 60 percent

Investigational Same as Stage A-2.

STAGE C
These tumors have penetrated the prostate capsule and spread to nearby structures such as the seminal vesicles or fat next to the prostate gland.
This stage is further divided into:
◆ C-1, indicating spread just beyond the prostate;
◆ C-2, indicating spread still in the local area but involving more of the immediately surrounding tissues. Stage C-2 will often obstruct the flow of urine, producing voiding difficulties.
About half of Stage C-1 patients and 80 percent of Stage C-2 patients have unsuspected lymph node metastases when the tumor is detected.

Standard Treatment The approach to Stage C cancer depends on the extent of the tumor and the patient's medical condition.
Treatment can be directed toward curing the cancer if the tumor can be removed or seems able to be treated successfully and if the patient's medical condition permits.
If the tumor seems too large or if the patient is too old or not in good health, palliative therapy can be provided to slow tumor growth and reduce symptoms.

◆ *Treatment for Cure* External beam radiation therapy using the linear accelerator is the treatment of choice. Some experts, however, believe that a radical prostatectomy can be done successfully in certain cases of Stage C-1 cancers where the tumor is confined closely to the prostate and the surgeon can remove all the cancer with a margin of normal tissue. Some urologists will give hormonal agents to shrink the cancers before surgery. In these cases as always, lymph nodes are first sampled to be certain they have no cancer. If nodes are positive, the prostatectomy is not done. Interstitial implants using radioactive palladium have also been used.

◆ *Treatment for Palliation* Radiation therapy to the prostate can reduce the size of the tumor, but long-term effects in prolonging life are not well documented. This therapy can reduce obstructions and make urination easier.
A transurethral prostatectomy (TURP) will also help urination and is less burdensome than radiation therapy. But incontinence is more likely after if radiation therapy has been given, if cancer has spread to the urinary control zone, the urethral sphincter.
Hormonal therapy is the mainstay of palliative therapy for prostate cancer.

Five-Year Survival 50 to 55 percent for C-1, 40 to 45 percent for C-2

Investigational Same as Stage A-2.

STAGE D
The tumor has spread to lymph nodes and distant locations and is rarely curable. There are often symptoms of urinary obstruction or pain from metastases to bone.
This stage is further divided into:

◆ D-0. The tumor appears localized to the prostate as if it were Stage B, but the blood test tumor marker prostatic acid phosphatase is elevated, indicating that the tumor has spread to distant sites.

◆ D-1. Spread to lymph nodes in the pelvis.

◆ D-2. Spread to bone or distant organs.

◆ D-3. Patients with Stage D-2 disease who have relapsed after adequate hormonal therapy.

Standard Treatment Most treatment aims to control symptoms—relieving obstruction or pain—and tries to prolong life. Radical surgery is generally not useful.

The standard treatment is hormonal manipulation through hormonal therapy or removal of the testicles. Hormonal therapy includes giving estrogens (diethylstilbestrol), antiandrogens (flutamide), luteinizing hormone-releasing hormone (LH-RH) agonists such as leuprolide, and progestational agents (Megace).

Impressive improvement often follows hormonal treatment, with reduction in pain and improvement in overall well-being. Voiding symptoms sometimes disappear, although this effect may take several months to occur. Relief of pain is often dramatic after the testicles are removed. This procedure produces the quickest results and does not require the use of any further medication for tumor control.

◆ A chemotherapeutic-hormonal agent called estramustine phosphate concentrates in the prostate cancer tissue and is believed to have some direct action against the tumor. Whether this effect is because of the hormonal activity or antitumor activity is not well understood. The role of this agent is still uncertain and it is used mainly for patients who fail traditional hormone therapy measures.

◆ When voiding problems are severe and there is no time to wait, a transurethral prostatectomy (TURP) will produce immediate relief of urinary obstruction.

Incontinence (leakage of urine) is a risk in TURP because the tumor may extend to the urethral sphincter muscle and prevent the canal from closing properly.

◆ Pain in areas of bone involved by tumor and that does not respond to hormonal therapy is best treated by external beam radiation to the area of pain. Relief is often felt within days.

◆ Observation without further immediate treatment may be suitable for selected patients who have no symptoms.

◆ External beam irradiation for possible cure in highly selected Stage D-1 patients, since patients with this limited Stage D disease will occasionally respond to external beam radiation to the prostate and pelvic area. Cure is rare.

Five-Year Survival 55 percent for D-0, 40 percent for D-1, 35 percent for D-2 and D-3

Investigational

◆ Combination hormonal manipulation with LH-RH agonists and progestational agents.

◆ Chemotherapy protocols.

◆ Alternative forms of radiotherapy with neutron beams. New devices producing more powerful forms of external radiation using proton and neutron beams have been developed, and patients are being treated in clinical trials.

Most current investigational chemotherapy protocols employ standard chemotherapeutic agents in varying combinations. Unfortunately, they have not been promising. But breakthroughs may be possible in the coming years. While the prostate cancer cell itself may resist toxic chemicals, certain parts of its environment may be more amenable to attack. For example, certain growth factors are needed to stimulate prostate cancer cell growth. Drugs that alter the behaviour of these growth factors may inhibit the cancer's rate of progress. One drug now being investigated for its ability to do just this is Suramin. Although few studies have been done, there is reason to believe that Suramin may be helpful for some patients with advanced disease.

TREATING OTHER PROSTATE TUMORS

DUCTAL CARCINOMAS

These arise within the prostatic ducts and comprise less than 5 percent of prostate cancers. There are four types:

♦ transitional cell carcinoma;
♦ intraductal adenocarcinoma;
♦ mixed ductal carcinoma; and
♦ endometroid carcinoma.

Transitional cell and mixed ductal carcinomas are aggressive cancers that require complete removal of the prostate and bladder (cystoprostatectomy) if found while the tumor is still confined to the prostate. The outlook is not good for patients with these cancers.

Intraductal adenocarcinomas are treated by radical prostatectomy.

Endometroid carcinomas arise near a structure called the verumontanum and are similar to certain types of uterine cancers in women. If the tumors are confined to the prostate, the treatment of choice is the removal of the prostate and bladder. Some patients with advanced disease respond to external beam radiation therapy, hormonal treatment or chemotherapy with 5-fluorouracil and doxorubicin.

CARCINOSARCOMAS, RHABDOMYOSARCOMAS, CHONDROSARCOMA AND OSTEOSARCOMA

These make up the rest of the prostate tumor types. If found early, complete removal of the prostate, bladder and adjacent pelvic structures offers the best chance for cure.

Radiation, hormonal therapy and chemotherapy are not effective.

TREATMENT FOLLOW-UP

Prostate-specific antigen (PSA) is moni-

tored shortly after prostate surgery and at regular intervals following all therapy for prostate cancer. Cured patients will have no measurable PSA in their blood.

Regular examination, chest x-rays, bone scans and various blood tests are performed at frequent intervals to detect recurrence or spread as early as possible.

TREATING IMPOTENCE AND INCONTINENCE

Impotence is nearly always treatable. There are a variety of external appliances, surgical implants or penile injection techniques that function quite well. Over 85 percent of patients and their mates are satisfied with the results of these methods.

Patients who become incontinent after the surgical removal of the prostate or radiation therapy have a wide selection of incontinence aids—diapers, condom catheters and penile clamps, for example—to collect urine, protect the skin and maintain hygiene. Exercises to try to strengthen the urethral sphincter muscle are usually not helpful but are worth the try.

The leaking will often subside after 6 to 12 months. If not, surgically inserted sphincter implants are successful in about three-quarters of patients. Recent experiments with collagen and Teflon injections seem encouraging. Drugs such as Pro-Banthine or oxybutinine reduce bladder contraction and may control the wetness.

RECURRENT AND METASTATIC CANCER

The cure rate is low or non-existent for patients with metastatic disease, but hormonal therapy, external beam radiation, experimental chemotherapy and supportive measures can often extend life and well-being for years.

♦ Locally recurrent tumors in the pelvis are best treated by external beam or interstitial radiation therapy if radical prostatectomy was the initial form of treatment.

♦ Patients originally receiving external

beam radiation therapy usually cannot be given additional external beam treatments, but selected patients can undergo interstitial radiotherapy.

♦ As is the case for most cancer of the prostate, hormonal therapy is the mainstay for metastatic disease.

♦ Chemotherapy protocols are continuing, but there are no truly promising developments.

THE MOST IMPORTANT QUESTIONS YOU CAN ASK

♦ Is my cancer confined to the prostate and how can you tell?

♦ Do I need a radical prostatectomy?

♦ What is the difference in results between surgery and radiation? Are they the same?

♦ What are the advantages and disadvantages of various hormone treatments?

♦ What are the chances that I'll become incontinent or impotent?

♦ How might I choose between surgery, radiation, hormonal therapy and watchful waiting? Why is one or the other treatment best for me? Should more than one be used? If so, is there a preferred sequence?

♦ Is my surgeon a Board-certified urologist experienced in this kind of operation?

SARCOMAS OF BONE AND SOFT TISSUE

Frederick Eilber, MD, and Malin Dollinger, MD

———◇———

Sarcomas are uncommon malignant tumors that begin either in bones or in soft tissues such as muscles, cartilage, fat or connective tissue. There are about 6,000 cases of soft tissue sarcoma and 2,000 cases of bone sarcomas in the United States each year, making up about 1 percent of cancers in adults and 15 percent in children (*see also* "Childhood Cancer: Soft Tissue and Bone Sarcomas," "Kaposi's Sarcoma," "Mesothelioma" and "Uterus: Uterine Sarcoma").

Malignant bone tumors tend to affect certain age groups. Osteosarcoma primarily affects teenagers. Ewing's sarcoma tends to affect children (ages 5 to 9) and young adults (ages 20 to 30). Chondrosarcomas tend to affect the older age groups (50 to 60 years). For childhood soft tissue sarcomas (specifically rhabdomyosarcoma) the age group most affected is children aged 1 to 3 years. Most adults with soft tissue sarcoma are 40 to 60 years old.

Over the past 15 years there has been a major advance in the early diagnosis of these tumors with CT and MRI scanning, as well as a dramatic improvement in overall survival, mainly because of effective chemotherapy. The overall survival for people with soft tissue sarcomas rose from about 40 percent in 1968 to about 70 percent in 1989. In the same years, survival for sarcomas of bone rose from less than 20 percent to over 70 percent.

In 1968, the usual treatment for tumors that began in an arm or leg was amputation of the limb. Now it is possible to preserve the limb in more than 90 percent of sarcomas in an arm or leg by using limb-sparing surgery followed by radiotherapy (although for osteosarcomas, the possibility of sparing the limb is not as high).

Types There are at least 56 different types of soft tissue sarcomas named according to the normal tissue from which the tumor is derived. Many have characteristic patterns of growth and spread. Specialists use the specific type to help plan work-up, tests and treatment, but the likely behavior of the tumor is more often related to its grade. There are three tumor categories related to the tumor's grade or activity as defined by the percentage of dividing cells (mitotic rate)—low grade, intermediate grade and high grade. The last is the most highly malignant.

The four common types of bone sarcomas are osteosarcoma, Ewing's sarcoma, chondrosarcoma and fibrosarcoma. All are usually high grade except chondrosarcoma.

How It Spreads Sarcomas may spread early to adjacent tissues without being confined by a shell or capsule, as is common with other types of tumors. If this capsule were present, it would tend to delay local spread and also make surgery easier. They also spread to distant sites, especially the lungs, and some types of sarcomas spread to nearby lymph nodes.

What Causes It In most cases the cause is unknown, although some sarcomas are related to certain diseases or exposure to specific agents. Soft tissue sarcomas do not arise from benign tumors, but some apparently benign bone tumors—cartilage or benign giant cell tumors, for example—can become malignant. Malignant bone tumors are more common in adolescence, supporting the theory that these tumors may occur because of rapid growth.

RISK FACTORS

♦ About 10 percent of people with von Recklinghausen's disease, a rare genetic abnormality affecting nerves, will develop neurofibrosarcoma. Malignant schwannomas may also develop as part of the condition.

♦ Other genetically linked diseases that have a slightly increased incidence of associated sarcomas include Werner's syndrome, tuberous sclerosis, intestinal polyposis, basal cell nevus syndrome and Gardner's syndrome.

♦ Lymphangiosarcoma is associated with people who have chronic swelling of an arm or leg and rarely may develop after many years in a swollen arm after mastectomy.

♦ Fibrosarcomas may develop after high-dose radiation formerly given for benign conditions, such as tuberculosis of the joints or thyroid disease.

♦ The risk of angiosarcoma of liver increases with exposure to thorotrast (no longer in use), arsenic, vinyl chloride or in association with cirrhosis or hemochromatosis.

♦ The risk of osteosarcoma increases with radiation exposure, and sarcomas of both bone and soft tissue can occur many years after radiotherapy, especially if it was given in childhood. Radiation exposure causes less than 5 percent of osteosarcomas and fibrosarcomas, however. (Many years ago, exposure to radium caused osteosarcomas in painters of glow-in-the-dark watch faces.)

♦ Various causes of chronic irritation or stimulation to bones, including chronic

TYPES OF SARCOMAS

Tumor Type	Tissue of Origin
Bone	
Chondrosarcoma	Cartilage
Osteosarcoma	Bone
Ewing's sarcoma	Probably neural crest (primitive nerve)
Fibrosarcoma	Connective (fibrous) tissue
Soft Tissue	
Fibrosarcoma	Connective (fibrous) tissue
Liposarcoma	Fat
Rhabdomyosarcoma	Skeletal muscle
Synovial sarcoma	Membranes lining joints
Neurofibrosarcoma	Nerve structures
Angiosarcoma	Blood vessels
Leiomyosarcoma	Smooth muscle, such as found in the wall of the bowel
Mesenchymoma	Primitive connective tissue
Malignant fibrous histiocytoma	Primitive connective tissue
Epithelioid sarcoma	Unknown
Clear cell sarcoma	Unknown
Dermatofibrosarcoma protuberans	Connective tissue
Parosteal sarcoma	Bone surface
Malignant schwannoma	Nerve structures
Hemangiosarcoma	Blood vessels
Primitive neuroectodermal tumor	Nerve tissues
Lymphangiosarcoma	Lymph vessels
Alveolar soft part sarcoma	Unknown
Granular cell myoblastoma	Skeletal muscle
Hemangiopericytoma	Blood vessels

bone infection, fractures and Paget's disease increase the risk.

♦ Sarcomas have developed in old scars or areas of trauma, but any definite cause has not been proved.

♦ Many types of bone and soft tissue sarcoma have been found to have associated characteristic chromosome abnormalities. Some families appear to have an increased incidence of sarcomas. Another inherited genetic abnormality—deletion of the retinoblastoma gene—also increases risk.

♦ Some chemotherapeutic agents, particularly "alkylating" agents, increase risk.

SCREENING

Because these are rare tumors that can arise virtually anywhere in the body, there are no standard screening measures. Both bone and soft tissue sarcomas may appear silently with an enlarging mass or swelling that may not be apparent until it causes pain or pressure symptoms.

Early detection requires that all unexplained masses or lumps in the soft tissues be assessed clinically and, in some cases, with CT or MRI scans and that they be biopsied or removed. Early detection is often difficult, however, not only because these cancers grow without producing symptoms but also because they arise in inaccessible places.

COMMON SIGNS AND SYMPTOMS

The most common complaints are a swelling or mass, most often painless, or pain in an affected bone or joint, especially at night. There may rarely be general symptoms such as fever, malaise, weight loss or bleeding. Rarely, sarcomas may cause a low blood sugar, with symptoms of hypoglycemia. Malignant bone sarcomas cause pain as they become larger.

DIAGNOSIS

Blood and Other Tests
♦ Blood tests—including serum chemistry panel, LDH, serum protein electrophoresis, calcium, and acid and alkaline phosphatase levels—to aid in differential diagnosis.

Imaging
♦ X-rays will suggest a diagnosis and the most probable type of bone sarcomas, but soft tissue sarcomas do not show up well on regular x-rays.

♦ For soft tissue tumors, CT or MRI scans are useful for finding masses and determining their size and relationships to surrounding structures.

♦ Bone scans may add additional information about the tumor type and extent.

♦ Arteriography (x-rays of the tumor blood vessels) can outline tumor margins and help select a perfusion vessel for chemotherapy.

♦ Chest x-ray or CT to determine spread to lungs.

Biopsy
♦ Biopsy of the suspected lesion is essential. The type of biopsy procedure used has to take the possible surgical treatment into account. Definitive surgery may be done at the same time as the biopsy or later.

STAGING

Stage is determined by the tumor's size and grade and whether it has spread to nearby lymph nodes or distant sites. Several staging systems are used for adult soft tissue sarcomas, pediatric sarcomas and bone sarcomas.

The TNM system is useful to specialists, but a simplified staging system uses the grade of the tumor—the primary factor determining survival—to divide adult soft tissue sarcomas into four stages. Stages I, II and III, none of which involve spread to nearby lymph nodes or distant sites, are also divided into sub-stages A (tumors less than 2 in./5 cm in diameter) and B (tumors larger than that). Stage IV tumors have spread to regional lymph nodes (IVA) or to distant sites (IVB).

Grade is determined primarily by the percentage of dividing cells in the tumor. Grade 1 tumors are well-differentiated and have only a small chance of spreading to another site. Grade 2 tumors are moderately differentiated and have a less than 20 percent chance of spreading. Grade 3 tumors are poorly differentiated, meaning that they contain immature cells that divide rapidly. They have a greater than 50 percent chance of metastasizing.

Five-year survival is usually better than 75 percent for low-grade tumors and less than 25 percent for high-grade tumors.

ADULT SOFT TISSUE SARCOMAS: TREATMENT OVERVIEW

Sarcomas are best treated by an experienced team of specialists in surgical oncology (often orthopedic oncologists in the case of bone tumors), radiation oncology, medical oncology and often physical medicine and rehabilitation.

The initial biopsy must be carefully planned to ensure that enough tissue is available for diagnosis, but also to allow for subsequent surgery. This is especially important with sarcomas involving arms or legs, where the appropriate biopsy can make limb-sparing surgery more effective.

Prognosis is affected by a patient's age, the size of the primary tumor, grade and stage, degree of lymphatic and blood vessel invasion, the duration of symptoms and the location of the tumor on the arm, leg or trunk. Unfavorable prognostic signs include age over 60, a tumor larger than 2 in. (5 cm), a high-grade tumor, spread to lymph nodes or distant sites, a deep rather than a superficial malignancy, and symptoms lasting less than one year.

Low-grade tumors can usually be cured by surgery alone. Higher grade sarcomas have more tendency to recur in the same area or metastasize and so are often treated with surgery, radiotherapy and/or regional chemotherapy.

Many of these tumors are often treated by a combination of surgery, radiation therapy and chemotherapy to improve the possibility of cure. The prognosis for sarcomas involving the retroperitoneum (area in the back of the abdomen) is less favorable, since it is difficult to surgically resect all the tumor as well as to give higher-dosage radiotherapy.

 Surgery Surgery for these tumors often has to be extensive, with a wide margin of tissue around the tumor being removed. Sarcomas involving muscles require removal of the entire affected muscle group.

Bone sarcomas must be removed with a wide margin of apparently normal bone. Amputation can be avoided most of the time, as limb-salvage surgery is now often possible in selected patients.

After primary malignant tumors of bone are partially or completely removed, the bone may be reconstructed. This procedure may include bone grafts, but these are not always satisfactory. A more reliable method is custom-made metal bones with artificial joint replacement. Remarkable achievements have made it possible to avoid amputation by substituting a prosthetic bone tailored to the patient. In children, an arm or leg prosthetic bone can be lengthened as the child grows.

 Radiation Radiation therapy is used to prevent local recurrences of radiosensitive tumors and may be given either before or after surgery.

 Chemotherapy Several drugs have proven to be effective in treating bone and soft tissue sarcomas. The dosages required to provide a good chance for cure often produce significant side effects, though.

Effective single agents include doxorubicin (Adriamycin), cyclophosphamide, high-dose methotrexate (with leucovorin rescue), ifosfamide, dacarbazine (DTIC), vincristine, dactinomycin (Actinomycin D), etoposide and investigational agents.

Commonly used combinations include doxorubicin + cyclosphosphamide + methotrexate, CyVADIC (cyclophosphamide + vincristine + doxorubicin +

dacarbazine), ifosfamide + etoposide, doxorubicin + cyclophosphamide and doxorubicin + dacarbazine + cyclophosphamide. Other combinations have been used, chiefly of these drugs but also of others available for investigational use.

Chemotherapy is part of the standard and optimal initial treatment for Ewing's sarcoma and osteosarcoma. For Ewing's sarcoma, radiation therapy of approximately 4,500 cGy is added. Surgery then follows for all patients with osteosarcoma and most patients with Ewing's sarcoma. Additional chemotherapy is mandatory for both Ewing's sarcoma and osteosarcoma after surgery. In some centers, another tumor specimen is examined for significant tumor destruction to see if the same chemotherapeutic agent should be given again.

Adjuvant Chemotherapy Even if a bone or soft tissue sarcoma is apparently localized and could apparently be completely removed, there is a significant risk that tumor cells too small to detect have already spread to other places in the body. Additional treatment with chemotherapy (adjuvant) attempts to eliminate these tumor deposits.

Adjuvant chemotherapy is commonly used for certain sarcomas, especially childhood sarcomas (rhabdomyosarcoma and Ewing's sarcoma) and osteosarcoma. The use of adjuvant chemotherapy for other sarcomas is under clinical investigation.

The role of adjuvant chemotherapy for soft tissue sarcomas is not fully established. The combination of doxorubicin, high-dose cyclophosphamide and high-dose methotrexate may be of value. Several trials have shown a reduction in local recurrence if chemotherapy is combined with radiation or if radiation therapy is combined with surgery for the treatment of the primary tumor.

♦ **In Metastatic Disease** The treatment of metastatic disease in both bone and soft tissue sarcomas usually involves the use of chemotherapy. If tumors are confined to the lungs, an attempt may be made to surgically remove the metastatic deposits. Removal of only a small wedge or triangular-shaped portion of the lung may be needed, rather than the entire lung or a major portion of it. Chemotherapy is sometimes used preoperatively in an attempt to shrink the metastases.

Investigational
♦ Current investigational protocols for soft tissue sarcoma include the use of chemotherapy before surgery (neoadjuvant) in primary soft tissue sarcomas and trials of new drugs in advanced disease.
♦ There are investigational protocols for patients with high-risk Ewing's sarcoma (large tumors in the pelvis) that don't respond well to preoperative treatment. As well as the standard chemotherapy, radiation and surgery, patients are now being entered into trials of high-dose chemotherapy and autologous bone marrow transplantation.

ADULT SOFT TISSUE SARCOMAS: TREATMENT BY STAGE

(For treatment of soft tissue tumors and sarcomas of bone in children, *see* "Childhood Cancer: Soft Tissue and Bone Sarcomas.")

STAGE I
These are well-differentiated (low-grade) tumors that have not spread to nearby lymph nodes or other sites.

Standard Treatment The primary treatment is surgery, with wide (3/4 in./2 cm) margins free of tumor being essential. Radiotherapy is used for tumors that cannot be removed, when the tumor-free margins are uncertain and residual tumor cells are likely, or when wider resection would mean amputation or removal of a vital organ. Adjuvant therapy is generally used only in clinical trials.

Five-Year Survival Over 90 percent

STAGE II

These are moderately well-differentiated tumors (medium grade) that have not spread to nearby lymph nodes or to other sites. They are highly treatable and curable, but are more likely to spread than Stage I tumors.

Standard Treatment For sarcomas involving the arms or legs, limb-sparing surgery (wide local excision) is often combined with preoperative or postoperative radiotherapy. In some centers, intra-arterial chemotherapy is also given. Research is continuing on the best way to combine these treatments.

In some cases involving limbs, amputation may still be necessary if conservative surgery combined with radiotherapy is not possible. The use of adjuvant chemotherapy in this stage is still under investigation, but studies so far seem to show benefit.

Sarcomas of the trunk, head and neck, and abdomen are treated with surgery, often followed by high-dose radiotherapy. Preoperative radiotherapy sometimes permits more conservative surgery, with radiotherapy also given postoperatively. Again, the use of adjuvant chemotherapy is under investigation.

High-dose radiotherapy and chemotherapy are used for tumors that cannot be removed surgically (in the head and neck or abdomen, for example). In some centers, radiotherapy is given during surgery for abdominal sarcomas (intraoperative radiotherapy).

Five-Year Survival 70 percent

Investigational
♦ Preoperative regional chemotherapy, combined with limb-sparing surgery.
♦ Adjuvant chemotherapy following surgery.
♦ The use of various special types of radiotherapy beams.
♦ Radiotherapy after limb-sparing surgery.

STAGE III

These are poorly differentiated or undifferentiated (high-grade) tumors that have not spread to nearby lymph nodes or to distant sites. This stage is further divided into IIIA and IIIB according to the size of the primary tumor.

Standard Treatment Stage IIIA sarcomas are highly treatable and often curable but have an increased chance of metastatic spread. The standard treatment is surgery with radiotherapy or chemotherapy, or sometimes all three.

Sarcomas of the arms or legs are treated in a similar way to Stage II tumors. Sarcomas of the abdomen, trunk, and head and neck are treated with surgery followed by high-dose radiation. Radiotherapy is also sometimes given before surgery, and high-dose radiation sometimes combined with chemotherapy is given if the tumor cannot be completely removed surgically.

Stage IIIB sarcomas are treated much like Stage II and IIIA tumors. Because these tumors are larger, however, in many cases of tumors of the arms or legs amputation will be necessary. In some cases, preoperative radiotherapy or combination chemotherapy may allow tumors to be surgically removed when it would not have been otherwise possible.

Stage IIIB sarcomas of the abdomen, trunk, and head and neck are treated with surgery, often followed by high-dose radiotherapy. If the tumor cannot be completely removed, high-dose radiotherapy combined with chemotherapy may relieve symptoms.

Five-Year Survival 20 to 50 percent

Investigational
♦ Investigational treatments similar to those for Stage II.
♦ Intraoperative radiotherapy for Stage IIIA abdominal sarcomas.

STAGE IV

This stage is divided into two groups.

Tumors of any grade or size that have spread to regional lymph nodes but not to distant sites are Stage IVA. Tumors that have spread to distant sites beyond the lymph nodes draining the area of the cancer (most commonly to the lung) are Stage IVB.

Standard Treatment In Stage IVA, local control of the primary tumor is best obtained with surgery (including removal of lymph nodes) followed by radiotherapy. This may require amputation in some patients with sarcomas of the arm or leg. In some centers, radiotherapy is given both pre- and postoperatively. If the tumor cannot be surgically removed, radiotherapy and chemotherapy are used.

In Stage IVB, if the lung is the only site of spread, cure may be possible in up to 30 percent of patients by aggressive treatment of the primary tumor similar to earlier stages and removal of the lung metastases, even if there are several.

If lung metastases are not removed or there are other sites of metastasis, palliation may be provided by radiotherapy to the primary tumor combined with chemotherapy. Various combinations are used, generally containing doxorubicin and dacarbazine, sometimes with other agents as well. Combinations including ifosfamide are also used.

Standard therapy is not curative, so patients should be considered candidates for clinical trials.

Five-Year Survival Up to 20 percent

SUPPORTIVE THERAPY

Physical therapy with active and passive range-of-motion and strengthening exercises for the arms and legs is extremely important for people with primary bone and soft tissue tumors of the extremities. Exercise programs and elastic stockings can help prevent stiffness and swelling of the extremities.

TREATMENT FOLLOW-UP

Patients with malignant bone and soft tissue sarcomas have to be followed on a regular basis.

♦ Routine physical examinations look for any mass or recurrence of pain.

♦ X-rays and, in some cases, CT scans look for evidence of local tumor recurrence.

♦ Routine chest X-rays are done every two to three months for the first two years. Early detection of lung metastases is important because, occasionally, surgical removal of the metastases can be curative.

RECURRENT SOFT TISSUE SARCOMAS

Treatment depends on the initial situation and treatment. Local recurrences often require aggressive local therapy, which means more surgery and radiotherapy. A recurrence in the same area as the original tumor makes another recurrence even more likely.

♦ If previous treatment was aggressive, amputation may be needed for tumors of the arm or leg.

♦ If lung metastasis is the first area of recurrence, treatment is the same as for Stage IV disease.

♦ If tumors recur after chemotherapy treatment, clinical trials using new agents are appropriate.

THE MOST IMPORTANT QUESTIONS YOU CAN ASK

♦ What will my limitations be after treatment of the bone or soft tissue tumor?

♦ Can I save my limb?

♦ How sick will I become from chemotherapy? Will I lose my hair?

♦ What is my overall chance of survival?

♦ Will it be possible for me to have a family after this treatment?

SKIN

Jill R. Slater-Freedberg, MD, and Kenneth A. Arndt, MD

◇

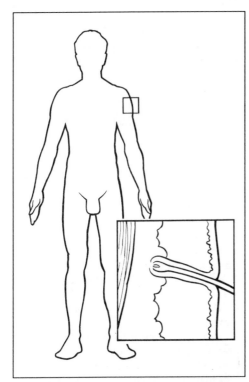

Skin cancer is the most common form of cancer found in humans. Over 600,000 cases are diagnosed in the United States each year, and the number is growing by 3.4 percent a year. One in every three new cancers is a skin cancer. It is estimated that 40 to 50 percent of fair-skinned people who live to be 65 years old will have at least one skin cancer (*see also* "Melanoma"). Ten years ago, skin cancer was unusual in those under 40, but now it is seen regularly in younger people. It is not uncommon in people in their twenties.

The most prevalent types of skin cancer—basal cell and squamous cell—are two to three times more common in men than in women. Both are almost always curable.

Types Basal cell cancer (BCC) is the most common form of all skin cancers, affecting more than 400,000 people each year. It develops in the outermost layer of the skin, the epidermis, on hair-bearing surfaces. The appearance of BCC can vary considerably. The most common type is the nodular basal cell carcinoma, a flesh-colored (cream to pink) round or oval translucent nodule with overlying small blood vessels and a pearly-appearing rolled border. This tumor slowly grows sideways. It may eventually ulcerate and form a crust over the center as it outgrows its blood supply.

A second type of BCC is the pigmented lesion. This is darker than the nodular type, appearing blue, brown or black. It may be similar in appearance to the very aggressive malignant melanoma tumor. Naturally, it is very important to distinguish between malignant melanomas and pigmented BCC.

A third type of BCC is the superficial type that appears as a red, often scaly, localized plaque. It is frequently confused with psoriasis or eczema. There is also a morphea or sclerosing type, a single, firm, ill-defined, slightly raised lesion that tends to be more subtle to recognize than the nodular, superficial and pigmented forms. If untreated, basal cell carcinomas may crust, ulcerate and sometimes bleed.

Squamous cell carcinoma (SCC) is the second most common form of skin cancer, affecting between 80,000 and 100,000 people each year in the United States. It arises from the cells that make the protective keratin of the epidermis (keratinocytes). These tumors usually occur in areas of sun-damaged skin and at sites of previous burns, scars or chronic ulcers. SCC usually appears as a red, scaling, well-defined plaque and may gradually develop an ulcer, a scaly crust or a wart-like surface. Eventually it can spread into the deeper or surrounding tissues.

Squamous cell cancers are considered superficial when the upper part of the dermis is involved and infiltrative when the lower dermis and fat tissues under the skin (subcutaneous) are invaded. These cancers are also described based on how differentiated the cells are—well-differentiated, moderately differentiated and poorly differentiated. The less differentiated the lesion, the least amount of normal tissue is preserved and the more aggressive the cancer.

Verrucous carcinoma is a cauliflower-like (fungating) type of SCC found in the mouth, on the membranes lining the anus and genitals or on the bottom surface of the foot. There are also a number of lesions that are precancerous. Actinic keratoses, for example, are red, scaly discolored areas on sun-exposed areas of fair-skinned individuals that tend to scratch off but come back. Cutaneous horns are hard, funnel-shaped lesions extending from a red base on the skin. Also potentially precancerous is leukoplakia, a white patch on the oral and genital membranes.

How It Spreads Basal cell cancer usually remains unchanged for years or grows very slowly. It rarely spreads to distant sites. One study reported less than 0.01 percent occurrence of metastatic disease. The lesions that tended to spread were large, involved the head and neck with extensive local invasion and had recurred after treatment. When metastatic disease occurs it spreads to local lymph nodes and less often to bone, the lungs and the liver. Survival is less than one year once such spread has been discovered.

Squamous cell cancer has a higher rate of metastatic disease, with studies reporting a 3 percent rate of spread to distant sites. The most likely lesions to spread are large, invasive, greater than 1/10 in. (4 mm) thick and poorly differentiated.

Squamous cell cancer spreads via the lymph system and can involve bone, liver and brain. Metastases increase to a rate of 11 percent when SCC involves the oral and genital membranes and to 10 to 30 percent when the lesions are on areas of the skin previously injured from burns.

What Causes It Most skin cancers are caused by excessive exposure to sunlight. Genetic background is also a factor, since light-skinned people suffer a more adverse reaction to the sun's ultraviolet radiation.

RISK FACTORS

The two major risk factors for developing skin cancers are the amount of exposure to ultraviolet light (usually as sunlight) and the individual's response to ultraviolet light, which depends on skin type and the amount of melanin skin pigment that protects against ultraviolet light absorption.

At Significantly Higher Risk
♦ People who live in areas with high sun exposure and at high altitudes.
♦ People with fair skin (with less melanin in their skin).
♦ Males have a slightly higher incidence than females.
♦ Squamous cell carcinoma is most prevalent in people over 55. Males predominate except on the lower leg sites, where women have a higher incidence.
♦ Outside workers, since most malignant skin tumors occur on sun-exposed areas of the body including the head, neck and the back of the hands.
♦ People with medical conditions involving suppression of the immune system—those infected with the HIV virus, people with cancer, those who have undergone an organ transplant and are taking immune-modulating drugs, those with debilitating chronic diseases, the malnourished, the elderly and patients receiving chemotherapy drugs and steroid hormones.
♦ Individuals with genetic skin disorders that predispose to skin cancer, such as basal cell nevus syndrome, xeroderma pigmentosum and albinism.

At Slightly Higher Risk

♦ Exposure to chemical carcinogens such as coal tar, arsenic in insecticides and nitrogen mustard (chemotherapy) ointment, viral carcinogens (some warts), ionizing radiation (x-rays), and chronic irritation and inflammation.

PREVENTION

People can protect themselves against ultraviolet light damage by taking simple precautions.

♦ *Using Sunscreens* A sunscreen of at least SPF (sunlight protection factor) 15 is recommended. The sunscreen preparation should be applied frequently, and more often with sweating and when swimming. Sunscreen use should begin in infancy.

Regular use of sunscreens with an SPF of 15 during the first 18 years of life can reduce the lifetime incidence of skin cancer by as much as 78 percent. One serious childhood or adolescent sunburn doubles the chances of developing skin cancer, especially malignant melanoma.

Most sunscreens absorb the ultraviolet light of the B wavelength and prevent it from penetrating the skin. The SPF number correlates with the amount of time one can spend in the sun before the skin becomes pink or red. For example, if an SPF 15 is worn, a person can remain exposed to the sun 15 times longer without the skin becoming pink.

The majority of sunscreens do not protect against penetration of longer wavelength ultraviolet light of the A type. The screens actually allow more exposure to the A type radiation by allowing a person to remain outside longer. There are new sunscreens that provide increased protection against ultraviolet light of the A and B types. *However, sun exposure should be kept to a minimum.*

♦ *Wearing Protective Clothing* People who work outside should wear clothing that protects their skin, including long-sleeved shirts, hats and pants. Outdoor recreational activities should be scheduled before 11:00 A.M. and after 2:30 P.M., when the concentration of ultraviolet light is decreased by 70 to 80 percent.

♦ *Avoiding Tanning Booths* Tanning booths have advertised that by using UVA (A type ultraviolet light) a "safe" tan is obtained. There is no such thing as a "safe" tan.

Tanning is a response of the skin to injury. UVA does cause less redness than UVB, but like UVB it may induce skin cancer and photoaging (drying, wrinkles and pigment changes). UVA is actually used experimentally to produce skin cancer in mice. Since 1986, about 2 million people a year have visited tanning booths. This will contribute to an increase in the number of skin cancers we will see over the next 10 to 20 years.

♦ *Being Aware of Skin Changes and Getting Early Treatment* Besides sunscreens, avoiding ultraviolet light and wearing protective clothing, preventive measures include early detection and swift removal of precancerous lesions.

SCREENING

The best screening test is an extensive examination of the skin. Part of a yearly physical should include a thorough examination of the skin including the mouth, behind the ears, around the nose, the scalp, the penis, the areas around the vagina and rectum, the palms of the hands and the soles of the feet. Lymph nodes should also be examined.

Everyone should be examined this way, especially fair-skinned, blond-haired, blue-eyed individuals and people who have had previous skin cancers. Special attention should be given to areas where a previous skin cancer was removed. These people should also examine themselves often to assess any change or development of new lesions to bring to the attention of a physician. If a skin lesion changes in any way, a dermatologist should be consulted.

COMMON SIGNS AND SYMPTOMS

The most common sign is simply a sore or mark on the skin that changes in size, color and shape. It may become itchy or painful and may start to bleed or ulcerate.

DIAGNOSIS

During the initial doctor's appointment, a medical history will be obtained with particular attention given to previous skin lesions, genetic skin disorders and exposure to chemical carcinogens or radiation. The history of the lesion in question should also be clarified—how long it has been present and how it has changed.

Imaging

♦ X-rays, like blood tests, are not usually necessary during the initial doctor visit. They may be necessary to look for signs of bone destruction, however, if there is evidence that the skin lesion is fixed to or invading the bone.

♦ Chest x-rays should be considered with advanced cancers to look for lung metastasis.

Endoscopy and Biopsy

♦ A biopsy should be performed on all suspicious lesions and the specimen sent to a qualified pathologist. The biopsy result will help the physician choose the appropriate treatment.

Four biopsy techniques are employed for skin cancer, with the type used depending on the size and location of the lesion, the equipment available and the experience of the physician.

♦ Shave biopsy uses a scalpel to remove a thin slice of an area in question. This procedure is used when the lesion extends above the skin and the underlying skin is smooth, open and convex.

♦ Punch biopsy uses a cylindrical instrument that is rotated into the skin and removes a cylindrical specimen. This method is used when tissue at a greater depth is required for diagnosis.

♦ Incisional biopsy removes a portion of the tumor with a scalpel.

♦ Excisional biopsy removes the entire lesion.

Because of the ease and minimal complications of these procedures, they can all be performed in the office, with local anesthesia being used to eliminate discomfort. Adverse effects include bleeding, infection, and scarring.

TREATMENT OVERVIEW

There are six widely used methods to treat skin cancer. Which method is chosen depends on the type of lesion, its size and location, the definition of its borders, how invasive it is, how long it has been present and whether more than one lesion is involved. The person's age and overall health are also considered, as is the potential effect of treatment on appearance.

All treatment methods have a cure rate of about 90 percent or more. Tumors that have less than a 90 percent cure rate include sclerosing or morpheaform basal cell cancers, poorly differentiated squamous cell cancers, lesions around the eye, nose and the forehead-temple region, tumors larger than 3/4 in. (2 cm), older lesions and recurrent cancers.

Basal cell and squamous cell cancers are treated using similar procedures. A larger amount of apparently normal tissue may have to be removed when cutting out a SCC, since there is a higher rate of metastasis than with BCC.

STANDARD TREATMENTS

Curettage with or without Electrodesiccation (C&E) This is a two-step procedure in which a curet (sharp-tipped instrument) removes the softer cancer tissue from normal tissue and bleeding is controlled by a chemical agent or by electrical current. This cycle is repeated two to four times. Nodular and superficial BCC and non-invasive SCC can usually be treated effectively with C&E.

C&E is ideal for small tumors with distinct borders, for primary lesions and for lesions on surfaces with minimal excess tissue. It is not recommended for large tumors, tumors invading dermis or fat, lesions with poorly defined borders, poorly differentiated squamous cell carcinomas, recurrent lesions or lesions at certain anatomic sites that have lower cure rates.

C&E is a low-risk procedure that can be performed on an outpatient basis. In contrast to surgical excision, an open wound is left that can then bleed, become infected and form a scar. The site may take one to three months to heal and appear acceptable.

 Cryosurgery This technique uses liquid nitrogen at very low temperatures to freeze the skin. The nitrogen is applied with an aerosolized spray to achieve tissue temperatures below –58°F (–50°C). The tissue is then allowed to thaw for about two minutes. This cycle is repeated two to three times.

Like C&E, cryosurgery is a low-risk procedure. It can, therefore, be used for people who cannot tolerate surgery and is also useful for anyone who is having treatment to prevent blood clotting (anticoagulation therapy).

Cryotherapy is effective for removing lesions where there is minimal excess tissue and can be used for large primary tumors. It is not useful with poorly defined lesions, poorly differentiated SCC, morpheaform BCC, recurrent lesions, lesions in areas of decreased cure rates or on the extremities (arms and legs) where there is decreased blood flow.

As in C&E, cryotherapy leaves an open wound that takes three to ten weeks to heal. The wound may "weep" for two or three weeks after the procedure. Antibiotic creams or ointments are often used to avoid infection. Nodular, superficial BCC and noninvasive SCC can usually be treated effectively with cryotherapy.

 Radiation Treatment with radiation has a reported cure rate of 89 to 95 percent. Various programs include one to five doses.

Radiation is useful for older people who cannot tolerate surgery, for multiple lesions or large superficial lesions and for lesions that are too inaccessible to be removed surgically. It is particularly useful in lesions of the eyelids, nose, lips and ears. It can also be used as a palliative measure rather than for cure on excessively large cancers.

It should not be used for patients under 50 years old because of the possibility of causing new cancers at the radiation site. Treated areas become inflamed (acute radiation dermatitis). This resolves in four to six weeks, but results in loss of skin pigment and thinning, which may worsen in time. Therefore, long-term cosmetic results may not be as good as with other treatments. Another major risk is that recurrences may be more difficult to wipe out.

For patients over 50, radiation therapy can be used to treat nodular, superficial BCC and all SCC. It is primarily used for patients with multiple superficial lesions.

 Chemotherapy 5-fluorouracil (5-FU) is a chemotherapeutic agent that blocks DNA synthesis, thereby preventing normal cell growth and ultimately causing cell death. 5-FU is available as a 5 percent cream and a 2 percent and 5 percent solution. It is applied directly to the skin twice a day for four weeks or more. As it works it causes an inflammatory reaction, which heals after the treatment is stopped.

Advantages of 5-FU are that it is easy to use and has minimal adverse effects. Disadvantages are that it may cause redness and a change in the pigment of the skin. After treatment with 5-FU, the tumor may be controlled on the surface but may continue to invade at the base. Recurrence rates are estimated to be 20 to 50 percent, so follow-up is important.

Intravenous 5-FU has been used for skin cancers that have spread to distant sites, but few data are available on how effective this is because of the limited number of cases involved.

Masoprocol Cream Masoprocol cream 10 percent is a new topical therapeutic agent used to treat actinic keratoses. It is applied twice a day for four weeks. It is easy to use. Adverse reactions include erythema, scaling and itching.

Surgery Excision is a surgical procedure that removes the entire lesion with an appropriate margin of apparently normal tissue. The area is then closed with sutures.This is a more invasive procedure than C&E. The sutures help the healing process as well as produce excellent cosmetic results. This procedure can be used effectively for all skin cancers.

Mohs Micrographic Surgery This technique was first described in 1936 by Dr. Frederick Mohs. It involves removing successive horizontal layers of the skin cancer and any surrounding tissue that may be involved. Each layer is microscopically examined and the section that involves tumor is marked. Subsequent horizontal layers remove the areas of tumor involvement, sparing the normal skin tissue.

Mohs surgery has the highest cure rate of all treatment methods. It is, therefore, recommended for poorly differentiated SCC, morpheaform BCC, invasive tumors, recurrent lesions, lesions with indistinct borders, large primary tumors of long duration, lesions at sites of decreased cure rate and in patients with nevoid basal cell syndrome.

The disadvantages of Mohs surgery are that a great deal of expertise is required by the physician, the procedure is time-consuming and it requires more equipment than the other methods. The resulting wound may be closed with stitches, often followed by plastic reconstruction.

INVESTIGATIONAL

Although the treatments now most widely used have greater than a 90 percent cure rate, other therapies are being investigated that may be more practical, effective and cosmetically elegant. Examples of the newer methods of treatment include:

Retinoids These are synthetic and natural derivatives of vitamin A. Patients with vitamin A deficiency may have an increased susceptibility to skin cancer. This deficiency causes a premalignant change of the skin that can be reversed by applying vitamin A.

Retinoids induce differentiation (maturing) of tumor cells derived from surface tissues (epithelium). Recent investigations have used the retinoids to treat premalignant and malignant skin cancers. Use of the locally applied (topical) and internal (systemic) forms have demonstrated a fair cure rate when treating basal cell cancers. Limited information exists for use in SCC, but one study reported a 70 percent response rate.

Interferons Interferons are proteins produced by human cells in response to a viral infection. Interferons have an antiviral activity, they inhibit the growth of malignant cells and they promote cell maturation. There are three interferons—alpha, beta and gamma.
♦ Interferon-alpha is found in T and B lymphocytes and in macrophages.
♦ Interferon-beta is found in fibroblasts (connective tissue producing cells).
♦ Interferon-gamma is found in activated T cells.

Interferon-alpha has been the most frequently studied interferon for use with skin cancers as well as other types of cancer. Preliminary reports have shown significant results in short-term remission of basal cell carcinomas when interferon-alpha is injected into the tumor (intralesional injection). Interferon is also effective given as nine intralesional injections over three weeks or, in a sustained-release form, as one or three intralesional injections per week.

Interferon leaves no surgical wound, has good cosmetic results and avoids bleeding and infection. Short-term side effects include fever, chills, muscle aches, headaches and nausea.

Photodynamic Therapy (PDT) This treatment uses visible light in combination with a photosensitizer, a compound that attracts light. The photosensitizer now being used is a hematoporphyrin derivative, HPD.

Approximately 48 to 72 hours after HPD is intravenously injected, most of the compound is cleared by the normal skin and selectively retained in the cancerous cells. Upon exposure to different colors of light, HPD undergoes a photodynamic reaction that damages the tumor cells and spares the uninvolved tissue. In practice, HPD is given as an intravenous injection and is followed 48 to 72 hours later by irradiation with red or blue-green light.

There are no well-controlled studies using HPD, but encouraging preliminary results have been reported in treating basal and squamous cell carcinomas.

A disadvantage of photodynamic therapy with HPD is that levels of HPD may stay in the normal skin for three to six weeks after the injection. During this time, patients need protection from all bright light, since exposure to light can result in severe redness and swelling of the skin. This adverse effect would be eliminated if an effective photosensitizer could be applied only to the affected area of skin.

 Laser Therapy The carbon dioxide laser may be used as a cutting instrument, much like a scalpel. It is useful for removing superficial basal and squamous cell carcinomas in patients with bleeding disorders or who have tumors in locations that tend to be bloody, such as the scalp. The wound remaining after the procedure is similar to that left by a scalpel excision. When a defocused beam is used to remove lesions, the cosmetic result appears similar to the wound made by electrodesiccation and curettage.

The most appropriate method of curing a specific skin cancer is the most effective, least toxic, most efficient and most cosmetically elegant therapy, which may be a combination of any of these standard or investigational treatments.

TREATMENT FOLLOW-UP

Twenty percent of people with a single basal cell cancer will develop a second one at another site within a year. If there were two basal cell cancers, there is a 40 percent chance of developing a new one within one year. People who have had a skin lesion removed should, therefore, see their doctor twice a year for the first three years after treatment, followed by yearly visits.

THE MOST IMPORTANT QUESTIONS YOU CAN ASK

◆ What are the most important things I can do to lower my risk of getting skin cancers?
◆ Will my physician be carefully and regularly examining all my skin surface to look for any premalignant and malignant lesions?
◆ Has the biopsy been reviewed by a pathologist with special training in skin tumors?
◆ Which method of treatment will give me the best results?
◆ What is the chance of recurrence or spread with this lesion and your recommended treatment?

SMALL INTESTINE

Ernest H. Rosenbaum, MD

◇

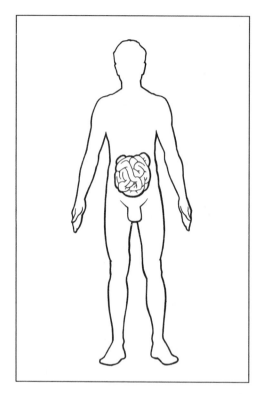

The small intestine is the longest segment of the gastrointestinal tract, making up three quarters of its total length. Yet malignant tumors are much less common in this organ than they are in the esophagus, stomach and large bowel. Of all the gastrointestinal tumors diagnosed, only 1.5 percent are found in the small intestine. About 260 new cases of and 110 deaths from cancer of the small intestine are seen annually. Most are patients over 45, and men account for 60 percent.

There are many reasons for the lower incidence. Cancer-causing agents have less contact with the surface membranes because of the rapid transit time of food through the small bowel compared with the colon. And, since the stool is still liquid, there is less mechanical injury to the membranes.

The inner surface of the small intestine secretes a large amount of gamma globulin that protects the lining against disease. Benzpyrene hydrolase, which can detoxify carcinogens, is found in large amounts in the lining (mucosa) of the small intestine. Finally, the contents of the small bowel are alkaline, which reduces the production of carcinogens from bile and prevents the formation of nitrosamines, environmental carcinogens that are formed only under acidic conditions.

Malignancies of the small bowel are almost always treatable and some may be curable. Their prognosis and treatment depend on the cellular origin.

Types Small intestinal malignancies are generally adenocarcinomas, sarcomas, carcinoid tumors and lymphomas.

The most common of all—half of small intestine tumors—are adenocarcinomas that develop in glandular tissue. Most people with adenocarcinomas have metastases to the lymph nodes, liver or peritoneum (abdominal lining) at the time of diagnosis.

Sarcomas are slow-growing tumors that account for 11 percent of small bowel cancers. Sarcomas can develop in any soft tissue such as fat cells (liposarcoma), blood vessels (angiosarcoma) or nerves (neural sarcomas, neurofibrosarcomas or malignant schwannomas, which develop from the nerve sheath, most commonly in the ileum). But 75 percent of the sarcomas, called leiomyosarcomas, originate in the smooth muscles encircling the bowel. These malignancies may reach a large size before diagnosis (many are larger than 2 in. (5 cm)). Only a third of smooth muscle tumors are malignant.

Carcinoid tumors account for 30 percent of small bowel malignancies. They are often small (usually 1/2 to 1 1/2 in./1 to 5 cm in diameter) and slow growing. There may be multiple lesions and may be present for years (*see* "Carcinoids of the Gastrointestinal Tract").

Lymphomas arising from lymphoid tissues in the wall of the small bowel make up 14 percent of small bowel tumors. They may occur in any part of the small intestine and 20 percent of them develop in multiple sites. Of all the lymphomas that start someplace other than in lymph nodes (extranodal lymphomas), 33 percent do so in the gastrointestinal tract, 10 percent in the small bowel. Most of these lesions are non-Hodgkin's lymphomas.

How It Spreads Small bowel cancers can spread directly through the bowel wall to adjacent tissues. Leiomyosarcomas grow in the muscle wall and extend to the surface (serosa). Sarcomas spread directly to the tissues supporting the bowel (mesentery), the retroperitoneum or the adjacent bowel. These cancers also spread through the lymphatic system and bloodstream to regional lymph nodes or to the liver, lungs or bone.

What Causes It There is an association with some inherited cancers and inflammatory bowel disease (Crohn's disease and celiac disease) and neurofibromatosis. Lymphomas are associated with immune deficiencies and celiac disease.

RISK FACTORS

At Higher Risk
♦ People older than 60, expecially those with a history of bowel disease.
♦ People with changes in the small intestine acidity, rapid transit and nitrosamine exposure.

♦ Those with inherited gastrointestinal disorders—Peutz-Jeghers syndrome, familial polyposis, inflammatory bowel disease, Crohn's disease and neurofibromatosis.
♦ Those with increased lymphoid deposits in the ileum and immune deficiency diseases are at a higher risk for lymphomas.
♦ A history of or the presence of a *Helicobacter pylori* infection may lead to small bowel inflammation that may lead to the initiation of a lymphoma.

SCREENING

There are no general screening methods available, but if a tumor is suspected because of abdominal pain, anemia or some other symptom, a test for hidden blood in the stool is recommended.

COMMON SIGNS AND SYMPTOMS

Ten percent of people with small intestinal cancers have no symptoms. Most have abdominal pain or distention because of a partial or complete obstruction of the small bowel. There may also be weight loss, nausea and vomiting, fever, change in bowel habits and a general malaise, or weakness that may result from anemia caused by bleeding or malabsorption. The bowel may also become perforated, which can cause acute symptoms. With adenocarcinomas, jaundice may appear when the tumor is in the mid-duodenum, blocking drainage of the common bile duct. Blockage of the bowel may also be caused by what is called pseudolymphoma, a benign overgrowth of the lymph nodes.

DIAGNOSIS

Physical Examination
♦ Abdominal mass or painful distension.
♦ Rectal bleeding—possibly caused by ulcerations in the gastrointestinal tract—which may result in anemia.

♦ A partial or complete obstruction of the intestinal tract.
♦ Jaundice, which may be due to a tumor in the duodenum or to liver metastasis.
♦ Bowel kinking (intussusception).
♦ Often fatty fluid (chylous ascites) can collect in the abdomen.

Blood and Other Tests
♦ Blood counts usually show iron deficiency anemia when bleeding occurs.
♦ The level of carcinoembryonic antigen (CEA) in the blood is often elevated with adenocarcinomas.

Imaging
♦ The most useful x-rays are an upper gastrointestinal and a small bowel series. These can detect a small cancer (often a "napkin ring" deformity) or a polyp.
♦ X-rays showing small bowel thickening with ulceration may indicate a lymphoma.
♦ An abdominal CT scan can help identify lesions outside the bowel, including metastases.
♦ Angiography is helpful for evaluating the abdominal tumor blood vessels, displaced vessels and new blood vessels (neovascularization).
♦ A small bowel x-ray may locate a tumor. This procedure involves passing a small plastic tube through the nose to the duodenum and injecting barium and air to provide contrast.

Endoscopy and Biopsy
♦ Fiberoptic endoscopy is rarely possible unless it is done during surgery.
♦ A small part of the terminal ileum can be seen during a colonoscopic evaluation.
♦ Small bowel endoscopy is useful during surgery for additional evaluation.

STAGING

There is no staging system for primary small intestine cancer except for lymphomas. Cell type rather than stage is the major factor in prognosis and treatment decisions.

TREATMENT OVERVIEW

As in other gastrointestinal cancers, the standard treatment is to remove the tumor surgically whenever possible.

 Surgery The best chance for cure is offered by the surgical removal of a part of the small bowel with a wide margin around the tumor, along with the attached tissues supporting the bowel (mesentery) and its lymphatic drainage. If this cannot be done, surgical bypass and radiation can be considered as palliative measures for residual disease.

 Radiation The bowel is extremely sensitive to radiation, which limits the usefulness of this therapy. It may be poorly tolerated and may result in weakness, nausea, vomiting, and diarrhea with small bowel inflammation. It may lead to occasional remissions for sarcomas, but is usually used for relief of pain and obstructions. Small bowel lymphomas are highly responsive to radiation.

Radiation can complement surgery and is often recommended in lymphomas. Intraoperative radiotherapy (IORT) to the tumor or the tumor bed and area at risk may be done, because normal tissues can be moved aside and protected.

 Chemotherapy Like radiotherapy, chemotherapy is a less effective therapy than surgery and is recommended only for disease that can't be surgically removed or for metastases.

TREATMENT BY TUMOR TYPE

ADENOCARCINOMA
Standard Treatment If the tumor can be completely removed, radical surgery may lead to a cure. Simple excision of the

tumor might be adequate for small malignancies, but for larger tumors the recommended procedure requires a segment of the bowel with wide margins to be removed. If the cancer arises in the first part of the small bowel (duodenum), it should be noted that the duodenum is in a difficult location. It is behind the liver, pancreas and stomach, and the Whipple surgical procedure—involving the removal of the pancreas and duodenum—may be necessary.

Palliation If surgical removal of the tumor is impossible, the symptoms of the disease may be relieved by a surgical bypass or palliative radiation therapy.

Five-Year Survival 20 percent (for resectable adenocarcinoma)

Investigational
♦ Radiation therapy with radiosensitizers and with or without chemotherapy.
♦ Various chemotherapy combinations have been tried such as 5-FU + leucovorin, 5-FU + streptozocin or 5-FU + BCNU. Biologic response modifiers such as interferon are being evaluated.

SMALL INTESTINE LEIOMYOSARCOMA
Standard Treatment If the primary tumor can be removed, radical surgery similar to that for adenocarcinomas may lead to a cure. Isolated metastases in the liver and lung can also be removed.

If the primary tumor cannot be removed, any tumor that is obstructing the bowel can be surgically bypassed. Tumors that can't be removed may also respond to high-dose radiation therapy, occasionally with long-term survival.

Palliation A combined approach using surgery and radiotherapy can help relieve symptoms of pain and obstruction in patients when metastases can't be removed.

Palliative chemotherapy with doxorubicin, cisplatin, ifosfamide, vincristine or dacarbazine (DTIC) can have response rates of up to 65 percent. Adjuvant chemotherapy may also be given after surgery if the tumor is high-grade, there is a high risk for local recurrence or there is a significant risk of metastasis (lymphatic or blood vessel involvement).

Five-Year Survival About 50 percent if the tumor can be removed surgically

Investigational
♦ Clinical trials are evaluating the value of new anticancer drugs and biologicals.
♦ Adjuvant radiotherapy in combination with chemotherapy is being studied.

SMALL INTESTINE CARCINOID
(*See* "Carcinoids of the Gastrointestinal Tract")

Five-Year Survival 54 percent

SMALL INTESTINE LYMPHOMA
Standard Treatment It is unusual to find a single lymphoma as a primary small bowel tumor, so it is mandatory that the standard lymphoma staging work-up be done to look for evidence of other areas of disease. The work-up will include abdominal and pelvic CT scans, a chest x-ray and bone marrow aspiration and biopsy. Depending on the stage and cell type, the standard treatment options include surgery, radiation and combination chemotherapy, all of which may lead to a cure.

For disease that is localized to the bowel wall or has gone beyond the wall (local extension), surgical removal of the tumor alone may be adequate if 12 or more nearby lymph nodes are removed and show no evidence of disease (a 40 percent five-year survival). But the addition of combination chemotherapy or radiation should also be considered. Radiation may lead to a cure, control tumor growth or relieve symptoms.

For disease that extends into the regional lymph nodes, the tumor should be removed at the time of diagnosis. Combination chemotherapy is then the treatment of choice (*see* "Lymphomas: Non-Hodgkin's").

Combination chemotherapy is also the treatment of choice for disease that is extensive or cannot be removed surgically. Radiation therapy is often also used to eliminate any potential residual tumor cells, often in conjunction with chemotherapy.

Recent reports associate the infection *Helicobacter pylori* with small bowel lymphomas. Eradication of the bacteria with antibiotics may lead to a regression of lymphomas in some cases.

 Palliation Radiation therapy can relieve the symptoms associated with large lymphomas that cannot be removed, often in combination with chemotherapy. Single liver metastases may respond well to radiation (survival chances decrease as the number of metastases increase).

Five-Year Survival 25 percent for diffuse lymphoma, 50 percent or more for nodular lymphoma

Investigational
◆ Adjuvant radiotherapy and chemotherapy are being studied.

SUPPORTIVE THERAPY

Nutritional support may be necessary after treatment of small intestinal cancers. This is especially so after a major portion of the small bowel has been removed or if the duodenum or terminal ileum have been removed or bypassed. These procedures result in poor absorption of iron, calcium, folate, vitamin B_{12}, fat and fat-soluble vitamins and pancreatic/biliary digestive secretions, leading to deficien-

cies in essential nutrients. Nutritional replacement programs can correct these deficiencies (*see* Chapter 18).

RECURRENT OR METASTATIC CANCER

Tumors may come back in the small bowel after treatment or may metastasize from cancers arising elsewhere, especially cancers of the colon, kidney, pancreas or stomach, which may extend directly into the small bowel. Symptoms include intestinal obstruction or bleeding from the tumor.

◆ If possible, surgery may be attempted for locally recurrent small intestine cancer, with removal of the lymph nodes if that is appropriate. Clinical trials are now evaluating ways of improving local control, such as the use of radiation therapy with radiosensitizers with or without chemotherapy.

◆ There is no standard chemotherapy for recurrent metastatic adenocarcinoma or leiomyosarcoma of the small intestine. Patients may be considered candidates for standard combination chemotherapy programs, or clinical trials evaluating the use of new anticancer drugs or biologicals in Phase I or Phase II trials.

THE MOST IMPORTANT QUESTIONS YOU CAN ASK

◆ What is the role of surgery for small bowel tumors?
◆ How do you tell the difference between benign and malignant tumors of the small bowel?
◆ How are small bowel lymphomas evaluated?
◆ Is there a role for radiotherapy?
◆ How does one select a chemotherapy program for small bowel cancer?
◆ What is the role for supportive nutritional therapy?

STOMACH

Ernest H. Rosenbaum, MD, and Malin Dollinger, MD

◇

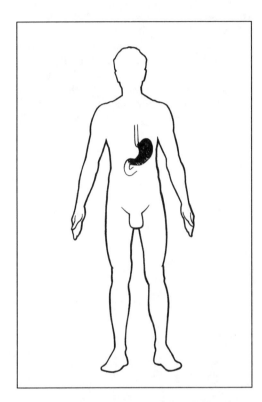

Cancer of the stomach—also called gastric cancer or gastric carcinoma—is a treatable disease that can often be cured when it is found and treated at a local stage. Unfortunately, the general outlook for this type of cancer is poor because 80 percent of the cases diagnosed in the United States are already at an advanced stage, having spread to nearby or distant organs. In 1994, 24,000 Americans will be diagnosed with gastric cancer, and 14,000 of them will die because of the disease.

A more encouraging fact about this cancer, however, is that the death rate has dramatically decreased, falling approximately 60 percent between 1930 and 1970.

Stomach cancer was the leading cause of cancer deaths in the United States between 1900 and 1945, but is now the eighth most common cause of cancer deaths. The exact reason for the decline—which is greatest among the elderly and whites—is not understood, although dietary changes have been considered.

Types Stomach cancers are classified according to what sort of tissues they start in. The most common type arises in the glandular tissue lining the stomach. These tumors are called adenocarcinomas and account for over 95 percent of all stomach tumors. One particular form of this cell type, unusual in the United States but more common in Japan, is the superficial spreading adenocarcinoma that essentially replaces the lining (mucosa) of the stomach with sheets of malignant cells. Another rare subtype is scirrhous carcinoma (linitis plastica), a poorly differentiated mixture of mucin-producing carcinoma cells that infiltrates the muscle wall and turns it into rigid, leatherlike scar tissue that can't stretch or move during the normal digestive process (peristalsis).

Occasionally, a cancer may develop in lymph tissue (gastric lymphoma) or from the smooth muscles of the stomach wall (leiomyosarcoma). Carcinoids and plasmacytomas can also develop in the stomach.

How It Spreads The disease can spread directly through the stomach wall into adjacent organs and through the lymph system to nodes in the abdomen, the left side of the neck and the left armpit. Metastases through the bloodstream can spread to the liver, lungs, bone and brain. Metastases are also found in the lining of the abdominal cavity (peritoneum) and around the rectum.

What Causes It The exact cause is unknown, but most gastric cancers are believed to be caused by carcinogens, with diet as a major factor. Nitrites found in smoked meats, fish and other foods and the nitrates used as food preservatives have been implicated, along with aflatoxin, a carcinogenic fungus contaminant that is present in some foodstuffs such as peanuts.

Various medical conditions are also associated with the development of stomach cancer. A history of or the presence of a *Helicobacter pylori* infection may lead to stomach inflammation that can induce mutations and DNA damage. This may deactivate suppressor genes and may lead to cancer. The lack of acid in stomach secretions (achlorhydria), for example, means that the bacteria responsible for converting nitrates to carcinogenic nitrosamines are not destroyed. About 5 to 10 percent of people with pernicious anemia will develop gastric cancer. And the chronic backup, or reflux, of stomach

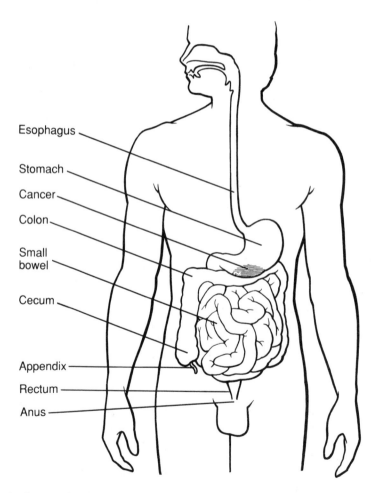

Esophagus

Stomach

Cancer

Colon

Small bowel

Cecum

Appendix

Rectum

Anus

Gastrointestinal tract, showing stomach cancer

acids into the esophagus can irritate the glandular tissue at the junction of the stomach and esophagus, which may lead to cancer. Gastric polyps are another possibility, since they may become malignant.

RISK FACTORS

At Slightly Higher Risk
♦ People with type A blood and achlorhydria (lack of stomach acid).
♦ Males living in colder climates.
♦ Those who have had part of the stomach removed because of peptic ulcers, leading to a decrease in stomach acids. There is a 6.5 percent incidence of tumors in the remaining stomach (gastric stump).
♦ Older people whose stomach lining produces less acid as it ages (atrophic gastritis).
♦ Peptic ulcer and atrophic gastritis associated with *Helicobacter pylori* infection (for carcinoma and lymphoma).
♦ Slightly increased risk with alcohol or tobacco use.

At Significantly Higher Risk
♦ Those aged between 50 and 59.
♦ Twice as frequent in lower socio-economic groups in North America and Western Europe.
♦ Workers in various industries—coal mining, nickel refining (in Soviet Europe), rubber and timber processing.
♦ Workers exposed to asbestos fibers.
♦ People with pernicious anemia are 5 to 10 percent more likely to develop gastric cancer.
♦ People whose diet contains smoked, highly salted and barbecued foods. Japanese immigrants have a decreased incidence of this cancer when they adopt an American diet and lifestyle, a tenfold drop after two generations.

SCREENING

Screening would be helpful for finding early tumors that do not reach the outer wall of the stomach (serosa) or penetrate the serosa but have not spread to lymph nodes. By looking at the stomach through a lighted tube (fiberoptic endoscopy) or by using x-rays of the upper gastrointestinal tract, smaller tumors can be detected. These tests are especially pertinent for people with gastric complaints.

Although screening programs are available in countries such as Japan with high gastric cancer rates, they are not common in the United States. Screening is not cost-effective, given the dramatic decline in the incidence of stomach cancer. Upper gastrointestinal x-rays, for example, discover cancer in only 0.15 percent (1 in 600) of apparently healthy people.

COMMON SIGNS AND SYMPTOMS

The symptoms of stomach cancer are similar to the symptoms of a hiatal hernia or peptic ulcer, namely a vague pain aggravated by food, nausea, heartburn and indigestion. These symptoms are often thought to be due to stress and are treated with antacids or H-2 blockers. Unfortunately, the temporary relief this treatment brings often delays the tests that could diagnose cancer.

Loss of appetite, feelings of fullness after even a small meal and weight loss are common (upper abdominal pain, vomiting after meals and weight loss are seen in 80 to 90 percent of cases). There may also be mild anemia, weakness, gastrointestinal bleeding (40 percent of cases) and vomiting of blood. Both vomiting blood and rectal bleeding are seen in peptic ulcer disease, esophageal varices (varicose veins in the esophagus that grow and burst, a disease common in drinkers) and occasionally leiomyosarcomas.

DIAGNOSIS

Gastric cancers often seem to be benign ulcers, which are like pits in the stomach lining. Larger ulcers—more than 3/4 in. (2 cm) in diameter—that have borders raised above the level of the surrounding stomach are more likely to be malignant.

Physical Examination

There are few specific findings on a physical examination, and they generally indicate an advanced tumor.

♦ Enlarged lymph nodes above the left collarbone (supraclavicular node).

♦ Nodal masses around the rectum, inside the navel or in the abdomen (involving the ovary).

♦ Enlarged liver (hepatomegaly).

♦ Increased fluid in the abdomen (ascites).

Blood and Other Tests

♦ Test for hidden blood in the stools.

♦ Complete blood count (CBC), which may indicate anemia from gastrointestinal bleeding.

♦ Serum chemistry profile to evaluate abnormal liver and bone chemistry enzymes, including tests for elevated levels of carcinoembryonic antigen (CEA) and levels of serum ferritin to indicate iron deficiency.

♦ Analysis of gastric acid to detect achlorhydria.

Imaging

♦ X-rays of the upper gastrointestinal tract (UGI series) by standard and double-contrast methods may find larger ulcer lesions.

♦ Chest x-rays.

♦ CT scan of the abdomen.

♦ Bone scan if the bone enzyme alkaline phosphatase is elevated in the serum.

♦ Ultrasound to help measure tumor size and predict recurrence.

Endoscopy and Biopsy

♦ Examination of the stomach through a gastroscope inserted through the esophagus (fiberoptic endoscopy) may find ulcers and masses. It is the most definitive test for diagnosing stomach cancer. Seventy percent of early malignant ulcers may look benign and even heal, but are usually positive on biopsy.

♦ A small piece of tissue may be removed from any suspicious area for biopsy analysis by a pathologist, or a brush can be passed through the gastroscope to obtain cells in a way similar to a Pap smear. Tissue and brush biopsies can diagnose 98 percent of cases.

STAGING

Stages are defined according to the TNM classification. The major factor in defining the primary tumor is how deeply it invades through the stomach wall and whether it invades adjacent structures such as the spleen, small intestine or colon, liver, diaphragm, pancreas, kidney, adrenal gland or the abdominal wall. The stage is important in determining the initial treatment options as well as the prognosis.

TREATMENT OVERVIEW

Stomach cancer is a somewhat treatable disease, with over half the patients with early stage disease being curable. Localized distal gastric cancer is 50 percent curable, although localized proximal gastric cancer has only a 10 to 15 percent five-year survival. Early-stage disease accounts for only 10 to 20 percent of all cases diagnosed in the United States, however. Five-year survival for more advanced cancers range from around 20 percent for those with regional disease to almost nil for those with distant metastases. Treatment for metastatic cancer can relieve symptoms and sometimes prolong survival, but long remissions are not common. There is a need for new active treatment programs for gastric cancer.

Radical surgery is the only treatment that can lead to a cure, though lesser surgical procedures can play a significant role in therapy designed to relieve symptoms. Radiation and chemotherapy are also treatment options. Neither has been shown to improve the outlook for those with advanced tumors generally, although some patients with responsive tumors may benefit.

Surgical procedures for stomach cancer

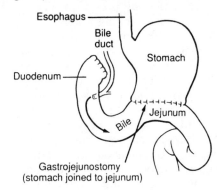

Partial Gastrectomy with Gastrojejunostomy (Billroth II)

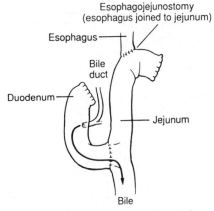

Total Gastrectomy Reconstruction with a "Roux-en-Y" Procedure to Prevent Bile from Entering the Esophagus

Surgery The ideal treatment is radical surgery, meaning that most or all of the stomach is removed (subtotal or total gastrectomy) along with the surrounding lymph nodes. In early-stage disease (10 to 20 percent of all cases) over 50 percent are curable. But one-third of stomach cancers are inoperable at the time of diagnosis and require follow-up therapy with radiation and/or chemotherapy. About one-third can potentially be cured with surgery, although very radical operations may just increase the number of complications without increasing survival.

The decision about whether to remove the stomach depends on whether the tumor has invaded the adjacent bowel above and below the stomach, the lower part of the stomach near the duodenum or the junction of the esophagus and the upper part of the stomach. If it doesn't, up to 85 percent of the stomach is removed, along with the first portion of the small bowel (duodenum), nearby lymph nodes and the pad of fat (omentum) between the bowel and the lining of the abdominal cavity.

A CT scan may be helpful in detecting the margins of the cancer and lymph node involvement. Since it may seem to indicate more extensive disease than is really present, the CT result alone should not be a reason to avoid surgery.

This is major surgery. The incision may run from the chest down to the navel. All of the stomach must be removed if there is extensive stomach involvement. The esophagus may have to be connected to the mid-small bowel (esophagojejunostomy) and a gastric pouch constructed. With a total gastrectomy, 5 to 15 percent of patients may not survive the operation and there may be significant complications. One major complication is that the connection constructed during the esophagojejunostomy may break down. The surgical margin should be greater than 2 1/2 in. (6 cm) beyond the gross tumor. (A frozen section should be done to confirm that the margin has no cancer.)

When extensive surgery for cure is impractical or impossible, part of the stomach might still be removed as a palliative measure. Sometimes the tumor causes recurrent bleeding or becomes so large that it obstructs the gastrointestinal tract and causes nausea, vomiting or stomach distention. A partial gastrectomy can temporarily improve the quality of life, although total gastrectomies have a high rate of complications and have little benefit when all the tumor cannot be removed. If up to four liver metastases are found by CT or at surgery, they are sometimes removed.

 Radiation The role of radiation therapy is mainly to relieve symptoms, not cure the cancer. Doses between 5,000 and 5,500 cGy can possibly help control tumors that can't be removed. Sometimes palliation is attempted over three to four weeks with 3,500 to 4,000 cGy, with infusions of 5-fluorouracil used as a radiation sensitizer during the first and often the fourth week. This combined therapy can increase survival. One study shows 23 percent of high-risk patients who had 5-FU and radiation following complete resection were still alive after five years while only 4 percent of those who had just radiation were still alive. Studies using 5-FU at the beginning of, during and after radiation therapy suggest possible advantages in response and an improved survival of from 6 to about 14 months in one study.

Preoperative Radiation One Japanese trial showed that radiation given two weeks before surgery reduced the size and involvement of lymph nodes and improved survival by 12 percent. Another study showed that radiation before surgery increased the number of tumors that could be removed from 76 percent to 85 percent, although there was no increase in survival.

Intraoperative Radiation (IORT) Giving radiation therapy directly to the tumor area during surgery for biopsy-proven residual cancer has been evaluated and shows survival increases. Some clinical trials with IORT added external radiation therapy with or without chemotherapy. Some studies have shown five-year survival increases from nil to 50 percent.

 Chemotherapy While chemotherapy is occasionally useful in shrinking potentially operable tumors, its main role is in the treatment of advanced or metastatic disease. For almost 30 years, 5-fluorouracil (5-FU) has been the most common single drug used to treat advanced stomach cancer, with about 20 percent of patients responding to the treatment. Around the early 1980s, there were suggestions that using drug combinations instead of single drugs was to become the "gold standard" of treatment, but results from recent trials question the value of routine combination chemotherapy.

One problem with combination chemotherapy is the poor complete response rate for *all* drug programs, with average survival varying between four and nine months. A second problem is that there has been little overall difference in survival for those receiving 5-FU alone or in combinations. The response rate may be higher for a combination, but the toxicity of the programs has to be assessed in light of the overall failure of chemotherapy to improve survival.

The standard combination recently had been FAM (5-FU + Adriamycin + mitomycin-C), with a response rate of about 20 to 30 percent with little survival advantage and rare complete remission. Other combinations using 5-FU and a variety of drugs—including etoposide, Adriamycin and cisplatin (EAP)—have higher reported response rates. Reports from Europe showed that other combinations were superior to FAM in both response and survival. Some of these are the FAMtx combination (5-FU + Adriamycin + high-dose methotrexate with leucovorin rescue), EAP (etoposide + Adriamycin + Platinol), which has a high toxicity, ELF (etoposide + leucovorin + 5-FU) and FAP (5-FU + Adriamycin + Platinol).

Investigational Combinations Some new combinations show promise. EAP, for example, was reported to have a 57 percent response rate with 15 percent complete responses. For metastatic disease, the response rate is about 40 percent with 8 percent complete response. The EAP response rate in recent studies has decreased to about 40 percent, with moderately severe toxicity. The average survival is about 12 to 17 months for those with a complete response.

EAP is considered effective for locally advanced cancer, since, if shrinkage occurs, it offers a surgical option to many who otherwise wouldn't have been able to have an operation.

Another effective and less toxic combination is ELF (etoposide + leucovorin + 5-FU). Response rates of 53 percent (12 percent complete) have been obtained for locally advanced disease, 49 percent (10 percent complete) for metastatic disease. Another combination EFP (etoposide + 5-FU + cisplatin) is being administered pre- and postoperatively with a reported increase in the surgical cure rate (including unresectable local/regional stomach cancers).

The combinations EAP, ELF, EFP and FAMtx have proven to be of greater value than 5-fluorouracil alone, and chemotherapy modulators such as leucovorin may have the potential of improving drug effectiveness. Trials are ongoing comparing EAP, FAMtx and other combinations, for advanced gastric cancer. Additional combinations being studied in clinical trials include methotrexate + leucovorin + platinum, infusions of 5-FU + carboplatin, and chemoimmunotherapy protocols ELFI (etoposide + leucovorin + 5-FU + interferon) or PALA + 5-FU + leucovorin. Unfortunately, there has been little improvement in the survival rate.

Whatever drugs are used, chemotherapy should start as soon as possible. Waiting 40 to 60 days allows the tumor cell population to double. Primary stomach cancer appears to be more responsive to chemotherapy than metastatic cancer.

Adjuvant Chemotherapy Despite many ongoing American clinical trials evaluating the use of chemotherapy as an adjuvant therapy after surgery, there is not yet any conclusive proof of its effectiveness, although early results suggest that further clinical trials should be conducted to improve response and survival.

The Japanese have reported major benefits in adjuvant programs, but stomach cancer is different in Japan. The cancer is less differentiated and the surgery is more aggressive. Patients usually have fewer tumor cells left after the operation, which may explain the better results of adjuvant therapy.

 Biological Therapy Trials evaluating the use of radioactive tagged monoclonal antibodies or toxins such as ricin to kill cancer cells while sparing normal tissues are underway. Results so far have not been encouraging and more studies will have to be done to discover whether there is any benefit. The use of interferon or PALA in combination with chemotherapy merits further clinical trials, and some of the preliminary results are encouraging.

TREATMENT BY STAGE

STAGE 0
TNM Tis, N0, M0
An in situ tumor has not spread beyond the limiting membrane of the top level of the stomach lining (the mucosa).

Standard Treatment Experience in Japan, where this stage is diagnosed often, indicates that almost all patients who undergo a gastrectomy will survive beyond five years. An American series has recently confirmed these results.

Five-Year Survival Over 90 percent

STAGE I

TNM T1, N0, M0 (Stage IA)
T1, N1, M0 or T2, N0, M0 (Stage IB)
The cancer is confined to the stomach wall and no lymph nodes are involved.

Standard Treatment Surgery is the treatment of choice, although how extensive the operation has to be depends on the tumor's location and how much of the stomach is involved.

If the lesion is not in the area where the stomach joins the esophagus and does not diffusely involve the stomach, about three-quarters of the lower part of the stomach is removed (a radical subtotal gastrectomy). This treatment is associated with improved survival over other procedures.

When the lesion does involve the top of the stomach (cardia), cure may be attempted by removing most or all of the stomach, along with a sufficient length of the esophagus.

If the lesion diffusely involves the stomach, the entire stomach has to be removed along with, at a minimum, the greater and lesser omentum (fatty tissue) and nearby lymph nodes and the valve between the stomach and the duodenum (pylorus).

Five-Year Survival 52 to 85 percent for distal cancers (stomach outlet); 10 to 15 percent for proximal cancers (stomach entry)

Investigational
♦ Clinical trials of adjuvant combination chemotherapy and/or radiotherapy are appropriate whenever the tumor invades to the serosa or local lymph nodes either grossly or microscopically (Stage IB) to try to improve the survival. One adjuvant mitomycin-C trial has shown improved survival.

Neoadjuvant therapy is being evaluated for proximal cancers (stomach entry). A novel postoperative adjuvant intraperitoneal chemotherapy program for high-risk patients, to prevent tumor spread and recurrent disease in the abdomen, uses mitomycin-C and 5-FU. An intraperitoneal catheter is placed at surgery for the intraperitoneal infusion chemotherapy.

STAGE II

TNM T1, N2, M0 or T2, N1, M0 or T3, N0, M0
The cancer is confined to the stomach wall and does not involve adjacent tissues. The lymph nodes very close to the tumor or in the region around the stomach may be involved.

Standard Treatment This stage is sometimes curable with surgery. As in Stage I, the surgical procedure depends on the location and extent of the tumor. Procedures are the same as for Stage I cancers.

Five-Year Survival T1 or T2, N1 or N2, M0 over 20 percent
T3, N0, M0 under 20 percent

Investigational Same as Stage I (adjuvant chemotherapy and/or radiotherapy).

STAGE III

TNM T2, N2, M0 or T3, N1, M0 or T4, N0, M0 (Stage IIIA)
T3, N2, M0 or T4, N1, M0 (Stage IIIB)
The cancer involves tissues adjacent to the stomach and/or the lymph nodes very close to the tumor or in the region around the stomach.

Standard Treatment Cancer at this stage is treatable but not usually curable. All patients whose tumors can be removed should have surgery, but radical surgery for cure is limited to those who do not have extensive lymph node involvement at the time of exploratory surgery. Up to 17 percent of selected patients can be cured by surgery alone if the lymph nodes involved are confined to the immediate vicinity of the tumor (N1).

Overall survival is poor with either single or combined approaches to treatment, so all newly diagnosed patients with Stage

III cancer should be considered candidates for clinical trials of new treatments.

Five-Year Survival 17 percent for distal cancers

Investigational
♦ Radiation therapy and/or adjuvant chemotherapy is being evaluated in patients with known residual disease or if the tumor invades the serosa.
♦ Adjuvant chemotherapy with 5-FU and other chemotherapy combinations is being studied for those with no known residual disease who have a high risk of recurrence.

STAGE IV
TNM T4, N2, M0 (Stage IVA)
Any T, any N, M1 (Stage IVB)
The cancer has spread to adjacent tissue and to lymph nodes in the region around the stomach or has spread to distant sites, most commonly the liver or other organs.

Standard Treatment Because survival is so poor with all available single and combined treatment methods, no one approach can be considered state-of-the-art. Palliative surgery, combination chemotherapy and occasionally radiotherapy are all options.

When it is possible to remove the primary tumor, palliative surgery will at least reduce the risk of bleeding or obstruction and may lead to a longer survival.

When the tumor is so large that it blocks the entrance from the esophagus to the stomach, a gastroscope can be passed down the esophagus and a temporary hole created by using a laser beam or cauterization. A plastic tube can then be inserted through the hole to maintain a swallowing passage (*see* Chapter 9).

Chemotherapy—with 5-FU, FAMtx, EAP or ELF—can offer significant palliation to some patients and long-term remissions are sometimes possible.

Five-Year Survival Less than 5 percent

Investigational
♦ Neoadjuvant chemotherapy to shrink the tumor before surgery may make surgery possible. An occasional patient with Stage IV (T4, N3) cancer might be cured surgically. Investigational programs should be considered.

TREATING OTHER TUMOR TYPES

GASTRIC LYMPHOMAS
These tumors, which may imitate primary adenocarcinomas of the stomach, are uncommon, making up only about 5 percent of gastric malignancies. These tumors are becoming more common, however.

A recent association has been shown between gastric lymphomas and ulcers and an infection with *Helicobacter pylori*. Eradication of the infection with antibiotics may lead to a regression of the lymphoma in some cases.

Patients with gastric lymphoma should have a general lymphoma evaluation including a chest x-ray, chest, pelvic, and abdominal CT scans, bone marrow biopsies.

Standard Treatment Removing part of the stomach, if possible, may be the ideal treatment. In one series of 50 consecutive cases, a survival of 90 percent was obtained when the tumor involved only the mucosa, 80 percent when it involved the submucosa. A study for Stages IE and IIE (local tumor extension) lymphoma showed that patients who had four courses of CHOP (Cytoxan + Adriamycin + Oncovin + prednisone) followed by radiation therapy and then additional chemotherapy did as well as patients who had surgery.

When the lymphoma fully penetrates the gastric wall and the lymph nodes in the region become involved, the survival is decreased to about 25 percent.

Radiation after surgery helps reduce the chance for local recurrences and is appropriate adjuvant therapy, especially for IE and IIE tumors. The radiation therapy port usually covers the upper abdomen as well as the regional lymph nodes, and is given over several weeks. Combination chemotherapy is being studied following surgery and merits further investigation.

LEIOMYOSARCOMAS

These tumors that start in the smooth muscles of the stomach wall account for only 1 to 3 percent of all gastric malignancies. Bleeding is common and five-year survival is about 45 percent.

Standard Treatment The primary treatment is partial removal of the stomach, taking out just the area of the tumor and a rim of normal surrounding tissue. Radiation therapy and chemotherapy may be used after surgery or for metastatic disease. The most common chemotherapy combinations now used are Adriamycin + dacarbazine (DTIC) or Adriamycin + cisplatin. Ifosfamide may also be effective.

SUPPORTIVE CARE

Removing part or all of the stomach naturally produces many problems that require medical attention.

♦ Iron deficiency anemia often develops after a gastrectomy, since iron is absorbed mainly in the duodenum and stomach acids play a role in the process.

♦ Monthly doses of vitamin B_{12} should be given after a few years to prevent pernicious anemia.

♦ The dumping syndrome—with symptoms such as abdominal fullness, nausea, vomiting, a rapid heartbeat, weakness and dizziness—is quite common after surgery because food passes through the system so quickly that there is little time for absorption. The dumping syndrome often resolves with time. Many treatments, including smaller meals and a lower-carbohydrate diet, and no chocolate or peppermint, can help. No food or fluid after 7:00 or 8:00 P.M. may help too.

♦ Symptoms of upset stomach (gastritis) may be related to the alkaline backup, or reflux, of bile and intestinal secretions into the esophagus. Symptoms can be controlled by antacids such as Maalox, Mylanta or Riopan, by sucralfate, which coats the stomach lining, or by a bile blocker such as Questran.

♦ Walking or simply staying upright after meals as well as sleeping with the head elevated can help control reflux by improving the drainage of the gastric pouch and help reduce symptoms.

♦ If the antrum—the gastrin-producing part of the stomach—is removed, there will be little need for gastric acid blockers. But if acid is still being produced, H-2 blockers such as Tagamet, Zantac, Pepsid or Prilosec will help.

♦ Bacteria can grow in the loop of the duodenum bypassed by a connection of the stomach to the small bowel, producing what is called the blind loop syndrome. This bacteria breaks down bile and the acids pouring in from the pancreas, resulting in diarrhea and poor absorption of fats. The blind loop syndrome can be treated with oral antibiotics.

RECURRENT CANCER

Survival is very poor with all available single and combined approaches to treatment, although an occasional patient might have a remission lasting several months or even a few years.

♦ All patients with recurrent stomach cancer should be considered candidates for Phase I and Phase II clinical trials testing anticancer drugs or biologicals. New agents such as triazinate and cisplatin analogues are being developed. There are also investigational programs using complex drug combinations and sequences (pharmacologic modulation).

♦ Standard treatment options are palliative chemotherapy with 5-FU, FAM, EAP, ELF, FAP, ELFI, and FAMtx.

♦ For the patient with either local disease that couldn't be removed or local recurrent or residual disease after surgery, the use of radiation therapy in combination with chemotherapy has been considered the best palliative treatment, not only in helping to prevent and occasionally relieve an obstruction but also in reducing and controlling pain. This treatment has had no major benefits for survival, however.

One study of patients treated with 3,500 to 4,000 cGy with or without intravenous 5-FU during the first three days of radiation therapy showed an average survival of 12 months for the combination therapy versus 5.9 months for radiation therapy alone. The radiation therapy group had no five-year survivals, while 12 percent of the patients with the combination survived five years. Another study showed a combination of radiation therapy and methyl-CCNU + 5-FU had a disease-free interval of more than four years, which exceeds that of chemotherapy alone.

More recent programs under evaluation include a "sandwich" approach—giving chemotherapy such as 5-FU infusion during the initial week of radiotherapy as well as during the fourth week—and, if surgery is done, intraoperative radiation therapy with or without chemotherapy.

THE MOST IMPORTANT QUESTIONS YOU CAN ASK

♦ How do you tell a benign ulcer from a malignant one?
♦ What is the best way to cure my gastric cancer? Does the stage make a difference?
♦ What disability might I have after surgery?
♦ Is there any role for radiation and/or chemotherapy? Before or after surgery?
♦ What is a good program for palliation and support if that is needed?

TESTIS

Alan Yagoda, MD

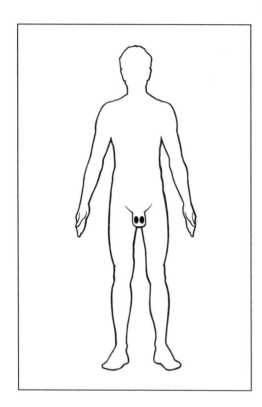

Testis cancer—also called germ cell tumors—accounts for about 1 percent of all male cancers, about 6,800 cases in the U.S. in 1994. Yet only 325 men will die of the disease because of earlier diagnosis and effective cisplatin-based chemotherapy.

In the past 35 years, the five-year survival rate has increased from 63 percent to more than 91 percent. This improvement reflects not only advances in treatment but also the fact that less than 15 percent of patients are now first seen with distant disease while more than 60 percent have only a testicular mass.

Types Testis cancers are broadly divided into two types—seminoma and non-seminoma. This arbitrary division was based on the better response and cure rates for seminoma resulting from radiation therapy, but with chemotherapy treatments this distinction is no longer of much importance.

Seminoma Pure seminoma, which makes up 25 to 35 percent of all testis tumors, is divided into three types—anaplastic, classic and spermatocytic. Anaplastic and classic seminomas seem to have a similar prognosis for each stage. Spermatocytic seminomas, a tumor frequently found in dogs, is a rare variety occurring in elderly men. It almost never spreads.

Seminoma is discovered generally in the fourth decade of life and has on occasion been confused with histiocytic lymphoma (the testis is the most frequent site of lymphomas that do not start in lymph nodes).

Non-seminoma Men with non-seminomatous testis tumors have an average age 10 years younger than that for seminoma, the mid-thirties. These tumors are composed of various cell types as seen under the microscope—embryonal carcinoma, teratoma, yolk-sac or endodermal sinus carcinoma and choriocarcinoma.

More than 90 percent of non-seminomatous germ cell tumors have more than one cell type in them—embryonal cell carcinoma with or without seminoma, embryonal cell carcinoma with or without yolk-sac tumor and with or without teratoma, and so on. Pure embryonal carcinoma, pure teratoma and pure yolk-sac tumor each account for 2 to 3 percent and pure choriocarcinoma for 0.03 percent.

Embryonal cell carcinoma, a primitive cell type having the capacity to change into all the cell varieties listed above, is an aggressive tumor. But it is less aggressive than the choriocarcinoma variety, which is full of blood vessels and, therefore, spreads quickly by the bloodstream. Rapidly multiplying tumors like seminoma, embryonal cell and, to a lesser extent, teratocarcinoma are more solid masses that can outgrow their blood supply, producing cystic or "dead tissue" areas inside the tumor.

Teratocarcinoma is a mixture of embryonal cell carcinoma and teratoma, while so-called mature teratoma implies that embryonal cell carcinoma must have been present but has changed to a more mature (differentiated), more normal-appearing and less malignant cell form either spontaneously or because of therapy. There is also a very rare and aggressive teratocarcinoma variety called sarcomatous teratocarcinoma, which is not very responsive to the chemotherapy now available and is categorized as a poor-risk cancer.

Pure yolk-sac tumors are extremely rare and more frequently observed in the chest (mediastinum), except in children under 15, where it accounts for 90 percent of testis cancers. The testes, which are derived from the yolk sac early in the embryo's development, move to an area called the urogenital ridge. Since the embryonic germ cells from this ridge travel almost the whole length of the developing body to their destination in the scrotum, bits of primitive tissue called embryonic rests can be left behind during the migration. This explains why some germ cell tumors are found in non-testicular (extragonadal) sites in the chest or abdomen.

How It Spreads There is a difference in the way cancers of the testis spread. Right-testis tumors spread by the spermatic cord and its associated blood and lymph vessels into lymph glands surrounding and between the large blood vessels, the aorta and the inferior vena cava (interaortocaval).

Left-testis tumors drain via the spermatic cord vessels into the left kidney artery and venous lymphatic areas and to lymph nodes just below the left kidney. They generally are not found in the interaortocaval nodal system as frequently observed with right-side tumors. Unless surgery has disturbed the scrotum—to remove the testis or repair an undescended testis through a scrotal incision—testis tumors always drain directly into the abdominal lymph nodes and not into the groin lymph nodes.

The most frequent site of organ metastases is the lungs, although in advanced cases the liver, bones and brain can be involved, particularly in cases of choriocarcinoma and, to a lesser extent, embryonal cell carcinoma.

What Causes It Unknown. There is no firm evidence that heredity is a factor, although a number of father and son cases have been described. There has been some association with a few uncommon genetic diseases such as hermaphroditism (mixture of male/female development) and Klinefelter's and Turner's syndromes.

The failure of the testis to descend into the scrotum (cryptorchidism) accounts for 10 percent of testicular cancers. But it is not known whether cryptorchidism is due to some underlying testicular abnormality that prevented the testicle's migration into the scrotum or to an anatomic abnormality that made an otherwise normal testis remain within the abdominal cavity, thereby leading to a cancerous change by, for example, raising the temperature of the testicle.

Other postulated causes are excessive maternal bleeding during pregnancy, testicular injury, mumps, HIV infection and the use of the synthetic female hormone diethylstilbestrol (DES) usually taken during pregnancy to prevent miscarriage.

Each testis is surrounded by a thick fibrous capsule (tunica albuginea), lies in the scrotum and is composed of many small, thin, coiled tubes (called seminiferous tubules) packed into over 250 sections, or lobules.

Sperm is formed within these coiled tubules, then migrates to enter the straight tubules that make up the rete testis and the epididymis. These straight tubes then converge into one larger tube, the spermatic cord. From its attachment to the upper end of the testis, the spermatic cord travels upward to enter into the body cavity through an opening called the inguinal ring (the area where inguinal hernias occur). From there the cord goes through the prostate, where it ends in the penile section of the urethra.

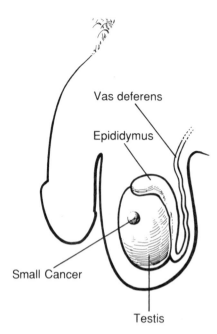

Vas deferens

Epididymus

Small Cancer

Testis

Cancer on the surface of testis

(DES has been implicated in the development of vaginal cancer.)

RISK FACTORS

At Significantly Higher Risk
♦ For men between 20 and 34 years old, testis tumors make up 22 percent of all cancers and rank first in cancer incidence. It is the second most common cancer for men aged 35 to 39 years and third for those 15 to 19.
♦ American white males have a rate four times that of black males.

At Slightly Higher Risk
♦ Uncommonly, tumors are found in men with fertility problems. About 5 percent of men cured of testis cancer are at risk to develop another in the remaining testis within 25 years.

SCREENING

Testicular ultrasound is an accurate way to detect masses, but sonograms are too expensive to be used for screening. The most cost-effective screening method is simple physical examination of the testicles. Although a program has been developed in the Scandinavian countries to educate men about self-examination (similar to that for breast cancer in women), it has not gained acceptance in the United States. At the very least, men who have already had a testis cancer and those who had an undescended testicle should learn self-examination and intermittently undergo sonograms.

COMMON SIGNS AND SYMPTOMS

Swelling of the testicles, discomfort or masses are present in over 90 percent of cases. Such symptoms are sometimes ignored or misdiagnosed as being caused by an injury, as an inflamation of the testis (orchitis) or spermatic cord (epididymitis) requiring only antibiotic therapy, or as enlarging veins of the spermatic cord.

Breast tenderness or enlargement because of high levels of HCG (human chorionic gonadotropin), and abdominal pain or cough with blood-tinged sputum, can be the main complaints, due to metastases.

TESTIS TUMOR MARKERS

Testis cancers produce hormones that can be measured in the blood. These measurements are extremely reliable tumor markers. The three main markers are HCG, lactate dehydrogenase (LDH) and alpha-fetoprotein (AFP). They are so dependable that any increase above normal blood levels indicates a testis tumor recurrence. This is true even if there is no evidence of cancer by physical examination and x-ray examinations.

The Uses of Tumor Markers These markers are used to monitor the response to therapy. If the tumor markers decrease or return to normal levels after treatment, there is obviously a response. An increase is a sign of disease progression or failure to respond.

If the levels increase, signifying relapse, chemotherapy or sometimes surgery is needed (the cure rate for "marker relapse" is excellent, approaching 100 percent). But normal levels do not guarantee the complete absence of testis cancer, since microscopic deposits may still exist. This is why follow-up requires chest x-rays and CT scans. When masses are seen on CT scans and x-rays, particularly in the abdomen when measuring more than 1.2 in. (3 cm), they are likely to be malignant. Smaller masses when accompanied by an increase in the marker level also indicate that more treatment is necessary. If the markers are normal, small masses may well be only remaining scar tissue or benign teratoma.

The rate of disappearance of a marker from blood can also be predicted by its "half-life"—the time it takes for the amount of a marker in the bloodstream to be reduced by half. The half-life for HCG is about 30 hours, and five to seven days for AFP. Physicians using these formulas can determine to some degree whether the tumor is responding to treatment completely or partially. Studies in the United States use this information to plan for aggressive chemotherapy combined with autologous bone marrow transplantation.

Markers and Particular Tumor Types Seminoma can have HCG and LDH, and about 80 percent of men with non-seminomatous germ cell cancer have an abnormality in one or more of the three markers.

HCG About 10 percent of patients with pure seminoma have a high HCG level, but never to the extent observed for those with choriocarcinoma or embryonal cell carcinoma.

HCG is produced by embryonal cells, by choriocarcinoma and by a tissue called syncytiotrophoblast found in seminomas, as well as in the normal placenta during pregnancy. In fact, HCG is used for pregnancy tests because it increases early within the first trimester.

It is a rather specific testis tumor marker associated with breast enlargement and nipple tenderness in males when markedly increased. Some unusual lung, liver and pancreatic cancers also can increase HCG levels although these are uncommon. One caution in using this marker is that marijuana smokers have increased HCG blood levels. So marijuana should not be used as an antinausea drug, since elevations that are not tumor-related may confuse physicians evaluating their patients after chemotherapy.

LDH This hormone—more specifically LDH-1, since there are five LDH enzymes—is increased in more than half of men with seminoma, but it is not as specific for testis cancer as HCG and AFP.

AFP This is called an oncofetal protein because it originates from the fetal liver and gastrointestinal tract and from the yolk sac of the embryo. AFP increases in a mother's blood during the second and third trimesters and disappears from a baby's bloodstream shortly after birth. AFP is found in 20 to 70 percent of testis tumor cases. Repeated AFP testing is sufficiently accurate to monitor yolk sac tumors in 90 percent of children. [It is also seen in 70 percent of patients with a primary liver cancer (hepatoma).]

New markers are being evaluated; none have proved accurate.

DIAGNOSIS

Physical Examination
♦ A testicular mass that can be felt, particularly a painless mass or one that does not completely clear within two weeks of antibiotic therapy, requires further tests. Some doctors now feel that all masses should be investigated by ultrasound.
♦ Enlarged lymph nodes in the abdomen and neck.

Blood and Other Tests
♦ Blood tests for markers such as LDH, AFP and HCG.
♦ Blood counts, biochemical screening profile, serum magnesium and urine collection for a creatinine clearance to evaluate kidney function.
♦ If bleomycin is to be used, lung function tests are performed as a baseline for future comparisons before additional treatment (bleomycin can cause lung scarring).
♦ Analysis of sperm and so-called sperm banking should be considered in most patients, since treatment can result in infertility. This might be the result of chemotherapy-induced toxicity or by loss of ejaculation if the surgical removal of lymph nodes requires cutting the nerves that control this function.

Imaging
♦ Ultrasound is extremely accurate, and any solid mass found on ultrasound should be considered cancerous until proven otherwise.
♦ Chest x-rays to evaluate lung metastases. Many oncologists advise obtaining a baseline CT of the chest, even with a normal chest x-ray, to aid in follow-up.
♦ CT scans of the abdomen and pelvis are part of the staging procedure to evaluate the abdominal (retroperitoneal) and pelvic lymph nodes. Some physicians now use MRI instead of CT scans.
♦ Lymphangiography may help in about 10 percent of cases, but it is no longer routinely used because CT scans are more accurate. Sometimes it is still used to plan radiation therapy ports.
♦ X-ray tomograms of the chest have been largely replaced by the more accurate chest CT scan.
♦ Radionuclide bone and brain CT scans have to be done only when there are symptoms, although some doctors routinely order these scans for men with pure choriocarcinoma.

Biopsy
♦ The removal of the testicle (orchiectomy) through an incision in the groin—never a scrotal incision or an aspiration biopsy—is required for diagnosis. Even when metastatic disease is found, the testis where the cancer started still has to be removed because the primary tumor does not always respond fully to chemotherapy.
♦ A recently recognized chromosomal abnormality found in many poor-risk non-seminomatous tumors is the presence of multiple copies of the short section (arm) of chromosome 12 (i12p). If a poor-risk case is suspected, fresh tumor may be sent for chromosome analysis. Such cases may require a more aggressive investigational approach to treatment.

STAGING

Several staging divisions are used for testis cancer, including the AJCC, based on the TNM classification. The stage depends on whether the primary tumor involves the testis, epididymis, spermatic cord and scrotum, whether a single node of various sizes or multiple nodes are involved and whether there are distant metastases to other organs, the most common being the lungs or lymph nodes above the diaphragm.

TREATMENT OVERVIEW

Surgery is necessary in all cases because the removal of the affected testicle is required for diagnosis. The use of further surgery, radiation and chemotherapy depends on the stage of the disease.

 Surgery For local tumors, the first step is to remove the testis, epididymis and spermatic cord (radical orchiectomy), performed by an inguinal approach, meaning that it is removed through the groin. This is never done through an incision in the scrotum because that would open up new lymph drainage areas to the groin.

When the cancer diagnosis is confirmed after orchiectomy, another operation is done to remove the lymph nodes in the back of the abdomen. This standard operation is known as a retroperitoneal lymph node dissection. Although recent studies suggest that in highly selected cases—those with small (T1) tumors and without spermatic cord or lymphatic and blood vessel invasion or embryonal components—simple surveillance can be used after the orchiectomy (in other words, watch until a relapse occurs), retroperitoneal lymph node dissection remains the "gold-standard" for treatment.

New surgical techniques have resolved many quality-of-life issues raised by this operation. The procedure is now much more acceptable, since the ability to have children is preserved in over 60 percent of cases. What is needed is more precise information to determine which tumors will ultimately relapse and then to evaluate by means of clinical trials the question of which patients need surgery or chemotherapy.

 Radiation For localized seminoma, radiation therapy to the pelvis and retroperitoneal lymph node areas is used as a preventive measure. Since most Stage I seminoma cases will probably never relapse, an investigational question is whether radiation (or even chemotherapy) is needed at all.

Chemotherapy There are many commonly used chemotherapy regimens for Stage III and, to some extent, for Stage II cases. Each agent has been found to be active against testis tumors when given alone, but prolonged, complete disappearance of tumors is best when other drugs are combined with cisplatin.

CHEMOTHERAPY COMBINATIONS USED FOR TESTIS CANCER	
PVB	Cisplatin + vinblastine + bleomycin
VAB-6	Cisplatin + vinblastine + bleomycin + actinomycin + cyclophosphamide
BEP	Cisplatin + etoposide + bleomycin
VPV	Cisplatin + etoposide + vinblastine
EP	Cisplatin + etoposide
IEC	Cisplatin + etoposide + ifosfamide
VIP	Cisplatin + vinblastine + ifosfamide

The earlier regimens of PVB and VAB-6 have mostly been replaced by PEB and EP. There is some controversy concerning the need for bleomycin, since one study reported that the relapse rate is higher when this drug is not included in etoposide and cisplatin (or carboplatin) combinations.

While the older combinations are still sometimes given as so-called salvage therapy in relapsing cases, the ones containing ifosfamide (IEC and VIP), a derivative of cyclophosphamide, are the new salvage therapies. Because ifosfamide is a urinary bladder irritant that can produce blood in the urine, uroprotective drugs such as Mesna and NAC are required to prevent this complication. Such drugs do not affect the antitumor activity of ifosfamide.

Another role for this drug, as well as for etoposide and carboplatin, particularly in very high dosage, is in combination with autologous bone marrow transplantation as salvage therapy or as the primary treatment for very poor risk cases.

Bone Marrow Transplatation This procedure is replacing much more toxic salvage chemotherapy such as high-dose cisplatin and a combination named POMP/ACE. With complete responses seen in 20 to 40 percent of heavily pretreated men given bone marrow transplantation combinations, this therapy is sometimes being used for early relapse after one or two programs containing cisplatin have failed, as well as immediately after one relapse or with less than expected decrease in markers in poor-risk cases.

TREATMENT BY STAGE

STAGE I

TNM Tis–T3, N0, M0

The tumor is limited to the testis (Tis, T1) or the epididymis (T2). There are no lymph nodes involved nor distant metastases. In the AJCC staging system, spermatic cord (T3) involvement is placed together with scrotal (T4) invasion into Stage II.

Standard Treatment Radical (inguinal) orchiectomy—removal of the testis, epididymis and spermatic cord.

For pure seminoma, prophylactic radiation therapy is given to a total dose of 2,500 to 3,000 cGy to the pelvic and abdominal lymph node areas on the same side as the tumor.

For non-seminomatous germ cell tumors, retroperitoneal lymph node dissection is done to guarantee Stage I status. When Stage I is proved by surgery, the node dissection becomes both a diagnostic and prophylactic measure. Removal of microscopically involved nodes (really a Stage II case) is not only diagnostic but also therapeutic, for cure follows in almost all cases.

Five-Year Survival 95 to 100 percent

Investigational The concept of surveillance only—without lymph node surgery—has been investigated for non-seminomatous tumors because 60 to 80 percent of Stage I cases will never relapse and effective cisplatin-based chemotherapy will cure almost all early relapses. At this time, surveillance must still be considered investigational; it is not offered to patients with seminoma.

In a recent study, the relapse rate varied from 20 to 40 percent. However, for good-risk patients or those with a true T1, N0, M0 tumor, the rate decreased to 15 to 25 percent.

In contrast, the relapse rate increased significantly to over 50 percent for poor-risk Stage I cases having tumor invasion of the epididymis, spermatic cord and lymphatic and/or blood vessels, particularly for the embryonal cell carcinoma variety. Surveillance should not be offered for such poor-risk cases.

If surveillance is the form of therapy chosen for good-risk cases, it should be realized that this demands very careful follow-up, every four to six weeks for at least one to two years. Although almost all relapses will be found within the first

10 to 12 months, tumors have recurred as late as three years after diagnosis. With careful follow-up and starting chemotherapy immediately after detection of a relapse, less than 1 to 2 percent of men will die. For men not willing to make this type of follow-up commitment, the correct choice is surgery.

STAGE II

TNM Any T, N1–3, M0

The tumor involves the retroperitoneal lymph nodes either in a single node measuring 3/4 in. (2 cm) or less (N1), in a single node 3/4 to 2 in. (2 to 5 cm) or with multiple nodes all less than 2 in. (5 cm) (N2), or in any node larger than that (N3).

Stage II is also divided into non-bulky and bulky. Bulky disease indicates extensive retroperitoneal lymph node involvement with more than five nodes generally greater than 3/4 in. (2 cm), one node more than 2 in. (5 cm), or tumor that has spread to the fat surrounding the lymph node.

In the AJCC staging system, Stage III means only N1, M0 with Stage IV being N2, M0 or N3, M0 or any T, any N, M1 (organ invasion).

Standard Treatment Radical inguinal orchiectomy followed by therapeutic doses of radiation therapy (at least 4,000 cGy) will cure more than 90 percent of non-bulky seminoma cases. Because of the potential need for chemotherapy at relapse and the questionable benefit of preventive radiation to the chest and neck, further radiation therapy is not recommended.

For bulky Stage II seminoma (greater than 4 in./10 cm), chemotherapy is preferred since older studies find the cure rate to be about 70 percent (admittedly, newer techniques and radiation equipment may produce better results).

Men with non-seminomatous germ cell Stage II cancer always used to have retroperitoneal lymph node dissection, but major controversies now exist as to the best form of therapy. For truly bulky masses (greater than 2 in./5 cm), chemotherapy may be a much better approach, with surgery as the salvage treatment for any remaining masses.

Surgery is appropriate for tumors less than 1 1/4 in. (3 cm) on abdominal and pelvic CT scans, but the value of prophylactic chemotherapy has to be discussed with each patient. One trial compared no additional immediate therapy versus only two courses of PVB (BEP can be substituted) or VAB-6 (EP can be substituted) after surgery. Half of the patients with no additional therapy relapsed with tumor while less than 5 percent of those given two courses of prophylactic chemotherapy did so. Almost all relapsing cases completely responded when given the standard four courses of chemotherapy. What this means is that delayed chemotherapy given at relapse did not jeopardize curability, since overall survival was identical for both groups.

Relapse rates are very low for Stage II cases in whom there are only a few positive lymph nodes found at surgery, with none greater than 3/4 in. (2 cm). Consequently, chemotherapy can be withheld in such cases until relapse is found.

For non-seminomatous Stage II tumor masses between 1 1/4 and 2 in. (3 to 5 cm), urologists prefer surgery while some medical oncologists prefer chemotherapy, indicating that there are two possible and acceptable methods of treatment and we are not yet sure which is preferable. Both are correct choices. In any case, surgery is required for all patients who continue to show evidence of remaining masses after initial treatment with chemotherapy. However, for children with yolk-sac tumors, radiation after chemotherapy is preferred for residual masses.

Five-Year Survival 90 to 95 percent

Investigational
♦ Prophylactic chemotherapy.

STAGE III
TNM Any T, any N, M1

The tumor invades other organs, most commonly the lungs or lymph nodes above the diaphragm.

Standard Treatment Radical orchiectomy followed by chemotherapy for both seminoma and non-seminomatous tumors.

The most frequently used drug combinations are cisplatin and etoposide (EP), each day for five consecutive days repeated every three weeks for four doses or cycles, or BEP, which uses the same doses and schedule of five days but adds bleomycin weekly for three cycles.

Fluids are given by vein to prevent cisplatin-induced kidney toxicity. Drugs are given by the same route to stop or minimize nausea and vomiting. A total of three to four cycles are given at no more than three- to four-week intervals, since it is harmful to space therapy at longer intervals. Only complete response is acceptable, and surgery is required when CT scans of the chest, abdomen and pelvis find any remaining disease, indicating a partial response.

If the remaining mass is less than 1 1/4 in. (3 cm), only scar tissue or benign teratoma may be found in the pathological specimen and no further treatment will be required because the relapse rate is less than 10 percent. But the relapse rate increases to 20 to 30 percent in men found to have viable (living) tumor (it is not unusual to find small areas of viable tumor in larger masses). In these cases, more chemotherapy, with a salvage regimen, must be given. Thereafter, careful follow-up is required.

Five-Year Survival More than 70 to 90 percent

Investigational
♦ The etoposide + carboplatin + bleomycin combination is now being evaluated.

♦ Depending on the definition used for poor risk, no more than 25 to 50 percent, at best, will attain complete response. For patients not attaining a complete response and whose AFP and HCG markers are not decreasing at the normal half-life rate, consideration should be given to autologous bone marrow transplantation, which can cure at least 30 percent of heavily pretreated cases.

TREATMENT FOLLOW-UP
Follow-up is an integral part of testis cancer therapy, particularly since most relapses occur quickly within the first year.

♦ Marker levels (some doctors also include a complete blood and platelet count) and chest x-rays should be taken monthly—definitely no later than at six-week intervals—with CT scans at three- to four-month intervals during the first year.

♦ If abdominal or chest surgery has been performed, a repeat CT scan to serve as a new anatomic baseline can be done six weeks after the operation. Similar tests are then repeated every 8 to 12 weeks during the second year. Since relapse is very uncommon after two years, the same tests can be done every three to four months for the third year, every four months during the fourth year and every six months during the fifth year. Some doctors also do yearly examinations after that, but the value of such testing is uncertain.

♦ All men should be taught how to examine the remaining testicle and have a sonogram when any change is found.

Long-Term Toxicity With almost all men being cured and having the expectation of a normal lifespan, therapy has been closely studied to evaluate any long-term toxicities.

♦ During therapy, nausea and vomiting can generally be prevented or minimized. Alopecia (hair loss) will occur but hair will return—sometimes thicker, darker and less wavy—within two to six months after chemotherapy is stopped.

♦ Low blood potassium, calcium and magnesium levels may be found but can generally be easily corrected and disappear after therapy.

♦ Lung scarring can occur when bleomycin is used, so pulmonary function tests are used to monitor any change. If lung function decreases, the drug must be stopped. It is rarely fatal or produces symptoms with present doses.

♦ There have been rare reports of heart attacks and high blood pressure with some older combinations, but the newer regimens that are given for a much shorter time—only three to four months—should alleviate this uncommon toxicity.

♦ The question of very delayed high blood pressure (hypertension) because of magnesium and renin imbalance has not yet been resolved, so blood pressure should be monitored at each follow-up. Since one study noted an increase in serum cholesterol, a lipid profile should be checked yearly.

♦ Following some chemotherapy combinations, particularly PVB, there have been reports of a chronic vascular disorder called Raynaud's phenomenon in 10 to 20 percent of cases. Again, this issue should be minimized with newer combinations and a smaller total bleomycin dose.

♦ Sex drive (libido) is not changed by treatment and neither are erections. Chemotherapy may temporarily or permanently decrease the sperm count. Male hormone replacement is needed in men having orchiectomy for bilateral testicular cancers.

♦ There is absolutely no evidence of any increased risk of abnormalities in children fathered by men who have had testis chemotherapy. Basically, either the sperm works or it doesn't. But it has been found that some men who have a testis cancer have low or zero sperm count before therapy, so a count should be done to document fertility *before* treatment is started and re-evaluated thereafter.

RECURRENT OR NEW CANCER

Since a few patients may get another testis tumor, observation combined with self-examination and/or a baseline testicular sonography should always be done.

A new testicular cancer is treated according to the stages listed earlier. A relapse indicated only by an increasing HCG or AFP marker requires a completely new work-up.

♦ When the tumor is documented by CT scan, particularly in late relapsing cases, surgical debulking may be warranted to identify the type of tumor that recurred, followed by salvage chemotherapy.

♦ When markers are positive yet cancer cannot be found by any diagnostic test (including MRI), salvage chemotherapy should be started, since it is generally very successful in such cases. Some doctors, however, may recommend exploratory surgery first.

♦ For metastases to the spinal cord and bone, radiation therapy is the treatment of choice to control local symptoms. Brain metastases may be removed surgically, if possible, and should be followed by therapeutic full-dose radiation therapy.

THE MOST IMPORTANT QUESTIONS YOU CAN ASK

♦ What type of testis cancer do I have? What is the stage?

♦ Am I in the good-risk or poor-risk group?

♦ Will nerve-sparing surgery be possible?

♦ When should I sperm bank?

♦ What are the toxic effects and risks of chemotherapy?

♦ What are my tumor markers? What other tests are needed for follow-up?

♦ What is my chance of cure?

THYMUS

Malin Dollinger, MD, and Ernest H. Rosenbaum, MD

◇

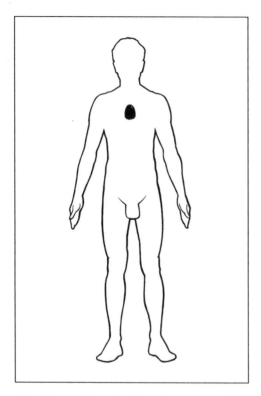

The thymus is a gland in the center of the chest (mediastinum) that has the important function during embryonic life of producing lymphocytes for the immune system. These thymus-derived, or T lymphocytes, are a major part of our immune system (cellular immunity) for our entire lives. Although these T lymphocytes look fairly similar under the microscope to the other major class of lymphocytes, B lymphocytes, they perform specialized immunologic functions to protect us from foreign organisms.

A variety of cancers can develop in the thymus. The most common tumor is malignant thymoma, which originates in the covering, or epithelium, of the thymus gland. All other tumor types are uncommon. These include lymphomas, germ cell tumors, carcinoids, carcinoma and thymolipomas.

Types Under the microscope, there are a number of cell sub-types of thymoma, but it is difficult to relate this microscopic appearance to how a tumor behaves. Some thymomas are non-invasive and appear to behave like benign tumors; others have all of the invasive characteristics of malignancy. So whether the tumors are called malignant depends not on their appearance but on their behavior (whether they have invasive characteristics). In the absence of invasion, the presence of a clearly defined covering, or "capsule," tends to classify the tumor as benign. But since all thymomas can become invasive and extend beyond the capsule, they should all be considered potentially malignant.

How It Spreads Most malignant thymomas grow slowly and have a tendency to recur in the chest at the site of origin. They seldom spread elsewhere, but if they do metastasize they often spread to the heart or lungs, especially to the coverings over the heart (pericardium) and lungs (pleura).

What Causes It The cause is unknown, but a number of systemic conditions, or syndromes, are associated with thymoma. Associated immune disorders include low red blood counts (pure red cell aplasia), low gamma globulins, signs and symptoms of connective tissue disorders, thyroiditis, ulcerative colitis, pernicious anemia, enteritis, sarcoid and, especially, a special type of muscle weakness called myasthenia gravis.

Various endocrine disorders are associated with thymoma, including hyperthyroidism, adrenal insufficiency (Addison's disease) and hypopituitarism.

RISK FACTORS

None known.

SCREENING

There are no general screening procedures for apparently healthy people. About a third of all thymoma cases are discovered during a routine or diagnostic chest x-ray. Myasthenia gravis, characterized by ever-worsening muscle weakness, is associated with a thymoma in up to 50 percent of cases. Removing the tumor will produce a complete remission of the myasthenia gravis in about one-third of patients, and at least half will improve.

COMMON SIGNS AND SYMPTOMS

People with thymoma often have no symptoms but may have chest-related complaints such as a cough, shortness of breath, difficulty swallowing and chest pain or tightness. If the tumor is very large, the neck and face may be swollen because of an obstruction of the superior vena cava (superior vena caval syndrome).

The associated diseases or syndromes also produce a variety of symptoms. The predominant symptom of muscle weakness found with myasthenia gravis is especially noted in the eyelids. Severe depression of the red cells (pure red cell aplasia) in 5 percent of patients with thymoma leads to severe anemia, and 5 to 10 percent have a low gamma globulin level. Signs and symptoms of other autoimmune or endocrine disorders can lead to the diagnosis.

DIAGNOSIS

A thymoma can be suspected in a patient with myasthenia gravis or one of the other autoimmune or endocrine disorders noted above.

Imaging
♦ A thymoma can be strongly suspected if a mass is seen on a chest x-ray in the location of the thymus in the center of the chest.

Endoscopy and Biopsy
♦ The biopsy needed for a definite diagnosis may sometimes be obtainable with a fine needle aspiration (FNA) but may also require definitive surgery.

STAGING

The most useful staging system defines four stages according to whether the tumor has remained within the capsule (limited), has broken through the capsule and spread either into adjacent tissues confined to the mediastinum or beyond these areas.

TREATMENT BY STAGE

STAGE I
The tumor cells remain confined within the capsule, which is intact.

Standard Treatment A non-invasive malignant thymoma is treated by the surgical removal of the tumor. Very specific and special precautions are needed for patients with myasthenia gravis because of the possibility of respiratory problems. Anesthesiologists experienced in this problem can dramatically reduce the rate of operative mortality.

If there is absolutely no evidence of spread through or beyond the capsule, no further therapy is needed. But if follow-up cannot be counted on, radiation therapy, possibly with adjuvant chemotherapy, may be given after surgery to try to improve the chances for long-term control.

There is a difference of opinion about the role of adjuvant radiotherapy for patients with encapsulated non-invasive thymomas. Since the recurrence rate is extremely low (about 2 percent), some physicians prefer to avoid the risks of radiation therapy. Others believe that radiotherapy is an essential part of treatment, and can help prevent local recurrence, especially for larger tumors.

If, as sometimes happens, the mass is discovered at surgery to have invaded adjacent organs, radiation therapy is used in addition to or instead of surgery.

Five-Year Survival 83 percent (70 percent for people with myasthenia gravis, 90 percent for those without)

STAGES II, III AND IV
The tumor has grown around the capsule into the adjacent fat or membrane (pleura) (Stage II), directly into surrounding organs (Stage III) or elsewhere in the chest or body (Stage IV).

Standard Treatment Invasive malignant thymoma is treated with surgical removal of the tumor if possible.

Radiation therapy is given postoperatively whether of not the tumor has been apparently completely removed. Fairly substantial doses, usually 3,500 to 4,500 cGy, are given and special techniques are necessary because of the large radiation ports required.

Drug therapy for locally invasive or advanced thymomas include the use of steroid hormones such as prednisone. These have caused regression of some thymomas that could not be removed and did not respond to radiotherapy.

Five-Year Survival 54 percent

Ten-Year Survival 30 percent

Investigational
♦ Chemotherapy is under clinical evaluation, and a variety of drugs have been found to be useful in patients who have residual or recurrent disease following surgery or radiation therapy. The combination of cisplatin + doxorubicin + vincristine + Cytoxan produced a 91 percent response rate (47 percent complete) in one study.
♦ In one trial, almost half of the patients treated with a four-drug combination of vincristine + Cytoxan + lomustine + prednisone had complete responses. The combination of cisplatin + Adriamycin + Cytoxan has produced a 70 percent remission rate.

TREATMENT FOLLOW-UP
♦ Periodic physical examinations, initially every two months during the first year.
♦ Routine x-rays and CT scans of the chest at intervals to detect recurrences.
♦ Routine blood chemistry tests are done every four to six months.
♦ Infections with unusual bacteria or fungi may occur, even if steroid hormones (prednisone) were not given. (These drugs impair the immune response.)

RECURRENT CANCER
While the rate of recurrences is less than 2 percent for non-invasive tumors, it is 20 to 50 percent for invasive malignancies.

Local recurrences can be treated with repeat surgery, radiation therapy, drug therapy with corticosteroids (such as prednisone) or chemotherapy.

Chemotherapy programs include the multiple drug combinations mentioned above.

THE MOST IMPORTANT QUESTIONS YOU CAN ASK
♦ How safe is surgery? Are there special precautions?
♦ Do I need radiation therapy? What are the side effects?
♦ Should chemotherapy be used?
♦ If my tumor recurs, can I be cured?

THYROID

Malin Dollinger, MD, and Orlo H. Clark, MD

◇

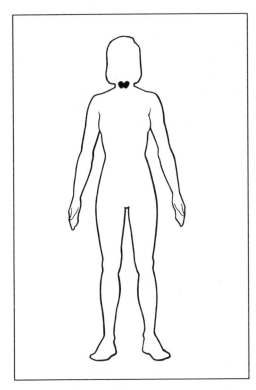

Cancer of the thyroid is the most common endocrine malignancy but is an uncommon cancer, comprising only about 1 percent of invasive cancers. It is estimated that there will be about 13,000 new cases in 1994, 9,600 in women and 3,400 in men. People with these malignancies are usually treated successfully.

Although invasive thyroid cancer is uncommon, doctors often have to diagnose and treat thyroid nodules, since about 4 percent of adults develop them. Thyroid cancer commonly appears as a "cold" nodule, meaning that it does not take up radioactive iodine. About 20 percent of cold nodules are cancer.

Most cases occur between 25 and 65 years of age, and the age at diagnosis is one of the most important factors in predicting prognosis. Men under 40 and women under 50 have significantly lower rates of recurrence and better survival rates than older patients.

Types About 90 percent of thyroid cancers develop from the follicular cells. Some develop from the parafollicular cells or C cells (medullary). Patients with well-differentiated tumors generally have a good prognosis. Those with undifferentiated or anaplastic tumors do not.

Papillary carcinomas are generally slow growing, with an 80 percent overall survival at 10 years. Even when tumors spread to regional lymph nodes or the lungs, survival may be more than 10 years. Tiny, clinically insignificant papillary carcinomas are found in 5 to 10 percent of thyroid glands examined at routine autopsies.

Follicular carcinomas occur in patients about 10 years older than those who get papillary carcinomas. Although these tumors are also usually slow growing, they behave somewhat more aggressively than papillary carcinomas and are more likely to spread to the lungs or bones. Hurthle cell cancers are generally included with follicular cancers, but are more likely to be multi-focal and involve regional lymph nodes. In contrast to follicular cancers, Hurthle cell tumors also do not take up radioactive iodine.

Three percent of thyroid cancers are undifferentiated (anaplastic) carcinomas. They occur in older patients, grow rapidly, behave aggressively and respond poorly to treatment.

Medullary carcinomas make up about 5 percent of thyroid cancers. These tumors secrete calcitonin, a tumor marker that is helpful in diagnosis and follow-up and also in screening relatives of those affected, since this tumor may occur on a familial, or inherited, basis. In the syndromes of multiple endocrine neoplasia (MEN), the cancer may be associated with tumors in other endocrine organs, such as pheochromocytoma of the adrenals, parathyroid tumors and islet cell cancer (*see* "Adrenal Gland," "Parathyroid" and "Islet Cell and Other Pancreatic Carcinomas").

Unusual tumors that can arise in the thyroid gland include sarcomas, lymphomas, epidermoid carcinomas and teratomas. The thyroid gland can also be a site of metastasis from other cancers, especially cancers of the lung, kidney, breast, and melanoma.

How It Spreads Papillary carcinomas spread to nearby lymph nodes and the tissues in the neck, with metastatic lesions to the lungs and bones. With follicular carcinomas, local spread to lymph nodes is less common. These tumors spread through the bloodstream, with metastasis occurring more often to bone. Anaplastic carcinoma usually extensively invades surrounding tissue. Medullary carcinoma spreads to lymph nodes and may invade blood vessels with metastases to the liver.

What Causes It Thyroid cancer is associated with significant excess or deficiency of iodine in the diet, some inherited diseases and especially with exposure to radiation. There is an increased incidence of thyroid cancer among survivors of the atomic blasts in Japan.

The risk of radiation exposure to the neck is now well known, and radiation therapy to treat benign conditions of the head and neck—a common practice in the first half of this century—fortunately has been abandoned. This should eventually lead to a decrease in the incidence of thyroid cancer, but there is a long period between radiation exposure and the development of a tumor.

One new method of preventing thyroid cancer was used on a wide scale with children in the Chernobyl region of Russia after the nuclear reactor accident. Potassium iodide was given to some children in an attempt to block thyroid uptake of radioactive iodine in the fallout. It will probably take at least 30 years to know if this approach was effective. Unfortunately, 200 cases of childhood thyroid cancer have already been diagnosed.

RISK FACTORS

At Significantly Higher Risk
♦ Exposure to radiation therapy, especially between 1920 and 1950, for enlarged lymph nodes in the neck, mastoiditis, tonsils, whooping cough, acne, enlarged thymus gland, keloids and fungal infections. The incidence directly relates to the amount of radiation given and inversely with the age of the person at the time of exposure. It generally takes 10 to 30 years after radiation exposure for a tumor to develop.

Thyroid cancer will develop in about 5 percent of children treated with low-dose radiation to the head and neck. Four percent of thyroid cancer patients have a history of such radiation therapy. Factors for increasing the risk after radiation exposure include female sex, younger age at exposure and a longer interval after radiation.

Forty percent of patients with thyroid nodules and a history of exposure to external radiation have thyroid cancer.

At Slightly Higher Risk
♦ Papillary carcinoma is increased in people with familial colon polyposis (multiple polyps of the colon), deficiency in the blood clotting Factor XI, and several other rare diseases.
♦ Risk for medullary carcinoma is inherited from one parent (autosomal-domi-

nant) in 50 percent of patients.

♦ More anaplastic and follicular carcinomas develop in people from areas with endemic goiter. Eighty percent of patients with anaplastic carcinoma have a history of nodular goiter.

♦ Iodine deficiency is associated with follicular carcinoma, which is more common in iodine-deficient areas such as Germany.

♦ Iodine abundance is associated with papillary carcinoma, more common in areas using iodized salt (United States) or a high-iodine diet (Iceland).

♦ Patients with Hashimoto's thyroiditis have an increased incidence of lymphoma of the thyroid gland.

♦ There is a slight increased risk of thyroid cancer in patients with chronic TSH (thyroid-stimulating hormone) elevation, usually as a congenital defect, or other thyroid abnormalities.

SCREENING

Physical examination is the best way to identify early-stage thyroid cancer. Two groups of people need special screening procedures:

♦ Those with a family history of thyroid cancer or multiple endocrine neoplasia (MEN II). Serum thyroglobulin is useful in the former and serum calcitonin and carcinoembryonic antigen (CEA) are important tumor markers in the latter.

♦ Those who have had radiation therapy to the neck and who have no visible thyroid lumps should be examined at least every two years. A lump in the thyroid of

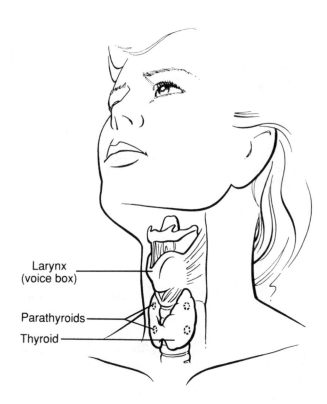

Larynx (voice box)

Parathyroids

Thyroid

Thyroid and parathyroid glands

these people generally suggests that the thyroid gland should be removed, since 40 percent will have cancer. To avoid surgery, nodules less than about 1/2 in. (1 cm) are sometimes treated with thyroid hormone for six months to see if they will regress.

Patients with enlargement of the entire thyroid, without specific lumps or nodules, should have thyroid function tests and an ultrasound scan. If the thyroid is not overactive, thyroid hormone is given for six months. If a nodule grows, the thyroid lobe with the nodule is removed surgically. Otherwise, thyroid hormone treatment is continued. The risk of cancer in an enlarged thyroid with many nodules is significantly lower than in a thyroid with a single nodule.

COMMON SIGNS AND SYMPTOMS

An enlargement of the entire thyroid, part of the thyroid or a lump or nodule is sometimes noticed while looking in the mirror while applying makeup or shaving. There may be enlarged lymph nodes in the neck that can be felt and there may be pain in the thyroid (especially with anaplastic carcinoma). Thyroid cancers also rarely occur at the base of the tongue.

Pressure symptoms, including airway obstruction, hoarseness or difficulty swallowing, develop in fewer than 5 percent of patients.

DIAGNOSIS

The most cost-effective way to evaluate a patient with a thyroid nodule is to have a sensitive thyroid-stimulating hormone (TSH) blood test to document normal thyroid function and to perform a fine needle aspiration (FNA) biopsy to determine whether the nodule is benign, suspicious or malignant. Patients with benign nodules are treated with thyroid hormone to suppress TSH; about 50 percent of these nodules will shrink. Malignant nodules should be removed, as should solitary

"cold" nodules. FNA is usually repeated after six months if the nodule has not decreased in size.

Physical Examination
♦ Careful examination of the thyroid gland and adjacent lymph nodes.

Blood and Other Tests
Blood tests are not generally useful to determine if a thyroid nodule is benign or malignant.
♦ Serum thyroglobulin levels are elevated in most patients with well-differentiated thyroid cancers, but the level cannot indicate whether a lump is benign or malignant. The presence of thyroglobulin after a total thyroidectomy (surgical removal of the thyroid gland) or the recurrence of a high level after surgery suggests recurrent or metastatic disease.
♦ An elevated serum calcitonin after total thyroidectomy and a modified radical neck dissection for medullary carcinoma suggests persistent disease. Families of all patients with medullary carcinoma should also be screened.
♦ CEA (carcinoembryonic antigen) levels are useful in predicting prognosis and discovering persistent disease in patients with medullary thyroid carcinoma.
♦ Blood tests, including serum alkaline phosphatase, are done to look for metastatic disease in the liver or bone. An elevated alkaline phosphatase level could suggest either liver or bone metastasis, leading to liver and bone scans. Selective venous catheterization for serum calcitonin is sometimes helpful for locating metastatic tumors.

Imaging
♦ Images of the thyroid can be taken after injection of a radioactive iodine tracer or of technetium 99m. Because thyroid cancers do not generally take up as much iodine as normal thyroid tissue, a cancer appears as a cold area on a scan. Only about 15 percent of cold nodules are can-

cer, however, and "warm" nodules are rarely malignant. Though used extensively in the past to classify nodules as hot or cold, thyroid scans are used less and less because more information is provided by FNA.

♦ Ultrasound is a safe and simple way of determining if a mass is solid or filled with fluid (cystic). It can also detect multiple nodules where only one may be felt. High-resolution ultrasound can find nodules as small as 3 mm in diameter. It cannot distinguish benign from malignant tumors. Since it is non-invasive and sensitive, it is the most accurate way to measure and follow a suspicious nodule in a patient given thyroid hormone in an attempt to suppress the nodule. It may also be used to guide biopsy procedures.

♦ Standard x-rays, such as chest x-ray to look for metastases.

Endoscopy and Biopsy

♦ Indirect or direct laryngoscopy if there is hoarseness, difficulty swallowing, coughing of blood (hemoptysis), shortness of breath or if the patient has had a previous neck operation.

♦ Fine needle aspiration (FNA) biopsy is the initial step in evaluating thyroid nodules in patients who do not have a history of exposure to low-dose radiation therapy, as it provides more information than any other diagnostic technique. It is over 90 percent accurate for benign lesions and about 99 percent accurate for malignancies. FNA is not recommended for those with a history of radiation therapy because they usually have many nodules, only 40 percent have cancer, and the wrong nodule may be aspirated.

FNA is also very useful in selecting patients for surgery. Only about 3 percent of patients with benign findings on FNA will have thyroid cancer, so surgery can be postponed in these patients while the thyroid suppression trial is done. The TSH level must be suppressed by the dosage of thyroid hormone. If the nodule decreases, thyroid hormone is continued. If the nodule does not change after six months, aspiration is repeated. Malignant FNA results should lead to immediate surgery.

♦ Lesions larger than 1 1/4 in. (3 cm), especially rapidly growing ones, are more likely to be lymphoma or anaplastic thyroid carcinoma. FNA may be satisfactory for diagnosis of anaplastic cancer, but the diagnosis of lymphoma of the thyroid usually requires a larger cutting needle or open biopsy.

STAGING

The TNM staging system is useful but has not been uniformly accepted because it is more complex than other staging systems. Many clinicians use the DeGroot system, which classifies tumors according to Class 1 (confined to the thyroid), Class 2 (involving regional nodes), Class 3 (locally invasive) and Class 4 (distant metastases). Others use the AGES (age, grade, extent and size) or AMES (age, metastases, extent and size) classifications to predict the tumor's aggressiveness. Staging systems have been designated for papillary and follicular carcinoma. There are no generally accepted staging systems for medullary carcinoma or anaplastic carcinoma.

TREATMENT OVERVIEW

A number of factors affect the prognosis for papillary and follicular thyroid cancers. A better prognosis can be expected with a pure papillary carcinoma in younger patients (women under 50 and men under 40), a tumor smaller than 3/4 in. (2 cm), small diffuse metastases, female sex and low-grade lesions.

A worse prognosis is related to age over 40, the degree of invasion (vascular and thyroid capsule) in follicular carcinoma, distant metastasis, a large tumor (especially over 1 1/2 in./5 cm), large nodular metastases, male sex and high-grade lesions (aneuploid).

Surgery The primary treatment of thyroid cancer is surgery, but there are some differences in opinion about the extent of thyroid resection required for the best prognosis. A near-total thyroidectomy—removing almost all the thyroid—offers the best chance for cure, especially if the cancer is in several places within the gland. The removal of all functioning thyroid tissue also makes it possible to scan for metastatic disease with radioactive iodine and to use serum thyroglobulin values to detect persistent disease.

One of the risks of a total thyroidectomy is the inadvertent removal of the parathyroid glands, which are situated, two on each side, at the edge of the thyroid. When a total thyroidectomy is done, an attempt is usually made to leave all four parathyroid glands in place. The surgeon must maintain an adequate supply of blood to the parathyroid glands to prevent the symptoms and signs of hypoparathyroidism or parathyroid hormone deficiency. Thyroid operations also have some risk of damage to the nerves in the neck that supply the larynx (voice box).

Removing one side of the thyroid (called a lobectomy) has fewer complications because only one nerve and two parathyroids are at risk. It is useful in selected cases with small papillary cancers or follicular cancers with only minimal invasion. Tumor might remain, however, in a few patients.

The surgeon may select a procedure depending on the type of thyroid cancer as well as the size of the nodule and his or her own experience.

Radioactive Iodine Therapy It has been standard practice in many reputable cancer treatment centers to give radioactive iodine after surgery. Assuming that a scan demonstrates that the tumor takes up iodine, as occurs in about two-thirds of cases, there is general agreement that this therapy is useful in patients over 45 years with papillary and follicular cancers if their tumors are multiple, locally invasive, larger than 1 in. (2.5 cm) or are associated with local or distant metastases.

This therapy has side effects, including temporary bone marrow suppression, inflammation of salivary glands, nausea and vomiting, scarring of the lung, pain in areas of metastasis and, rarely, leukemia.

The radioactive iodine is given when the patient is hypothyroid in preparation for the scan. A serum thyroglobulin level should also be obtained since persistent disease is present when it is elevated. After scanning or treatment, patients are again placed on thyroid hormone in order to avoid hypothyroidism and to suppress the TSH levels, which might stimulate residual tumor cells to grow. Some patients will require retreatment with radioactive iodine if the serum thyroglobulin level again becomes elevated or recurrent disease becomes evident.

TREATMENT BY TYPE AND STAGE

PAPILLARY THYROID CANCER
STAGE I
Tumor is confined to the thyroid gland. If it is on one side, it is considered Stage IA. If on both sides or there is more than one lump, it is Stage IB.

Standard Treatment The standard surgical procedure is removal of one side of the thyroid (lobectomy), but about 20 percent of patients will have a recurrence. Enlarged lymph nodes are also removed. Thyroid hormone is then given to suppress the thyroid-stimulating hormone (TSH) from the pituitary gland, which decreases the chance of recurrence.

Other options are a near-total or total thyroidectomy. The rationale for this is that there is an increased chance of multiple tumors in both lobes and any tumor left behind could change into the highly malignant (anaplastic) form. More important, scanning for metastases is possible once the thyroid is removed.

Five-Year Survival Over 95 percent

STAGE II

Cancer has spread to lymph nodes (IIA if to nodes on one side, IIB if to both sides or the mediastinal nodes—those in the center of the upper chest).

Standard Treatment The treatment is virtually identical to that for Stage I. The only difference between the two stages is the spread to lymph nodes. Removal of these metastases usually by a functional or modified radical neck dissection reduces the chance of local recurrence and minimally improves survival.

Five-Year Survival Over 95 percent

STAGE III

The tumor has invaded the tissues of the neck.

Standard Treatment Total thyroidectomy, plus removal of all apparent areas of cancer that have spread to the neck (debulking). After surgery, radioactive iodine should be given if the tumor takes up this isotope. If the uptake is minimal or absent, external radiation may be given.

Five-Year Survival 60 percent

STAGE IV

There are distant metastases, usually to lungs, bone and distant lymph nodes.

Standard Treatment Patients who have only distant lymph node metastasis may often be cured by radioactive iodine after a total thyroidectomy.

Solitary lung or bone metastases should be surgically removed, if possible. A therapeutic dose of radioactive iodine is then given; if there is no uptake, external radiation therapy is given to the area

involved. Taking thyroid hormone to suppress TSH may be effective in many metastatic tumors that are not sensitive to radioactive iodine.

Chemotherapy has produced occasional long-term remission.

Ten-Year Survival Less than 20 percent

FOLLICULAR THYROID CANCER
STAGE I

The tumor is localized to the thyroid gland (IA if on one side, IB if on both sides or there are multiple lesions).

Standard Treatment Either a near-total thyroidectomy or a lobectomy may be done. This type of cancer has a higher risk of metastasis to lung and bone. One disadvantage of leaving a remnant of thyroid is the difficulty in subsequent scanning with radioactive iodine (I-131). The residual thyroid rather than the metastasis will take up the isotope.

Sometimes, I-131 is used to eliminate any remaining thyroid tissue. Similarly, when therapeutic doses of I-131 are planned, all or almost all of the thyroid gland should be removed first.

Less extensive operations such as lobectomy have fewer complications, but 5 to 10 percent of patients will have a recurrence in the thyroid. Metastatic disease also cannot be treated with I-131 until the normal thyroid tissue has been removed.

As with papillary carcinoma, enlarged lymph nodes discovered at surgery, although less frequently involved, should be removed without extensive surgery. In patients who have a limited surgical procedure (lobectomy), thyroid hormone is given postoperatively to suppress TSH and decrease the chance of recurrence.

Five-Year Survival 70 to 90 percent

STAGE II

The tumor has spread to lymph nodes

(IIA if on one side, IIB if on both sides or to the mediastinal nodes—those in the center of the chest).

Standard Treatment Treatment is similar to that for Stage I. The only difference is the involvement of nearby lymph nodes, which increases local recurrence but only minimally influences survival.

Options include total or near-total thyroidectomy or lobectomy. The same considerations about hypoparathyroidism and distant metastases apply.

Five-Year Survival 50 to 70 percent

STAGE III
The tumor invades the tissues of the neck.

Standard Treatment Total thyroidectomy and removal of local areas of tumor spread (debulking). If the tumor takes up radioactive iodine (I-131), the isotope is given in an attempt to treat all potential residual disease. When the I-131 uptake is low, external radiotherapy is given to the neck.

Five-Year Survival 20 to 60 percent (worse if blood vessels are invaded)

STAGE IV
There are distant metastases, usually to lungs and bone.

Standard Treatment Treatment is usually not curative but may produce significant palliation.

The treatment options are similar to Stage IV papillary thyroid cancer, and include therapeutic doses of radioactive iodine if the metastases take up this isotope or external radiotherapy for localized lesions that do not respond to radioactive iodine. Tumors in many patients can be suppressed with thyroid hormone. A number of investigative chemotherapy protocols are being developed for patients with metastatic disease that does not respond to these treatment programs.

Five-Year Survival Unusual

MEDULLARY THYROID CARCINOMA
In the sporadic form, the tumor is usually on only one side of the thyroid. In the inherited (familial) form, the tumor is almost always on both sides. It is usually a hard mass situated in the lateral portion of the thyroid lobe at the level of the cricoid cartilage.

Prognosis depends upon the size of the primary tumor, the involvement of nearby lymph nodes and whether the tumor can be completely removed and whether there are distant metastases.

Standard Treatment A total thyroidectomy is done, with a thorough central neck cleanout, meaning that all fibrofatty and lymphoid tissue is removed. If regional nodes are involved and the primary tumor is larger than 3/4 in. (2 cm), a modified radical neck dissection is done on the same side.

If the tumor is confined to the thyroid gland, almost all patients will be cured. In general, there is no benefit to radioactive iodine therapy, radiotherapy or chemotherapy, although occasional responses to these treatments are seen in metastatic disease.

Treatment for metastatic disease has generally been unsatisfactory, pointing up the need for detection and diagnosis while the tumor is confined to the thyroid and can be cured surgically. Patients with metastatic disease benefit from palliative surgery. They may have significant symptoms, especially severe diarrhea, related to the hormone produced by the tumor. This usually responds to treatment with somatostatin or nutmeg.

Five-Year Survival 40 to 95 percent. Survival is best in familial medullary thyroid cancer without other aspects of MEN, and intermediate for sporadic and for MEN IIA. It is worst for patients with MEN IIB, that is in patients with a marfanoid habitus, mucosal neuromas, pheochromocytomas and ganglioneuromatosis.

ANAPLASTIC THYROID CARCINOMA

There are large cell and small cell types. Both grow rapidly and extend beyond the thyroid.

Standard Treatment Patients with this tumor have an extremely poor prognosis, most patients not surviving even one year after diagnosis.

After the diagnosis is established by FNA or a cutting needle biopsy, aggressive radiation therapy and chemotherapy is recommended for three weeks. No treatment is given for the following two weeks, then a thyroidectomy is performed. Radiation and chemotherapy are resumed two weeks after the operation. This treatment is usually not curative, but it appears to offer the best palliation and the best hope for survival.

Five-Year Survival About 5 percent, the average survival being less than six months

PRIMARY LYMPHOMA OF THE THYROID

Standard Treatment These patients have a rapidly enlarging thyroid mass, often with pressure symptoms. At least a third have thyroiditis (Hashimoto's disease) and most have limited-stage disease. The prognosis depends on the lymphoma subtype as well as on the stage.

Treatment is similar to that for any B-cell lymphoma arising outside lymph nodes. Since most patients have diffuse lymphomas, they tend to be treated after diagnosis by open biopsy with aggressive third-generation combination chemotherapy programs (*see* "Lymphomas: Non-Hodgkin's").

TREATMENT FOLLOW-UP

For well-differentiated thyroid cancers (papillary and follicular carcinoma), follow-up should include:
♦ Periodic physical examination, especially of the thyroid and cervical lymph nodes.
♦ Serologic marker (thyroglobulin).
♦ Scanning with radioactive iodine and treatment with 30 MCi (millicuries) (low-risk patients) or 100 MCi (high-risk patients if they have had a total or near-total parathyroidectomy).
♦ Periodic ultrasound examinations of the neck to identify recurrence in the thyroid area or lymph node metastases.
♦ Chest x-ray to detect metastases.
For medullary thyroid cancer, follow-up should include:
♦ Serum calcitonin level and CEA level every six months.
♦ Physical examination, emphasizing the thyroid, although calcitonin level is more accurate than physical examination for following persistent disease.
♦ CT or MRI scan of neck and mediastinum.
♦ Chest x-ray every six months until stable.
♦ Chemistry panel every six months.

RECURRENT AND METASTATIC DISEASE

When thyroid carcinoma is recurrent or metastatic and is also widespread or can't be removed, it is treated with radioactive iodine. If it does not take up radiaoctive iodine, it should be treated with radiation therapy.
♦ For the papillary and follicular types, an effort is made to scan for metastatic disease with radioactive iodine. After the thyroid gland is removed and thyroid hormone is stopped for an appropriate time, a tracer dose of radioactive iodine is given. If hot spots appear at sites outside the thyroid area, suggesting metastases, a therapeutic dose of radioactive iodine is given. Radioactive iodine effectively irradiates

microscopic metastases. Larger metastases should be removed surgically before radioactive iodine is given. The thyroglobulin level should be determined, since if it is detectable or elevated after a total thyroidectomy, residual tumor is present.

♦ External radiation is used in patients whose tumors do not take up radioactive iodine or are undifferentiated.

♦ Some patients respond to chemotherapy, with regimens containing doxorubicin having the highest response rate. The combination of cisplatin and doxorubicin may produce some complete and partial remissions in metastatic thyroid cancer. In a few cases, the complete responders survived more than two years. Another combination (doxorubicin + bleomycin + vincristine + melphalan) was reported to show responses in about one-third of patients.

♦ In patients with anaplastic thyroid cancer, chemotherapy is occasionally effective and is usually combined with external radiation.

♦ Patients with metastatic thyroid carcinoma, especially if unsuitable or unresponsive to radioactive iodine, should be considered for entry into clinical trials in the hopes of finding a more effective chemotherapy program.

THE MOST IMPORTANT QUESTIONS YOU CAN ASK

♦ How extensive should my surgery be?

♦ What is the chance of complications of surgery, especially damage to the parathyroid glands and the risk of nerve malfunction?

♦ Why do I need to take thyroid hormone after surgery?

♦ Will I need radioactive iodine?

♦ What follow-up do I need?

♦ What is my chance of cure, and when can you be sure?

TROPHOBLASTIC DISEASE

Jeffrey L. Stern, MD

◇

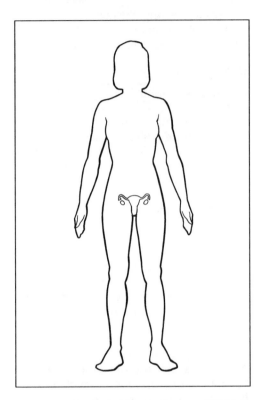

Gestational trophoblastic disease (GTD) is a rare cancer that develops from an abnormal fertilized egg. Of all the cancers that afflict women, it is one of the most commonly cured. Even when it is metastatic, the survival rate is extremely high.

The cure rate depends on the cell type, the extent of disease, the duration of time from the onset of the initial pregnancy to the start of therapy, the sites of metastases, the type of pregnancy before the development of GTD and earlier therapy. In some cases, it can also depend on the degree of elevation of the serum beta human chorionic gonadotropin (βHCG), a protein produced by a normal pregnancy as well as by all the different GTD cell types. It can be detected in the blood and urine and is an extremely sensitive tumor marker for GTD. It is measured often during both therapy and follow-up to measure the response to treatment and to detect recurrent disease.

Types There are three types of gestational trophoblastic disease—hydatidiform mole (also called a molar pregnancy), invasive mole (chorioadenoma destruens) and gestational choriocarcinoma, which is further divided according to whether it is metastatic or non-metastatic.

♦ A hydatidiform mole is essentially an abnormal embryo that contains many fluid-filled cysts. There are two types of hydatidiform moles, complete and incomplete (partial). The diagnosis of a complete hydatidiform mole is usually made during the first half of a pregnancy and is recognized by the health care provider about 50 percent of the time before the tumor cysts are expelled. A variety of clinical conditions may be confused with a molar pregnancy, but these can usually be distinguished on the basis of medical history, a physical exam and an ultrasound examination.

In contrast to a complete mole, a partial mole is associated with a fetus. It occurs much less frequently than a complete mole. The fetus usually dies within nine weeks after the last menstrual period although occasionally it can survive to term. Partial moles are rarely associated with multiple ovarian cysts (thecolutein cysts), high βHCG titers and other accompaniments of a complete mole. There is also a lower incidence of malignant behavior (5 to 10 percent).

♦ An invasive mole (chorioadenoma destruens) is defined as a hydatidiform mole that invades the wall of the uterine muscle. It develops in 15 to 30 percent of all molar pregnancies.

♦ Choriocarcinoma is a very rapidly growing malignancy that tends to spread quickly. About 50 percent of all cases of gestational choriocarcinoma follow a hydatidiform mole, 25 percent follow a spontaneous abortion or tubal pregnancy and 25 percent follow a normal pregnancy. Choriocarcinoma follows a normal-term pregnancy in 1 in 40,000 pregnancies. GTD after a normal pregnancy is always a choriocarcinoma, never a mole or an invasive mole.

What Causes It A complete hydatidiform or invasive mole occurs when a single sperm fertilizes an egg without a nucleus. The chromosomes in the sperm duplicate, resulting in an abnormal embryo that has only male genetic material. A mole can also occur when two sperm fertilize a single egg. A mole develops from the abnormally fertilized egg and is characterized by a lack of a normal fetus and by many small fluid-filled cysts.

The cause of choriocarcinoma is uncertain. It can arise from a normal pregnancy, a miscarriage, a tubal pregnancy or from either type of mole.

How It Spreads Hydatidiform moles generally stay confined to the endometrial cavity. When it begins to invade the wall of the uterus, it is called an invasive mole. Occasionally a hydatidiform mole and an invasive mole can spread to distant sites, most typically to the lung.

An invasive mole can penetrate the full thickness of the uterine wall and rupture, resulting in severe intra-abdominal or vaginal bleeding. Invasive moles can also metastasize, most commonly to the vagina and lung. This may be confusing since women with proven invasive moles who have metastases may also have choriocar-cinoma. Although an invasive mole is locally more aggressive than a non-invasive mole, it is no more likely to be complicated by choriocarcinoma.

Choriocarcinoma can spread virtually anywhere in the body but most commonly spreads to the lung, the lower genital tract (cervix, vagina and vulva), the brain, liver, kidney and the gastrointestinal tract.

RISK FACTORS

Gestational trophoblastic disease occurs only in women of reproductive age. An invasive mole develops in 15 to 30 percent of all complete moles and 5 to 10 percent of all partial moles. Choriocarcinoma develops in 3 percent of complete moles but rarely in partial moles.

At Significantly Higher Risk

Risks for the development of a hydatidiform or invasive mole or choriocarcinoma include:

♦ A prior mole (30 times the risk).

♦ Maternal age greater than 40 years (5 times) or less than 20 years (1.5 times).

♦ A previous spontaneous abortion (twice the risk).

At Slightly Lower Risk

♦ Eating a diet high in vitamin A and having one or more children without having a previous abortion is statistically correlated with a lower than average risk of developing a complete mole.

At Risk for Developing an Invasive Mole or Choriocarcinoma

For women with a molar pregnancy, there are several risk factors associated with the subsequent development of an invasive mole and choriocarcinoma. These include delayed hemorrhage after a dilation and curettage procedure (D&C), large ovarian cysts, acute pulmonary failure at the time of the D&C, a large uterus before the D&C, a serum βHCG level greater than 40,000 mIU/mL, a history of a previous mole and maternal age over 40.

SCREENING

Since it is so rare, GTD is not routinely screened for.

COMMON SIGNS AND SYMPTOMS

A molar pregnancy is usually associated with bleeding in the first half of a pregnancy, an absent fetal heartbeat, pain in the lower abdomen, and occasionally with high blood pressure before 24 weeks of pregnancy, excessive nausea or vomiting, a uterus larger than normal for the gestational age (50 percent of all cases) and the expulsion of cysts.

Eighty to 90 percent of women with partial moles have abnormal uterine bleeding, a smaller than expected uterus for the gestational age of the pregnancy or the signs and symptoms of a spontaneous abortion.

The most common symptoms of choriocarcinoma are lack of a menstrual period, symptoms of pregnancy, abnormal vaginal bleeding or pelvic pain. Women with liver metastases may have bleeding within the abdomen because of a ruptured liver. Those with metastases to the lung may have a dry cough, cough up blood and have chest pain or shortness of breath. Spread to the intestinal tract may be associated with chronic blood loss and anemia or with massive hemorrhage. Brain metastases are often associated with symptoms that suggest a brain tumor or stroke.

DIAGNOSIS

The diagnosis is usually suspected after an ultrasound examination of the uterus, but absolute diagnosis of a mole is made by examining the cysts under a microscope. A serum βHCG level far in excess of that of a normal pregnancy would support the diagnosis of a hydatidiform mole.

An invasive mole is seldom diagnosed definitively without a hysterectomy. The diagnosis is usually made after a hydatidiform mole is removed and there is a persistently elevated βHCG titer without evidence of metastases.

Confirmation of choriocarcinoma by removing cells for pathological analysis is not required and may be hazardous since this tumor bleeds easily. The diagnosis is made by the presence of metastases and an elevated βHCG level or, occasionally, on a D&C specimen.

Physical Examination
♦ When GDT is suspected or diagnosed, the physical examination pays particular attention to the pelvis, abdomen (specifically the liver), the lungs and the brain.

Blood and Other Tests
♦ Complete blood count.
♦ Tests for liver enzymes and kidney function.
♦ Serum chemistries.
♦ Serum βHCG.
♦ Thyroid function tests.

Imaging
Studies before evacuation of a hydatiform mole include:
♦ Pelvic ultrasound.
♦ Chest x-ray.

STAGING

Gestational trophoblastic disease is not staged but is divided into non-metastatic or metastatic. Non-metastatic choriocarcinoma is defined as having no disease outside the uterus and has a survival rate of 100 percent. Metastatic choriocarcinoma is further divided into low-risk (good prognosis) and high-risk (poor prognosis) based on several factors.

TREATMENT OVERVIEW

Before starting chemotherapy for invasive mole or for non-metastatic and metastatic choriocarcinoma, certain diagnostic tests should be performed including a chest x-ray and a CT scan of the abdomen, pelvis and head. Even when the chest x-ray is normal, a CT scan of the lungs may reveal small metastases in up to 40 percent of women. These women have a 50 percent failure rate with single drug chemotherapy. A complete blood count, platelet count and kidney and liver function tests are also required before initiating chemotherapy.

An important aspect of treating women with GTD is to start therapy as quickly as possible after the diagnosis is made. It is also important to give chemotherapy as often as possible until the serum βHCG titers return to normal. A course of chemotherapy is generally given every 14 to 21 days, depending on the drug regimen used.

Depending on the extent of the disease, most physicians give one to three cycles of chemotherapy after the first normal βHCG level, then follow the titers monthly for 6 to 24 months after treatment. All women are advised to use oral contraceptives for one to two years after therapy.

TREATMENT BY TYPE AND STAGE

HYDATIDIFORM MOLE (MOLAR PREGNANCY)

Complications associated with a molar pregnancy include anemia because of blood loss, severe high blood pressure, an overactive thyroid gland, heart failure, hemorrhage, infection and acute pulmonary failure.

Standard Treatment As soon the diagnosis is made, a therapeutic suction dilatation and curettage (D&C) is performed in the operating room under anesthesia. For women who have completed childbearing, the removal of the uterus and cervix (a hysterectomy) is also an option.

Rhogam is given to women with Rh negative blood to prevent Rh sensitization. In about a third of women with a molar pregnancy, there may be enlargement of one or both ovaries because of multiple (thecolutein) cysts caused by the high levels of βHCG. Occasionally the cysts can rupture, bleed or become infected. In the vast majority of cases, these cysts do not have to be surgically removed because they resolve with time, although sometimes it can take several weeks or months for them to disappear completely.

Chemotherapy may be given after the removal of the mole if there is a tissue diagnosis of choriocarcinoma, if the serum βHCG rises for two successive weeks or plateaus for three weeks or more (in the vast majority of women, the βHCG level plateaus or rises by seven weeks after the D&C), if metastases are found, if the serum βHCG rises again after reaching a normal level or if there is a hemorrhage not related to an incomplete D&C.

Five-Year Survival 100 percent

NON-METASTATIC GTD

Non-metastatic disease may be either an invasive mole or choriocarcinoma and is defined as having no disease outside the uterus.

Standard Treatment Chemotherapy for an invasive mole and non-metastatic choriocarcinoma is the same. All cases of non-metastatic GTD are considered curable, even if there is extensive local disease. If chemotherapy fails, a hysterectomy is usually performed.

The standard treatment is with a single chemotherapeutic drug. Most physicians use methotrexate if the liver functions are normal or actinomycin-D if they are aren't. Methotrexate is given daily, either by injection into a muscle or intravenously, for five days. This schedule is repeated every 14 days until the βHCG level returns to normal. Three to four courses are usually required.

Methotrexate may also be given on days 1, 3, 5 and 7 with leucovorin given on Days 2, 4, 6 and 8. When used in this fashion, only one course of treatment is given (with a cure rate of around 80 percent). A second or third course is given only if the βHCG titer does not return to normal.

Actinomycin-D is usually given intravenously for five consecutive days and repeated every two weeks. If treatment with methotrexate fails to bring about titer remission, then actinomycin-D is given (or vice versa).

Five-Year Survival 100 percent for both invasive mole and non-metastatic choriocarcinoma

LOW-RISK METASTATIC GTD

Metastatic choriocarcinoma is considered low-risk when it is diagnosed less than four months after the onset of the pregnancy, when the βHCG titer is less than 40,000 mIU/ml, when there are no liver or brain metastases and when there has been no previous treatment with chemotherapy.

Standard Treatment Therapy for women with low-risk metastatic GTD is usually with a single chemotherapeutic drug as for non-metastatic disease. But many physicians use only single-agent chemotherapy for women who have an abnormal postmolar βHCG titer. All other cases with good prognostic features are treated with a combination of methotrexate + actinomycin-D + Cytoxan (MAC).

Those who fail chemotherapy with methotrexate alone (approximately 20 percent) are then treated with actinomycin-D or with MAC. MAC is given intravenously for five consecutive days every two to three weeks until the βHCG titer returns to normal.

Five-Year Survival 97 to 100 percent

HIGH-RISK METASTATIC GTD

Metastatic choriocarcinoma is considered high-risk when it is diagnosed more than four months after the onset of pregnancy, associated with a serum βHCG titer greater than 40,000 mIU/mL, liver or brain metastases, a history of chemotherapy or if it occurs after a full-term pregnancy.

Standard Treatment Poor-risk metastatic disease has to be treated as soon as possible with aggressive chemotherapy. Women with brain or liver metastases are often treated with radiation therapy to the brain or liver. Women with liver metastases have the worst prognosis.

Standard chemotherapy has been with MAC, but recently there has been a trend toward using a regimen known as EMA-CO, which includes the drugs etoposide, methotrexate, actinomycin-D, vincristine and Cytoxan.

Other drugs used in women who fail to respond to MAC and/or EMA-CO include vinblastine, cisplatin, bleomycin and ifosfamide. Once a negative βHCG level is obtained, most women are treated with three more courses of chemotherapy and are then followed with monthly βHCG titers for two years.

Five-Year Survival 75 percent

TREATMENT FOLLOW-UP

Regular measurements of the serum βHCG levels are the most important part of the follow-up surveillance for molar pregnancies. The levels are monitored weekly until normal—usually, the level progressively declines to normal within 14 weeks after the D&C—then monthly for 6 to 12 months.

◆ A gynecologic examination and careful physical examination is done one week after the D&C and then every four weeks until the βHCG titer returns to normal or unless symptoms develop.

◆ Contraception (preferably oral contraceptives) should be used for 6 to 12 months after the D&C.

The serum βHCG levels are also monitored for other types of GTD. Once the βHCG titer returns to normal after treatment, the levels should be measured monthly for one year in the case of non-metastatic disease or two years for metastatic disease.

Pregnancy After GTD Treatment No significant side effects of chemotherapy for GTD affect future pregnancies. There does not seem to be a higher infertility rate, a lower chance for a successful term pregnancy or a higher rate of spontaneous abortion. But there is a higher incidence of subsequent GTD.

Most physicians recommend avoiding pregnancy for the first year after a hydatidiform mole is treated. This will prevent any confusion about the interpretation of elevated βHCG levels.

RECURRENT CANCER

Recurrent disease is usually treated with chemotherapy or occasionally surgery if the metastases are isolated. Chemotherapy for gestational trophoblastic disease automatically puts a woman in the high-risk group for recurrences.

Cure rates vary, depending on the site of metastases.

THE MOST IMPORTANT QUESTIONS YOU CAN ASK

♦ What type of gestational trophoblastic disease do I have, and what is its extent?

♦ What is the likelihood of cure?

♦ How was the chemotherapy decided upon?

♦ What are my prospects of having a normal pregnancy later on?

♦ Will a specialist in gynecologic oncology be involved in my care?

UTERUS:
ENDOMETRIAL CARCINOMA

Jeffrey L. Stern, MD

◇

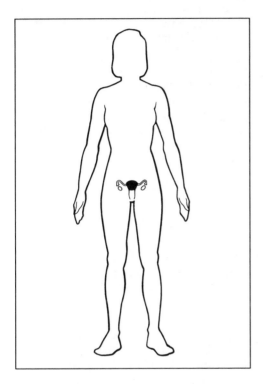

Endometrial cancer—carcinoma of the lining of the uterus—is the most common gynecologic malignancy and accounts for about 13 percent of all malignancies occurring in women. There are about 34,000 cases of endometrial cancer diagnosed in the United States each year but, encouragingly, there has been a significant decrease in the number of women who develop endometrial cancer each year since 1975.

Similarly, the death rate from endometrial cancer has steadily declined from 1950 to 1985, falling more than 60 percent. Since this cancer is usually diagnosed at an early stage, the cure rate is high, with a five-year survival of 83 percent in 1985.

Types All endometrial carcinomas arise from the glands of the lining of the uterus. Adenocarcinoma accounts for 75 percent of all endometrial carcinomas. Endometrial adenocarcinomas that contain benign squamous cells are known as adenoacanthomas and account for 17 percent of endometrial cancers.

The remaining three types of endometrial carcinoma have a poor prognosis. Approximately 15 percent of women have adenosquamous carcinoma, in which both the gland cells and squamous cells are malignant. Three percent have a clear cell carcinoma, and about 1 percent have a papillary carcinoma.

Uterine sarcoma is another kind of uterine malignancy. (*See* "Uterus: Uterine Sarcomas".)

How It Spreads From where it arises in the lining of the uterus, endometrial carcinoma eventually invades the wall of the uterus and may involve the cervix. With time, it can grow through the wall of the uterus into the surrounding tissues (the parametrium), the bladder and the rectum (*see* page 348).

It can also spread by the lymphatic system to the vagina, fallopian tubes, ovaries, the pelvic and aortic lymph nodes and to the lymph nodes in the groin and above the collarbone (supraclavicular). Like ovarian carcinoma, endometrial cancer can also spread throughout the abdominal cavity and occasionally through the bloodstream to the lung, liver and brain. How rapidly it spreads depends on the grade (histologic virulence) of the cancer.

Endometrial cancer is often associated

with a primary carcinoma of the ovary. (*See* "Ovarian Germ Cell Tumors.")

What Causes It Unknown.

RISK FACTORS

The use of birth control pills decreases the risk of developing endometrial cancer by half.

At Significantly Higher Risk
♦ Postmenopausal women.
♦ Menopause after age 52 (2.4 times as likely).
♦ Lack of children (twice as likely).
♦ Women with hypertension (twice as likely).
♦ Diabetics (2.8 times as likely).
♦ Women who do not ovulate, in other words those with polycystic ovaries (Stein-Leventhal syndrome).
♦ Estrogen replacement therapy without supplemental progesterone (seven times as likely).
♦ History of pelvic radiation therapy (eight times as likely).
♦ Obesity greater than 50 pounds (23 kg) over ideal body weight (10 times as likely).

SCREENING

Screening for endometrial carcinoma is not as satisfactory as screening for cancer of the cervix because of the inaccessibility of the uterine cavity. Pap smears detect only a small percentage of endometrial cancers.

There have been studies of other screening methods that can be performed in the doctor's office, with several showing the benefit of using endometrial biopsies to screen high-risk women who have no symptoms. This procedure is associated with some discomfort, however, and may not be cost-effective in the absence of risk factors. Routine annual screening for women without symptoms is not recommended by the American College of Obstetricians and Gynecologists.

COMMON SIGNS AND SYMPTOMS

In 90 percent of cases, there is abnormal uterine bleeding, from insignificant staining to a hemorrhage. There may also be pain in the pelvis, back or legs, bladder or rectal symptoms, weight loss and general weakness. Five percent of women will have no symptoms.

DIAGNOSIS

Physical Examination
♦ On a gynecologic examination, the external genitalia is usually normal. The cervix may be involved with cancer (Stage II), and the vagina may also be involved (Stage III).
♦ Occasionally the uterus will be enlarged or softened and masses may be detected in the pelvis (a rectal examination is an important aspect of the pelvic examination).
♦ Enlarged lymph nodes in the neck and groin.
♦ Enlarged liver, abdominal mass or excessive abdominal fluid (ascites).

Blood and Other Tests
♦ Complete blood count.
♦ Serum liver and kidney tests.
♦ Serum CA-125 is produced by a small percentage of women with endometrial carcinoma, which can be useful in follow-up to detect recurrences.

Imaging
♦ CT or MRI scan of the abdomen and MRI scan of the pelvis are both useful for determining the extent of cancer in the pelvis, the presence of ovarian disease and the presence of involved pelvic and aortic lymph nodes and liver metastases.
♦ Chest x-ray.

Endoscopy and Biopsy
♦ The definitive diagnosis is made on an endometrial biopsy, which involves a small scraping of the uterus and is usually

performed in the doctor's office. A dilation and curettage (D&C) is required for some women—those who have biopsy-proven endometrial hyperplasia (see below), who have an insufficient specimen on an office biopsy or who can't have an endometrial biopsy done in the office because of a small cervical opening or discomfort.

STAGING

Cancer of the uterus is surgically staged. Between 70 and 80 percent of all endometrial cancers are Stage I. In 1988, the International Federation of Gynecology and Obstetricians (FIGO) staging was revised to include the grade of the cancer (degree of virulence) as determined on microscopic examination. The cancers are divided into three grades, with Grade 1 (well-differentiated) having the best prognosis and Grade 3 (least-differentiated) having the poorest.

ENDOMETRIAL CANCER PRECURSORS

Endometrial hyperplasia, an overgrowth of the lining of the uterus, is a precursor to the development of cancer. This disorder tends to progress from a simple, benign hyperplasia confined to the lining of the uterus, to more severe forms of hyperplasia and eventually to an invasive malignancy. The risk factors for endometrial hyperplasia are similar to those of endometrial carcinoma.

Abnormal uterine bleeding is usually the first symptom. The diagnosis is made by evaluating the lining of the uterus by biopsy or dilation and curettage (D&C).

Treatment depends on the degree of hyperplasia, the age of the woman and her reproductive desires. Total abdominal hysterectomy and removal of both tubes and both ovaries is recommended for postmenopausal women and women who have completed childbearing. Women who want to keep their reproductive organs can be treated with oral progestational hormones for several months. The cure rate depends on the degree of hyperplasia and the sensitivity of the endometrium to the progestational therapy.

TREATMENT OVERVIEW

Treatment of endometrial carcinoma is based primarily on the stage and grade of the cancer.

The standard therapy is an abdominal hysterectomy with removal of both fallopian tubes and ovaries, selective removal of pelvic and aortic lymph nodes and washings from the abdominal cavity to look for malignant cells.

Most gynecologic oncologists also recommend obtaining a specimen from the cancer for analysis of its estrogen and progesterone receptor content. The receptor content has prognostic value and may be useful in the selection of hormone therapy for recurrent or metastatic cancer.

 Surgery Most gynecologic oncologists recommend a midline abdominal incision to gain access to the upper abdomen. Complications of surgery can include infection, bleeding and injury to the bladder, rectum or ureter causing a leak, although this is rare. There may also be blood clots in the legs, occasionally dislodging and traveling to the lungs (pulmonary embolism).

 Radiation Women who have Stages Ib, Ic or IIa uterine cancers are frequently treated two to six weeks after surgery with radiation to the entire pelvis and upper vagina. Total dose is 4,000 to 5,000 cGy in divided doses given daily, five days a week for four to five weeks. Although pelvic external beam radiation therapy will decrease the frequency of recurrences in the pelvis and vagina, it does not statistically improve the five-year survival rate.

Side effects of radiation can include diarrhea, nausea and vomiting, bleeding from the bladder or rectum, vaginal scarring, intestinal obstruction, or leaks (fistulas) in the urinary or intestinal tracts.

 Chemotherapy Treatment with chemotherapy after surgery is being evaluated for later stages of the disease.

TREATMENT BY STAGE

ENDOMETRIAL HYPERPLASIA

Total abdominal hysterectomy and removal of both tubes and both ovaries is the treatment of choice when fertility is no longer an issue or when progestational hormone therapy is contraindicated. For those women who desire more children or preservation of the uterus, a D&C, therapy with oral progestational agents, induction of ovulation and avoidance of postmenopausal estrogen therapy without progesterone is frequently effective. Careful follow-up with an endometrial biopsy or a D&C is necessary.

STAGE Ia

The tumor is limited to the endometrium.

Standard Treatment Regardless of the grade, standard therapy is removal of the uterus and both tubes and ovaries. Postoperative radiation therapy is not usually required.

Five-Year Survival 90 to 95 percent

Investigational
♦ The most significant study in progress is whether postoperative pelvic radiation therapy improves survival.

STAGE Ib

The tumor invades the uterine wall but through less than half of its thickness.

Standard Treatment The abdominal removal of the uterus, both tubes and ovaries and sampling the pelvic and para-aortic lymph nodes is all that is required under certain conditions—namely, that

the tumor is Grade 1 or 2, involves the upper two-thirds of the uterus, does not invade the blood vessels of the uterus, invades the wall of the uterus by less than one-third and the abdominal washings contain no malignant cells.

If the tumor (any grade) invades more than one-third of the uterine wall or significantly invades the blood vessels, external beam radiation therapy is usually given to the pelvis and upper vagina after surgery. The total dose is 4,000 to 5,000 cGy, given daily in divided doses, five days a week for four to five weeks.

Five-Year Survival Up to 80 percent

Investigational
♦ The most significant study in progress is whether postoperative pelvic radiation therapy improves survival.
♦ Studies are looking at the role of adjuvant chemotherapy with Adriamycin, mitoxantrone, cisplatin, Cytoxan, carboplatin or progestational hormones in various doses and regimens.

STAGE Ic

The tumor invades the uterine wall by more than half of its thickness.

Standard Treatment Almost all gynecologic oncologists recommend whole pelvis radiation after surgery to decrease the frequency of recurrent disease in the vagina and pelvis. Although it does not statistically improve the five-year survival rate, it is effective in decreasing the incidence of local recurrences in the field of radiation.

Five-Year Survival Up to 70 percent

Investigational *See* Stage Ib.

STAGE IIa

The glands that line the cervix are involved.

Standard Treatment This stage is generally treated like Stage Ic—surgery followed by radiation. Sometimes, however, radiotherapy is given before surgery, with radioactive cesium temporarily placed in the upper vagina two weeks after external radiation treatment is finished.

Five-Year Survival Up to 60 percent

Investigational See Stage Ib.

STAGE IIb
The tumor cells invade the cervix.

Standard Treatment Before surgery, whole-pelvis external beam radiation therapy (total dose of 4,000 cGy) is given in divided doses, five days a week, over five weeks. After a two-week break, this is followed by a three-day application of radioactive cesium to the upper vagina, cervix and uterus. Six weeks later, an abdominal hysterectomy is performed, along with removal of both tubes and ovaries, selective pelvic and aortic lymph node sampling and cytological assessment of the abdominal cavity.

Alternative therapy for younger, non-obese women in good medical condition is a radical abdominal hysterectomy, removal of the tubes and ovaries, removal of all the pelvic lymph nodes and surgical staging.

Five-Year Survival Up to 60 percent

Investigational
♦ Studies are looking at the role of adjuvant chemotherapy with Adriamycin, mitoxantrone, cisplatin, Cytoxan, carboplatin or progestational hormones in various doses and regimens.

STAGE IIIa
This stage is defined by involvement of the uterine surface and/or the tubes and ovaries and/or the presence of malignant cells in the abdominal fluid (positive peritoneal washings).

Standard Treatment After surgery, any additional treatment is controversial and

should be considered investigational. The chance of malignant cells being present within the abdominal cavity (Stage IIIa) increases with higher grades of cancer and with deeper invasion of the tumor into the uterine wall.

There is some controversy over the significance of malignant cells floating in the abdominal cavity, but most gynecologic oncologists recommend treatment with radiation therapy to the entire abdomen, intra-abdominal radioactive substances such as chromic phosphate, progestational hormone therapy or combination chemotherapy.

Which treatment is the most appropriate remains controversial because there is not enough information about the risk for recurrence and the prognosis.

Five-Year Survival Up to 30 percent

Investigational
♦ Postoperative pelvic radiation.
♦ Pelvic and whole-abdomen radiation.
♦ Intra-abdominal radiation (radioactive phosphate).
♦ Pelvic radiation and intravenous combination chemotherapy with cisplatin or carboplatin + Adriamycin or mitoxantrone + Cytoxan.
♦ Intravenous combination chemotherapy alone.
♦ Intra-abdominal chemotherapy (cisplatin or carboplatin).
♦ Occasionally high-dose progestational hormones.

STAGE IIIb
Vaginal metastases.

Standard Treatment This stage is generally treated by abdominal hysterectomy, removal of the tubes and ovaries on both sides, thorough staging and, occasionally, surgical excision of the metastases.

These cases are then usually treated with external beam radiation therapy to the pelvis and vagina (total dose 4,000 to

5,000 cGy given in divided doses five days a week for four to five weeks). This is followed by either a temporary cesium insertion or the placing of radioactive iridium directly into the cancer (interstitial implant). Sometimes radiation therapy precedes surgery.

Endometrial cancer that extends locally outside the uterus is usually treated with radiation therapy—five weeks of external radiation therapy to the pelvis followed by two temporary cesium insertions two weeks apart or by a radioactive iridium interstitial implant—followed by surgery, if possible.

Five-Year Survival Up to 30 percent

Investigational See Stage IIb.

STAGE IIIc
Metastases to the pelvic and/or para-aortic lymph nodes.

Standard Treatment After surgery, women with positive pelvic and negative aortic lymph nodes receive external beam pelvic radiation therapy. If the para-aortic lymph nodes are involved, most gynecologic oncologists recommend radiation therapy to the aortic region as well.

Many gynecologic oncologists also recommend adjuvant chemotherapy such as cisplatin or carboplatin, Adriamycin or Cytoxan for women with positive aortic node metastases.

Five-Year Survival Up to 30 percent

Investigational See Stage Ib.

STAGE IVa
The tumor invades the bladder or rectum.

Standard Treatment Treatment of cancer involving the bladder or rectum is usually by external radiation therapy to the pelvis followed by two insertions of radioactive cesium or interstitial radiation with iridi-

um inserted directly into the tumor.

Whole-pelvis radiation therapy followed by the surgical removal of the uterus, vagina, bladder and/or rectum (pelvic exenteration) is another acceptable therapy.

Five-Year Survival Up to 5 percent

Investigational
♦ Studies are looking at the role of adjuvant chemotherapy with Adriamycin, mitoxantrone, cisplatin, Cytoxan, carboplatin, ifosfamide or progestational hormones in various doses and regimens.

STAGE IVb
Distant metastases, intra-abdominal spread or disease in the lymph nodes of the groin.

Standard Treatment Treatment is based on the location of the distant metastasis, with the most common sites being the lungs or liver. Therapy is rarely curative and is usually palliative.

There is a 20 to 30 percent response rate to progestational hormones. If the metastatic cancer or the initial uterine tumor is sensitive to progestational hormones, as shown by the number of progesterone receptors it contains, then the response rate to hormone therapy will be significantly higher. The most commonly used progestational agent is Megace. Similarly, if the tumor contains many estrogen receptors, then antiestrogen therapy with tamoxifen may be effective with a response rate of 20 to 30 percent. Sometimes the two hormones are used together.

Chemotherapy with cisplatin + Adriamycin + Cytoxan every three to four weeks has been shown to be effective in some patients, with response rates in the range of 30 percent.

Chemotherapy is frequently given with hormones to many women and is given alone to those women whose tumors are estrogen or progesterone receptor negative. Women with intra-abdominal metastases can be treated with intra-abdominal chemotherapy (cisplatin or carboplatin).

Occasionally, palliative radiation therapy may be given to a localized distant metastasis.

Five-Year Survival Up to 5 percent

Investigational
♦ Chemotherapeutic drugs given in various doses and combinations are being studied. These include cisplatin, carboplatin, Adriamycin, mitoxantrone, Cytoxan, ifosfamide, 5-fluorouracil, methotrexate and Taxol with or without progestational hormones or antiestrogenic drugs.

TREATMENT FOLLOW-UP

Most gynecologic oncologists recommend a general physical and pelvic examination including a Pap smear every three months for the first two years, then every six months for another three years.
♦ The serum CA-125 level can be monitored if it was elevated before therapy.
♦ X-ray studies are done whenever specific signs and symptoms warrant.

RECURRENT CANCER

Approximately 70 percent of recurrences take place within three years of the initial therapy. Symptoms of recurrent cancer may include vaginal bleeding or discharge, pain in the pelvis, abdomen, back or legs, leg swelling (edema), weight loss and chronic cough.

Local recurrences—those in the pelvic wall, vagina and the tissue surrounding the cervix and uterus (parametrium)—are the most common sites in women who have not received pelvic radiation; distant metastases to the lung, liver or abdominal cavity are more common in women who have.

Radiation therapy, if not given previously, may cure those women with a vaginal or parametrial recurrence. In women who have a localized vaginal recurrence involving the bladder or rectum, the removal of the bladder and/or rectum and vagina (total pelvic exenteration) can be curative in 40 to 50 percent of cases.

Unfortunately, most women with recurrent endometrial cancer outside the pelvis cannot be cured. But symptoms may be relieved with progestational therapy, antiestrogen therapy or chemotherapy as noted above.

THE MOST IMPORTANT QUESTIONS YOU CAN ASK
♦ What qualifications do you have for treating cancer? Will a specialist in gynecologic oncology be involved in my case?
♦ Why do I need radiation therapy?
♦ Is chemotherapy of any benefit?
♦ Can I take estrogen replacement therapy?
♦ What symptoms of recurrent cancer should I be looking for after treatment?

UTERUS: UTERINE SARCOMAS

Jeffrey L. Stern, MD

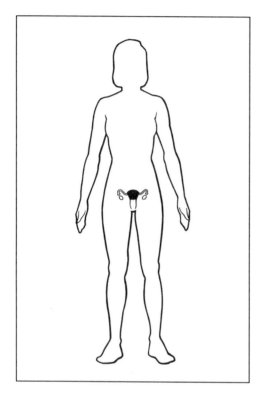

Uterine sarcomas are very rare. They are responsible for only 1 to 5 percent of all malignancies of the uterus (*see* "Uterus: Endometrial Carcinoma" for the much more common cancer of the uterus) and account for less than 1 percent of all gynecologic malignancies (*see* page 348).

Uterine sarcomas are treated like other uterine cancers, but the rate of cure is not high—50 to 75 percent for early-stage disease and less than 10 percent for advanced sarcomas.

Symptoms are similar to those of endometrial carcinoma, but some women are first diagnosed as having a benign uterine tumor called a fibroid. After this rapidly growing, presumably benign fibroid is surgically removed, the pathologist finds that it is a cancerous tumor.

Types There are two general categories of tumors, pure and mixed. Those pure tumors arising from the smooth muscle of the uterine wall or from a benign fibroid are known as leiomyosarcomas and account for about 30 percent of all uterine sarcomas. Leiomyosarcomas are considered benign if there are less than 5 dividing cells on microscopic examination and malignant if there are more than 10 dividing cells. If there are between 5 to 10 dividing cells, they are considered low-grade malignancies.

Another 15 percent of uterine sarcomas arise from the supporting stromal cells that surround the glands within the lining of the uterus (the endometrium) and are known as pure endometrial stromal sarcomas. They are classified according to grade, from the less virulent low-grade tumors to the extremely virulent high-grade tumors.

The most common type of uterine sarcomas—half of all cases—arise from both the endometrial glands *and* the supporting stromal cells of the endometrium. These are known as mixed mesodermal sarcomas, and are further subdivided into homologous and heterologous tumors. The homologous variety—also known as carcinosarcomas—contain malignant cells transformed from cells normally found in the uterus. The heterologous type—called malignant mixed mesodermal tumors—contain cellular elements not normally found in the uterus, including malignant bone, fat, cartilage and striated muscle.

Heterologous mixed mesodermal

tumors are the most common type of uterine sarcoma and account for 1 to 3 percent of all uterine cancers. Homologous tumors are much less common.

How It Spreads Uterine sarcomas can grow locally to involve the tissue surrounding the uterus and cervix, to the rectum and bladder, to the groin, pelvic and aortic lymph nodes, to the surfaces of the abdominal cavity and distantly to the liver, lung and brain (*see* page 348).

Leiomyosarcomas spread by direct local extension, abdominal implantation or via the bloodstream. The lung is the most common site of metastases, followed by the liver, brain and bone.

Low-grade stromal sarcomas are usually slow growing and tend to remain confined to the uterus in about 70 percent of cases. Spread beyond the uterus occurs via the lymph system or via the bloodstream. High-grade stromal sarcomas spread in similar ways, but they behave much more aggressively and are usually advanced at the time of diagnosis.

What Causes It The exact cause is unknown. Like the more common endometrial carcinoma, heterologous mixed mesodermal tumors appear to be associated with diabetes, hypertension and obesity. There is also a significant association with previous pelvic radiation (10 to 30 percent of cases). The average time interval between pelvic radiation and the development of the sarcoma is 15 to 20 years.

Unlike other uterine sarcomas, leiomyosarcomas have no association with previous pelvic radiation.

RISK FACTORS

Heterologous mixed mesodermal tumors can occur in any age group, including infants, but they most commonly occur in postmenopausal women with a median age of 65. Homologous mixed mesodermal tumors can also occur in all age groups, but the median age is 57 years.

For leiomyosarcomas, the average age at diagnosis is 53.

Low-grade stromal sarcomas occur much more frequently in premenopausal women, with 70 percent occurring in women under 50. High-grade stromal sarcomas most commonly occur in postmenopausal women.

At Significantly Higher Risk
♦ Previous pelvic radiation.
♦ Women who are diabetic, hypertensive or obese.

SCREENING
—*See* "Endometrial Carcinoma"

COMMON SIGNS AND SYMPTOMS
—*See* "Endometrial Carcinoma"

DIAGNOSIS
—*See* "Endometrial Carcinoma"

Imaging
♦ Chest x-ray.
♦ Pelvic and abdominal CT scans to detect pelvic extension of tumor, pelvic and aortic lymph nodes and liver metastases.
♦ Pelvic MRI.

STAGING
—*See* "Endometrial Carcinoma'

TREATMENT OVERVIEW
—*See* "Endometrial Carcinoma"

TREATMENT BY CELL TYPE
MIXED MESODERMAL SARCOMAS
The prognosis depends mainly on the stage of the cancer. There does not seem to be any difference in survival between

homologous and heterologous mixed mesodermal tumors.

Standard Treatment Hysterectomy, removal of tubes and ovaries on both sides, washings to check for malignant cells in the abdominal cavity and sampling of the pelvic and aortic lymph nodes on both sides.

After surgery, most women are treated with radiation therapy (total dose 4,000 to 5,000 cGy given in divided doses five days a week for five weeks) to the entire pelvis, including the upper vagina.

Chemotherapy is often used as an adjuvant therapy, although there is no documented proof of its benefit.

Investigational
♦ A clinical trial now being done by the Gynecologic Oncology Group is comparing ifosfamide with cisplatin versus ifosfamide without cisplatin for the treatment of mixed mesodermal tumors. Thirty-five percent of women respond to intravenous ifosfamide alone.
♦ Adriamycin in combination with DTIC or Cytoxan has been shown to be more effective than Adriamycin alone for advanced disease.
♦ Vincristine and Cytoxan have also been used in combination with actinomycin-D or Adriamycin, with or without DTIC, with some effectiveness.
♦ Mitoxantrone, a drug similar to Adriamycin, with ifosfamide is being studied.

LEIOMYOSARCOMA
Good prognostic factors for this tumor type include the presence of a small tumor, a tumor arising from a benign uterine fibroid (5 to 10 percent of all cases), a low number of dividing cells and being premenopausal.

Standard Treatment Abdominal hysterectomy, removal of the tubes and ovaries, washings to check for malignant cells in the abdominal cavity and selective sampling of the pelvic and aortic lymph nodes.

Any additional treatment for women with early-stage disease and less than 5 dividing cells per microscopic field has not been shown to be beneficial.

Women with 5 to 10 dividing cells are *sometimes* treated with postoperative pelvic radiation or adjuvant chemotherapy, while women with more than 10 dividing cells are *usually* given these treatments.

Postoperative whole-pelvis external beam radiation therapy (total dose 4,000 to 5,000 cGy given in divided doses five days a week for five weeks) is sometimes given to decrease the local recurrence rate in early-stage disease.

Although postoperative pelvic radiation and/or chemotherapy are often given, they have not been shown conclusively to increase survival. The most commonly used chemotherapeutic drugs include vincristine + Adriamycin or actinomycin-D + Cytoxan + DTIC.

Advanced leiomyosarcoma is treated with radiation therapy and/or chemotherapy.

Investigational
♦ Current studies include comparing postoperative pelvic radiation therapy versus no treatment, and chemotherapy.
♦ Cisplatin has been shown not to be of benefit.
♦ For women with advanced disease, Adriamycin in combination with DTIC or Cytoxan has been shown to be no more effective than Adriamycin alone.
♦ Vincristine has been used with actinomycin-D or Adriamycin and Cytoxan with or without DTIC with some effectiveness in advanced disease.
♦ Mitoxantrone, a drug similar to Adriamycin, and ifosfamide are being studied.

LOW-GRADE ENDOMETRIAL STROMAL SARCOMA
Standard Treatment As with the other types, the standard treatment for these sar-

comas usually includes a hysterectomy, removal of the tubes and ovaries on both sides, selective pelvic and aortic node sampling and abdominal cytologic washings.

Early-stage disease can also be treated by a radical hysterectomy, removal of the pelvic lymph nodes and sampling of the aortic nodes, removal of the tubes and ovaries and abdominal cytologic washings.

Postoperative radiation therapy to the pelvis (4,500 to 5,000 cGy given in divided doses, five days a week for five weeks) is often given to decrease the chance of a pelvic recurrence. The frequency of recurrence depends primarily on the depth of uterine invasion.

Since these tumors frequently contain progesterone and/or estrogen receptors, hormone therapy with progestins or the antiestrogen tamoxifen is often given.

Investigational
♦ Various types and doses of progestins and antiestrogens are being studied.

HIGH-GRADE ENDOMETRIAL STROMAL SARCOMA
Standard Treatment For high grade stromal sarcomas, standard therapy is a hysterectomy, removal of the tubes and ovaries, selective pelvic and aortic node sampling and washings from the abdominal cavity to look for malignant cells.

For early-stage cancer, postoperative pelvic radiation therapy (total dose of 4,000 to 5,000 cGy given in divided doses, five days a week for five weeks) is recommended because it decreases the chance of a pelvic recurrence.

Adjuvant chemotherapy is sometimes given, but it should be considered experimental.

Investigational
♦ Since pelvic and distant recurrences are common and the prognosis of this malignancy is poor, many gynecologic oncologists and medical oncologists recommend adjuvant chemotherapy even though it has not yet been shown to be effective.

♦ Adriamycin in combination with DTIC or Cytoxan has been shown to be no more effective than Adriamycin alone.
♦ Vincristine and Cytoxan in combination with actinomycin-D or Adriamycin with or without DTIC may be somewhat effective.
♦ Mitoxantrone, a drug similar to Adriamycin, and ifosfamide are being studied.

TREATMENT BY STAGE

STAGE I—See "Endometrial Carcinoma"

Five-Year Survival 75 percent for Stage Ia, 50 percent for Stages Ib and Ic

STAGE IIa—See "Endometrial Carcinoma" The tumor involves the endocervical glands.

Five-Year Survival 50 percent

STAGE IIb—See "Endometrial Carcinoma" Cervical stromal invasion.

Five-Year Survival 50 percent

STAGE IIIa—See "Endometrial Carcinoma"

Five-Year Survival 0 to 20 percent

STAGE IIIb—See "Endometrial Carcinoma" There are vaginal metastases.

Five-Year Survival 0 to 10 percent

STAGE IIIc —See "Endometrial Carcinoma" Metastases to the pelvic and para-aortic lymph nodes.

Five-Year Survival 0 to 10 percent

Investigational See adjuvant chemotherapies under "Treatment by Cell Type."

STAGE IVa—See "Endometrial Carcinoma" The tumor invades the bladder or rectum.

Five-Year Survival 0 to 5 percent

STAGE IVb
There are distant metastases, with spread to organs within the abdomen and/or disease in the groin lymph nodes.

Standard Treatment Metastatic sarcomas are usually treated with chemotherapy. Commonly used drugs include Adriamycin or ifosfamide alone and the combinations of vincristine + actinomycin-D or Adriamycin + Cytoxan + DTIC.

Five-Year Survival 0 to 5 percent

Investigational
♦ Various doses and combinations of chemotherapy drugs are being evaluated.
♦ Mitoxantrone, a drug similar to Adriamycin, is being studied.

TREATMENT FOLLOW-UP

—*See "Endometrial Carcinoma"*

RECURRENT CANCER

Uterine sarcomas usually recur within three years of treatment and may develop in the vagina, pelvis, lymph nodes, liver and lungs. Recurrences of leiomyosarcomas are usually distant, with only 5 percent confined to the pelvis. Recurrences of low-grade stromal sarcomas can occur late, sometimes 10 years after initial treat-ment. Although pelvic recurrences are the most common, it can recur in the abdominal cavity or in the lungs.

Common symptoms of recurrent cancer include vaginal bleeding or discharge, pain in the pelvis, abdomen, back or legs, swelling in the legs or abdomen, chronic cough or weight loss.

Treatment There is no standard therapy for recurrent disease.
♦ Chemotherapy has been used with variable effectiveness but rarely leads to a cure.
♦ Women with localized disease in the pelvis sometimes benefit from radiation therapy and occasionally by the removal of the pelvic organs (pelvic exenteration).
♦ Women with low-grade endometrial stromal sarcomas might benefit from progestational hormone or antiestrogen therapy.

THE MOST IMPORTANT QUESTIONS YOU CAN ASK

♦ What qualifications do you have for treating cancer? Are you a specialist in gynecologic oncology?
♦ What kind of sarcoma do I have?
♦ What is the stage?
♦ What benefit is there to having radiation therapy after surgery?
♦ Is there any benefit from chemotherapy?

VAGINA

Jeffrey L. Stern, MD

◇

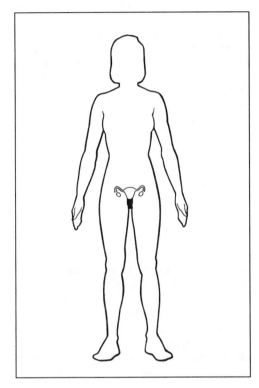

Carcinoma of the vagina is a relatively uncommon disease, affecting only about 2,000 women in the United States each year. It accounts for only 1 to 2 percent of all gynecologic malignancies and occurs primarily in postmenopausal women. Cancer arising in another organ that spreads to the vagina is much more common.

Types The most common type of vaginal cancer develops in the surface (squamous) cells lining the vagina. About 85 percent of all vaginal cancers are squamous cell tumors. About 5 percent develop in glan-

dular tissues (adenocarcinoma). Other cell types include melanoma (3 percent), sarcomas (3 percent) and endodermal sinus tumor (1 percent).

Squamous cell carcinomas, leiomyosarcomas and melanomas generally arise in older women. Adenocarcinomas and rhabdomyosarcomas usually occur during adolescence. The very rare sarcoma botryoides and endodermal sinus tumors most frequently occur in infants.

How It Spreads Squamous cell carcinomas that originate in the skin lining of the vagina can remain confined to the lining for some time. At this stage it is known as vaginal intraepithelial neoplasia (VAIN) or dysplasia. Eventually it will invade the vaginal wall. With time, the tumor can extend directly to the tissue surrounding the vagina, the pelvic walls, the bladder or the rectum. (*See* page 348.)

Lymphatic invasion and metastases is another avenue of spread. Carcinomas arising in the upper vagina can spread to the pelvic lymph nodes, and those in the lower vagina can spread to the lymph nodes in the groin.

Adenocarcinomas spread in a similar fashion, but they may have a higher incidence of metastases to the pelvic lymph nodes.

What Causes It The human papilloma virus (HPV), a sexually transmitted virus responsible for genital warts, is believed to cause vaginal intraepithelial neoplasia and invasive squamous cell carcinoma of the vagina. The time from infection to the development of an invasive cancer is thought to be from 5 to 10 years.

Most cases of adenocarcinoma of the vagina used to be associated with exposure to diethylstilbestrol (DES) in embryonic life. DES was given in the 1950s to women who were thought to be at risk for a miscarriage. The incidence of DES-related adenocarcinoma is highest for those women who were exposed during the first three months of their mother's pregnancy. The peak incidence is between age 17 and 21. The incidence of this disease peaked in the early 1970s and is now uncommon, since DES use during pregnancy fell out of favor during the 1960s and was banned in the early 1970s.

What causes the other vaginal malignancies is not clear.

RISK FACTORS

Squamous cell carcinoma of the vagina is associated with a previous history of genital warts or of intraepithelial or invasive carcinoma of the cervix or vulva. In 10 to 20 percent of women with squamous cell carcinoma of the vagina, there is a history of vaginal radiation therapy, usually for a cervical cancer.

SCREENING

Screening for malignancies of the vagina is similar to screening for cervical cancer. A careful annual pelvic examination and Pap smear is recommended. Women who have been exposed to DES are followed more carefully with twice-yearly pelvic examinations, Pap smears of the cervix and vaginal wall and colposcopic (magnification) examination of the vagina.

COMMON SIGNS AND SYMPTOMS

The most common symptoms are abnormal vaginal bleeding and a foul-smelling vaginal discharge. There may be pain in the pelvis, back or legs, as well as leg swelling (edema).

DIAGNOSIS

Physical Examination
◆ A careful gynecologic, pelvic and rectal examination is performed to assess the local spread of the cancer.
◆ Examination of the lymph nodes in the groin and neck and an abdominal examination are important to detect masses.

Blood and Other Tests
◆ Complete blood count (CBC).
◆ Serum carcinoembryonic antigen (CEA).
◆ Serum squamous cell carcinoma antigen (SCCA).
◆ Serum alpha-fetoprotein (for an endodermal sinus tumor).
◆ Serum kidney and liver function tests.

Imaging
◆ Chest x-ray.
◆ CT scan of the pelvis and abdomen.
◆ MRI of the pelvis.

Endoscopy and Biopsy
◆ Cystourethroscopy.
◆ Proctosigmoidoscopy.
◆ The cancer is confirmed by a vaginal biopsy.

STAGING

Vaginal carcinoma is staged by either the FIGO system (International Federation of Gynecology and Obstetricians) or the TNM classification. In the TNM system, N1 indicates pelvic lymph node metastases when the upper two-thirds of the vagina is involved or groin node metastases on one side when the lower two-thirds of the vagina is involved. N2 indicates groin node metastases on both sides.

TREATMENT OVERVIEW

Several factors are considered in choosing

the most appropriate way to manage vaginal cancer, including the cell type, stage, size, location of the lesion, presence or absence of the uterus and whether the woman has had previous radiation to the pelvis.

Early carcinomas are generally treated with either surgery or radiation therapy—external radiation and one or two insertions of radioactive cesium placed against the cancer (intracavitary) or radioactive iridium placed directly into the cancer (interstitial radiation). The total dose of 4,000 to 5,000 cGy is given in divided doses to the pelvis five days a week for five weeks.

Advanced cancers are treated with radiation therapy alone or with the simultaneous administration of combination chemotherapy.

If the serum CEA, SCCA or AFP (for endodermal sinus tumors) was elevated before therapy, it can be checked periodically to assess response to treatment or detect recurrent disease.

TREATMENT BY STAGE

STAGE 0 (squamous cell carcinoma)
TNM Tis, N0, M0
Carcinoma in situ or intraepithelial carcinoma.

Standard Treatment There are a number of effective treatments, including the partial or complete removal of the vagina (vaginectomy), which occasionally requires a skin graft. The tumor may also be treated with laser therapy, intravaginal chemotherapy with 5-fluorouracil cream or intracavitary radiation with a cesium implant.

Five-Year Survival 100 percent

Investigational None.

STAGE I (squamous cell carcinoma or adenocarcinoma)
TNM T1, N0, M0
The carcinoma is limited to the vaginal wall.

Standard Treatment Young women with lesions involving the upper third of the vagina can be treated by a radical vaginectomy, radical hysterectomy and removal of the pelvic lymph nodes on both sides.

Equally effective for all Stage I tumors, regardless of age and site, are external beam radiation therapy and intracavitary or interstitial radiation therapy. Smaller lesions are sometimes treated with only intracavitary or interstitial radiation therapy.

Five-Year Survival 70 to 80 percent

Investigational
♦ Meticulous surgical staging before radiation therapy.
♦ Chemotherapy given simultaneously with radiation therapy. Chemotherapeutic regimens under investigation include mitomycin-C + 5-fluorouracil (5-FU) with or without cisplatin.
♦ Radiation therapy with heat (hyperthermia).

STAGE II *(squamous cell carcinoma and adenocarcinoma)*
TNM T2, N0, M0
The carcinoma involves the adjacent vaginal tissue but has not extended to the pelvic wall.

Standard Treatment External beam radiation and interstitial or intracavitary radiation.

Five-Year Survival About 50 percent

Investigational Same as Stage I.

STAGE III and STAGE IVa
(squamous cell carcinoma and adenocarcinoma)
TNM T3 (or less), N1, M0 or T3, N0, M0
(Stage III)
The carcinoma has extended to the pelvic wall.

TNM Any T, N2, M0 or T4, N0, M0 (Stage IVa)

The carcinoma has extended beyond the true pelvis or involves the lining of the bladder or rectum.

Standard Treatment These carcinomas are generally treated with external beam, intracavitary or interstitial radiation therapy. Surgery is an option in selected cases.

Five-Year Survival About 30 percent for Stage III, about 10 percent for Stage IVa

Investigational Same as Stage I.

STAGE IVb
TNM Any T, any N, M1
There is spread to distant organs.

Standard Treatment Neither radiation nor surgery can cure women with distant metastases, but both are used for local relief of symptoms.

A number of chemotherapy regimens that are effective in the treatment of metastatic cervical cancer are also used to treat metastatic vaginal cancers—cisplatin, carboplatin and the combinations of mitomycin-C + vincristine + bleomycin + cisplatin and cisplatin + ifosfamide + etoposide.

Five-Year Survival Less than 10 percent

Investigational
◆ Various doses and combinations of chemotherapeutic drugs are being evaluated, including cisplatin, carboplatin, ifosfamide, etoposide, mitomycin-C, 5-FU, vincristine, vinblastine, mitoxantrone, bleomycin and methotrexate.

TREATING OTHER CELL TYPES

Endodermal Sinus Tumors These are extremely rare and are treated with surgery and combination chemotherapy programs such as cisplatin + bleomycin + etoposide.

Vaginal Sarcomas Sarcomas of the botryoid type are treated with chemotherapy, including vincristine, actinomycin-D, Cytoxan and dacarbazine (DTIC) or Mesna + ifosfamide + adriamycin + DTIC followed by surgery or radiation therapy.

Malignant Melanoma These tumors are generally treated by aggressive surgery, but the overall survival rate is extremely poor—less than 15 percent. Advanced melanomas are treated with chemotherapy regimens including dacarbazine (DTIC) + cisplatin + Cytoxan + tamoxifen (*see* "Melanoma").

TREATMENT FOLLOW-UP

After therapy, women are followed every three months with a careful general physical examination, pelvic examination and Pap smear.
◆ A chest x-ray or an abdominal or pelvic CT scan may be obtained if symptoms warrant.
◆ If the serum CEA and/or AFP were elevated before therapy, they can be followed to detect recurrent disease.

RECURRENT CANCER

Vaginal cancer can recur in the vagina, pelvis, liver, lungs and lymph nodes. Symptoms of recurrent disease include weight loss, vaginal or rectal bleeding, bleeding from the urinary tract, pain in the pelvis, back or leg, leg swelling and the development of a chronic cough.
◆ If the tumor is confined to the vagina, bladder and/or rectum, a recurrent vaginal carcinoma may be treated by the removal of the vagina, bladder and/or rectum (pelvic exenteration).
◆ Locally recurrent unresectable and/or metastatic disease is treated with single chemotherapeutic drugs such as cisplatin or

carboplatin, or combination chemotherapeutic drug regimens such as mitomycin-C + vincristine + bleomycin + cisplatin, or carboplatin/or cisplatin + ifosfamide + etoposide.

Investigational

♦ Various doses and combinations of the different chemotherapeutic drugs are being studied, including cisplatin, carboplatin, ifosfamide, etoposide, mitomycin-C, 5-FU, vincristine, vinblastine, mitoxantrone, bleomycin and methotrexate.

THE MOST IMPORTANT QUESTIONS YOU CAN ASK

♦ What qualifications do you have for treating cancer?
♦ Will a gynecologic oncologist be involved in my care?
♦ What stage of cancer do I have?
♦ What is the cell type?
♦ Was the cancer related to DES (diethylstilbestrol)?
♦ Will concurrent chemotherapy be of value in the treatment of my cancer?
♦ What signs and symptoms should I look for after I've been treated?

VULVA
Jeffrey L. Stern, MD

◇

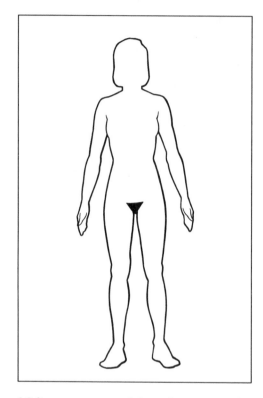

Malignant tumors of the vulva account for 3 to 5 percent of all cancers of the female genital tract and are easily cured when diagnosed at an early stage. And, because of better access to routine gynecologic care, these cancers are being diagnosed at an earlier stage.

Surgery has long been the mainstay of treatment, but views about the extent of surgery have changed over the years. In the 1940s, it was noted that the failure rate was much higher with conservative surgical measures. Since then, more radical operations have been performed with a marked improvement in the survival rate. But recently, as younger women with earlier disease are diagnosed with vulvar cancer, there has been a trend toward more conservative surgery with a greater emphasis on limiting the psychosexual consequences of therapy and preserving the normal female genital anatomy. Similarly, there has been a recent trend toward using local radiation therapy with chemotherapy in advanced cases either to reduce the amount of surgery needed or to improve the chance that the tumor can be removed.

Types Squamous cell carcinomas account for about 86 percent of all vulvar malignancies. Melanoma accounts for another 6 percent, adenocarcinoma of the Bartholin's gland for 4 percent, sarcomas for 2 percent, basal cell carcinoma for 2 percent and Paget's disease for 0.5 percent of all vulvar cancers.

Some physicians believe that the grade of the tumor cells as seen under the microscope is also significant. Immature, or undifferentiated, cells are more virulent and aggressive. Grade 1 (mature, or well-differentiated) cancers have a better prognosis than Grade 3 (poorly differentiated) tumors.

How It Spreads Squamous cell carcinoma arises in the skin of the genitalia and stays confined to the skin for an estimated 1 to 10 years. (At this stage, it is referred to as a carcinoma in situ or vulvar intraepithelial neoplasia—VIN.) Eventually it becomes invasive. With time it becomes locally destructive, growing to involve the urethra, vagina and the anus. It can also spread through the lymphatic system to the lymph nodes in the groin, then to the lymph nodes in the pelvis. Distant metastases, most frequently to the lungs and liver, are relatively rare (*see* page 348).

What Causes It Like carcinoma of the cervix, the risk factors for the development of vulvar cancer are primarily related to the likelihood of exposure to the sexually transmitted human papilloma virus (HPV).

RISK FACTORS

♦ The vast majority of women with invasive vulvar carcinoma are post-menopausal. But there has been a definite trend over the past two decades of an increasing incidence of carcinoma in situ and invasive squamous cell carcinoma in younger women. Forty percent of women with carcinoma in situ are under 40 years old.

♦ Five to ten percent of women with invasive vulvar carcinoma have a history of genital warts, and 15 percent have a history of or subsequent diagnosis of a cancer confined to the skin (carcinoma in situ) or invasive carcinoma of the cervix.

♦ Approximately 80 percent of the invasive squamous lesions of the vulva are associated with human papilloma virus types 16 or 18.

♦ Other sexually transmitted diseases such as syphilis, lymphogranuloma venereum and herpes simplex virus II also increase the risk for vulvar carcinoma.

♦ There is a higher incidence in women from lower socioeconomic groups, women with multiple partners and women with a history of infectious vulvitis or a history of vulvar dystrophy (abnormal benign or premalignant skin changes).

SCREENING

Careful visual and manual inspection of the external genitalia during an annual gynecologic examination is important. Women with a diagnosis of an HPV-related infection of any portion of the lower genital tract should undergo a careful col-poscopic (magnification) examination of the entire lower genital tract.

COMMON SIGNS AND SYMPTOMS

The most common signs and symptoms are a lump or an ulcer, itching, pain, burning, bleeding and discharge. Unfortunately, many women do not get medical attention when these signs appear. At the time of diagnosis, two out of three women with vulvar carcinoma have had symptoms for more than six months and one out of three has had symptoms for more than a year.

DIAGNOSIS

Physical Examination

♦ Careful visual and manual inspection of the external genitalia, anus and groin lymph nodes is crucial.

♦ Because of the association with precancerous and cancerous lesions of the cervix and vagina, a careful pelvic examination is also necessary.

♦ The majority of squamous cell carcinomas arise on the labia majora and minora and are frequently associated with vulvar dystrophy. The clitoris, outer vagina and the skin between the vagina and anus (perineum) may also be involved

Endoscopy and Biopsy

♦ The definitive diagnosis is made on a biopsy, sometimes under colposcopic direction (magnification) for smaller lesions.

♦ Upon diagnosis, a metastatic work-up is done, including a chest x-ray, CT scan of the pelvis and abdomen (occasionally), cystoscopy and proctoscopy (occasionally), a complete blood count and serum liver and kidney function tests.

STAGING

Staging is based on physical findings and x-ray results. Both the FIGO (International

Federation of Gynecology and Obstetricians) and the TNM classifications are used to stage vulvar cancer.

TREATMENT OVERVIEW

The prognosis for vulvar cancer depends on several factors—cell type, stage (which emphasizes local tumor extent), the presence or absence of groin node metastases, the size of the lesion, the depth of invasion, whether blood or lymphatic vessels are involved, the grade of the tumor and the pattern of invasion.

At diagnosis, about 35 percent of all vulvar carcinomas are Stage I, 30 percent of women have Stage II, 25 percent have Stage III and 10 percent have Stage IV disease. The overall five-year survival rate for all women with invasive squamous cell carcinoma of the vulva is 69 percent.

Surgery The standard therapy for the past four decades has been radical surgical excision of the vulva and the removal of the lymph nodes in the groin and, occasionally, the pelvis. External beam radiation therapy is frequently given to the groin and pelvis after surgery to women with positive groin and/or pelvic lymph nodes on one or both sides.

Over the past 15 years, less radical surgery and the removal of the groin nodes on one side has been shown to be equally effective in small, early-stage disease. Despite this trend toward conservative therapy, experience has taught that limiting surgery because of advanced age or frailty can result in overwhelming problems with locally advanced recurrent cancer in women who have lived longer than expected.

A radical vulvectomy and groin dissection is extraordinarily well tolerated and can be done in phases if the patient's medical condition warrants. Whether sexual function returns depends on the extent of surgery and radiation therapy. Sexual function is also surprisingly more satisfactory than one would think.

Complications of radical surgery for vulvar cancer include wound breakdown or infection, chronic leg swelling, collection of lymphatic fluid in the groin (lymphocyst), scarring of the vaginal opening, vaginal or uterine prolapse, loss of urine when coughing (stress incontinence), blood clots in the leg that can dislodge and go to the lung (pulmonary embolism, which occurs in 1 to 3 percent of women), and death (approximately 1 to 2 percent).

 Chemotherapy and Radiotherapy In recent years, chemotherapy has been used in combination with local external beam radiation therapy and occasionally with interstitial radiation, in which radioactive iridium is temporarily placed directly into the cancer. This treatment has been used for women with advanced cancers, allowing subsequent surgical removal of the tumor or the preservation of the bladder or anus.

Currently, there is no standard chemotherapy for advanced or recurrent cancer, but drugs that are sometimes effective for other squamous cell carcinomas of the genital tract—such as cisplatin, mitomycin-C, 5-fluorouracil (5-FU), Cytoxan and bleomycin—have been used with some success.

TREATMENT BY STAGE

STAGE 0
TNM Tis, N0, M0
Vulvar carcinoma in situ, also known as intraepithelial carcinoma.

Standard Treatment Standard therapy has been either wide local excision or laser therapy. Occasionally a partial or total vulvectomy is performed with or without skin grafting.

Five-Year Survival 100 percent

Investigational None.

STAGE I
TNM T1, N0, M0
The tumor is confined to vulva and/or perineum, is less than 3/4 in. (2 cm) in diameter and there are no nodal metastases.

Standard Treatment For Grade 1 lesions with less than 2 mm of invasion or Grade 2 lesions with less than 1 mm of invasion and no vascular involvement, a wide local excision is adequate therapy.

For lesions that are clearly on one side of the vulva, a radical local excision with a complete groin node dissection on the same side is performed.

For other Stage I cancers involving the skin between the vaginal opening or the anus or clitoris, a radical vulvectomy and groin lymph node dissection on both sides is performed.

Five-Year Survival Over 90 percent

Investigational
♦ Conservative surgery.
♦ Treatment with radiation therapy with or without chemotherapy (5-FU + mitomycin-C + cisplatin).

STAGE II
TNM T2, N0, M0
The tumor is confined to the vulva and/or perineum and is more than 3/4 in. (2 cm) in diameter but has not spread to lymph nodes.

Standard Treatment Radical vulvectomy with removal of the groin lymph nodes on both sides.

Five-Year Survival 80 percent, up to 90 percent for those patients with surgically negative groin nodes

Investigational Same as Stage I.

STAGE III
TNM T3 or less, N1 or less, M0
The tumor may be of any size with either adjacent spread to the vagina, urethra or anus or metastases to the groin lymph nodes on one side.

Standard Treatment Radical vulvectomy with groin lymph node dissection on both sides is the standard therapy. Sometimes, a pelvic lymph node dissection is done at the time of surgery if the groin lymph nodes are positive.

External beam radiation therapy is frequently given postoperatively to the groin and pelvis if there are groin lymph node metastases. With two or more pathologically positive groin nodes, there has been a significantly better survival rate with pelvic radiation than with pelvic lymph node dissection in a study conducted by the Gynecologic Oncology Group.

Women with large vulvar lesions who have only a small margin of normal tissue around the tumor on microscopic examination of the surgical specimen may be treated with postoperative external beam radiation therapy to the remaining genital skin.

Five-Year Survival About 50 percent

Investigational
♦ Preoperative external beam and interstitial radiation therapy (radioactive substances inserted directly into the tumor for one to two days) with or without chemotherapy (5-FU + mitomycin-C + cisplatin).
♦ Radiation therapy and heat (hyperthermia) have been used to improve resectability and to decrease the amount of surgery necessary in women with large cancers or cancers involving the urethra or anus.

STAGE IVa
TNM Any T, N2, M0 or T4, N0, M0
The tumor may involve the upper urethra, the bladder mucosa, the rectal mucosa, the

pelvic bone, and/or there are bilateral groin node metastases.

Standard Treatment Options include:
♦ Radical vulvectomy, removal of the lymph nodes on both sides and removal of the vagina, bladder and/or rectum (pelvic exenteration).
♦ Surgery followed by radiation therapy in those with close surgical margins.
♦ Radiation therapy with combination chemotherapy (5-FU + mitomycin-C + cisplatin), occasionally followed by radical surgery.

Five-Year Survival About 15 percent

Investigational
♦ External beam radiation therapy and interstitial radiation therapy with or without heat (hyperthermia) and with or without various doses and kinds of chemotherapeutic drugs are being evaluated.

STAGE IVb
TNM Any T, any N, M1a or M1b.
There are distant metastases including pelvic lymph nodes.

Standard Treatment Vulvar cancer that has spread to distant sites is treated with chemotherapy, but there is no standard chemotherapeutic regimen. Cisplatin, carboplatin, methotrexate, vincristine and bleomycin are all commonly used drugs.

Usually palliative local surgical removal or radiation therapy to the vulva is done for local symptom relief.

Women with metastases to the pelvic nodes are treated with pelvic external beam radiation therapy.

Five-Year Survival From 5 percent (metastases to the lungs or liver) to 25 percent (metastases to the pelvic lymph nodes)

Investigational
♦ Ifosfamide, carboplatin, 5-FU, mitomycin-C, methotrexate, vincristine,

bleomycin and cisplatin in various combinations and doses are being investigated.

RECURRENT CANCER

Recurrences are more common in women with large lesions or if treatment involved limited surgery. They usually occur within the first three years after treatment. The recurrence may be anywhere on the remaining external genitalia, in the groin or pelvic nodes or at distant sites. Symptoms of recurrent cancer may include bleeding, pain in the genitals, groin, pelvis or legs, leg swelling (edema), weight loss, chronic cough and chest pain.

Treatment options include wide local excision (for a local recurrence), radical local excision, pelvic exenteration, external beam radiation therapy, interstitial radiation therapy and chemotherapy.

TREATING OTHER VULVAR MALIGNANCIES

MALIGNANT MELANOMA OF THE VULVA

Although relatively rare, this is the second most common type of vulvar cancer. It occurs most commonly in women around the age of menopause and in postmenopausal women.

More than 80 percent of melanomas arise from the labia minora and clitoris. Most women seek medical attention because of itching, bleeding or a lump. Superficially spreading melanomas and mucocutaneous melanomas account for approximately 60 percent and 10 percent respectively of all vulvar melanomas and are somewhat slow growing until invasion occurs. Thirty percent are nodular melanomas, which behave much more aggressively.

Standard Treatment Radical vulvectomy and bilateral groin node dissection is the standard therapy, although over the past few years there has been a trend toward more conservative surgery.

Melanomas that are less than 0.7 mm in thickness without vascular space involvement can be treated by a wide local excision with a 3/4 in. (2 cm) skin margin, without a groin dissection.

The role of a pelvic lymph node dissection has not been determined, but if the groin nodes are involved, a pelvic lymph node dissection may be performed. The prognosis and survival is determined in large part by the depth of invasion and whether there are metastases.

Five-Year Survival 40 to 80 percent depending on the stage and the depth of invasion

BASAL CELL CARCINOMA

This type of vulvar cancer invades adjacent tissues but rarely metastasizes. It has an excellent cure rate and is managed with only a wide local excision.

ADENOCARCINOMA OF THE VULVA

This is a rare tumor and generally arises from the Bartholin's gland, located at the opening of the vagina. Survival is related to stage. Treatment is usually radical vulvectomy and bilateral groin node dissection.

PAGET'S DISEASE

This occurs most commonly in post-menopausal white women. Intense itching is the most common symptom.

About 30 percent of Paget's disease is associated with an underlying invasive adenocarcinoma, and for these the prognosis is quite poor. But Paget's disease confined to the vulvar skin has an excellent prognosis with only rare instances of subsequent invasion or death.

If there is no underlying adenocarcinoma, a wide local excision or total vulvectomy is all that is required.

If there is an underlying adenocarcinoma, radical vulvectomy and bilateral groin dissection is usually performed.

VULVAR SARCOMAS

These account for only 1 to 2 percent of all vulvar malignancies. The majority of vulvar sarcomas arise from the smooth muscle and are known as leiomyosarcomas.

Treatment is usually radical surgery followed by radiation therapy.

THE MOST IMPORTANT QUESTIONS YOU CAN ASK

♦ What type of cancer do I have?
♦ Is a radical vulvectomy and removal of the groin lymph nodes on both sides necessary if I have Stage I disease?
♦ Is there a role for radiation therapy with or without chemotherapy for my cancer?
♦ What is my prognosis?
♦ What qualifications do you have for treating cancer? Will a gynecologic oncologist be involved in my care?

GLOSSARY OF MEDICAL TERMS

Malin Dollinger, MD

───────◇───────

A

Absolute neutrophil count (ANC)
The actual count of the white blood cells (also called polys or granulocytes) that engulf and destroy bacteria. There is some concern about infection if the count is less than 1,000.

Acupressure
The use of finger pressure over various points on the body (the same points used in acupuncture) to treat symptoms or disease.

Adenocarcinoma
Cancer that arises from glandular tissues. Examples include cancers of the breast, lung, thyroid, colon and pancreas.

Adenoma
A benign (non-malignant) tumor that arises from glandular tissues, such as the breast, lung, thyroid, colon and pancreas.

Adjuvant chemotherapy
Chemotherapy used along with surgery or radiation therapy. It is usually given after all visible and known cancer has been removed by surgery or radiotherapy, but is sometimes given before surgery (*See* Neoadjuvant chemotherapy). Adjuvant chemotherapy is usually used in cases where there is a high risk of hidden cancer cells remaining and may increase the likelihood of cure by destroying small amounts of undetectable cancer.

Alkaline phosphatase
A blood enzyme commonly used in medical diagnosis. It is elevated in cases of bile obstruction (liver disease or cancer involving the liver) and in various bone diseases, including cancer involving bone. A variation of this test can distinguish between elevations due to bone and liver disease.

Alkylating agents
A family of anticancer drugs that combine with a cancer cell's DNA to prevent normal cell division.

Allogeneic transplant
A form of transplantation or transfer of a tissue—bone marrow, for example—from one individual to another. It is preferable that the tissue types match, but this is not always possible.

Alopecia
Partial or complete loss of hair. This may result from radiotherapy to the head (hair may not completely return after therapy) or from certain chemotherapeutic agents (hair always returns).

Alpha-fetoprotein
A protein that is elevated in the blood of patients with certain forms of cancer, such as liver or testis.

Ambulatory care
The use of outpatient facilities—doctors' offices, home care, outpatient hospital clinics and day-care facilities—to provide modern medical care without the need for hospitalization.

Ambulatory infusion
The administration of chemotherapy by a small pump device usually worn under the clothes. The pump delivers anticancer drugs slowly and gradually, with minimal or no side effects. Since there is no need to remain in the hospital or even at home, this method allows patients to work and carry on with their normal activities.

Amenorrhea
The temporary or permanent lack of menstrual periods. This may be a normal part of the menopause or is sometimes brought on by severe physical or emotional stresses. Some anticancer drugs can produce amenorrhea, especially if the woman is near the age when menopause would normally occur.

Amino acids
The building blocks of proteins, analogous to the freight cars making up a train.

Analgesic
A drug that relieves pain. Analgesics may be mild (aspirin or acetaminophen), stronger (codeine) or very strong (morphine). There are also a large number of mild, moderate or strong synthetic analgesics.

Anaplastic
A tumor that appears "wild" under the microscope, having no resemblance to the normal tissue of the organ involved. It is usually possi-

ble to tell where anaplastic tumors originate only by where the biopsy was taken or, knowing the area of involvement, by inference.

Anastomosis
The point where two organs are joined together. In cancer therapy it usually refers to joining two portions of the bowel after a segment containing cancer has been removed.

Androgens
Male sex hormones. Testosterone is produced naturally and there are several synthetic ones used in treatment.

Anemia
Having less than the normal amount of hemoglobin or red cells in the blood. This may be due to bleeding, lack of blood production by the bone marrow or to the brief survival of blood already manufactured. Symptoms include tiredness, shortness of breath and weakness.

Aneuploid
Tumor cells that do not have the normal number of chromosomes—46—in a human cell. Tumor cells that do have 46 chromosomes are called euploid. Aneuploid tumors often have a worse prognosis.

Angiography
The taking of x-ray pictures of blood vessels by injecting a radio-opaque contrast agent into the blood vessel. Angiograms may be taken to determine a tumor's blood supply before surgery, to place a catheter or infusion pump or to determine the site for other intra-arterial procedures.

Antibody
A protein (gamma globulin) made by the body in response to a specific foreign protein, or antigen. The antigen may result from an infection, a cancer or some other source. If the same alien substance attacks again, the white blood cells are able to recognize it and reproduce the specific antibody to fight it.

Antiemetics
Drugs given to prevent or minimize nausea and vomiting.

Antigens
Substances that cause activation of the immune system.

Antimetabolites
A family of antitumor drugs that resemble normal vitamins or building blocks of metabolism. They bind to the tumor's enzymes and chemical pathways. The tumor cells "think" they are getting the real vitamin or building block and starve to the point where they can't grow or multiply.

Asbestosis
Scarring of the lungs and the lining of the chest cavity from the inhalation of asbestos dust. This increases the risk of lung cancer and cancer of the chest cavity lining (mesothelioma).

Ascites
An abnormal fluid collection in the abdomen from cancer or other causes.

Aspiration
Removal of fluid or tissue, usually with a needle or tube, from a specific area of the body. This procedure may be done to obtain a diagnosis or to relieve symptoms.

Atrophy
A withering or reduction in size of a tissue or a part of the body. This may result from lack of use during immobilization or prolonged bedrest or from pressure from an adjacent tumor.

Atypical
Not usual or ordinary. For example, cancer is the result of atypical cell division.

Autoimmunity
A condition in which the body's immune system fights and rejects its own tissues.

Autologous transplant
Removal of a patient's own tissue, especially bone marrow, and its return to the same patient after chemotherapy. This might more correctly be called bone marrow reinfusion, or protection, rather than transplantation.

Autosomal
A non-sex-linked method of inheritance. The inherited characteristic does not depend on whether the person is male or female since the gene in question is not found on the sex (X or Y) chromosomes.

Axilla
The armpit. Lymph glands in the armpit are called the axillary nodes.

B

Barium enema
An x-ray study of the colon (large bowel) in which the patient is given an enema of a liquid barium mixture before the x-rays are taken. Laxatives and/or regular enemas are usually required beforehand.

Barium swallow
An x-ray study of the portion of the digestive canal between the throat and stomach (esophagus) in which the patient swallows a barium mixture while the radiologist watches for signs of narrowing, irregularity or blockage. No preparation is required except fasting. Sometimes, in a procedure called an upper gastrointestinal (UGI) series, the barium is also observed after it enters the stomach to check for stomach problems or ulcers.

Basal cell carcinoma
A form of skin cancer that grows very slowly and is curable in almost all cases by surgery or other local treatment. The growth may be so slow that malignancy is not at first suspected.

B cell
Lymphocytes are the cells in the body that are intimately involved in the immune response. They occur in the blood, in lymph nodes and in various organs. The two types of lymphocytes are B cells and T cells. Special techniques are needed to tell them apart because they look the same when viewed by ordinary methods under the microscope. It may be essential to make this distinction in cases of lymphomas, since the treatment and prognosis of B cell lymphomas may be very different than that of T cell lymphomas.

BCG
A material prepared from killed bird tuberculosis bacteria. This has been widely used, especially in Europe, to vaccinate health care workers who work closely with tuberculosis patients and has been used in cancer treatment to stimulate the immune system.

Bench surgery
Complete removal of a selected organ or tissue from the body during surgery in order to perform a separate, often delicate or complex, surgical procedure. The organ is then replaced into the body (in its original site; however, sometimes the location is changed). Bench surgery can allow: 1) better control for removal of a tumor, particularly in a vital organ which cannot or does not have to be totally sacrificed, 2) delicate surgery often requiring a microscope, 3) delineation of margins of resection to assure tumor is fully excised or to lessen spilling of cancer cells into the surrounding tissue or cavity, such as the peritoneum, and 4) cooling the organ to permit more time for surgery. A good example of bench surgery is in the treatment of kidney cancer, especially when it occurs in a patient with only one kidney or with boderline renal failure, and when the tumor is located in the center of the kidney. Blood vessels are disconnected temporarily, the kidney is completely removed to a separate operating table (bench), the tumor is removed with repair to the kidney, and then, using vascular surgical techniques, is replaced into the body.

Benign
A tumor that has no tendency to grow into surrounding tissues or spread to other parts of the body. In other words, it is not malignant. Under the microscope, a benign tumor does not resemble cancer.

Bilateral
Occurring on both sides of the body.

Biologic response modifiers
Substances and agents that may have a direct antitumor effect, and also affect tumors indirectly by stimulating or triggering the immune system to fight cancer. Examples include interferon, IL-2 and LAK cells.

Biopsy
The surgical removal of a small portion of tissue for diagnosis. In almost all cases a biopsy diagnosis of cancer is required before appropriate and correct treatment planning can take place. In some cases a needle biopsy may be enough for diagnosis, but in others the removal of a pea-sized wedge of tissue is needed. In many cases, the biopsy may be the first step of the definitive surgical procedure that not only proves the diagnosis but attempts to cure the cancer by completely removing the tumor.

Blastic
A bone lesion that appears on an x-ray to have more calcium (density) than normal.

Bleeding disorders
Blood clotting is a complex process involving the interaction of many substances in the blood that promote coagulation. A deficiency of any of these substances results in a bleeding disorder. Some disorders are inherited (hemophilia, for example) and some (such as liver disease) are acquired. A common disorder associated with cancer is a low platelet count (thrombocytopenia), which sometimes results from chemotherapy or radiotherapy and may make platelet transfusions necessary until the process subsides. Sophisticated tests are often needed to diagnose bleeding disorders.

Blood-brain barrier
A microscopic structure in the brain that separates blood capillaries from nerve cells. This prevents some substances from entering the brain. Many cancer chemotherapeutic agents, for example, cannot be used to treat brain tumors because they cannot pass through the barrier. Some others (CCNU, BCNU) are designed to penetrate it. There are techniques that can eliminate the barrier temporarily to allow the use of other antitumor drugs.

Blood cells
The red cells, white cells and platelets that make up the blood. They are made in the bone marrow.

Blood chemistry panel
Multiple chemical analyses prepared by an automatic apparatus from a single blood sample. These panels often include measurements of electrolytes (minerals) and proteins as well as tests of liver, kidney and thyroid function. The advantages of panels include less cost and greater accuracy and speed, with results often available the same or the following day.

Bolus (or "push") chemotherapy
Administration of intravenous chemotherapy over a short time, usually five minutes or less. The other method is called infusion chemotherapy, which may last from 15 minutes to several hours or days.

Bone marrow
A soft substance found within bone cavities. Marrow is composed of developing red cells, white cells, platelets and fat. Some forms of cancer can be diagnosed by examining bone marrow.

Bone marrow examination
The process of removing bone marrow by withdrawing it through a needle for pathological examination. It is usually withdrawn from the breast bone (sternum) or the hip bone. Both these bones are just under the skin, making the removal of marrow easy, safe and only momentarily uncomfortable with a local anesthetic. The procedure takes about ten minutes—nine and a half minutes for the anesthetic to take effect and 30 seconds for the actual procedure.

Bone marrow suppression
A decrease in one or more of the blood counts. This condition can be caused by chemotherapy, radiation, disease or various medications.

Bone scan
A picture of all of the bones in the body taken about two hours after injection of a radioactive tracer. "Hot spots" indicate areas of bone abnormality that may indicate tumors, although they can also be due to other causes such as arthritis. No preparation is required and the test is easy. The main problem is lying still on a hard table for 15 minutes. This test can help determine if cancer has spread to the bones, if therapy is working and if damaged bony areas are healing.

Brachytherapy
The use of a radioactive "seed" implanted directly into a tumor. This allows a very high but sharply localized dose of radiation to be given to a tumor while sparing surrounding tissues from significant radiation exposure.

Brain scan
A picture of the brain taken after the intravenous injection of a radioactive tracer. CT and MRI scans have in most cases replaced such brain scans, since CT and MRI tend to discover smaller lesions and are more useful for following up the effects of therapy.

Bronchogenic carcinoma
Carcinoma of the lung.

Bronchoscopy
Inspection—and often biopsy—of the breathing tubes (bronchi) going to the lungs by means of a long tube inserted through the mouth or nose. The instrument usually used is a fiber-optic bronchoscope that is flexible and allows excellent visualization around corners. The procedure is often done on an outpatient basis after local anesthesia and sedation.

Bypass
A surgical procedure to "go around" an organ or area affected by cancer and allow normal flow or drainage to continue. In cancer of the pancreas, for example, the bile ducts may be blocked. A bypass procedure will allow the bile to drain into the small bowel, as it should.

C

Cachexia
The wasting away of the body, often due to malnutrition, disease or cancer.

Calcium
An important body mineral that is a vital component of bone. The calcium level may be elevated if tumors involve bone.

Candidiasis (Moniliasis)
A common fungal infection often seen as white patches on the tongue or the inside of the mouth.

Carcinogenesis
The development or production of cancer.

Carcinoma
A form of cancer that develops in the tissues covering or lining organs of the body such as the skin, uterus, lung or breast (epithelial tissues). Eighty to 90 percent of all cancers are carcinomas.

Carcinoma in situ
The earliest stage of cancer, in which the tumor is still confined to the local area, before it has grown to a significant size or has spread. In situ carcinomas are highly curable.

Cardiomyopathy
A condition in which the heart muscle is diseased. It may develop because of the toxic effect of a few anticancer drugs.

CAT scan
See CT scan

Catheter
A tube made of rubber, plastic or metal that can be introduced into a body cavity such as the bladder to drain fluid or to deliver fluids or medication.

Catheterization
The process of introducing a catheter. The term is also used when a tube is placed into an artery or a vein to take x-rays.

CEA (carcinoembryonic antigen)
A "tumor marker" in the blood that may indicate the presence of cancer. It may be elevated in some cancers, especially of the breast, bowel and lung. By monitoring the amount of CEA, doctors can detect the presence of these cancers and assess the progress of treatment.

Cell cycle
Each cell in the body, including a cancer cell, goes through several stages every time it divides. Various anticancer drugs affect the cell at different stages of this cell cycle.

Cell-cycle specific
Chemotherapeutic drugs that kill only cells that are dividing rather than resting.

Cell surface markers
Special proteins on the surface or edge of cells that can be used to identify them or their characteristics.

Cells
The fundamental unit, or building blocks, of human tissues.

Cellular immunity
Immunity brought about by the action of immune cells such as lymphocytes.

Cellulitis
Inflammation of the skin and underlying tissues.

Centigray (cGy)
A unit of measurement of radiation therapy that is replacing the older term *rads*.

Cervical dysplasia
The presence of abnormal—and possibly precancerous—cells in the mouth of the uterus (cervix).

Cervical (lymph) nodes
The lymph nodes in the neck.

Cervix
The lower portion of the uterus, which protrudes into the vagina and forms a portion of the birth canal during delivery. The Pap test is designed to check this area for cancer.

Chemoprevention
Attempting to prevent cancer through drugs, chemicals, vitamins or minerals.

Chemotherapy
The treatment of cancer by chemicals (drugs) designed to kill cancer cells or stop them from growing.

Choriocarcinoma
A carcinoma composed of cells arising in the placenta or the testes.

Chromosomes
The fundamental strands of genetic material (DNA) that carry all our genes. There are 23 pairs in each cell. Tumor cells sometimes have more or fewer than 23 pairs (*see* Aneuploid).

Clinical
Refers to the treatment of humans, as opposed to animals or laboratory studies. Also refers to the general use of a treatment by a practicing physician, as opposed to research done in cancer research centers ("preclinical").

Clinical trials
The procedure in which new cancer treatments are tested in humans. Clinical trials are conducted after experiments in animals and preliminary studies in humans have shown that a new treatment method might be effective.

Clone
A strain of cells—whether normal or malignant—derived from a single original cell.

Clonigenic assay

A test done by growing tumor cells in the laboratory and identifying which chemotherapy agents will prevent their growth. This information is sometimes useful in deciding which drugs to use or not to use in treatment.

Cobalt; cobalt treatment

A radiotherapy machine using gamma rays generated from the radioisotope cobalt 60.

Coin lesion

A single "spot" on a chest x-ray that may be a tumor, infection or other lesion. Given this name because it resembles the shadow of a coin.

Colonoscopy

A procedure to inspect the rectum and colon by means of a long fiber-optic telescope that is lighted and flexible. Biopsy specimens of suspicious tissue can also be obtained.

Colony stimulating factor (CSF)

A substance that stimulates the growth of bone marrow cells. Current clinical trials are using CSF to try to increase the dosage of chemotherapy that can be given safely.

Colostomy

An artificial opening in the abdominal wall created so that feces drains from the colon into a bag. A colostomy is sometimes necessary after the removal of a diseased section of the large intestine, and can be either temporary or permanent (*see* Ostomy).

Colposcopy

A way to detect small lesions by inspecting the cervix with special binocular magnifying instruments after applying a solution to stain cancer tissue.

Combination chemotherapy

The use of several anticancer drugs at the same time. Most chemotherapy is now given this way, since it is a much more effective method.

Combined modality therapy

Treatment with two or more types of therapy—surgery, radiotherapy, chemotherapy and biological therapy. These may be used at the same time or one after the other. Surgery, for example, is often followed by chemotherapy to destroy random cancer cells that may have spread from the original site.

Computerized tomography

See CT scan

Cone biopsy

Removal of a ring of tissue from the opening of the cervix.

Congestive heart failure

Weakness of the heart muscle usually due to heart disease, but sometimes due to other causes, causing a buildup of fluid in body tissues.

Consolidation

A second round of chemotherapy to further reduce the number of cancer cells.

Contralateral

On the opposite side of the body. In cancer therapy it refers to a tumor or a site of disease. (*see also* Ipsilateral)

Cooperative groups

Clinical trials of new cancer treatments require many patients, generally more than any single physician or hospital can see. A number of physicians and/or hospitals form a cooperative group to treat a large number of patients in the same way so that the effectiveness of a new treatment can be evaluated quickly.

Cortisone

A natural hormone produced by the adrenal glands. The term is also loosely used to designate synthetic forms of the hormone (such as prednisone) that are used to treat inflammatory conditions and diseases, including certain cancers.

Cranial irradiation

The delivery of radiation to the brain to treat brain tumors.

Creatinine clearance

A sensitive test of kidney function that requires a 24-hour urine sample and a blood sample. The test is often required to make sure it is safe to give anticancer drugs that may be toxic to the kidneys.

Cruciferous vegetables

Vegetables such as cauliflower and Brussels sprouts that are high in beta carotene and are thought to help protect against colon cancer.

Cryosurgery

The use of a special cold probe as a surgical instrument. It is used to destroy cancer tissues.

CT scan

A CT (computerized tomography) scan creates cross-section images of the body, which may show cancer or metastases earlier and more accurately than other imaging methods. This type of x-ray machine has revolutionized the diagnosis of cancer and other diseases.

Cushing's syndrome

A condition characterized by swelling of the face and back of the neck and purple lines over the abdomen. It results from an excess of cortisone or hydrocortisone caused either by disease or by the administration of these substances or their synthetic derivatives.

Cyst
A fluid-filled sac of tissue that is usually benign but can be malignant. Cysts are sometimes removed just to be sure they are benign. Lumps in the breast are often found to be harmless cysts rather than cancer.

Cystitis
An inflammation and irritation of the bladder caused by bacterial infection, chemotherapy or radiation treatments. Symptoms include a burning sensation when urinating or a frequent urgent need to urinate.

Cytogenetics
Laboratory study or analysis of the chromosome pattern of a cell.

Cytokine
A substance secreted by immune system cells, usually to send "messages" to other immune cells.

Cytology
The study under a microscope of cells that have been cast off or scraped off organs such as the uterus, lungs, bladder or stomach. Also called exfoliative cytology (*see* Pap smear).

Cystoscopy
Inspection of the inside of the bladder by means of a telescope. During the procedure a catheter may also be placed, biopsies taken or tissue removed.

D

Debulking
A procedure that removes a significant part or most of a tumor in cases where it is not possible to remove all of it. This may make subsequent radiotherapy or chemotherapy easier and more effective.

Differentiation
The process of maturation of a cell line of cancer cells. When they are fully differentiated or well-differentiated, they more closely resemble the normal cells in the tissue of origin.

Diuretics
Drugs that increase the elimination of water and salts in the urine.

DNA (deoxyribonucleic acid)
The building block of our genetic material. DNA is responsible for the passing of hereditary characteristics and information on cell growth, division and function.

Dose limiting
A side effect, complication or risk that makes it impossible or unwise to exceed a specific dose of a chemotherapeutic agent. A total dosage of bleomycin of more than 400 units, for example, may produce severe lung scarring. Lung toxicity is, therefore, dose limiting.

Drug resistance
The development of resistance in cancer cells to a specific drug or drugs. If resistance develops, a patient in remission from chemotherapy may relapse despite continued administration of anticancer drugs.

Dysphagia
Difficulty in swallowing; a sensation of food sticking in the throat.

Dysplasia
Abnormal developments or changes in cells, which are sometimes an indication that cancer may develop.

Dyspnea
Shortness of breath.

Dysuria
Difficult or painful urination; burning on urination.

E

Edema
The accumulation of fluid within tissues.

Effusion
A collection of fluid inside a body cavity, such as around the lungs (pleural), intestines (peritoneal) or heart (pericardial). This can be caused by cancer invading the cavity.

Electrolytes
Certain chemicals—including sodium, potassium, chloride and bicarbonate—found in the tissues and blood. They are often measured as an aid to patient care.

Electron beam
A form of radiotherapy in which the beam does not penetrate completely through the body as ordinary x-rays do. It is used for treating the skin or lesions beneath the skin.

Electrophoresis
See Serum protein electrophoresis

Emboli
Pieces of tissue, usually blood clots but sometimes tumor cells, that travel in the circulatory system until they lodge in a small artery or capillary, often in the lungs.

Embolization
A method of treating tumors in a localized area by blocking the blood vessels to the area. This is done by inserting a thin tube (catheter) into an artery and injecting tiny pellets or other materials, which then travel "downstream" and block the smaller arteries. The pellets may also carry chemotherapeutic agents for release in the area ("chemoembolization").

Emesis
A fancy word for vomiting.

Endemic
Refers to a disease process that is common in a particular community or population.

Endocrine glands
Glands—such as the pituitary, thyroid, ovaries and testes—that secrete hormones to control digestion, reproduction, growth, metabolism or other body functions.

Endometrial carcinoma
A cancer of the inner lining (endometrium) of the uterus.

Endoscope
An instrument (telescope) designed to allow examination of hollow organs or body cavities. There are many specialized types such as the cystoscope for the bladder, colonoscope for the colon, gastroscope for the stomach and bronchoscope for the lungs.

Endoscopy
Examination of interior body structures with an endoscope. The physician is able to take photographs, obtain small samples of tissue or remove small growths during the procedure.

Enteral feeding
Administration of liquid food (nutrients) through a tube inserted into the stomach or intestine.

Enterostomal therapist
A medical professional specializing in the care of artificial openings in the abdominal wall and elsewhere—ileostomies, gastrostomies or colostomies, for example.

Enterostomy
The opening used for enteral feeding or for drainage if the bowel is obstructed.

Enzymes
Proteins that play a part in specific chemical reactions. The level of enzymes in the blood is often measured because abnormal levels may be a sign of various diseases.

Epidermoid carcinoma
A cancer arising from surface cells in an organ and resembling skin ("epidermis") when viewed under the microscope.

Epidural
The space just outside the spinal cord. Plastic catheters may be inserted in the space to deliver anesthetics or morphine for pain control.

Epstein-Barr (EB) virus
A virus known to cause infectious mononucleosis and associated with Burkitt's lymphoma and certain cancers of the head and neck.

ERCP (endoscopic retrograde cholangiopancreatography)
A specialized procedure in which a catheter is introduced through a gastroscope into the internal bile ducts.

Esophageal speech
A way of speaking used by people who have had their larynx (voice box) removed. As air is expelled from the esophagus, the walls of the pharynx and esophagus vibrate to produce sound.

Esophagitis
Soreness and inflammation of the esophagus due to infection, toxicity from radiotherapy or chemotherapy or some physical injury.

Estrogen
The female sex hormone produced by the ovaries. Estrogen controls the development of physical sexual characteristics, menstruation and pregnancy. Synthetic forms are used in oral contraceptives and in various therapies.

Estrogen-receptor (ER) assay
A test that determines whether the breast cancer in a particular patient is stimulated by estrogen.

Excision
Surgical removal of tissue.

Extravasation
Leakage into the surrounding tissues of intravenous fluids or drugs—especially cancer chemotherapeutic agents—from the vein being used for injection. Extravasation may damage tissues.

F

Familial polyposis
A hereditary condition in which members of the same family develop intestinal polyps. Also called Gardner's syndrome, it is considered a risk factor for colorectal cancer.

Fiber-optics
Flexible tubes that transmit light by means of

glass fibers. They are used to inspect and treat internal parts of the body. Various types of endoscopes use fiber-optic technology.

Fibrocystic breasts
A condition, which may come and go in relation to the menstrual cycle, in which fluids normally absorbed by breast tissue become trapped and form cysts. There may be difficulty distinguishing between cysts and breast cancer.

Fine needle aspiration (FNA)
A simple and painless way to obtain small bits of tissue for diagnosis. After local anesthesia, a small needle is inserted through the skin directly into a tumor and a sample of tissue is drawn up inside the needle. In some cases—thyroid cancer, for example—FNA has become an integral part of the early diagnostic process. But the amount of tissue obtained this way may not be enough to diagnose lymphomas and some other cancers.

Fissures
Cracks or a splitting in the skin or an internal membrane.

Fistula
An abnormal opening between the inside of the body and the skin or between two areas inside the body.

Frozen section
A procedure done by the pathologist during surgery to give the surgeon an immediate answer as to whether a tissue is benign or malignant. Tissue is removed by biopsy, frozen, cut into thin slices, stained and examined under a microscope. This information is vital in helping the surgeon decide the most appropriate course of action.

G

Gamma globulin
Proteins in the blood that contain antibodies, part of the body's defense against infection.

Gamma rays
The form of electromagnetic radiation produced by certain radioactive sources. They are similar to x-rays but have a shorter wavelength.

Gene
A biological unit of DNA capable of transmitting a single characteristic from parent to offspring.

Grade of tumor
A way of describing tumors by their appearance under the microscope. Low-grade tumors are slow to grow and spread, while high-grade

tumors grow and spread rapidly.

Graft-versus-host disease
After bone marrow transplantation or blood transfusion, immune cells in the donated (grafted) material may identify the patient's tissues (the host) as foreign and try to destroy them.

Granulocyte
The most common type of white blood cell. Its function is to kill bacteria (also called neutrophil, poly, PMN).

Guaiac test
A test to see if there is hidden blood in the stool. A positive result may be a sign of cancer, but many benign conditions also cause bleeding.

Gynecomastia
Swelling of the breast tissues in men. Although this can be caused by medications and other diseases, in the cancer field it is caused by certain cancers of the testis or by female hormones used to treat prostate cancer.

H

Hematocrit
A way of measuring the red cell content of the blood. The normal level is about 40 to 45 in men and from 37 to 42 in women. A low hematocrit is a sign of anemia.

Hematologist
A physician (internist) who specializes in blood diseases.

Hematoma
A blood lump under the skin that appears like a "black and blue" mark.

Hematopoietic
Pertaining to the blood-forming organs such as the bone marrow.

Hematuria
Blood in the urine. This may be obvious (gross hematuria) or hidden (microscopic hematuria).

Hemoglobin
A way of measuring the red cell content of the blood. The normal value in men is about 13 to 15 grams, in women from 12.5 to 14 grams.

Hemolytic anemia
Anemia resulting from the breakdown of red blood cells in the bloodstream before the end of their usual life span of 120 days.

Hemorrhagic cystitis
A bladder irritation, which may be caused by the anticancer drugs cyclophosphamide (Cytoxan) or ifosfamide.

Hepatic
Pertaining to the liver.

Hepatotoxicity
Adverse effects of drugs on the liver indicated by abnormal blood tests of liver function. It is also sometimes associated with jaundice.

Herpes simplex
A common acute viral inflammation of the skin or mucous membranes characterized by the development of blisters. This infection around the mouth is commonly called a cold sore.

Herpes zoster (shingles)
A painful eruption in the skin caused by a virus infection that affects nerves. The same virus that causes shingles causes chicken pox.

Histology
The appearance of tissues, including cancers, under the microscope.

Hormonal anticancer therapy
A form of therapy that takes advantage of the tendency of some cancers—especially breast and prostate cancers—to stabilize or shrink if certain hormones are administered.

Hormones
Naturally occurring substances that are released by the endocrine organs and circulate in the blood. Hormones control growth, metabolism, reproduction and other functions, and can stimulate or turn off the growth or activity of specific target cells. Some hormones are used after surgery to treat breast, ovarian, prostate, uterine and other cancers.

Hospice
A facility and a philosophy of care that stress comfort, peace of mind and the control of symptoms. Hospice care, provided on either an outpatient or inpatient basis, is generally invoked when no further anticancer therapy is available and life expectancy is very short. Hospice also helps family and friends to care for and cope with the loss of a dying loved one.

Humoral immunity
Immunity mediated by substances such as proteins (gamma globulins) produced by the immune system.

Hyperalimentation
Artificial feeding—temporary or permanent—by means of concentrated protein and fat solutions delivered intravenously. A special catheter is usually needed.

Hypercalcemia
High levels of calcium in the blood. It is a sign of some forms of cancer or of cancer spreading to bone and also occurs in some benign conditions.

Hyperthermia
Increased body temperature. Generally used to mean the use of special devices to raise body temperature as a way of treating cancer. It is usually used along with radiation therapy.

Hypothermia
Excessively low body temperature.

Hysterectomy
Surgical removal of the uterus.

I

IL-2
See Interleukins.

Ileostomy
An artificial opening in the skin of the abdomen, leading to the small bowel (ileum) (*see* Ostomy).

Iliac
The part of the lower abdomen just above the hip bone on each side of the body. Also refers to the iliac bone just above the hip joint.

Immune/immunity
A state of adequate defense against infections or foreign substances. Some cancers are also believed to produce immune responses.

Immune system
The body mechanisms that resist and fight disease. The main defenders are white blood cells and antibodies, which, along with other specialized defenders, react to the presence of foreign substances in the body and try to destroy them.

Immunoelectrophoresis
A way to separate serum gamma globulins—called IgA, IgG and IgM—into groups according to their immunologic qualities.

Immunosuppression
The state of having decreased immunity and thus being less able to fight infections and disease.

Immunosuppressive drug
A drug that modifies the natural immune response so that it will not react to foreign substances. This type of drug is most commonly given after organ transplants so that the new organ will not be rejected.

Immunotherapy
A method of cancer therapy that stimulates the body's defense mechanism to attack cancer cells or combat a specific disease.

Incontinence
Inadvertent loss of urine or feces, usually due

to loss of nerve or muscle control.

Indirect laryngoscopy
Inspection of the lower throat, pharynx and larynx (voice box) by means of a small mirror placed in the back of the throat (*see* Laryngoscopy).

Induction
The initial treatment—usually of chemotherapy—to eliminate or control cancer. Usually applied to leukemia or lymphoma.

Induration
Firmness or hardness of tissues.

Inferior vena cava
The large vein draining the blood from the legs and abdomen back into the heart.

Infiltration
The leaking of fluid or medicines into tissues from a tube or needle. This can cause irritation or swelling (*see* Extravasation).

Inflammation
The triggering of local body defenses causing defensive white blood cells (leukocytes) to pour into the tissues from the circulatory system. It is characterized by redness, heat, pain and swelling.

Informed consent
A legal standard defining how much a patient must know about the potential benefits and risks of therapy before agreeing to receive it.

Infusion
Administration of fluids and/or medications into a vein or artery over a period of time.

Infusion pumps
Small, preloaded mechanical devices used to continuously administer intravenous chemotherapy over a designated time.

Inguinal
Pertaining to the groin, the common site for hernias and the location of the inguinal lymph nodes, an area where cancer may spread.

In situ
A very early stage of cancer in which the tumor is localized to one area.

Interferons
Natural substances produced in response to infections. They have been created artificially by recombinant DNA technology in an attempt to control cancer.

Interleukins
A group of cytokines produced by body cells that convey molecular messages between cells of the immune system. Interleukin-2 (IL-2), the best known of these, acts primarily on T-lymphocytes; it is being used in the treatment of cancer.

Intra-arterial
Drugs directed into an artery through a catheter.

Intracavitary therapy
Treatment directed into a body cavity via a catheter.

Intramuscular (IM)
The injection of a drug into the muscle, whence it is absorbed into the circulation.

Intraperitoneal
Delivery of drugs and fluids into the abdominal cavity.

Intrapleural
Delivery of drugs and fluids into the space around the lung. Often employed when fluid collects there as a result of cancer.

Intrathecal
Administration of drugs into the spinal fluid.

Intravenous (IV)
The administration of drugs or fluids directly into the vein.

Intravenous pyelogram (IVP)
An x-ray of the kidneys taken after the intravenous administration of a radiopaque dye that is concentrated and excreted by the kidneys. This makes the kidneys and drainage system visible on an x-ray.

Invasive cancer
Cancer that spreads to the healthy tissue surrounding the original tumor site.

Ipsilateral
On the same side of the body (*see also* Contralateral).

J

Jaundice
The accumulation of bilirubin, a breakdown product of hemoglobin, which results in a yellow discoloration of the skin and the whites of the eyes. Jaundice is a sign of liver disease or blockage of the major bile ducts.

K

Kidney failure (renal failure)
Malfunction of the kidneys due to disease or the toxic effects of drugs or chemicals. Urine volume may or may not be diminished.

L

Laparotomy
An operation in which the abdominal cavity is opened.

Large cell carcinoma
A type of cancer of the lung, although large cell cancers may occur in other organs.

Laryngectomy
The surgical removal of the larynx (voice box) resulting in the loss of normal speech. A laryngectomee is someone who has undergone this operation.

Laryngoscopy
Inspection of the lower throat, pharynx and larynx by means of a small mirror placed in the back of the throat (indirect laryngoscopy) or by direct examination under anesthesia (direct laryngoscopy).

Leukocyte
White blood cell.

Leukocytosis
An increase in the number of leukocytes in the blood.

Leukopenia
A decreased white blood cell count (below 5,000).

Leukopheresis
A washing procedure that removes white blood cells from the blood.

Leukoplakia
White plaque on the mucous membranes of the mouth and gums. This may be precancerous.

Linear accelerator
A radiation therapy machine that produces a high energy beam.

Liver function tests
A group—panel—of blood tests to check if the liver is healthy.

Lobectomy
Removal of one lobe of a lung; the right lung contains three lobes, the left lung contains two.

Localized
A cancer confined to the site of origin without evidence of spread.

Lumbar puncture
Removal of spinal fluid for examination. This simple procedure—also called a spinal tap—involves numbing the skin of the back with a local anesthetic and placing a needle into the numbed area to remove the spinal fluid.

Lumpectomy
The removal of a breast cancer (lump) and the surrounding tissue without removing the entire breast. It is a less radical procedure than mastectomy and is usually followed by radiation treatment.

LVN
Licensed vocational nurse. A nurse trained to do more limited tasks than a registered nurse (RN).

Lymph nodes
Oval-shaped organs, often the size of peas or beans, that are located throughout the body and contain clusters of cells called lymphocytes. They produce infection-fighting lymphocytes and also filter out and destroy bacteria, foreign substances and cancer cells. They are connected by small vessels called lymphatics. Lymph nodes act as our first line of defense against infections and the spread of cancer.

Lymphangiogram
An x-ray picture of the abdominal lymph nodes obtained by injecting a contrast substance under the skin on the feet. This test helps to determine if cancer has spread to the abdominal lymph nodes.

Lymphatic system
The system of lymph nodes and the lymphatic vessels that connect them.

Lymphedema
Swelling, usually of an arm or leg, caused by obstructed lymphatic vessels. It can develop because of a tumor or as an unusual late effect of surgery or radiotherapy.

Lymphocytes
A family of white blood cells responsible for the production of antibodies and for the direct destruction of invading organisms or cancer cells.

Lymphokine
A specific protein (cytokine) secreted by lymphocytes.

Lytic
A bone lesion that has less calcium than normal. It may appear to be a "hole" in the bone.

M

Macrophages
White blood cells that destroy invading organisms by ingesting them.

Malaise
Tiredness or lack of "drive."

Malignant
An adjective meaning cancerous. Two important qualities of malignancies are the tendency to sink roots into surrounding tissues and to break off and spread elsewhere ("metastasize").

Markers (tumor markers)
Chemicals in the blood that are produced by certain cancers. Measuring the markers is useful for diagnosis, but especially useful for following the course of treatment (*see* CEA).

Mediastinum
The central portion of the chest, comprising the heart, large blood vessels, esophagus, trachea and surrounding tissues.

Metaplasia
Cells that appear abnormal under the microscope and do not yet show signs of malignancy.

Metastasis
The spread of cancer from one part of the body to another by way of the lymph system or bloodstream. Cells in the new cancer are like those in the original tumor.

Methadone (Dolophine)
A synthetic narcotic pain reliever related to morphine.

Milligrams/meter squared (mg/m²)
A formula for calculating dosages of chemotherapy drugs according to the surface area of the body. Since the amount of skin is hard to determine exactly, it is closely estimated from height and weight. An average person might have 1.7 square meters of body surface area. If the standard drug dosage were 650 mg/m^2, then 650 x 1.7 = 1105 mg of drug to be given.

Mitosis
The process of cell reproduction or division. Cancer cells usually have higher rates of mitosis than normal cells. The number of divisions seen under the microscope reflects how aggressive the cancer is.

Modality
A general class or method of treatment. The basic modalities of cancer therapy include surgery, radiation therapy, chemotherapy and immunotherapy.

Monoclonal antibodies
Highly specific antibodies, usually manufactured in a laboratory, that react to a specific cancer antigen or are directed against a specific type of cancer. Current research is studying their role in therapy. One potential use is to deliver chemotherapy and radiotherapy directly to a tumor, thus killing the cancer cells and sparing healthy tissue. Studies are also trying to find out if monoclonal antibodies can be produced to detect and diagnose cancer cells at a very early and curable stage.

Monoclonal gammopathy
An elevation in gamma globulin in the blood caused by a single clone of plasma cells or lymphocytes. Such a protein pattern may be associated with multiple myeloma.

Morbidity
Sickness; illness; symptoms and signs of disease. Not to be confused with mortality.

Mortality
Death as a result of disease.

MRI (Magnetic Resonance Imaging)
A method of creating images of the body using a magnetic field and radio waves rather than x-rays. Although the images are similar to those of CT scans, they can be taken in all three directions (planes) rather than just in cross-sections. There is no x-ray exposure.

Mucosa (mucous membrane)
The inner lining of the gastrointestinal tract or other structures such as the vagina and nose.

Mucositis
Inflammation of the mucous membranes. Soreness—like "cold sores"—can develop in the mouth as a side effect of chemotherapy.

Multicentricity
A tumor that appears to start growing in several places at once.

Multimodality
Using a combination of two or more types of therapy—for example, radiotherapy plus chemotherapy, radiation plus surgery or chemotherapy plus surgery.

Mutation
A permanent change in a cell's DNA that alters its genetic potential. It may be a response to a chemical substance (mutagen) or result from a physical effect such as radiation. Sometimes the daughter cells may be cancerous.

Myelogram
An x-ray of the spinal cord after the introduction of radiopaque dye into the sac surrounding it. Used to see if a tumor involves the spinal cord or nerve roots.

Myeloma
A cancer of the protein-producing plasma cells of the bone marrow. Multiple bone lesions are common.

Myelosuppression
A fall in the blood counts caused by therapy, especially chemotherapy and radiotherapy.

N

Nadir
The lowest point to which white blood cell or platelet counts fall after chemotherapy.

Narcotics
A legal term defining euphoric and pain-relieving (analgesic) substances whose use is closely regulated by government. There are natural and synthetic types.

Nasopharynx
The part of the nasal cavity behind the nose and above the part of the throat that we can see.

National Cancer Institute
A highly regarded research center in Bethesda, Maryland, that conducts basic and clinical research on new cancer treatments and supervises clinical trials of new treatments throughout the United States.

National Surgical Adjuvant Breast/Bowel Project (NSABP)
A group of dedicated research and clinical physicians who have formed a large cooperative group to study new treatments. Many major advances in treatment are attributed to this group.

Necrosis
The disintegration of tissues caused by some physical or chemical agent or by lack of blood supply. Cancers treated effectively by chemotherapy, radiotherapy, heat or biological agents undergo necrosis.

Needle biopsy
Removing a tiny bit of tissue for diagnosis by placing a needle into a tumor. The procedure is usually done under local anesthesia. (*see* Fine needle aspiration)

Neoadjuvant chemotherapy
Chemotherapy given *before* the primary treatment, either surgery or radiation therapy, to improve the effectiveness of treatment. (*See* Adjuvant chemotherapy)

Neoplasm
A new abnormal growth. Neoplasms may be benign or malignant.

Nephrotoxic
Toxic to the kidneys. The term is generally used to refer to a drug's effect.

Nerve block
Removing pain by numbing a nerve temporari-ly (with a local anesthetic) or permanently (with an alcohol injection).

Neuropathy
Malfunction of a nerve, often causing numbness (sensory nerve) or weakness (motor nerve). It is sometimes a side effect of anti-cancer drugs.

Neurotoxicity
Toxic effects (usually of drugs) on the nervous system.

Neutrophils
One of the white blood cells that fights infection. Also called granulocytes, polys or PMNs.

Nitrosoureas
A class of chemical compounds that can enter the brain through the blood-brain barrier. The anti-cancer drugs BCNU, CCNU and methyl-CCNU are nitrosoureas. (*See* Blood-brain barrier)

"No code"
An order, written in a hospital chart after careful and considered discussions, to *not* attempt to resuscitate a patient if breathing and/or the heartbeat should stop. This is usually considered if the patient, after all reasonable therapeutic efforts have been made and have failed, is suffering greatly and rapidly failing from a far-advanced malignancy. Also "Do Not Rescuscitate" (DNR).

Nodes
See Lymph nodes

Nodule
A small lump or tumor that can be benign or malignant.

Non-cell-cycle specific
Chemotheraputic drugs capable of destroying cells that are not actively dividing.

Nuclear Magnetic Resonance (NMR)
An old term for MRI.

O

Oncogenes
Specific stretches of cellular DNA that, when inappropriately activated, contribute to the transformation of normal cells into malignant ones.

Oncologist
A physician who specializes in cancer therapy. There are surgical, radiation, pediatric, gynecologic and medical oncologists. The term *oncologist* alone generally refers to medical oncologists, who are internists with expertise in chemotherapy and the handling of the general medical problems that arise during the disease.

Oncology
The medical specialty that deals with the diagnosis, treatment and study of cancer.

Oophorectomy
The surgical removal of one or both ovaries.

Opportunistic infections
Many common fungi and bacteria and a few microscopic parasites do not ordinarily cause infections in healthy people. But such ordinarily harmless organisms can produce severe, life-threatening and hard-to-contol infections in cancer patients by taking advantage of the reduced immune response resulting from the disease or therapy.

Ostomy
A surgically created opening in the skin, leading to an internal organ, for purposes of drainage (*see* Colostomy; Ileostomy).

Ototoxicity
Toxic effects on the ears, generally resulting in a ringing in the ears or hearing loss.

P

Palate
The roof of the mouth. The hard palate is in front, the soft palate just behind.

Palliative
Treatment that aims to improve well-being, relieve symptoms or control the growth of cancer, but not primarily intended or expected to produce a cure.

Palpation
Examination by feeling an area of the body—such as the breast and prostate—with the fingers to detect abnormalities. A palpable mass is one that can be felt.

Paracentesis
Removing fluid from the abdomen by inserting a small needle through the skin. This is usually done under local anesthesia.

Paraneoplastic (syndrome)
Various symptoms and signs—changes in body minerals, nerve function or water balance, for example—that indicate the presence of a tumor in the body but are not related to direct pressure by the tumor.

Parenteral nutrition
Artificial feeding by the intravenous administration of concentrated amino acid, sugar and fat solutions (*see* Hyperalimentation; TPN).

Pathologic fracture
A fracture (break) in a bone through an area weakened by cancer. Usually little or no injury or trauma precedes the fracture, as is the case with the usual fracture of healthy bones.

Pathologist
A physician skilled in the performance and interpretation of laboratory tests and in the examination of tissues to provide a diagnosis.

Pathology
Study of disease through the examination of body tissues, organs and materials. Any tumor suspected of being cancerous must be diagnosed by pathologic examination. The physician who does this is called a pathologist.

PDQ (Physicians Data Query)
A comprehensive, up-to-date information service on state-of-the-art cancer treatment provided by the National Cancer Institute via computer or fax.

Percutaneous endoscopic gastrostomy
Placement of a feeding tube through the skin directly into the stomach. This employs a technique of shining a light inside the stomach, by means of a gastroscope, to identify the exact location to safely pass the feeding tube through the skin, using a small incision under local anesthesia.

Performance status
A measurement of how well a cancer patient is functioning. Index numbers from 0 to 100—increasing in steps of 10—are used to document and record functional status, as opposed to other measurements that indicate the size of a tumor. A person with a performance status of 80 functions better than one with a score of 50. Also called Karnofsky score.

Perineum
The part of the body between the anus and the genitals.

Perioperative
Occurring at or around the time of surgery. Often used with reference to chemotherapy or radiotherapy treatments.

Peritonoscopy
Inspection of the inside of the abdominal cavity by means of a telescope inserted under anesthesia through a tiny opening in the skin.

Petechiae
Tiny areas of bleeding under the skin usually caused by a low platelet count.

Phlebitis
Inflammation of the veins, often causing pain

and tenderness (*see* Pulmonary embolism; Thrombophlebitis).

Photodynamic therapy
The injection of a light-sensitizing chemical or dye and the subsequent application of light, usually laser, to a tumor. The chemical improves the effect of the laser treatment and thus minimizes or prevents damage to normal tissues.

Photosensitivity
Extreme sensitivity to the sun. Some medications—including a few anticancer drugs as well as tetracycline antibiotics—produce photosensitivity as a side effect, leaving the patient prone to sunburn.

Placebo
An inert substance, used in a research study or clinical trial, that resembles an actual medication. It is used to eliminate the improvement that may result from the *belief* that a medication is being given, rather than the actual effect of a medication.

Plasmapheresis
The replacement or "washing" of a patient's plasma by donor plasma or saline.

Platelet
One of the three kinds of circulating blood cells. The normal platelet count is about 150,000 to 300,000. Platelets are responsible for creating the first part of a blood clot. Platelet transfusions are used in cancer patients to prevent or control bleeding when the number of platelets has significantly decreased.

Plateletpheresis
Collection of platelets in a machine for transfusion into another person.

Pneumonectomy
Surgical removal of a lung.

Polycythemia
An excessively high red blood cell count. This may be caused by a primary blood disease or as a response to another type of disease.

Polyp
A growth that protrudes from mucous membranes, often looking like a tiny mushroom. Polyps may be found in the nose, ears, mouth, lungs, vocal cords, uterus, cervix, rectum, bladder and intestine. Some polyps occurring in the cervix, intestine, stomach or colon can eventually become malignant and should be removed.

Poorly differentiated
A tumor that under the microscope has little or only a slight resemblance to the normal tissue

from the same organ (*see* Undifferentiated; Well-differentiated).

Port (infusion)
A small disc with a soft center (about the size of a quarter) that is surgically placed just below the skin in the chest or abdomen. A tube coming out of the side is connected via a large vein directly into the bloodstream. By passing a small needle through the skin into the disc, fluids, drugs or blood products can be given without worrying about finding an adequate vein, making multiple venipunctures or causing leakage of the fluids into surrounding tissues.

Port-a-Cath
One type of infusion port, a venous access device that has nothing protruding from the skin. Injections are made into a chamber implanted just under the skin. (*see* Port)

Potassium
An important mineral in the body that is often lost during illness, especially with diarrhea. Low potassium levels can cause weakness.

Precancerous
Abnormal cellular changes or conditions—intestinal polyps, for example—that tend to become malignant. Also called premalignant.

Primary tumor
The place where a cancer first starts to grow. Even if it spreads elsewhere, it is still known by the place of origin. For example, breast cancer that has spread to the bone is still breast cancer, not bone cancer.

Proctoscopy
See Sigmoidoscopy

Progesterone
One of the female hormones (the other is estrogen). It causes the buildup of the uterine lining in preparation for conception and performs other functions before and during pregnancy. Certain synthetic forms of the hormone are used in cancer treatment.

Progesterone-receptor (PR) assay
A test that determines if the breast cancer in a particular patient is stimulated by progesterone.

Prognosis
A statement about the likely outcome of disease in a particular patient. In cancer, it is based on all available information about the type of tumor, staging, therapeutic possibilities, expected results and other personal or medical factors. For example, breast cancer

patients who are diagnosed early usually have a good prognosis.

Progression
The growth or advancement of cancer, indicating a worsening of the disease.

Prophylactic
Treatment designed to prevent a disease or complication that is likely to develop but has not yet appeared. Also may be called adjuvant treatment.

Prostate Specific Antigen (PSA)
A substance in the blood derived from the prostate gland. Its level may rise in prostatic cancer and is useful as a marker to monitor the effects of treatment.

Prosthesis
An artificial replacement or approximation of a body part—such as a leg, breast or eye—that is missing because of disease or treatment.

Protocol
A carefully designed and written description of a cancer treatment program. It includes dosages and formulas for any drugs to be administered.

Pulmonary embolism
A life-threatening condition in which a blood clot travels to the lungs from veins in the legs or pelvis, often from thrombophlebitis. The clots are diagnosed with a lung scan and treated with anticoagulants.

R

Radiation oncologist; radiotherapist
A physician who specializes in the use of radiation to treat cancer.

Radiation therapy
See Radiotherapy

Radical mastectomy
Removal of the entire breast along with underlying muscle and the lymph nodes of the armpit (axilla). In a *modified* radical mastectomy the underlying (pectoral) muscles are left in place.

Radical neck dissection
An extensive surgical operation to remove all of the lymph glands on one side of the neck, usually in association with surgery to remove a primary tumor that may have spread to the lymph glands in the neck.

Radical surgery
An extensive operation to remove the site of cancer and the adjacent structures and lymph nodes.

Radioactive implant
A source of high-dose radiation that is placed directly into and around a cancer to kill the cancer cells.

Radioactive isotope
A radioactive substance used for diagnosis (tracer dose used for scans) or treatment (therapeutic dose).

Radiologist
A doctor who specializes in the use of x-rays as well as other imaging techniques such as ultrasound, MRI and radioactive tracers to diagnose and investigate disease. New radiology techniques are also used for treatment in some cases ("interventional radiology").

Radiosensitive
A cancer that usually responds to radiation therapy. The opposite is radioresistant.

Radiosensitizer
A drug or biological agent that is given together with radiation therapy to increase its effect.

Radiotherapy
The use of high-energy radiation from x-ray machines, cobalt, radium or other sources for control or cure of cancer. It may reduce the size of a cancer before surgery or be used to destroy any remaining cancer cells after surgery. Radiotherapy can be helpful in treating recurrent cancers or relieving symptoms.

Rads
An obsolete unit measuring radiation dosage, now replaced by the centigray (cGy).

Recurrence
The reappearance of a disease after treatment had caused it to apparently disappear.

Red blood cells
Cells in the blood that bring oxygen to tissues and take carbon dioxide from them.

Regional involvement
The spread of cancer from its original site to nearby surrounding areas. Regional cancers are confined to one general location in the body.

Regression
The shrinkage of a cancer usually as the result of therapy. In a complete regression, all tumors disappear. In a partial regression, some tumor remains.

Rehabilitation
Programs that help patients adjust and return to a full productive life. Rehabilitation may involve physical measures such as physical therapy and prostheses, as well as counseling

and emotional support.

Remission
The partial or complete shrinkage of cancer usually occurring as the result of therapy. Also the period when the disease is under control. A remission is not necessarily a cure.

Renal
Pertaining to the kidney.

Resection
The surgical removal of tissue.

Residual disease; residual tumor
Cancer left behind after surgery or other treatment.

Resistance
Failure of a tumor to respond to radiotherapy or chemotherapy. The resistance may be evident during the first treatment (primary) or, after an initial response, during the subsequent treatment (secondary).

Retroperitoneum
The area of the abdomen near the back, behind all the organs, including the bowel.

Reverse isolation
Isolation to prevent visitors or hospital staff from carrying an infection into a patient's room. This usually means that everyone must wear a gown, mask and gloves.

Ribonucleic acid (RNA)
A nucleic acid present in all cells and similar to DNA. It is the biochemical blueprint for the formation of protein by the cells.

Risk factors
The habits or conditions that promote the development of many cancers. Cigarette smoking, for example, is the major risk factor for lung cancer. The major risk factor for skin cancer is overexposure to the sun.

Risk reduction
Techniques used to reduce the chances of developing cancer. High-fiber diets, for example, may help reduce the risk of colon cancer.

RNA
See Ribonucleic acid

S

Salvage
The attempt to cure a patient by a second, third or later alternative treatment program after the first-line treatment has failed to produce a cure.

Sampling
Removal of a portion of a tissue for diagnostic tests.

Sarcoma
A cancer of supporting or connective tissue such as cartilage, bone, muscle or fat. Sarcomas are often highly malignant but account for only 2 percent of all human cancers.

Scans (radioisotope)
Diagnostic procedures for assessing organs such as the liver, bone or brain. Radioactive tracers are introduced intravenously and if a malignant tumor or other foreign material is present pictures of the organ will show abnormalities that may indicate the presence of a tumor. There is no significant risk with this small, brief radiation exposure.

Screening
The search for cancer in apparently healthy people who have no cancer symptoms. Screening may also refer to coordinated programs in large populations.

Second-look surgery
Sometimes the only way to determine if aggressive therapy has worked is to explore the patient surgically some time after initial therapy. Second-look surgery can discover if there is any residual or recurrent cancer, which may help decide whether treatment is complete or if more radiotherapy or chemotherapy is needed. Residual tumor may also be removed during the operation.

Seizure (convulsion)
Shaking of a part or all of the body, often with loss of consciousness. This can be caused by an injury, a benign condition (such as idiopathic epilepsy) or a brain tumor.

Selective angiography
X-ray pictures of an organ taken after a catheter is passed through the artery to the organ and a dye, which shows on x-rays, is injected.

Sepsis (septicemia, bacteremia)
Bacterial growth within the bloodstream. This is a very serious situation and usually requires hospitalization for intravenous antibiotics.

Serum protein electrophoresis (SPEP)
A laboratory testing method that separates serum proteins into different groups—albumin, alpha globulin, beta globulin and gamma globulin. The different patterns produced are characteristic of various diseases.

Shingles (*see* Herpes zoster)

Sigmoidoscopy

An examination of the rectum and lower colon with a hollow lighted tube called a sigmoidoscope. It is used to detect colon polyps and cancer, to find the cause of bleeding and to evaluate other bowel diseases. A newer instrument using fiber-optics—the flexible sigmoidoscope—permits easier, safer and more extensive examination. Also called a proctoscopy. (*See also* Colonoscopy)

Sodium

An important mineral in the body that helps maintain fluid balance. It is measured as part of an electrolyte panel.

Sonography

The use of ultrasound pictures in diagnosis.

Sphincter

A circular muscle that tightens around an organ or cavity to close it and to regulate the flow of material. If the sphincter around the rectum and the mouth of the bladder aren't functioning properly, for example, urine and stool might be lost involuntarily.

Spleen

An organ adjacent to the stomach, composed mainly of lymphocytes, which removes worn-out blood cells and foreign materials from the bloodstream.

Sputum

Material coughed up from the lungs. Also called phlegm.

Squamous cell (epidermoid) carcinoma

Cancer arising from the skin or the surfaces of other structures, such as the mouth, cervix or lungs.

Staging

An organized process of determining how far a cancer has spread. Staging involves a physical exam, blood tests, x-rays, scans and sometimes surgery. Knowing the stage helps determine the most appropriate treatment and the prognosis.

Stereotactic needle biopsy

A procedure often used in the diagnosis of brain tumors. A specialized "frame" is used to hold a patient's head or other body part stationary while the biopsy needle is directed to exactly the right spot. Usually a CT scanner or other computer-associated equipment is used to find the correct position. This method has also been applied recently to very small breast cancers.

Steroids

A class of fat-soluble chemicals—including cortisone and male and female sex hormones—that are vital to many different functions within the body. Some steroid derivatives are used in cancer treatment.

Stoma

A surgically created opening in the skin for elimination of body wastes. A stoma is made in the abdominal wall for elimination of wastes, for example, when the colon and/or rectum can no longer perform this function (*see* Colostomy).

Stomatitis

Inflammation and soreness of the mouth. This is sometimes a side effect of chemotherapy or radiotherapy.

Stool

Feces or bowel movement.

Stool for occult blood

A test to determine if bleeding has occurred. This may show signs of bleeding that are too mild to see with the naked eye (*see* Guaiac test).

Superior vena cava

The large vein draining the blood from the head, neck and arms back into the heart.

Suppository

A way to administer medications by absorbing the drug into a wax preparation, then inserting it into the rectum or vagina. Suppositories are used to treat local conditions such as vaginitis or hemorrhoids and are also used when pills cannot be swallowed or kept down because of nausea, sore mouth or narrowing of the esophagus. Antinausea suppositories such as Compazine and Tigan are often used to combat this side effect of chemotherapy.

Systemic disease

Disease that involves the entire body rather than just one area.

T

T cell

See B cell

Teratogenic

A drug or toxin that, if taken during pregnancy, can cause the fetus to be malformed.

Terminal

This term has a number of definitions. Some people use it when cure is not possible, even if treatment can add years to the patient's life. Others say a patient is terminal when he or she has a specific short life expectancy, perhaps six months or one month. Still others mean that no other treatment can be given and "nature will take its course." If this term comes up, discuss with your doctor exactly what is meant by it.

Thoracentesis
Insertion of a needle or tube between the ribs and into the chest cavity to remove fluid. The procedure is done for diagnostic or treatment reasons and is performed under local anesthesia.

Thoracic
Pertaining to the thorax or chest.

Thoracotomy
A surgically created opening into the chest.

Thrombocytopenia
An abnormally low number of platelets (thrombocytes)—less then 150,000—due to disease, reaction to a drug or toxic reaction to treatments. Bleeding can occur if there are too few platelets, especially if the count falls to less than 20,000.

Thrombophlebitis
Inflammation of veins with blood clots inside the veins. Usually associated with pain, swelling and tenderness (*see also* Phlebitis; Pulmonary embolism).

Thrombosis
Formation of a blood clot within a blood vessel.

Tissue
A collection of cells of the same type. There are four basic types of tissues in the body: epithelial, connective, muscle and nerve.

TNM classification
A complex and exact system for describing the stage of development of most kinds of cancer. This system is not used for lymphomas, leukemias or Hodgkin's disease.

TPN (Total Parenteral Nutrition)
The use of complex protein and fat solutions to supply enough calories and nutrients to sustain life. The solutions are delivered intravenously.

Tracheostomy
An artificial opening in the neck leading to the windpipe (trachea). The opening is created surgically to allow breathing when the trachea is blocked.

Tumor
A lump, mass or swelling. A tumor can be either benign or malignant.

Tumor necrosis factor
A natural protein substance produced by the body, which may make tumors shrink.

U
Ulcer
A sore resulting from corrosion of normal tissue by some irritating process or substance such as stomach acid, chemicals, infections, impaired circulation or cancerous involvement.

Ultrasound
The use of high-frequency sound waves to create an image of the inside of the body. Also called ultrasonography.

Undifferentiated
A tumor that appears "wild" under the microscope, not resembling the tissue of origin. These tumors tend to grow and spread faster than well-differentiated tumors, which do resemble the normal tissue they come from (*see* Anaplastic; Poorly differentiated; Well-differentiated).

Unilateral
On one side of the body.

Urostomy
A surgical procedure in which the ureters that carry urine from the kidneys to the bladder are cut and connected to an opening on the skin outside the abdomen. This allows urine to flow into a collection bag (*see* Stoma).

Uterus
The female reproductive organ, located in the pelvis; the womb in which an unborn child develops until birth.

V
Venipuncture
Inserting a needle into a vein in order to obtain blood samples, start an intravenous infusion or give a medication.

Ventricles
Four fluid-filled cavities in the brain all connected with each other. There are two lateral ventricles in the top part of the brain—one on each side—with the third and fourth ventricles in the center of the brain. Obstruction of the connections or the outflow tract leads to swelling (hydrocephalus). Also refers to the chambers in the heart.

Vesicant drugs
Chemotherapeutic agents that can cause significant tissue irritation and soreness if they leak outside the vein after injection.

Virus
A tiny infectious agent that is smaller than bacteria. Many common infections such as colds

and hepatitis are caused by viruses. Viruses invade cells, alter the cells' chemistry and cause them to produce more virus. Several viruses produce cancers in animals. Their role in the development of human cancers is now being studied.

W

Well-differentiated
A tumor that under the microscope resembles normal tissue from the same organ (*see* Poorly differentiated; Undifferentiated).

White blood cells
Cells in the blood that fight infection. These are composed of monocytes, lymphocytes, neutrophils, eosinophils and basophils. The normal count is 5,000 to 10,000. It may be elevated or depressed in a wide variety of diseases. Chemotherapy and radiotherapy usually cause low white counts.

Z

Zoster
See Herpes zoster.

ANTICANCER DRUGS AND THEIR SIDE EFFECTS

Adrenocorticosteroids (Prednisone) (Dexamethasone) (Decadron), others
Type of Cancer Acute and chronic lymphocytic leukemias, Hodgkin's and non-Hodgkin's lymphoma, myeloma, breast, brain metastases
Route Administered Oral, Intravenous, Intramuscular
Precautions Use of antacids, H-2 blockers, check for increased blood sugar (for diabetes), interferes with immune function, infection precautions, low salt diet, do *not* stop taking large doses abruptly
Side Effects Could lead to peptic ulcer or mood changes, pancreatitis, edema (fluid and salt retention), headaches, sleeplessness, vertigo, psychiatric problems, muscle weakness (low potassium), osteoporosis, bone damage to hips, increased hair growth, increased blood sugar (diabetes), cataracts, malaise, increased infections

Altretamine (Hexamethylmelamine) (Hexalen)
Type of Cancer Ovary
Route Administered Oral
Side Effects Hair loss, rash, nausea and vomiting, appetite loss, diarrhea, abdominal cramps, bladder irritation, muscle weakness, tingling or numbness, unsteady gait, low blood counts

Aminoglutethimide (Cytadren)
Type of Cancer Breast, prostate, and adrenal
Route Administered Oral
Precautions Add salt to diet; you may receive hydrocortisone to take concurrently
Side Effects Unstable balance (ataxia), uncoordinated eye motion, sleepiness, lethargy, somnolence, dizziness, skin rash, low blood counts, eyelid swelling, low adrenal gland function (need cortisone replacement), loss of appetite, nausea, vomiting, constipation, gastric discomfort

Amsacrine (m-AMSA) (Group C investigational)
Indications Acute leukemia
Route Administered Intravenous
Precautions Maintain good mouth hygiene

Side Effects Nausea, vomiting, burning or stinging at injection site, sore mouth, transient yellowing of skin, decreased blood counts.

Androgens (Testosterone) Fluoxymesterone (Halotestin)
Type of Cancer Breast
Route Administered Oral, Intramuscular
Side Effects Loss of menstrual periods, masculinization, hoarseness, acne, clitoral enlargement, increased hair growth, jaundice, leg swelling (edema), nausea, intestinal upset, fluid and mineral imbalance

Asparaginase (Elspar)
Type of Cancer Acute lymphoblastic leukemia and lymphomas
Route Administered Intravenous, Intramuscular
Precautions Test dosage before treatment to assess for allergic reactions. Use antihistamines, corticosteroids (have epinephrine available in case of allergy). Retreatment at later time requires special precautions
Side Effects Fever, allergic reaction (anaphylaxis), neurologic problems (seizures, reduced level of consciousness, drowsiness), stroke, liver malfunction, weakness, increased blood sugar, pancreatitis, kidney failure, loss of appetite, nausea, vomiting, abdominal discomfort, sore mouth, malabsorption

BCG (Bacille Clamette-Guérin)
Type of Cancer Bladder
Route Administered Instilled into bladder
Precautions Acetaminophen and bedrest to minimize flu-like symptoms; notify your physician if this persists
Side Effects Fever, malaise, vomiting, myalgia, headache, chills, bladder irritation

Bleomycin (Blenoxane)
Type of Cancer Squamous carcinoma of head and neck, Hodgkin's and non-Hodgkin's lymphoma, testis, anus, vulva, uterus, cervix, malignant pleural effusions
Route Administered Intramuscular, Subcutaneous, Intravenous, Intracavitary

Precautions Allergic reactions (antihistamines), lung function tests to detect malfunction early, kidney failure requires reduced dose
Side Effects Darkening of skin, rash and thickening of skin of palms and fingers, lung scarring and decreased breathing function (limited life-time dosage), cough, shortness of breath, joint swelling, fever after first dose (test dose often used), sore mouth, anorexia, nausea/vomiting, difficulty swallowing, weight loss

Busulfan (Myleran)

Type of Cancer Chronic myelogenous leukemia, bone marrow transplantation
Route Administered Oral
Precautions Lung function tests
Side Effects Anemia, low blood counts, lung scarring (fibrosis), shortness of breath, loss of menstrual periods, impotence, fever, bruising, skin pigmentation, weakness, enlarged breasts, cataracts, anorexia, nausea, vomiting, diarrhea, dry mouth, sore mouth, increased uric acid (gout)

Carboplatin (Paraplatin)

Type of Cancer Ovary, cervix, small cell lung, head and neck, bladder, testis, mesothelioma, brain
Route Administered Intravenous
Precautions Hydration
Side Effects Anemia, low blood counts, nerve toxicity, decreased hearing, kidney toxicity, nausea, vomiting, loss of appetite, diarrhea, constipation, sore mouth, altered taste

Carmustine (BCNU) (BiCNU)

Type of Cancer Brain, Hodgkin's disease, lymphomas, myeloma, melanoma, lung, gastrointestinal
Route Administered Intravenous
Precautions May add local anesthetic to minimize pain on injection. Pulmonary evaluation if cough or difficulty breathing
Side Effects Anemia, low blood counts, pulmonary fibrosis, occasional liver toxicity, dizziness, loss of balance, skin darkening, vision changes, nausea, vomiting, pain on injection, pigmentation along vein

Chlorambucil (Leukeran)

Type of Cancer Chronic lymphatic leukemia, Hodgkin's and non-Hodgkin's lymphoma, breast, ovary
Route Administered Oral
Side Effects Anemia, low blood counts, rash, hair loss, lung fibrosis (cough), joint pains, loss of menstrual periods, low sperm count, nausea, vomiting, increased uric acid (gout), secondary malignancies

Chlorodeoxyadenosine (Leustatin)

Type of Cancer Hairy cell leukemia, lymphomas, chronic lymphocytic leukemia, cutaneous T cell lymphoma (mycosis fungoides)
Route Administered Intravenous
Precautions Nausea program, skin reaction with intravenous leak, monitor kidney function
Side Effects Low blood counts, nausea, vomiting, irritation at injection site, weakness, headache, kidney damage, fever, chills

Cisplatin (Platinol)

Type of Cancer Testis, ovary, head and neck, Hodgkin's and non-Hodgkin's lymphoma, sarcomas, bladder, lung, stomach, cervix, myeloma, prostate, mesothelioma, breast
Route Administered Intravenous
Precautions Nausea program, watch for hearing loss, hydration to prevent kidney failure
Side Effects Anemia, low blood counts, nerve toxicity (numbness, tingling, hearing loss) wheezing, reduced blood pressure, fast heart rate, nausea, vomiting, anorexia, mineral imbalance, increased uric acid (gout), loss of taste

Cyclophosphamide (Cytoxan)

Type of Cancer Hodgkin's and non-Hodgkin's lymphoma, multiple myeloma, sarcomas, leukemias, neuroblastoma, breast, lung, testis, endometrium, mycosis fungoides
Route Administered Oral, Intravenous
Precautions Increased fluid intake, bladder emptying
Side Effects Hair loss, bladder irritation or hemorrhage, anemia, low blood counts, immunosuppression, water overload (antidiuretic effect), sterility, lung scarring,

increased skin pigmentation, loss of appetite, nausea, vomiting, sore mouth (stomatitis), diarrhea, gastrointestinal ulcers, increased uric acid (gout), secondary malignancies

Cytarabine (Ara-C) (Cytosar)

Type of Cancer Acute leukemia, lymphomas, head and neck
Route Administered Intravenous, Subcutaneous, Spinal (intrathecal)
Side Effects Anemia, low blood counts, immunosuppression, liver malfunction with jaundice, dizziness, lethargy, rash, weakness, neuritis, imbalance (cerebellar toxicity), eye irritation (high dosage), nausea, vomiting, loss of appetite, sore mouth, diarrhea, difficulty swallowing, increased uric acid (gout)

Dacarbazine (DTIC)

Type of Cancer Hodgkin's disease, malignant melanoma, sarcomas, carcinoid, islet cell, medullary thyroid
Route Administered Intravenous
Precautions Nausea program, severe skin reactions with IV leak
Side Effects Anemia, low blood counts, liver toxicity, light-headedness, nerve tingling, rash from sun (photosensitivity), hair loss, itching, rash, anorexia, nausea, vomiting, sore mouth (stomatitis), diarrhea, metallic taste

Dactinomycin (Actinomycin D)

Type of Cancer Testis, melanoma, choriocarcinoma, Wilms' tumor, neuroblastoma, retinoblastoma, Kaposi's sarcoma, sarcomas
Route Administered Intravenous
Precautions Severe skin reaction with IV leak
Side Effects Anemia, low blood counts, hair loss, skin lumps, increased skin sensitivity if given with or after x-ray therapy, weakness, sleepiness, nausea, vomiting, loss of appetite, sore mouth, diarrhea, inflamed tongue, sores in corner of mouth

Daunorubicin (Cerubidine)

Type of Cancer Acute lymphoblastic and myelogenous leukemias
Route Administered Intravenous
Precautions Severe skin reaction with IV leak, monitor heart function
Side Effects Anemia, low blood counts,

red coloration of urine, cardiac toxicity (limited lifetime dosage), increased sensitivity to radiation, joint pain, nausea, vomiting, sore mouth, diarrhea

Doxorubicin (Adriamycin)

Type of Cancer Lung, breast, bladder, prostate, pancreas, stomach, ovary, thyroid, endometrium, sarcoma, leukemias, Hodgkin's and non-Hodgkin's lymphoma, mesothelioma, myeloma, cancer of unknown primary site, Wilms' tumor
Route Administered Intravenous
Precautions Severe skin reaction with IV leak, monitor effects on heart with special studies
Side Effects Hair loss, anemia, low blood counts, red coloration of urine, cardiac toxicity (limited lifetime dosage), skin cracking and increased nailbed pigmentation, increased skin toxicity when given with or after radiation, nausea, vomiting, sore mouth, diarrhea, iron loss, loss of appetite

Epirubicin

Type of Cancer Breast, stomach, lymphomas, ovary
Route Administered Intravenous
Precautions Severe skin reaction with IV leak, monitor heart function
Side Effects Hair loss, anemia, low blood counts, red coloration of urine, cardiac toxicity (limited lifetime dosage), skin cracking and increased nailbed pigmentation, increased skin toxicity when given with or after radiation, nausea, vomiting, sore mouth, diarrhea, iron loss, loss of appetite

Estramustine (Emcyt)

Type of Cancer Metastatic prostate
Route Administered Oral
Precautions May irradiate male breast to minimize swelling
Side Effects Headaches, loss of coordination, liver enzyme elevation, enlarged tender breasts, anemia, low blood counts, heart failure, strokes, thrombosis and embolism, fluid retention, nausea, vomiting, diarrhea

Estrogens (Diethylstilbestrol) (DES)

Type of Cancer Prostate, breast metastases (women 5 or more years postmenopausal and receptor positive)

Route Administered Oral
Precautions Take multivitamins and iron, avoid constipation, use low salt diet. Fluid retention may aggravate heart disease. May irradiate male breast to minimize swelling
Side Effects Increased clotting, enlarged breasts, testicle atrophy, loss of libido, edema (fluid retention), water-soluble vitamin deficiency, iron deficiency, gall stones, sugar intolerance, increased serum calcium, constipation, loss of appetite, nausea, vomiting

Etoposide (VP-16) (Vepesid)

Type of Cancer Acute non-lymphocytic leukemia, lymphoma, head and neck, testis, lung
Route Administered Intravenous, Oral
Precautions Monitor blood pressure during infusion
Side Effects Low blood counts, nerve numbness and tingling, wheezing, shortness of breath (bronchospasm), rapid heart rate, hair loss, low blood pressure if IV rate too rapid, loss of appetite, altered taste and smell, nausea, vomiting, sore mouth, diarrhea, loss of fluids and electrolytes

Fludarabine (Fludara)

Type of Cancer Chronic lymphocytic leukemia, lymphomas
Route Administered Intravenous
Precautions Nausea program
Side Effects Low blood counts, tiredness, sore mouth, diarrhea, abdominal cramps, hair loss, rash, rare nausea and vomiting

Fluorouracil (5-FU)

Type of Cancer Breast, stomach, colon, liver, pancreas, ovary, bladder, prostate. Topical use in skin cancer (ointment)
Route Administered Intravenous, Topical
Precautions Reduce dosage if liver failure
Side Effects Rash, photosensitivity (sun rash), rare heart toxicity, hair loss, anemia, low blood counts, skin dryness, nail cracking and loss, increased tears (tear duct narrowing), hand foot syndrome, (redness of skin), eye irritation, loss of appetite, nausea, vomiting, sore mouth and throat, diarrhea, bile salt loss, thiamine and niacin deficiency

Flutamide (Eulexin)

Type of Cancer Prostate
Route Administered Oral
Side Effects Hot flashes, loss of libido and potency, enlarged tender breasts, liver toxicity, anorexia, nausea, vomiting, diarrhea (if lactose deficiency)

5-FUDR (Floxuridine)

Type of Cancer Liver (primary or metastatic), head and neck, kidney
Route Administered Arterial infusion
Precautions Four times more active than 5-FU, if liver failure occurs, reduce dose
Side Effects Hair loss, rash, anemia, low blood counts, loss of appetite, nausea, vomiting, sore mouth and throat, diarrhea, bile salt loss, thiamine and niacin deficiency

Goserelin (Zoladex)

Type of Cancer Prostate
Route Administered Subcutaneous
Precautions Temporary increased bone pain, use flutamide (Eulexin) to improve results and help prevent flare reaction
Side Effects Hot flashes, enlarged swollen and tender breasts, skin rash, testicular atrophy, peripheral edema, dizziness, headaches, tingling in extremities, loss of appetite, nausea, vomiting, constipation, diarrhea, difficulty swallowing, elevated blood pressure

Hydroxyurea (Hydrea)

Type of Cancer Chronic myelogenous leukemia, head and neck, kidney, brain, melanoma, ovary
Route Administered Oral
Precautions Drink extra fluids
Side Effects Low blood counts, nausea, vomiting, diarrhea, iron loss, loss of appetite, sore mouth, constipation, increased uric acid (gout)

Idarubicin (Idamycin)

Type of Cancer Acute non-lymphocytic leukemia
Route Administered Intravenous
Precautions Nausea program, skin reaction if intravenous leak, cardiac monitoring studies
Side Effects Decreased blood counts, nausea, vomiting, diarrhea, sore mouth, hair loss, local irritation if leaks outside vein, heart toxicity after extended use

Ifosfamide (Ifex)

Type of Cancer Non-Hodgkin's lymphomas, lung, ovary, testis, sarcomas, melanoma, chronic lymphocytic leukemia
Route Administered Intravenous
Precautions Requires uroprotector (Mesna); bladder catheter often needed during treatment
Side Effects Bladder bleeding and inflammation, cystitis, kidney malfunction, low blood counts, sleepiness and confusion, hair loss, liver malfunction, phlebitis, antidiuretic effect (water overload), lung scarring, nausea, vomiting

IL-2 (Proleukin, Aldesleukin)

Type of Cancer Kidney cancer, melanoma
Route Administered Intravenous
Precautions Treatment conducted usually in hospital (often in intensive care unit); also given in lower dosage as outpatient. Multidisciplinary team oversees all aspects of administration. Complex and continuous monitoring, clinical evaluation, and laboratory/x-ray studies are needed to minimize risk of therapy.
Side Effects Many adverse effects: leakage of fluid from small blood vessels, low blood pressure, rapid heartbeat, edema, weight gain, shortness of breath, cough, temporary kidney impairment, nausea, vomiting, diarrhea, sore mouth, neurologic changes, disorientation, decreased blood counts, abnormal liver tests, hair loss, rash, itching, fatigue, fever, chills, muscle aching

Interferon-alpha
Intron-A
Roferon-A

Type of Cancer Melanoma, kidney, myeloma, chronic myelogenous leukemia, hairy cell leukemia, Kaposi's sarcoma, lymphoma, others
Route Administered Intramuscular
Side Effects Sweating, fever, nerve numbness and tingling, arthralgias, dizziness, rash, skin itching, high blood pressure, flu syndrome, muscle aching, weight loss, loss of appetite, nausea, vomiting, diarrhea, altered taste and smell, sore mouth

Leucovorin (Folinic acid)

Type of Cancer To reverse clinical toxicity of methotrexate and to potentiate and modulate 5-FU
Route Administered Oral, Intramuscular, Intravenous
Precautions May counteract antiepileptic effect of phenobarbital
Side Effects Will increase symptoms of pernicious anemia, allergic reactions, nausea, vomiting

Leuprolide (Lupron)

Type of Cancer Prostate
Route Administered Subcutaneous
Precautions Temporary increased bone pain, use flutamide (Eulexin) to improve results and help prevent flare reaction
Side Effects Hot flashes, enlarged swollen and tender breasts, skin rash, testicular atrophy, peripheral edema, dizziness, headaches, tingling in extremities, loss of appetite, nausea, vomiting, constipation, diarrhea, difficulty swallowing, elevated blood pressure

Levamisole (Ergamisole)

Type of Cancer Colon
Route Administered Oral
Precautions Has been reported to produce "antabuse-like" effects when given concomitantly with alcohol. No alcohol on days one takes levamisole
Side Effects Mild diarrhea, nausea, vomiting, stomatitis (sore mouth), altered taste and smell, abdominal discomfort and diarrhea (especially when combined with 5-FU), low blood counts, fatigue, weakness, and flu-like symptoms. Occasional headaches, confusion, insomnia, excitement and convulsions

Lomustine
CCNU

Type of Cancer Hodgkin's and non-Hodgkin's lymphoma, brain, melanoma, kidney, lung
Route Adminstered Oral
Precautions Nausea program
Side Effects Low blood counts, hair loss, confusion, liver toxicity (jaundice), lung toxicity (cough, shortness of breath), skin rash, itching, pre-leukemia and bone marrow scarring, loss of appetite, nausea, vomiting, diarrhea, sore mouth

Mechlorethamine (Mustargen) (Nitrogen mustard)

Type of Cancer Hodgkin's and non-Hodgkin's lymphoma, malignant pleural effusions, lung, mycosis fungoides

Route Administered Intravenous, Intracavitary, topical (skin ointment)

Precautions Antinausea program, severe reaction with IV leak

Side Effects Low blood counts, thrombophlebitis, tissue reaction, second malignancies, hair loss, skin rash (rare), sterility, anorexia, nausea, vomiting, gastrointestinal bleeding and ulcers, increased uric acid (gout), secondary malignancies

Melphalan (Alkeran)

Type of Cancer Multiple myeloma, ovary, breast

Route Administered Oral.

Side Effects Low blood counts, second malignancies, pulmonary scarring, loss of menstrual periods, low sperm count, dermatitis, nausea, vomiting, sore mouth, increased uric acid (gout)

Mercaptopurine (Purinethol) (6-MP)

Type of Cancer Acute leukemia, chronic myelogenous leukemia, immunosuppression

Route Administered Oral

Precautions Reduce dosage if allopurinol also given

Side Effects Low blood counts, liver scarring and abnormal function, lung scarring, shortness of breath, cough, pneumonia, kidney failure, headaches, stroke, mental changes, hair loss, loss of appetite, nausea, vomiting, diarrhea, sore mouth, abdominal discomfort, increased uric acid production (gout)

Mesna (Mesnex)

Type of Cancer To prevent bladder irritation (hemorrhagic cystitis) from ifosfamide and high-dose Cytoxan

Route Adminstered Intravenous

Side Effects Nausea, vomiting, diarrhea

Methotrexate (Mexate)

Type of Cancer Acute leukemia, sarcoma, choriocarcinoma, head and neck, breast, lung, stomach, esophagus, testis, lymphoma, mycosis fungoides

Route Administered Oral, Intravenous, Intramuscular, Subcutaneous, Spinal (intrathecal)

Precautions Maintain good fluid intake, alkaline urine, good oral hygiene, minimize sun exposure, use sun screen

Side Effects Low blood counts, skin rash, liver enzyme abnormalities and jaundice, kidney toxicity, lung scarring, shortness of breath, seizures, coma, dizziness, confusion, tiredness, joint pains, anorexia, nausea, vomiting, diarrhea, gastrointestinal bleeding and ulcers, lactose intolerance, iron and protein loss, fat-soluble vitamin loss

Mitomycin-C (Mutamycin)

Type of Cancer colon, stomach, pancreas, esophagus, anus, breast, lung, cervix, bladder

Route Administered Intravenous

Precautions Take care not to leak outside of vein, vitamin B6 (pyridoxine) will reduce tissue damage from extravasation, infections, bleeding

Side Effects Weakness, lung scarring (interstitial pneumonitis), renal failure with severe blood platelet reaction (hemolytic-uremic syndrome), hair loss, liver toxicity, synergistic heart toxicity with doxorubicin, loss of appetite, nausea, vomiting, diarrhea, sore mouth, loss of protein and salts, severe skin reaction with IV leak

Mitotane (Lysodren)

Type of Cancer Adrenal cortical carcinoma

Route Administered Oral

Side Effects Lethargy, sleepiness, dizziness, vertigo, skin rash, headaches, high blood pressure, blurred vision, bladder bleeding, anorexia, nausea, diarrhea

Mitoxantrone (Novantrone)

Type of Cancer Acute leukemia, breast, ovary, lymphomas

Route Adminstered Intravenous

Side Effects Low blood counts, heart toxicity, muscle damage, heart failure, liver toxicity, nausea, vomiting, diarrhea, sore mouth, gastrointestinal bleeding and ulcers, urine may turn green

Pentostatin (Deoxycoformycin)

Type of Cancer Hairy cell leukemia, lymphomas, cutaneous T cell lymphoma (Mycosis fungoides)

Route Administered Intravenous

Precautions Nausea program, monitor liver function
Side Effects Decreased blood counts, cough, shortness of breath, fever, chills, muscle aching, abnormal liver tests, confusion, headache, fatigue, nervous disturbances, nausea, vomiting, sore mouth, diarrhea

Procarbazine

Type of Cancer Hodgkin's disease, occasionally used in other cancers
Route Administered Oral
Precautions Avoid alcohol, old cheeses, red wine, yogurt, liver
Side Effects Rash, skin pigmentation, nausea, unsteady gait, decreased blood counts, mood changes, insomnia, tingling of toes and fingers

Progestins (Megace, Provera)

Types of Cancer Breast, prostate, uterus, kidney; to treat weight loss (cachexia)
Route Administered Oral, Intramuscular
Precautions History of thrombophlebitis, contraindicated in the first four months of pregnancy, low salt diet (fluid retention), which may worsen pre-existing epilepsy, migraine, asthma, cardiac or renal problems
Side Effects Vaginal bleeding, spotting and change in menstrual cycle, lack of menstrual periods, edema, (diuretics may be necessary), jaundice, allergic rash, itching, nausea, vomiting, weight gain and mental depression. When used in combination with estrogens, increased cerebral thrombosis and embolism. Occasional glucose intolerance. Increased excretion of salt: a sodium restricted diet may be essential

Streptozocin

Type of Cancer Pancreas (islet cell), small bowel
Route Administered Intravenous
Side Effects Severe skin reaction with IV leak, nausea and vomiting, diarrhea, nail changes, low blood counts, kidney or liver toxicity

Tamoxifen (Nolvadex)

Type of Cancer Breast, endometrial, ovary, melanoma, prostate (under investigation)
Route Administered Oral

Side Effects Hot flashes, low blood counts, vaginal bleeding, itching, anorexia, nausea, vomiting, taste changes, weight gain, dehydration, blood clots, uterine polyps, rare eye toxicity, low risk of uterine cancer. Bone pain initially may signify response

Taxol (Paclitaxel)

Type of Cancer Ovary, breast, lung, head and neck
Route Administered Intravenous
Precautions Hypersensitivity reaction; pretreat with steroids, H2 blockers, and antihistamines. Longer infusion times minimize this. Electrocardiogram monitoring, nausea program
Side Effects Decreased blood counts, sore mouth, complete hair loss, nerve damage, muscle and joint aching, slow heartbeat, abnormal heart rhythms, fatigue, headache, rare nausea and vomiting

Teniposide (VM-26)

Indications Acute leukemia, neuroblastoma, non-Hodgkin's lymphoma, small cell cancer
Route Administered Intravenous
Precautions Monitor blood pressure during infusion
Side Effects Nausea and vomiting, diarrhea, low blood counts, hair loss, allergic reactions, severe skin reaction with IV leak

Thioguanine

Type of Cancer Acute non-lymphocytic leukemia
Route Administered Oral.
Side Effects Low blood counts, liver failure (jaundice), bleeding, rash, anorexia, nausea, vomiting, diarrhea, increased uric acid (gout), niacin and amino acid deficiency

Thiotepa (Triethylenethiophosphoramide)

Type of Cancer Breast, bladder, ovary, Hodgkin's disease, bone marrow transplantation
Route Administered Intravenous
Side Effects Low blood counts, headaches, fever, bronchoconstriction, dizziness, local pain., loss of appetite, nausea, vomiting, potential secondary malignancies

Vinblastine (Velban)

Type of Cancer Hodgkin's disease, choriocarcinoma, testis, breast, lung, Kaposi's sarcoma

Route Administered Intravenous

Precautions Take care not to leak from IV site, constipation program

Side Effects Severe skin reaction with IV leak, low blood counts, peripheral neuropathies, headache, rash, hair loss, anorexia, nausea, vomiting, sore mouth or throat, constipation, abdominal discomfort

Vincristine (Oncovin)

Type of Cancer Acute lymphocytic leukemia, Hodgkin's and non-Hodgkin's lymphoma, neuroblastoma, testis, sarcomas, lung, breast, cervix, Wilms' tumor

Route Administered Intravenous

Precautions Take care not to leak from IV site (irritating), constipation program

Side Effects Severe reaction with IV leak, numbness, tingling fingers and feet, hair loss, loss of nerve function (foot drop and partial paralysis), low blood counts, nausea, vomiting, constipation, sore mouth and throat, difficulty chewing or swallowing, dry mouth, altered taste and smell, increased uric acid (gout)

RESOURCES

◇

DIRECTORY OF CANCER ASSOCIATIONS AND SUPPORT GROUPS

American Academy of Pain Medicine
5700 Old Orchard Road
Skokie, IL 60077
(708) 966-9510

American Cancer Society
National Headquarters
1599 Clifton Road N.E.
Atlanta, GA 30329
(800) ACS-2345

American Brain Tumor Association
3725 North Talman Avenue
Chicago, IL 60618
(312) 286-5571
(800) 886-2282

American Melanoma Foundation
c/o Malcolm Mitchell, MD
Center for Biological Therapy and
Melanoma Research
University of California, San Diego
9500 Gilman Drive
La Jolla, CA 92093

American Pain Society
5700 Old Orchard Road
Skokie, IL 60077
(708) 966-5595

Biological Therapy Institute Foundation
P.O. Box 681700
Franklin, TN 37068
(615) 790-7535

Bone Marrow Transplant Family Support Network
P.O. Box 845
Avon, CT 06001
(800) 826-9376

Breast Cancer Advisory Center
11426 Rockville Pike, Suite 406
Rockville, MD 20859
(301) 984-1020

CanCare
2929 Selwyn Avenue
Charlotte, NC 28209
(704) 372-1232
(one-to-one support services)

Cancer Guidance Institute
5604 Solway Street
Pittsburgh, PA 15217
(412) 521-2291 or 782-4023

Cancer Information Service
National Cancer Institute
Bethesda, MD
(800) 4-CANCER

Cancer Support Network
802 East Jefferson
Bloomington, IL 61701
(309) 829-2273

Candlelighters Childhood Cancer Foundation
7910 Woodmont Avenue, Suite 460
Bethesda, MD 20814
(301) 657-8401
(800) 366-2223

Children's Hospice International
1101 King Street, Suite 131
Alexandria, VA 22314
(703) 684-0330
(800) 242-4453

Choice in Dying
200 Varick Street
New York, NY 10014
(212) 366-5540

Colon Cancer Support Group
c/o Andrew Kneier
UCSF/Mt. Zion Cancer Center
2356 Sutter Street
San Francisco, CA 94120
(415) 885-7546

Corporate Angel Network
Westchester County Airport, Building 1
White Plains, NY 10604
(914) 328-1313
(long distance transportation service)

Encore
YWCA of the U.S.A.
726 Broadway, 5th Floor
New York, NY 10003
(212) 614-2700
(exercise and discussion program for
women with breast cancer)

The Helping Hand Melanoma Newletter
12 Arlington Avenue
Portland, ME 04101

Hospicelink
Hospice Education Institute
5 Essex Square, Suite 3-B
P.O. Box 713
Essex, CT 06426-0713
(203) 767-1620
(800) 331-1620

**International Association for
Enterostomal Therapy**
505-A Tustin Avenue, Suite 282
Santa Ana, CA 92705
(714) 972-1725

**International Association of
Laryngectomees**
1599 Clifton Road N.E.
Atlanta, GA 30329
(404) 329-7650

International Myeloma Foundation
2120 Stanley Hills Drive
Los Angeles, CA 90046
(213) 654-3023
(800) 452-CURE

Let's Face It
Box 711
Concord, MA 01742
(508) 371-3186
(for people who have facial disfigure-
ments)

Leukemia Society of America
600 Third Avenue
New York, NY 10016
(212) 573-8484
(800) 284-4271

The Lost Chord
(Contact a local chapter of the American
Cancer Society)

Make Today Count
c/o Mid-America Cancer Center
1235 East Cherokee
Springfield, MO 65804-2263
(417) 885-3324
(800) 432-2273

Make-a-Wish Foundation of America
1624 East Meadowbrook
Phoenix, AZ
(602) 248-9474

Melanoma Foundation
c/o Richard Sagebiel, MD
UCSF/Mt. Zion Medical Center
2356 Sutter Street, 5th Floor
San Francisco, CA 94120
(415) 885-7546

National Cancer Institute
Building 31, Room 10A19
9000 Rockville Pike
Bethesda, MD 20892
(800) 4-CANCER

**National Coalition for Cancer
Survivorship**
1010 Wayne Avenue, 5th Floor
Silver Spring, MD 20910
(301) 650-8868

National Hospice Organization
1901 N. Moore Street, Suite 901
Arlington, VA 22209
(703) 243-5900
(800) 658-8898

National Leukemia Association, Inc.
585 Stewart Avenue, Suite 536
Garden City, NY 11530
(516) 222-1944

**Patient Advocates for Advanced Cancer
Treatments**
1143 Parmelee N.W.
Grand Rapids, MI 49504
(616) 453-1477

PDQ (Physician Data Query)
(800) 4-CANCER

Planetree Health Resource Center
2040 Webster Street
San Francisco, CA 94115
(415) 923-3680

R.A. Bloch Cancer Foundation, Inc.
The Cancer Hotline
4410 Main Street
Kansas City, MO 64111
(816) 932-8453

Ronald McDonald Houses
Golin/Harris Communications, Inc.
500 North Michigan Avenue
Chicago, IL 60611
(312) 836-7384

Share
817 Broadway, 6th Floor
New York, NY 10003
(212) 260-0580
(self-help for women with breast cancer)

Skin Cancer Foundation
245 Fifth Avenue, Suite 2402
New York, NY 10016
(212) 725-5176

The Skin Cancer Fund
Box 561
New York, NY 10156

Sunshine Foundation
4010 Levick Street
Philadelphia, PA 19135
(215) 335-2622
(800) 767-1976

Sunshine Kids
2902 Ferndale Place
Houston, TX 77098
(713) 524-1264

Susan G. Komen Breast Cancer Foundation
5005 LBJ Freeway, Suite 370
Dallas, TX 75244
(800) I'M AWARE

United Ostomy Association
36 Executive Park, Suite 120
Irvine, CA 92714
(714) 660-8624

US-TOO
P.O. Box 7173
Oakbrook Terrace, IL
(800) 82-US-TOO

Wellness Community National Headquarters
2200 Colorado Avenue
Santa Monica, CA 90404-3506
(310) 453-2300
(800) PRO-HOPE

Y-ME
National Organization for Breast Cancer Information and Support, Inc.
18220 Harwood Avenue
Homewood, IL 60430-2104
(708) 799-8338
(800) 221-2141

CANCER INFORMATION SERVICE OFFICES

Comprehensive Cancer Center
University of Alabama at Birmingham
1918 University Boulevard, Room 108
University Station
Birmingham, AL 35294
(205) 934-6614

Jonsson Comprehensive Cancer Center/UCLA
1100 Glendon Avenue, Suite 711
Los Angeles, CA 90024
(213) 206-0278

Penrose Cancer Hospital
P.O. Box 7021
Colorado Springs, CO 80933
(719) 630-5271

Yale Comprehensive Cancer Center
Office of Cancer Communications
333 Cedar Street, LEPH 139
P.O. Box 3333
New Haven, CT 06510-8027
(203) 785-6347

Sylvester Comprehensive Cancer Center
Jackson Towers
1500 NW 12th Avenue, Suite 1004
Miami, FL 33136
(305) 548-4821

Illinois Cancer Council
36 South Wabash, Suite 700
Chicago, IL 60603
(312) 346-9813, Ext 351

University of Kansas Medical Center
Student Center, Room 203
39th and Rainbow Boulevard
Kansas City, KS 66103
(913) 588-4570

Markey Cancer Center
Roach Building, Room 170
800 Rose Street
Lexington, KY 40536-0093
(606) 257-3601

Kentucky Cancer Program
University of Louisville
529 South Jackson Street
Louisville, KY 40292
(502) 588-6318

Johns Hopkins Cancer Information Service
550 North Broadway, Room 307
Baltimore, MD 21205
(410) 955-3636

Dana-Farber Cancer Institute
44 Binney Street
Boston, MA 02115
(617) 732-3214

Michigan Cancer Foundation
110 E. Warren Avenue
Detroit, MI 48201
(313) 833-0710, Ext 432

Albert Einstein Cancer Center
Montefiore Medical Center
111 East 210th Street
Bronx, NY 10467
(212) 920-4826

Albert Einstein Cancer Center
Weiler Hospital
1825 Eastchester Road
Bronx, NY 10461
(212) 904-2754

Memorial Sloan-Kettering Cancer Center
Office of Cancer Communications
1275 York Avenue
New York, NY 10021
(212) 639-3540

Roswell Park Memorial Institute
Elm and Carlton Streets
Buffalo, NY 14263
(716) 845-3115

Duke Comprehensive Cancer Center
Erwin Square, Suite 10
2020 West Main Street
Durham, NC 27705
(919) 286-5515

Ireland Cancer Center
University Hospitals of Cleveland
Case Western Reserve University
2074 Abington Road
Cleveland, OH 44106
(216) 844-5432

Ohio Cancer Information Service
168 Upham Hall
473 West 12th Avenue
Columbus, OH 43210
(614) 293-4600

Fox Chase Cancer Center
510 Township Line Road
Cheltenham, PA 19012
(215) 728-3690

The Thompson Cancer Survival Center
1915 White Avenue, Suite 107
Knoxville, TN 37916
(615) 541-1318

M.D. Anderson Cancer Center
1515 Holcombe Boulevard, #229
Houston, TX 77030
(713) 792-3363

University of Utah Health Sciences Center
AB 15
50 North Medical Drive
Salt Lake City, UT 84132
(801) 581-5052

Fred Hutchinson Cancer Research Center
Mailstop MP-243
1124 Columbia
Seattle, WA 98104
(206) 467-4675

Mary Babb Randolph Cancer Center
West Virginia University
510 Medical Center Drive
Morgantown, WV 26506
(304) 293-2370

All these centers can also be reached by dialing (800) 4-CANCER.

NATIONAL CANCER INSTITUTE DESIGNATED COMPREHENSIVE CANCER CENTERS

University of Alabama at Birmingham Comprehensive Cancer Center
Basic Health Sciences Building, Room 108
1918 University Boulevard
Birmingham, AL 35294
(205) 934-6612

University of Arizona Cancer Center
1501 North Campbell Avenue
Tucson, AZ 85724
(602) 626-6372

Jonsson Comprehensive Cancer Center
University of California at Los Angeles
200 Medical Plaza
Los Angeles, CA 90027
(213) 206-0278

Kenneth T. Norris Jr. Comprehensive Cancer Center
University of Southern California
1441 Eastlake Avenue
Los Angeles, CA 90033-0804
(213) 226-2370

Penrose Cancer Hospital
P.O. Box 7021
Colorado Springs, CO 80933
(719) 630-5271

Yale University Comprehensive Cancer Center
333 Cedar Street
New Haven, CT 06510
(203) 785-6338

Lombardi Cancer Research Center
Georgetown University Medical Center
3800 Reservoir Road N.W.
Washington, DC 20007
(202) 687-2192

Sylvester Comprehensive Cancer Center
University of Miami Medical School
1475 Northwest 12th Avenue
Miami, FL 33136
(305) 548-4800

Johns Hopkins Oncology Center
600 North Wolfe Street
Baltimore, MD 21205
(410) 955-8638

Dana-Farber Cancer Institute
44 Binney Street
Boston, MA 02115
(617) 732-3214

University of Michigan Cancer Center
101 Simpson Drive
Ann Arbor, MI 48109-0752
(313) 936-9583

Meyer L. Prentis Comprehensive Cancer Center of Metropolitan Detroit
110 East Warren Avenue
Detroit, MI 48201
(313) 745-4329

Mayo Comprehensive Cancer Center
200 First Street S.W.
Rochester, MN 55905
(507) 284-3413

Norris Cotton Cancer Center
Dartmouth-Hitchcock Medical Center
One Medical Center Drive
Lebanon, NH 03756
(603) 646-5505

Albert Einstein Cancer Center
Weiler Hospital
1825 Eastchester Road
Bronx, NY 10461
(212) 904-2754

Albert Einstein Cancer Center
Montefiore Medical Center
111 East 210th Street
Bronx, NY 10467
(212) 920-4826

Roswell Park Cancer Institute
Elm and Carlton Streets
Buffalo, NY 14263
(716) 845-4400

Columbia University Comprehensive Cancer Center
College of Physicians and Surgeons
630 West 168th Street
New York, NY 10032
(212) 305-6905

Memorial Sloan-Kettering Cancer Center
1275 York Avenue
New York, NY 10021
(800) 525-2225

Kaplan Cancer Center
New York University Medical Center
462 First Avenue
New York, NY 10016-9103
(212) 263-6485

UNC Lineberger Comprehensive Cancer Center
University of North Carolina School of Medicine
Chapel Hill, NC 27599
(919) 966-4431

Duke Comprehensive Cancer Center
P.O. Box 3814
Durham, NC 27710
(919) 286-5515

Cancer Center of Wake Forest University at the Bowman Gray School of Medicine
300 South Hawthorne Road
Winston-Salem, NC 27103
(919) 748-4354

Ohio State University Comprehensive Cancer Center
300 West 10th Avenue
Columbus, OH 43210
(614) 293-5485

Fox Chase Cancer Center
7701 Burholme Avenue
Philadelphia, PA 19111
(215) 728-2570

University of Pennsylvania Cancer Center
3400 Spruce Street
Philadelphia, PA 19104
(215) 662-6364

Pittsburgh Cancer Institute
200 Meyran Avenue
Pittsburgh, PA 15213-2592
(800) 537-4063

The University of Texas M.D. Anderson Cancer Center
1515 Holcombe Boulevard
Houston, TX 77030
(713) 792-3245

Vermont Regional Cancer Center
University of Vermont
1 South Prospect Street
Burlington, VT 05401
(802) 656-4580

Fred Hutchinson Cancer Research Center
1124 Columbia Street
Seattle, WA 98104
(206) 667-4675

Mary Babb Randolph Cancer Center
West Virginia University
510 Medical Center Drive
Morgantown, WV 26506
(304) 293-2370

The University of Wisconsin Comprehensive Cancer Center
600 Highland Avenue
Madison, WI 53792
(608) 263-8600

CLINICAL CANCER CENTERS

City of Hope National Medical Center
Beckman Research Institute
1500 East Duarte Road
Duarte, CA 91010
(818) 359-8111, Ext 2292

University of California at San Diego
Cancer Center
225 Dickinson Street
San Diego, CA 92103
(619) 543-6178

University of Colorado Cancer Center
4200 East 9th Avenue, Box B190
Denver, CO 80262
(303) 270-7235

University of Chicago Cancer Research
Center
5841 South Maryland Avenue, Box 444
Chicago, IL 60637
(312) 702-6180

Albert Einstein College of Medicine
1300 Morris Park Avenue
Bronx, NY 10461
(212) 920-4826

University of Rochester Cancer Center
601 Elmwood Avenue, Box 704
Rochester, NY 14642
(716) 275-4911

Ireland Cancer Center
University Hospitals of Cleveland
Case Western Reserve University
2074 Abington Road
Cleveland, OH 44106
(216) 844-5432

Roger Williams Cancer Center
Brown University
825 Chalkstone Avenue
Providence, RI 02908
(401) 456-2071

St. Jude Children's Research Hospital
332 N. Lauderdale Street
Memphis, TN 38101-0318
(901) 522-0306

Institute for Cancer Research and Care
4450 Medical Drive
San Antonio, TX 78229
(512) 616-5580

Utah Regional Cancer Center
University of Utah Health Sciences Center
50 North Medical Drive, Room 2C110
Salt Lake City, UT 84132
(801) 581-4048

Massey Cancer Center
Medical College of Virginia
Virginia Commonwealth University
1200 E. Broad Street
Richmond, VA 23298
(804) 786-9641

CONSORTIA

Drew-Meharry-Morehouse Consortium
Cancer Center
1005 D.B. Todd Boulevard
Nashville, TN 37208
(615) 327-6927

CLINICAL TRIALS
COOPERATIVE GROUPS

Brain Tumor Cooperative Group
12501 Prosperity Drive, Suite 200
Silver Spring, MD 20904
(301) 680-9770

Cancer and Leukemia Group B
CALGB Central Office
444 Mount Support Road, Suite 2
Lebanon, NH 03766
(603) 646-6333

Children's Cancer Study Group
University of Southern California
199 North Lake Avenue, 3rd Floor
Pasadena, CA 91101-1859
(213) 681-3032

Eastern Cooperative Oncology Group
Wisconsin Clinical Cancer Center
University of Wisconsin
Medical Science Center, Room 4725
420 North Charter Street
Madison, WI 53706
(608) 263-6650

Gynecologic Oncology Group
GOG Headquarters
1234 Market Street, 19th Floor
Philadelphia, PA 19107
(215) 854-0770

Intergroup Rhabdomyosarcoma Study
Department of Pediatrics
Virginia Commonwealth University
Medical College of Virginia
MCV Box 646
Richmond, VA 23298
(804) 786-9602

National Surgical Adjuvant Project for Breast and Bowel Cancers
University of Pittsburgh
914 Scaife Hall, 3550 Terrace Street
Pittsburgh, PA 15261
(412) 648-9720

National Wilms' Tumor Study Group
Children's Cancer Research Center
Children's Hospital of Philadelphia
3400 Civic Center Boulevard, 9th Floor
Philadelphia, PA 19104
(215) 387-5518

North Central Cancer Treatment Group
Room 75 - Damon
Mayo Clinic
200 First Street S.W.
Rochester, MN 55905
(507) 284-4972

Pediatric Oncology Group
The Edward Mallinckrodt Department
of Pediatrics
Washington University School of
Medicine
4949 West Pine Street, Suite 2A
St. Louis, MS 63108
(314) 367-3446

Radiation Therapy Oncology Group
RTOG Headquarters
American College of Radiology
1101 Market Street, 14th Floor
Philadelphia, PA 19107
(215) 574-3195

Southwest Oncology Group
Cancer Therapy and Research Center
5430 Fredericksburg Road
San Antonio, TX 78229-3533
(512) 366-9300

SUGGESTED READINGS

◇

BOOKS FOR THE PUBLIC

Breast Cancer: The Complete Guide. Y. Hirshaut and P. Pressman, Bantam, 1993.

Can You Prevent Cancer? E.H. Rosenbaum, Mosby Medical Library, 1983.

Cancer and Hope: Charting a Survival Course. Judith Garrett Garrison, Comp. Care Publishing, 1989.

The Cancer Conqueror: An Incredible Journey to Wellness. Greg Anderson, Andrews and McMeel, Kansas City, 1990.

Cancervive: The Challenge of Life After Cancer. Susan Nessim and Judith Ellis, Houghton-Mifflin, 1991.

Choices: Realistic Alternatives in Cancer Treatment. Marion Morra and Eve Potts, Avon, 1987.

Choices in Healing: Integrating the Best of Conventional and Complementary Approaches to Cancer. Michael Lerner, MIT Press, 1994.

A Comprehensive Guide for Cancer Patients and Their Families. E.H. Rosenbaum and I.R. Rosenbaum, Bull Publishing, 1980.

Coping with Chemotherapy. N. Bruning, The Dial Press, Rev. ed., 1993.

Decision for Life: Portrait of Living. E.H. Rosenbaum, Bull Publishing, 1980.

The Diagnosis is Cancer. E.J. Larschan and R.J. Larschan, Bull Publishing, 1986.

Dr. Susan Love's Breast Book. Susan Love, Addison-Wesley, 1990.

From Victim to Victor. H. Benjamin, Jeremy Tarcher, 1987.

Getting Well Again. O.C. Simonton and J.L. Creighton, Bantam, 1978.

Going Home - a Home Care Training Program. E.H. Rosenbaum and I.R. Rosenbaum, Bull Publishing, 1980.

In the Company of Others: Understanding the Human Needs of Cancer Patients. Jory Graham, Harcourt Brace Jovanovich, 1982.

Living with Cancer. E.H. Rosenbaum, Mosby Medical Library, 1982.

Living with Lung Cancer: a Guide for Patients and their Families. B.G. Cox, Triad Publications Co., 1987.

Love, Medicine and Miracles. B.S. Siegel, Harper and Row, 1986.

Nutrition for Cancer Patients. J. Ramstack, E.R. Rosenbaum and B. Carter, Bull Publishing, 1990.

Nutrition for the Cancer Patient. E.H. Rosenbaum, C.N. Stitt, H. Drasin and I.R. Rosenbaum, Bull Publishing, 1980.

The Ostomy Book: Living Comfortably with Colostomies, Ileostomies and Urostomies. Barbara Dorr Mullen and Kerry McGinn, Bull Publishing, 1992.

The Race is Run One Step at a Time. N. Brinker and C.E. Harris, Simon and Schuster, 1990.

The Road Back to Health: Coping with the Emotional Side of Cancer. Neil A. Fiore, Bantam, 1984.

When Bad Things Happen to Good People. Herbert Kushner, Simon and Schuster, 2d ed., 1989.

Young People with Cancer: a Handbook for Parents. Office of Cancer Communications, National Cancer Institute and National Candlelighters Foundation. Department of Health and Human Services, 1988.

MEDICAL BOOKS

The American Cancer Society Cancer Book: Prevention, Detection, Diagnosis, Treatment, Rehabilitation, and Cure. Arthur I. Holleb et al., ed. Doubleday, 1993.

Cancer Nursing: Principles and Practice. Susan L. Groenwald et al., ed. Jones and Bartlett, 3d ed., 1993.

Cancer: Principles and Practice of Oncology. Vincent T. DeVita, Jr. et al., ed. Lippincott, 4th ed., 1993.

Cancer Chemotherapy: Principles and Practice. Bruce A. Chabner et al., ed. Lippincott, 1990.

Cancer Chemotherapy Handbook. David S. Fischer and M. Tish Knobf, ed. Year Book Medical Publishers, 4th ed., 1993.

Cancer Medicine. James F. Holland et al. Lea & Febiger, 3d ed., 1993.

Cancer Pain. Richard B. Patt, ed. Lippincott, 1993.

Cancer Treatment. Charles M. Haskell, ed. W.B. Saunders, 3d ed., 1990.

Comprehensive Textbook of Oncology. A.R. Moosa et al. Williams & Wilkins, 2d ed., 1991.

Diagnosis and Management of Breast Cancer. Marc E. Lippman, MD, et al., ed. W.B. Saunders, 1988.

Handbook of Oncology Nursing. Bonny Libbey Johnson and Jody Gross. Wiley, 1985.

Handbook of Pediatric Oncology. Roberta A. Gottlieb and Donald Pinkel, ed. Little, Brown & Co., 1989.

Handbook of Psychooncology: Psychological Care of the Patient with Cancer. James C. Holland and Julia Rowland, ed. Oxford University Press, 1989.

Manual of Clinical Oncology. Dennis Albert Casciato and Barry Bennett Lowitz, ed. Little, Brown & Co., 2d ed., 1988.

Manual of Clinical Problems in Oncology. Carol S. Portlock and Donald R. Goffinet. 2nd edition. Little, Brown & Co., 1986.

Manual of Oncologic Therapeutics 1991/ 1992. Robert E. Wittes, ed. Lippincott, 1991.

Neoplastic Diseases of the Blood. P.H. Wiernik, G.P. Canellos, R.A. Kyle and C.A. Schiffer, ed. Churchill Livingstone, 1991.

Principles and Practice of Radiation Oncology. Carlos A. Perez and Luther W. Brady, eds. Lippincott, 2d ed., 1992.

Principles of Cancer Biotherapy. Robert K. Oldham, ed. Raven Press, 2d ed., 1991.

AUDIOTAPES

c/o Cancer Care Associates
3440 Lomita Boulevard
Torrance, CA 90505

Coping with Cancer. M. Dollinger. 1991.

Understanding Cancer. M. Dollinger. 1990.

INDEX

◇

A

Abdominal-perineal resection, 281-82, 344
Abortion, risk factor, 626
Acetaminophen, 151, 289
Achlorhydria, 593
Acquired Immune Deficiency
  Syndrome *see* AIDS
Acromegaly, 557
ACS *see* American Cancer Society
  (ACS)
ACTH-producing tumor, 557-58
Actinomycin-D, *see also*
  Dactinomycin
  for bone and soft tissue sarcomas, 575
  for Ewing's sarcoma, 375
  for ovarian cancer, 542-43
  for rhabdomyosarcoma, 373
  for testis cancer, 607
  for trophoblastic disease, 628-29
  for uterine cancer, 640-42
  for vaginal cancer, 646
Active-specific immunotherapy *see*
  Tumor vaccines, 507
Active stimulation immunotherapy, 68
Activity, *see also* Exercise, 122-24, 128, 139
Acupressure, 179-80
Acute leukemia
  defined, 451
  lymphoblastic, 355, 359-60, 457-58
  lymphocytic, 357, 451
  myeloblastic, 456-57
  non-lymphoblastic, 355, 360
  treatment, 455-58
Acyclovir, 132, 157
Addiction, 153
Addison's disease, 613
Adenocarcinoma
  anus, 277
  bile duct, 283
  bladder, 288-89, 296
  breast, 310
  cervix, 347, 349, 350-51
  colorectal, 377-78
  endometrium, 631
  esophagus, 395
  gall bladder, 404
  intraductal, 570
  kidney, 444
  liver, 462, 467

lung, 469
pancreas, 544
prostate, 559
small intestine, 586, 587-88
stomach, 591
unknown primary site, 335
vagina, 643-45
vulva, 648-49, 653
Adenoma
  adrenocortical, 271-72
  chromophobe, 557-58
  cortical, 271
  pituitary, 305
Adenosquamous carcinoma
  cervix, 347, 349
  endometrium, 631
  pancreas, 544
Adjunctive therapies, unproven, 98-99
Adjuvant therapy, *see also*
  Treatment *under specific cancers*
  after surgery, 56-57
  chemotherapy, 33-34, 61
  immunotherapy, 68
Adoptive immunotherapy, 68
Adrenal gland cancer
  child, 356
  diagnosis, 272-73
  follow-up, 275
  questions to ask, 276
  recurrence, 276
  risk factors, 272
  screening, 272
  spread, 272
  staging, 273
  symptoms, 272
  treatment, 273-75
  types, 271-72
Adrenal glands, diagram, 446
Adrenal insufficiency, 613
Adrenergic blockers, 344
Adrenocortical carcinoma, 271-73, 274-75
Adriamycin, *see also* Doxorubicin
  for anal cancer, 282
  for bladder cancer, 294, 296
  for bone and soft tissue sarcomas, 575
  for breast cancer, 323, 329-31, 334
  for esophageal cancer, 402
  for gastrointestinal cancer, 345
  for Hodgkin's disease, 489-90
  for islet cell carcinoma, 433
  for Kaposi's sarcoma, 441-42

for leukemia, 457
for liver cancer, 465-67
for lung cancer, 479
for lymphoma, 482, 498
for multiple myeloma, 527, 529
for ovarian cancer, 536, 538
for pancreatic cancer, 546-48
for stomach cancer, 596-97, 600
for thymus cancer, 614
for uterine cancer, 634-37, 640-42
for vaginal cancer, 646
side effects, 129, 139
Advance Directive, 221
Affirmation, 202
Age
  breast cancer, 311
  colorectal cancer, 378
  multiple myeloma, 524
  pancreatic cancer, 544-45
  penile cancer, 554
  prostate cancer, 561
  small intestine cancer, 587
  stomach cancer, 593
  testis cancer, 604
  treatment options, 35
  trophoblastic disease, 626
  uterine sarcoma, 639
AIDS, *see also* Human immunodeficiency virus (HIV)
  blood transfusion, 102, 106
  brain tumor, 299
  CNS lymphoma, 305
  Kaposi's sarcoma, 436-41
  lymphoma, 481-83
AIDS-related cancers, 7
Albinism, 580
Alcohol
  mouth irritant, 132
  risk factor, 7, 238, 395-96, 412, 545
  and sexual dysfunction, 169
Aldosteronoma, 271
Alkaloids, 58
Alkeran, *see also* Melphalan
  for breast cancer, 329
  for Hodgkin's disease, 489
  for multiple myeloma, 527
  for ovarian cancer, 538
  may cause bladder cancer, 289
  may cause nausea, 129
Alkylating agents, 57, 83, 291, 527
Allergic reaction, to biological therapy, 73
Allogeneic bone marrow transplantation, 87